MW01201112

NEUROPSYCHOLOGY OF DEPRESSION

Neuropsychology of
DEPRESSION

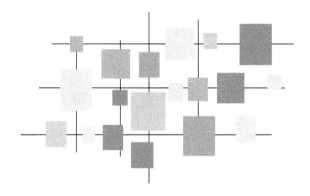

edited by
Shawn M. McClintock
Jimmy Choi

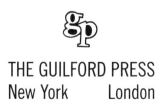

THE GUILFORD PRESS
New York   London

Library of Congress Cataloging-in-Publication Data
Names: McClintock, Shawn M., editor. | Choi, Jimmy (Editor), editor.
Title: Neuropsychology of depression / edited by Shawn M. McClintock, Jimmy
   Choi.
Description: New York : The Guilford Press, [2022] | Includes
   bibliographical references and index.
Identifiers: LCCN 2021047100 | ISBN 9781462549276 (cloth)
Subjects: LCSH: Depression, Mental. | BISAC: PSYCHOLOGY / Neuropsychology |
   PSYCHOLOGY / Psychopathology / Depression
Classification: LCC RC537 .N485 2022 | DDC 616.85/27071—dc23/eng/20211109
LC record available at *https://lccn.loc.gov/2021047100*

About the Editors

Shawn M. McClintock, PhD, MSCS, is Associate Professor and holds the Lydia Bryant Test Distinguished Professorship in Psychiatric Research in the Department of Psychiatry at The University of Texas (UT) Southwestern Medical Center. He is also Director of Research Training for the UT Southwestern Clinical Psychology Doctoral Program. Dr. McClintock is a globally recognized expert in the neurocognitive effects of depression and antidepressant neuromodulation therapeutics. Working on interdisciplinary health care teams, he has published numerous articles and book chapters on these topics. A recipient of the Robert A. and Phyllis Levitt Early Career Award from the Society for Clinical Neuropsychology, Dr. McClintock serves on the editorial boards of *Neuropsychology Review* and the *Journal of ECT*.

Jimmy Choi, PsyD, is a senior scientist at the Olin Neuropsychiatry Research Center in the Hartford Healthcare Behavioral Health Network and research neuropsychologist at The Institute of Living in Hartford, Connecticut. He directs the hospital network's cognitive rehabilitation service, which provides clinical assessment and treatment to children, adolescents, and adults. Dr. Choi has conducted research on cognitive recovery in neuropsychiatric disorders at VA Connecticut, Yale University, and Columbia University.

Contributors

Scott T. Aaronson, MD, Institute of Advanced Diagnostics and Therapeutics, Sheppard Pratt Health System, Baltimore, Maryland

Olusola Ajilore, MD, Department of Psychiatry, University of Illinois at Chicago, Chicago, Illinois

Shriya Awasthi, BS, Postbaccalaureate Intramural Research Training Program, National Institutes of Health, Bethesda, Maryland

K. Chase Bailey, PhD, ABPP-CN, Department of Psychiatry, Parkland Memorial Hospital, Dallas, Texas

Michael W. Best, PhD, Departments of Psychology and Psychological Clinical Science, University of Toronto Scarborough, Toronto, Ontario, Canada

Hannah R. Bogoian, MA, Department of Psychology, Georgia State University, Atlanta, Georgia

Kyle Brauer Boone, PhD, Department of Psychiatry, David Geffen School of Medicine, University of California, Los Angeles, Los Angeles, California

Christopher R. Bowie, PhD, Department of Psychology, Queen's University, Kingston, Ontario, Canada

Jenna E. Boyd, PhD, Anxiety Treatment and Research Clinic, St. Joseph's Healthcare Hamilton and Department of Psychiatry and Behavioural Neurosciences, McMaster University, Hamilton, Ontario, Canada

E. Sherwood Brown, MD, PhD, Department of Psychiatry, University of Texas Southwestern Medical Center, Dallas, Texas

Julia Browne, PhD, Center of Excellence for Psychosocial and Systemic Research, Department of Psychiatry, Massachusetts General Hospital, Boston, Massachusetts; Geriatric Research, Education, and Clinical Center, Durham VA Health Care System, Durham, North Carolina

Adam A. Christensen, PhD, Behavioral Health Program, Michael E. DeBakey VA Medical Center and Department of Psychiatry and Behavioral Sciences, Baylor College of Medicine, Houston, Texas

Paul Croarkin, DO, Department of Psychiatry and Psychology, Mayo Clinic, Rochester, Minnesota

Kathryn Cullen, MD, ABPP-CN, Department of Psychiatry and Behavioral Sciences, University of Minnesota Medical School, Minneapolis, Minnesota

C. Munro Cullum, PhD, Departments of Psychiatry, Neurology, and Neurological Surgery, University of Texas Southwestern Medical Center, Dallas, Texas

Zhi-De Deng, PhD, Noninvasive Neuromodulation Unit, Experimental Therapeutics and Pathophysiology Branch, National Institute of Mental Health, Bethesda, Maryland

Deanna Denman, PhD, Orthopedics & Sports Medicine, Novant Health, Charlotte, North Carolina

David A. Denney, PhD, Department of Psychiatry, University of Texas Southwestern Medical Center, Dallas, Texas

Sonya Dhillon, PhD, CPsych, Graduate Department of Psychological Clinical Science, University of Toronto, Toronto, Ontario, Canada

Vonetta M. Dotson, PhD, Department of Psychology and Gerontology Institute, Georgia State University, Atlanta, Georgia

Martha Finnegan, PhD, Department of Old Age Psychiatry, St James's Hospital, Dublin, Ireland

Alaina I. Gold, BA, Department of Psychology, University of Southern California, Los Angeles, California

Andrew M. Gradone, MA, Department of Psychology, Georgia State University, Atlanta, Georgia

Tracy L. Greer, PhD, MSCS, Department of Psychology, University of Texas at Arlington, Arlington, Texas; Department of Psychiatry, University of Texas Southwestern Medical Center, Dallas, Texas

Katherine Holshausen, PhD, Department of Psychiatry and Behavioural Neurosciences, McMaster University, Hamilton, Ontario, Canada

Laura Howe-Martin, PhD, ABPP, Department of Psychiatry, University of Texas Southwestern Medical Center, Dallas, Texas

Mustafa M. Husain, MD, Departments of Psychiatry, Neurology, and Biomedical Engineering, University of Texas Southwestern Medical Center, Dallas, Texas; Department of Psychiatry and Behavioral Sciences, Duke University School of Medicine, Durham, North Carolina

Jutta Joormann, PhD, Department of Psychology, Yale University, New Haven, Connecticut

Muzaffer Kaser, MD, PhD, Department of Psychiatry, University of Cambridge and Cambridgeshire and Peterborough NHS Foundation Trust, Cambridge, United Kingdom

Sara Kashani, MD, Department of Psychiatry, University of Illinois at Chicago, Chicago, Illinois

Brian Kavanaugh, PsyD, ABPP-CN, Department of Psychiatry and Human Behavior, E. P. Bradley Hospital/Warren Alpert Medical School, Brown University, Providence, Rhode Island

Bonnie Klimes-Dougan, PhD, Department of Psychology, University of Minnesota, Minneapolis, Minnesota

Tori Knox-Rice, PhD, Department of Psychosocial Oncology, Colorado Blood Cancer Institute, Presbyterian St. Luke's Medical Center, Denver, Colorado

Shellie-Anne Levy, PhD, Department of Clinical and Health Psychology, University of Florida, Gainesville, Florida

Sarah H. Lisanby, MD, Division of Translational Research and Noninvasive Neuromodulation Unit, Experimental Therapeutics and Pathophysiology Branch, National Institute of Mental Health, Bethesda, Maryland; Department of Psychiatry and Behavioral Sciences, Duke University School of Medicine, Durham, North Carolina

Donel M. Martin, PhD, School of Psychiatry, University of New South Wales, Sydney, Australia

Valeria Martinez-Kaigi, PhD, MS, Health Psychology Division, Institute of Living, Hartford Hospital, Hartford, Connecticut; Spine Wellness Center, Ayer Neuroscience Institute, Hartford Healthcare, Westport, Connecticut; Department of Psychiatry, Yale School of Medicine, New Haven, Connecticut

Declan M. McLoughlin, PhD, Department of Psychiatry and Trinity College Institute of Neuroscience, Trinity College Dublin, St Patrick's University Hospital, Dublin, Ireland

Margaret C. McKinnon, PhD, Department of Psychiatry and Behavioural Neurosciences, McMaster University, Hamilton, Ontario, Canada

Heather McNeely, PhD, Department of Psychiatry and Behavioural Neurosciences, McMaster University and Clinical Neuropsychology Service, St. Joseph's Healthcare Hamilton, Hamilton, Ontario, Canada

Melissa Milanovic, PhD, Department of Psychology, Queen's University, Kingston, Ontario, Canada

David Mischoulon, MD, Depression Clinical and Research Program, Massachusetts General Hospital, and Department of Psychiatry, Harvard Medical School, Boston, Massachusetts

Adriano Moffa, MPhil, School of Psychiatry, University of New South Wales, Sydney, Australia

Stevan Nikolin, PhD, School of Psychiatry, University of New South Wales, Sydney, Australia

Margaret O'Connor, PhD, Department of Neurology, Harvard Medical School, Boston, Massachusetts

Benjamin D. Pace, MS, Department of Psychiatry, University of Iowa Hospitals & Clinics, Iowa City, Iowa

Aamna Qureshi, MSc, Forensic Psychiatry, St. Joseph's Healthcare Hamilton, Hamilton, Ontario, Canada

Joshua Rosenblat, MD, Mood Disorders Psychopharmacology Unit, Toronto Western Hospital, and Department of Psychiatry, University of Toronto, Toronto, Ontario, Canada

Ashleigh V. Rutherford, MS, MPhil, Department of Psychology, Yale University, New Haven, Connecticut

Barbara J. Sahakian, PhD, Department of Psychiatry and Behavioural and Clinical Neuroscience Institute, University of Cambridge, Cambridge, United Kingdom

Haitham Salem, MD, MSc, PhD, Department of Psychiatry and Human Behavior, Warren Alpert Medical School, Brown University, Providence, Rhode Island

Jerome Sarris, PhD, NICM Health Research Institute, Western Sydney University, Penrith, Australia; Department of Psychiatry, Melbourne University, Parkville, Australia

Sudhakar Selvaraj, MBBS, DPhil, MRCPsych, Department of Psychiatry and Behavioral Sciences, McGovern School of Medicine, University of Texas Health Science Center, Houston, Texas

Hunter Small, PhD, Department of Psychiatry, University of Texas Southwestern Medical Center, Dallas, Texas

Jair C. Soares, MD, PhD, McGovern School of Medicine, University of Texas Health Science Center, Houston, Texas

Mariann Suarez, PhD, ABPP, Morsani College of Medicine, University of South Florida Health, Tampa, Florida

Michelle Thai, MA, Department of Psychology, University of Minnesota, Minneapolis, Minnesota

April D. Thames, PhD, Department of Psychiatry and Biobehavioral Sciences, University of California, Los Angeles, Los Angeles, California

Jeena Thomas, MS, Policy and Global Affairs, National Academies of Sciences, Engineering, and Medicine, Washington, DC

Tanya Tran, MS, Department of Psychology, Queen's University, Kingston, Ontario, Canada

Kayla Tureson, MS, Department of Psychology, University of Southern California, Los Angeles, California

Alik S. Widge, MD, Department of Psychiatry, University of Minnesota, Minneapolis, Minnesota

Konstantine K. Zakzanis, PhD, CPsych, Department of Psychology and Graduate Department of Psychological Clinical Science, University of Toronto, Toronto, Ontario, Canada

Preface

"A state of perpetual drifting" is how one patient described the seemingly endless experience of sadness, apprehension, and loss of interest. An experience we have all endured at some point in our lives, whether for moments, days, weeks, or months, or in some cases as an incessant undercurrent to our daily lives. An experience not constrained by place or time, but traversing history and culture with a binding familiarity—the lingering dark and heavy cloud that is more than a symbol to many of us.

Scientific attempts to lift this dark cloud must begin with a fundamental grasp of the nature of this experience—how it emerges and takes hold. On one end of the spectrum, depression can be conceptualized as an amorphous notion that only takes shape in the context of the historical glass that holds it. The authors of Chapter 1 lead off Part I, Scientific Foundations of Depression, by reaching far back into history to introduce Hippocratic deliberations on the imbalance of bodily fluids and the first explanation of depression based on humoral theory. On the other end of the spectrum, depression can be defined as a distinct neuroscientific phenomenon. The subsequent chapters in this section dive into the modern understanding of the morphology and cytoarchitecture of how depression exists in the brain (Chapter 2) and across the lifespan (Chapter 3), along with the profound impact it can have on quality of life and mental health (Chapter 4) as well as actual physical well-being (Chapter 5).

This capacious coverage from humoral theory to neural structure is a thoughtful tactic designed to capture a broad topic not easily pigeonholed by a monocular perspective. While the scientific foundation chapters describe the evolution of what we now call major depressive disorder, Part II, Neuropsychological Domains, focuses on the clinical neuropsychological framework of depression. Chapter 6 begins this process by looking through the lens of elemental cognitive functions and clinical neuropsychological theory and exploring the cognitive cache that is upstream to cognitive efficiency and intellectual capacity. This discussion is followed by delving into the complex interplay between learning, memory, and depression (Chapter 7) and how cognition is instrumental to perceiving and interpreting emotional experiences (Chapter 8) and functioning as the command "executive" center of a hierarchical organized brain system (Chapter 9).

At the heart of clinical neuropsychology is the practice of assessment. Part III, Clinical and Neuropsychological Assessment, provides a review of the metrics or measurement of depression in different contexts (Chapter 10) and the multiple factors that are paramount when evaluating people with depression (Chapter 11). Accurate cognitive results are, of course, a function of context. As such, the keys to proper interpretation, diagnostic formulation, and case conceptualization include symptom and performance validity (Chapter 12) as well as understanding the impact of culture and inclusion and diversity factors (Chapter 13). Indeed, inclusion and diversity are integral components of the clinical neuropsychological evaluation process that are essential to ensure the reliability and validity of the evaluation findings and successful enactment of therapeutic feedback. The last step in clinical neuropsychological assessment is effectively conveying the results to patients and their care partners and treatment programs alike. Chapter 14 provides invaluable information on how to do this by using motivational interviewing techniques.

While clinical neuropsychology helps us to understand and explore the cognitive underpinnings that play such a significant role in how people experience depression, just as importantly, it also informs the clinician on how to treat depression. For the clinician, the most up-to-date, modern information is essential, and the final section, Part IV, Neuropsychological Effects of Antidepressant Treatment, offers a comprehensive look at the crossroads of depression as a brain-based behavior illness and modern treatments that have emerged and been refined to treat it. Chapter 15 summarizes and compares antidepressant medications with a focus on their impact on cognition and also provides information about the validation of potential new pharmacological interventions. While antidepressant medications are the most widely used antidepressant method, Chapter 16 detours into the most uncommon, but still evidence-based, approach using select nutrient and herbal medicines that the scientific community endorses for the treatment of depression and as an aid to cognitive function. Chapters 17 and 18 combine to review distinct evidence-based psychological interventions from cognitive-behavioral therapy to cognitive training that specifically accommodate and target cognitive biases, inefficiencies, and impairments. Rounding out behavioral therapies is Chapter 19, which examines the neuropsychological evidence in support of physical exercise as a method to improve both cognition and depression. The subsequent chapters in this final section anchor the book by offering the latest on both established and more recently developed methods of antidepressant brain stimulation therapeutics, beginning with electroconvulsive therapy indications and administration (Chapter 20) to the more focal electric field induction method of magnetic seizure therapy (Chapter 21). Chapter 22 discusses vagus nerve and deep brain stimulation modalities, while Chapter 23 reviews repetitive transcranial magnetic stimulation as a noninvasive therapeutic intervention. Finally, Chapter 24 reviews the modern use of transcranial direct current stimulation, including the latest literature on the acute and cumulative cognitive benefits.

Clinical neuropsychology is a unique discipline that aims to establish and inform brain–behavior relationships. We are proud to have assembled a team of international experts who represent both the finest across multiple fields such as clinical neuropsychology, cognitive neuroscience, and psychiatry, as well as the diversity of our clinical and scientific fields in terms of age, gender, ethnicity, race, nationality, and sexual orientation. *Neuropsychology of Depression* provides cutting-edge and up-to-date information regarding the multiple facets of depression that encompasses knowledge spanning everything from diagnosis to treatment. To our knowledge, this is the first book to synthesize multiple aspects of the neuropsychology of depression, including current clinical diagnostic frameworks, assessment techniques, and mechanistic information. Moreover, the book includes comprehensive clinical neuropsychological evaluation protocol information and recommendations, therapeutic feedback and cognitive remediation strategies, performance and symptom validity information to ensure diagnostic accuracy, as well as inclusion and diversity factors to ensure accurate conceptualization and interpretation. As indicated above, the book provides current information on the neurocognitive effects across a spectrum of antidepressant therapeutics and emerging brain stimulation technologies. Collectively, for all health care clinical and research professionals who work with adults with depression, we hope that the scientific foundations and clinical applications provided in this comprehensive book create an invaluable resource that will lead to beneficial and meaningful change for the clinician, scientist, and, above all, adults with depression and their care partners.

A book of this nature is not written overnight, but rather spans days, weeks, and years. The concept of this book was formed early in our careers, and over our career development, the volume morphed, took shape, and became more solidified into what it is today. We are extremely thankful to our many mentors who throughout our career journey provided complete and unconditional support for us and our passions. To that end, it is only fitting that the book concludes on the topic of brain stimulation. Indeed, it was during both our times as early-career investigators at Columbia University and the New York State Psychiatric Institute under the guidance and mentorship of Chapter 21 author Sarah "Holly" Lisanby, in her Brain Stimulation and Therapeutic Modulation Division, that we first met and formed a solid friendship and collaboration that has led us here to this book.

We would like to express our gratitude to the editors at The Guilford Press for appreciating and recognizing the potential for this book and showing confidence in us to see it through to completion. We would like to specifically thank Rochelle Serwator, Senior Editor in Neuropsychology/Neuroscience, and Katherine Sommer, Associate Editor, for their continual encouragement, guidance, and wisdom. We are also very grateful to the authors from across the globe who represent an array of clinical and scientific disciplines and demographic backgrounds. They made this book possible by tirelessly punching out their chapters while wearing sweatpants (truly, that was our attire) at home during the worldwide COVID-19 pandemic. The breadth and richness of content covered are a testament to the incredible expertise of these authors who have pioneered, developed, and continued to refine our understanding of the neuropsychology of depression.

Contents

PART I

SCIENTIFIC FOUNDATIONS OF DEPRESSION

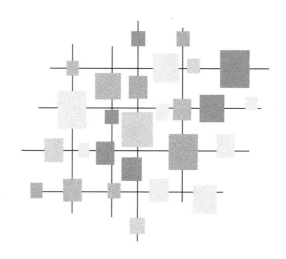

CHAPTER 1

Depression and Major Depressive Disorder
Evolution of Diagnosis and Symptomatology

Haitham Salem
Jair C. Soares
Sudhakar Selvaraj

EVOLUTION OF THE CONCEPT OF DEPRESSION

Depression is a common psychiatric illness with a fascinating history of origin. The earliest account of depression dates back to the second millennium B.C.E. in which depression was considered a demonic possession that was treated by priests. Herodotus, the Greek historian, wrote about a king in the fifth century who was driven mad by evil spirits. Early civilizations including Babylonian, Chinese, and Egyptian all considered mental illness as a form of demonic possession and used exorcism techniques designed to drive demons out of the afflicted person's body (Horwitz, Wakefield, & Lorenzo-Luaces, 2017). In contrast, early Roman and Greek doctors thought that depression was both a biological and psychological disease. The humoral theory developed by Hippocrates in his "Aphorisms" viewed depression as an imbalance of the four basic bodily fluids called humours. There were four humours: yellow bile, black pile, phlegm, and blood. Hippocrates thought that depression was caused by the presence of too much "black bile" in the human body, hence the name *melancholia*. The term *melancholia* is derived from the Ancient Greek words *melas*, which means "black," and *khole*, which means "bile" (Jackson, 1986; Liddell & Robert, 1980). Hippocrates remarkably described melancholia as fear of sadness that lasts a long time, associated with aversion to food, despondency, sleeplessness, irritability, and restlessness. To treat melancholia, Hippocrates recommended and used bloodletting, bathing, exercise, and dieting (Hippocrates, 1923–1931).

The humoral theory eventually fell out of favor after Artaeus Cappadocia (2nd century B.C.E.) started categorizing those with depression and described them as dull or stern, dejected, or unnecessarily torpid, without any manifest cause and distinguished them from those who experienced anger and grief, and sad dejection of mind. Similarly, during the same period, Galen noted such categorical distinctions in his case histories (Galen, 1929; Jackson, 1986; Radden, 2003).

In the 11th century, Persian physicians combined the two separate concepts of melancholia and phrenitis. Melancholia was described as a depressive type of mood disorder in which a person becomes suspicious and develops certain types of phobias. Avicenna's (Ibn Sina's) book *The Canon of Medicine* became the standard of medical thinking in Europe for centuries alongside Hippocrates' ideologies (Avicenna & Gruner, 1973; Haque, 2004; Jacquart, 2008; Safavi-Abbasi, Brasiliense, & Workman, 2007). Avicenna associated melancholia with the brain and classified its etiologies into intracerebral and extracerebral causes. Furthermore, he divided melancholia symptoms into early and chronic phases. He was also the first to introduce the benefit of music and lifestyle modification in ameliorating emotional distress (Khodaei et al., 2017; Shakeri, Sahebkar, & Javadi, 2016).

In the Renaissance period between the 14th and 17th centuries, there were contrasting views of how to describe mental illness. While witch-hunts and executions of the mentally ill were quite common, there began to emerge some acceptance of the idea that natural causes might be involved in mental illnesses and that mentally disturbed individuals required humane medical treatment. Robert Burton in the 17th century published his landmark book, *The Anatomy of Melancholy*, which comprehensively described for the first time three major components of depression: mood, cognition, and physical symptoms. Burton debated that only symptoms without cause could be considered evidence of what he labeled as the depressive disorder. Otherwise, he classified the symptoms as natural sorrow or fear. Burton suggested that treatment for melancholy should include diet, sleep, exercise, music, and distraction, as well as talking about the problem with a friend (Burton, 1621/2001; Jackson, 1983).

Until that moment in history, it is noteworthy that the prevailing view of depression remained the humoral theory. Humoral thought was foundational with diseases thought to always result from imbalances between the various humors. All interventions were designed to target and restore the balance to the body for appropriate equilibrium. Hippocratic preferences for altering lifestyles continued to prevail, intertwined with religious and magical methods, over more intensive medical interventions (Lagay, 2002).

In the 17th century, the term *depression* was used for the first time in literature by English authors to describe those who suffer from "a great depression of spirit" (Wolpert, 1999). The same term was later used in economics and physiology before it appeared in psychiatric symptomatology descriptions by the French psychiatrist Louis Delasiauve in 1856 (Berrios, 1988, 1996).

DEPRESSION IN THE LATE 19TH AND 20TH CENTURIES

By the turn of the 20th century, the German psychiatrist Emil Kraepelin may have been the first to use depression as the overarching term, as he referred to different kinds of melancholia as depressive states. Kraepelin identified depression and mania as parts of the manic–depressive condition and distinguished it from his second famous psychotic state, *dementia praecox* or *schizophrenia* (Davison, 2006; Kraepelin,1921). Despite acknowledging the psychogenic theory of mental illness as etiology, Kraepelin adopted the theory of organic etiology and pathology of psychiatric diseases. His approach was the inspiration for the American Psychiatric Association's *Diagnostic and Statistical Manual of Mental Disorders* (DSM) criteria (Kraepelin, 1903, 1915, 1917).

Unlike Kraepelin, who worked mainly with severely hospitalized patients, the Austrian neurologist and psychoanalyst Sigmund Freud (1856–1939) worked with patients with milder forms of psychiatric illnesses. In his paper "Mourning and Melancholia," Freud theorized that objective loss, albeit actual or symbolic, was the root cause of depression. In other words, he promoted the psychogenic etiology theory of depression (Freud, 1917/1957). American psychiatrist Adolf Meyer developed what became known as the Meyerian theory in which he moved from a clear-cut etiology of disease toward a mixed-origin etiology where all psychiatric diseases carry both a biological (organic) and social (psychological) framework (Meyer, 1922).

DEVELOPMENT OF THE DSM AND ICD CRITERIA

The first edition of the *Diagnostic and Statistical Manual of Mental Disorders* (DSM-I; American Psychiatric Association, 1952), presented the concept of depressive reaction, and the second edition, DSM-II (American Psychiatric Association, 1968), used the term "depressive neurosis," which was defined as an excessive reaction to internal conflict or an identifiable event, and also included a depressive type of manic–depressive psychosis within major affective disorders. Both DSM-I and DSM-II appeared to adopt a Kraepelinian style (e.g., organic etiology and pathology of disease). The diagnosis of depression was either based on biological conditions (endogenous factors) or described as a reaction to stressful events (exogenous factors) throughout the second half of the 20th century. This debate between endogenous and exogenous causal factors persisted for most of the 20th century over whether a unitary or binary model of depression represents a more accurate reflection of the syndrome. With the publishing of the third edition of the DSM, DSM-III (American Psychiatric Association, 1980), the psychiatric community began to accept the unitarian model of depression. Since that time, the psychiatry community has continued to adopt and affirm a definitive set of symptomatic criteria for depression that has remained stable until the present.

Unlike the DSM classification system that is mainly used in the United States, the *International Classification of Diseases* (ICD), published by the World Health Organization (WHO), is predominantly employed across European countries. The ICD was first adopted in 1948, and it defined three typical depressive symptoms that included depressed mood, anhedonia, and reduced energy, two of which are required for a diagnosis of depressive disorder (WHO, 1948a, 1948b). A significant difference from the previous versions and a particularly important feature of the most recent edition of the ICD (ICD-11) is the approach to describing the essential features of each disorder, representing those symptoms or characteristics that a clinician could reasonably expect to find in all cases of the disorder. At the same time, it avoids listing features in the guidelines that are superficially resembling diagnostic criteria, as well as avoiding arbitrary cutoffs and requirements (Evans et al., 2013; Gruenberg, Goldstein, & Pincus, 2005; Reed, Mendonça Correia, Esparza, Saxena, & Maj, 2011; Sadock, Sadock, & Kaplan, 2003). Unlike the ICD-10, the diagnostic guidelines for the depressive episode are one of the few places in ICD-11 where a minimal symptom count is required. This change is due to the long-standing research and clinical tradition of conceptualizing depression in this manner. A minimum of five of ten symptoms is required rather than the four of nine possible symptoms stipulated in ICD-10, thus increasing consistency with the current edition of DSM, DSM-5 (Reed et al., 2019).

In the early 1970s, studies demonstrated that earlier diagnostic approaches were unreliable. This observation ultimately led to the development of the Feighner diagnostic criteria and validation of 14 psychiatric disease diagnoses, including depression (Feighner et al., 1972).

To improve psychiatric diagnostic reliability and validity, Spitzer and colleagues modified the Feighner criteria with the addition of criteria for other psychiatric disorders in the Research Diagnostic Criteria (RDC; Spitzer, Endicott, & Robins,1978). To assist with diagnostic accuracy, the same team developed the clinician-administered, semistructured diagnostic interview, the Schedule for Affective Disorders and Schizophrenia (SADS; Endicott & Spitzer, 1978).

A dramatic shift in the U.S.-based psychiatric diagnostic nomenclature began with development of the DSM-III diagnostic criteria classification system (American Psychiatric Association, 1980). DSM-III diagnostic criteria, developed in light of the innovative Feighner criteria (Blashfield, 1982; Feighner et al., 1972), sought to improve reliability and validity that were highly criticized in the previous versions. DSM-III contained diagnostic criteria that specify the meaning of the categories. In addition, each category carried a description of the typical demographic profile of patients experiencing this disorder, a lengthy prose explanation of what the category meant, a description of how to differentiate the target category from any other category with which it might be confused, and a brief discussion of what was known about the course and onset of the disorder. Also, DSM-III established the multiaxial system of evaluation, in which Axis I describes the main psychopathological disorder, Axis II defines concomitant personality disorders or mental disabilities, Axis III identifies medical comorbidities, AxisIV defines psychosocial and environment issues (e.g., homelessness, legal issues), and Axis V calculates the global assessment of functioning.

On the other hand, the ninth edition of the ICD (ICD-9) contained no explicit criteria for a diagnosis of depression or a multiaxial system. Thus, DSM-III represented a dramatic shift away from the principles and diagnostic approaches used in ICD-9 (WHO, 1975). In DSM-III, both the depressive and bipolar disorders were distinguished by the presence or absence of manic/hypomanic symptoms. Overlapping affective conditions such as dysthymic disorder and cyclothymic disorder were included within the broad category of mood disorders. Depressive reaction and neurotic depression, which were included in DSM-I and DSM-II were removed from DSM-III. New to the DSM system in the third edition were the residual categories of bipolar disorder type II and atypical depression, which were regarded as conditions that did not meet the existing criteria for depression (major depressive disorder, bipolar disorder depressed, or dysthymic disorder). Following DSM-III, the WHO developed the clinical modification of ICD-9 (ICD-9-CM; WHO, 1979), which further described the clinical symptoms and signs rather than just presenting statistical groupings to improve the coding of conditions. ICD-9-CM went into effect in 1979 before DSM-III was published.

DSM-IV, published in 1994, did not represent a fundamental shift from the previous versions and made relatively few significant changes from the previous versions. Despite the conservative approach for change that the authors adopted while furnishing the DSM-IV, it included many more disorders than the previous version (DSM-III) had, mainly because many of the disorders from DSM-III were split apart into specific subtypes in DSM-IV (Rogler, 1997). A revised version, DSM-IV-TR, was released in 2000 to update the research literature between 1992 and 1998. That edition also left the criteria essentially untouched; it simply provided more details in the accompanying text on associated features of disorders and corrected the previous version's editing errors (Fischer, 2012).

DSM-5 CHANGES REGARDING DEPRESSIVE DISORDERS

Aside from the obvious change from a Roman to an Arabic numeral in the title (from DSM-IV-TR to DSM-5), DSM-5 developed significant updates for the depressive disorders section. Specifically, the chapter on Depressive Disorders, which had been part of the chapter "Bipolar and Related Disorders" in DSM-IV-TR, became a separate chapter in DSM-5. However, in the newly added specifier, depression with "mixed features" is considered a specifier that bridges the gap between the possibility of having unipolar depression with aspects of some bipolar disorder criteria. DSM-5 added disruptive mood dysregulation disorder (DMDD) as a new diagnosis for children up to 12 years of age who present with persistent irritability and frequent episodes of extreme behavioral abnormalities (Rao, 2014). Based on evidence collected over two decades that confirmed diagnostic criteria and treatment recommendations, the premenstrual dysphoric disorder diagnosis was moved from an appendix of DSM-IV-TR to Section II of DSM-5 (Epperson et al., 2012). The DSM-IV-TR diagnostic criteria for chronic major depression and dysthymia were merged into the new DSM-5 diagnosis of dysthymia or persistent depressive disorder, which is diagnosed in cases where the mood disturbance lasts at least 1 year in children or 2 years in adults.

CURRENT DIAGNOSTIC CRITERIA FOR DEPRESSION

DSM-5 Criteria

Depression is now defined as major depressive disorder (MDD), and the diagnosis is made by the presence of symptom clusters for a specified duration of time. Currently, to diagnose MDD according to DSM-5, five or more of the major symptoms (depressed mood, diminished interest, significant loss of appetite/weight loss, insomnia/hypersomnia, psychomotor retardation/agitation, loss of energy, diminished concentration, and recurrent suicidal ideations) should be present for a period of 2 weeks. Such symptoms have to adversely impact the social, occupational, and other vital functional areas of the individual, and should not be explained by substance abuse or other medical illnesses. A critical criterion for the diagnosis of MDD is the complete absence of an identifiable manic or hypomanic episode (American Psychiatric Association, 2013).

ICD-11 Criteria

According to the ICD-11 classification system, during a typical depressive episode, symptoms include low mood, low energy, and low activity. Moreover, common symptoms include reduced capacity for enjoyment, interest, and concentration, as well as marked tiredness. Sleep is usually disturbed, and appetite is diminished, with changes in body weight. Self-esteem and self-confidence are almost always reduced, and, even in a mild form, some ideas of guilt or worthlessness are often present. The lowered mood varies little from day to day, is unresponsive to circumstances, and may be accompanied by so-called somatic symptoms such as loss of interest and pleasurable feelings, early morning awakening, worsened mood in the morning, marked psychomotor retardation or agitation, loss of appetite, weight loss, and loss of libido. Depending on the number and severity of the symptoms, a depressive episode may be specified as mild, moderate, or severe.

For further categorization, in a "minor" episode, ICD-11 requires two or three of the depressive symptoms to be present as well as distress that accompanies daily life activities. For a "moderate" episode, four or more depressive symptoms are required, as well as significant difficulty in the performance of daily life activities. A "severe" episode requires several depressive symptoms to be present, as well as marked guilt, loss of self-esteem, and persistent suicidal ideations/attempts. If hallucinations or delusions occur with a severe episode, the episode is named severe depressive episode with psychotic symptoms. ICD-11 also identifies atypical depression episodes under other depressive episodes and depressive episode unspecified (WHO, 2019).

SPECIFIERS FOR DEPRESSIVE DISORDERS

DSM-IV included only four specifiers for MDD. With the advent of DSM-5, they were expanded to nearly double in number. Specifically, the depressive specifiers as noted in DSM-5 include:

- *With anxious distress:* Anxiety is a prominent feature of the major depressive episode (MDE). High anxiety levels have been associated with higher suicide risk, prolonged illness, and nonresponse to antidepressant treatment.

- *With mixed features:* This specifier is considered a bridge for those without an established manic episode that fulfills the bipolar disorder criteria, but who are likely to develop full-blown bipolar disorder at some point over time. The specifier requires that during at least 2 weeks of the MDE there are at least three manic or hypomanic symptoms, including elated or irritable mood, elevated self-esteem, increased motor activity or energy, reduced need for sleep, and increased goal-oriented activities. Many bipolar disorder illnesses begin with one or more MDEs.

- *With psychotic features:* This specifier describes those types of MDDs with psychotic features, typically delusions and hallucinations, that are either congruent or incongruent with the depressed mood. DSM-5 also notes that psychosis is part of the severity scale in which an MDE can be severe or severe with psychotic features.

• *With catatonia:* Catatonia is considered a form of severe psychomotor retardation. The symptoms are characterized by one or more of the following features: motor immobility, catalepsy, mutism, extreme negativism, posturing, stereotyped movements, grimacing, and repetition of another person's words or movements. The specifier is applied if catatonia is present during most of the MDE time frame.

• *With melancholic features:* The symptoms associated with melancholia include early morning awakening, worsened mood in the morning, marked psychomotor retardation or agitation, significant loss of appetite or weight loss, and excessive or inappropriate guilt. Another prominent feature is the near-complete absence of the capacity for pleasure and limited reactivity to pleasurable activities.

• *With atypical features:* Relative to melancholic features, this specifier is characterized by mood reactivity, which is the capacity to be cheered up (not being sad all the time) and reactive to positive or pleasurable events, as well as hypersomnia and hyperphagia. The mood may become euthymic for extended periods if the external circumstances remain favorable.

• *With peripartum onset:* As this specifier has had an important measurement and documentation problem, the current consensus is that this specifier is made if the MDE occurs during pregnancy or within 4 weeks postdelivery (Stuart-Parrigon & Stuart, 2014).

• *With seasonal pattern:* This specifier is confirmed if the onset and offset of the MDEs occur at specific times of the year. Depression onset during the winter season and remission of episodes must have occurred at a minimum during the prior two consecutive years, without any nonseasonal MDEs occurring during this period. Also, the seasonal MDEs must substantially outnumber any nonseasonal MDEs over the individual's lifetime.

DEPRESSIVE DISORDER SUBTYPES ACCORDING TO DSM-5 DIAGNOSTIC CRITERIA

Disruptive Mood Dysregulation Disorder

DMDD is a new psychiatric diagnosis that was introduced in DSM-5 to minimize the overdiagnosis of bipolar disorder in children (Rao, 2014). It is characterized by severe and recurrent (three or more times/week) temper outbursts that are inconsistent with developmental level, and such symptoms must be present for at least 12 months with no symptoms of free periods that last 3 or more months. The age at onset is usually before 10 years, and the diagnosis is typically made for the first time between the ages of 6 and 18 years.

Persistent Depressive Disorder (Dysthymia)

Persistent depressive disorder is a new label for what was once called dysthymic disorder. This diagnosis is characterized by the presence of a depressed mood nearly every day for at a minimum of 2 years. Symptom-free periods can be no more than 2 months at a time. For this diagnosis, there can be no manic or hypomanic episodes or cyclothymic disorder.

Premenstrual Dysphoric Disorder

Premenstrual dysphoric disorder is characterized by the occurrence of depressive symptoms in the week before the onset of menses, with symptoms typically improving within a few days after the onset of menses, till they become minimal or even absent postmenses. The depressive symptoms are usually associated with clinically significant distress or interference with employment, academic, social, and interpersonal activities. For this specifier, the depressive symptoms should occur during at least two menses cycles.

Substance/Medication-Induced Depressive Disorder

Substance/medication-induced depressive disorder is a new diagnosis in DSM-5. It is characterized by depressive symptoms that develop during or immediately after intoxication or withdrawal of a substance or medication that is capable of inducing depressive symptoms.

Depressive Disorder Due to Another Medical Condition

Depressive disorder due to another medical condition is characterized by prominent and persistent periods of depressed mood or markedly diminished interest or pleasure that predominates the clinical picture, with confirmed evidence that the disturbance is the direct pathophysiological consequence of another medical condition.

DIAGNOSTIC FEATURES OF DEPRESSION

Prevalence, Course, and Chronicity

Based on the United States National Comorbidity Survey that was conducted from 2001 to 2002 using the Composite International Diagnostic Interview and DSM-IV criteria for MDD, the 12 months and lifetime prevalence of MDD was estimated to be 6.6% and 16.2%, respectively. A National Epidemiologic Survey that was conducted from 2012 to 2013 with DSM-5 MDD criteria estimated 12 months and lifetime prevalence at 10.4% and 20.6%, respectively. Women relative to men were found to have a higher lifetime prevalence of depression (26.1% vs. 14.7%, respectively; Hasin et al., 2018). The prevalence in younger age groups was three times greater than in individuals ages 60 years or older. Hypersomnia and hyperphagia are more likely reported as predominant depressive symptoms in younger individuals, whereas melancholic symptoms are reportedly more common in older age groups (Brody, Pratt, & Hughes, 2018).

The course of MDD within individuals remains relatively stable across life development. However, across individuals, the course of MDD tends to be highly variable. As such, some patients may experience an MDE with full resolution of depressive symptoms, while others may spend much of their lives struggling with multiple MDEs composed of persistent and/or fluctuating symptoms (Chen, Eaton, Gallo, & Nestadt, 2000; Gilbody, Lightfoot, & Sheldon, 2007; Jabben, Penninx, Beekman, Smith, & Nolen, 2011). A longitudinal study of patients with MDD treated in primary care clinics found that 43% of the patients remitted after 39 months (Stegenga, Kamphuis, King, Nazareth, & Geerlings, 2010). However, a majority of patients (57%) had incomplete recovery from the MDE About 12% of patients with MDD had a chronic course (Judd, 1997; Kessler et al., 2003), with 60% of patients experiencing continued depression after 12 years (Judd et al., 1998). Chronicity of the depressive illness is often associated with higher depressive symptomatology, somatic symptoms, and substantial functional impairment (Stegenga et al., 2010). Hence, it is useful to ask individuals who present with depressive symptoms to identify the last period of at least two months during which they were entirely free of depressive symptoms.

A systematic review and meta-analysis of conversion from unipolar MDD to bipolar disorder found that approximately 12.9% of patients had converted to bipolar disorder after 10 years (Kessing, Willer, Andersen, & Bukh, 2017). A greater risk of conversion was found to occur in the first few years of the diagnosis. A large Danish epidemiological registry study that involved 91,587 individuals diagnosed with MDD reported a cumulative incidence of conversion to bipolar disorder at 8.7% in females and 7.7% in males (Musliner & Østergaard, 2018). A family history of bipolar disorder was the strongest predictor of conversion from MDD to bipolar disorder. These findings emphasize the importance of assessing mania or hypomania symptoms during all evaluations in patients who present with depressive symptoms.

Recovery and Recurrence

Typically, remission is reported to start as soon as 8 weeks, as shown in some prospective observational studies, until a full recovery is achieved, which can range from 3 months up to 1 year. The length of each MDE varies between 16 and 23 weeks, with a median of at least four MDEs in a lifetime (Cleare et al., 2015). Longer MDE duration, psychotic features, severe anxiety, preexisting comorbidities, and poor psychosocial functioning are all associated with higher MDE recurrence rates (Cleare et al., 2015). Factors that confer a greater risk of MDE recurrence include younger age, prior MDE that was severe in magnitude, and more than one historical MDE irrespective of severity. The risk of recurrence appears to be higher in the first few months after recovery from an MDE. In a prospective study of patients with MDD who recovered from a single MDE, 64% had at least one subsequent MDE with a median time of 3 years for the first recurrence (Solomon et al., 2000).

In a Dutch study (Hardeveld, Spijker, De Graaf, Nolen, & Beekman, 2013), the cumulative recurrence rate among those who had recovered from a single MDE was 13% at 5 years, 23% at 10 years, and 42% at 20 years. Clinical factors such as previous MDE and persistent subthreshold depressive symptoms were found to be related to the recurrence of major depressive illness (Hardeveld et al., 2013). A prior history of MDE recurrence is considered to be the most consistently identified risk factor for depressive relapse (Grilo et al., 2010).

FUTURE PROSPECTS IN THE EVOLUTION OF MDD

A substantial body of converging preclinical and clinical evidence, including genetic, molecular, postmortem, neuroimaging, and behavioral information, has yielded insights into the biological bases of MDD (Kaltenboeck & Harmer 2018; Pizzagalli, 2020; Sibille & French, 2013).

Despite these advances, MDD remains a common and inadequately treated illness, with few effective antidepressant strategies for prevention or cure. Many experts have proposed that a primary reason for the lack of prevention or cure is that current diagnostic standards have failed to take into account the heterogeneity and polymorphism of MDD (Holtzheimer & Nemeroff, 2006; Rush et al., 2004).

A pivotal article (Kapur, Phillips, & Insel, 2012) mentioned three additional reasons for the consistent failure to prevent and cure depression. First, the psychiatric community lacks a biological "gold-standard" diagnostic test for MDD. Second, the majority of neurobiological investigations, despite being statistically significant, had small or moderate effect sizes that limited translation to clinical practice. Third, replication studies in psychiatry have been scarce, as most studies focused on comparison of prototypical patients with MDD and "picture-perfect" healthy controls. This led to significant results that were difficult to replicate and lacked application in real life (Kapur et al., 2012).

To overcome the methodological limitations of prior research, in 2008, the National Institute of Mental Health (NIMH) announced that in the next few decades it would be essential to study the various biological, psychological, and social "signatures" of mental disorders, among which are the depressive disorders. The Research Domain Criteria (RDoC) framework was established in order to provide new ways to classify mental illnesses based on behavioral and neurobiological measures (Ivanets, Kinkulkina, Tikhonova, & Avdeeva, 2018; Kapur et al., 2012). The RDoC framework was launched in 2009 with the following four aims: (1) to identify fundamental behavioral components of mental health disorders via the integration of multiple scientific disciplines in a translational manner to reveal the link between observable behavior and neurobiological circuitry; (2) to describe the dimensions of these fundamental behavioral components that range from normal to abnormal; (3) to ultimately establish standardized, reliable, and valid measures of such components in order to facilitate continuity across research studies; and (4) to integrate the underlying "genetic, neurobiological, behavioral, environmental, and experiential components" that make up these disorders (Cuthbert & Insel, 2013).

The signature of the mental illness project launched by the NIMH uses a longitudinal approach to assess the biological, psychological, and social signatures of mental illness based on DSM-5 and RDoC dimensional approaches. The project has the potential to advance an understanding of mental illness that may go beyond the existing classification boundaries and revolutionize the field of mental health research (Lupien et al., 2017).

CONCLUSION

While depression is much better understood nowadays than it was in the past, the clinical and scientific community is still working to identify its components as a way of better understanding and, therefore, optimizing future treatment strategies. The current consensus is that depression is a combination of multiple biological, psychological, and social factors, many of which are yet to be fully elucidated. Further research is undoubtedly necessary not only to alleviate the depression symptoms but to enable functional recovery to improve the quality of life.

REFERENCES

American Psychiatric Association. (1952). *Diagnostic and statistical manual of mental disorders.* Washington, DC: Author.

American Psychiatric Association. (1968). *Diagnostic and statistical manual of mental disorders* (2nd ed.). Washington, DC: Author.

American Psychiatric Association. (1980). *Diagnostic and statistical manual of mental disorders* (3rd ed.). Washington, DC: Author.

American Psychiatric Association. (2013). *Diagnostic and statistical manual of mental disorders* (5th ed.). Arlington, VA: Author.

Avicenna. (1973). *The canon of medicine of Avicenna* (O. C. Gruner, Trans.). New York: AMS Press.

Berrios, G. E. (1988). Melancholia and depression during the 19th century: A conceptual history. *British Journal of Psychiatry.* 153 (3): 298–304.

Berrios, G. E. (1996). *The history of mental symptoms: Descriptive psychopathology since the nineteenth century.* Cambridge, UK: Cambridge University Press.

Blashfield, R. K. (1982). Feighner et al., invisible colleges, and the Matthew effect. *Schizophrenia Bulletin, 8*(1), 1–12.

Brody, D. J., Pratt, L. A., & Hughes, J. P. (2018). *Prevalence of depression among adults aged 20 and over: United States, 2013–2016.* NCHS Data Brief No. 303.

Burton, R. (2001). *The anatomy of melancholy.* New York: New York Review of Books. (Original work published 1621)

Chen, L., Eaton, W. W., Gallo, J. J., & Nestadt, G. (2000). Understanding the heterogeneity of depression through the triad of symptoms, course and risk factors: A longitudinal, population-based study. *Journal of Affective Disorder,* 59:1.

Cleare, A., Pariante, C. M., Young, A. H., Anderson, I. M., Christmas, D., Cowen, P. J., et al. (2015). Evidence-based guidelines for treating depressive disorders with antidepressants: A revision of the 2008 British Association for Psychopharmacology guidelines. *Journal of Psychopharmacology, 29*(5), 459–525.

Cuthbert, B. N., & Insel, T. R. (2013). Toward the future of psychiatric diagnosis: The seven pillars of RDoC. *BMC Medicine, 11*(1), 126.

Davison, K. (2006). Historical aspects of mood disorders. *Psychiatry, 5*(4), 115–118.

Endicott, J., & Spitzer, R. L. (1978). A diagnostic interview: The schedule for affective disorders and schizophrenia. *Archives of General Psychiatry, 35*(7), 837–844.

Epperson, C. N., Steiner, M., Hartlage, S. A., Eriksson, E., Schmidt, P. J., Jones, I., et al. (2012). Premenstrual dysphoric disorder: Evidence for a new category for DSM-5. *American Journal of Psychiatry, 169*(5), 465–475.

Evans, S. C., Reed, G. M., Roberts, M. C., Esparza, P., Watts, A. D., Correia, J. M., et al. (2013). Psychologists' perspectives on the diagnostic classification of mental disorders: Results from the WHO-IUPsyS Global Survey. *International Journal of Psychology: Journal international de psychologie, 48*(3), 177–193.

Feighner, J. P., Robins, E, Guze, S. B., Woodruff, R. A., Jr., Winokur, G., & Munoz, R. (1972). Diagnostic criteria for use in psychiatric research. *Archives of General Psychiatry, 26*(1), 57–63.

Fischer, B. A. (2012). A review of American psychiatry through its diagnoses: The history and development of the Diagnostic and Statistical Manual of Mental Disorders. *Journal of Nervous and Mental Disease, 200*(12), 1022–1030.

Freud, S. (1957). *Mourning and melancholia.* In J. Strachey (Ed. & Trans.), *Standard edition of the complete works of Sigmund Freud* (Vol. 14, pp. 237–258). London: Hogarth Press. (Original work published 1917)

Galen. (1929). On prognosis (A. J. Brock, Trans.). In A. J. Brock (Ed.), *Greek medicine, being extracts illustrative of medical writing from Hippocrates to Galen* (pp. 200–220). London: Dent.

Gilbody, S., Lightfoot, T., & Sheldon, T. (2007). Is low folate a risk factor for depression?: A meta-analysis and exploration of heterogeneity. *Journal of Epidemiology and Community Health, 61,* 631.

Grilo, C. M., Stout, R. L., Markowitz, J. C., Sanislow, C. A., Ansell, E. B., Skodol, A. E., et al. (2010). Personality disorders predict relapse after remission from an episode of major depressive disorder: A 6-year prospective study. *Journal of Clinical Psychiatry, 71,* 1629–1635.

Gruenberg, A. M., Goldstein, R. D., & Pincus, H. A. (2005). Classification of depression: Research and diagnostic criteria: DSM-IV and ICD-10. In J. Licinio & M.-L. Wong (Eds.), *Biology of depression. Biology of depression: From novel insights to therapeutic strategies* (pp. 1–12). Weinheim, Germany: Wiley-VCH Verlag.

Haque, A. (2004). Psychology from Islamic perspective: Contributions of early Muslim scholars and challenges to contemporary Muslim psychologists. *Journal of Religion and Health, 43*(4), 357–377.

Hardeveld, F., Spijker, J., De Graaf, R., Nolen, W. A., & Beekman, A. T. (2013). Recurrence of major depressive disorder and its predictors in the general population: results from the Netherlands Mental Health Survey and Incidence Study (NEMESIS). *Psychological Medicine, 43,* 39–48.

Hasin, D. S., Sarvet, A. L., Meyers, J. L., Saha, T. D., Ruan, W. J., Stohl, M., et al. (2018). Epidemiology of adult DSM-5 major depressive disorder and its specifiers in the United States. *JAMA Psychiatry, 75*(4), 336–346.

Hippocrates. (1923–1931). *Works of Hippocrates, Vol. I–IV* (W. H. S. Jones & E. T. Withington, Trans.). Cambridge, MA: Harvard University Press.

Holtzheimer, P. E., & Nemeroff, C. B. (2006). Future prospects in depression research. *Dialogues in Clinical Neuroscience, 8*(2),175–189.

Horwitz, A., Wakefield, J., & Lorenzo-Luaces, L. (2017). History of Depression. In R. J. DeRubeis & D. R. Strunk (Eds.), *The Oxford handbook of mood disorders* (pp. 11–23). New York: Oxford University Press.

Ivanets, N. N., Kinkulkina, M. A., Tikhonova, Y. G., & Avdeeva, T. I. (2018). [The current state and future prospects of depression research (clinical and classification problems).] *Zhurnal nevrologii i psikhiatrii imeni S.S. Korsakova, 118*(10), 76–81.

Jabben, N., Penninx, B. W., Beekman, A. T., Smith, J. H., & Nolen, W. A. (2011). Co-occurring manic symptomatology as a dimension which may help explaining heterogeneity of depression. *Journal of Affective Disorders, 131,* 224–232.

Jackson, S. W. (1983). Melancholia and mechanical explanation in eighteenth-century medicine. *Journal of the History of Medicine and Allied Sciences, 38*(3), 298–319.

Jackson, S. W. (1986). *Melancholia and depression: From Hippocratic times to modern times.* New Haven, CT: Yale University Press.

Jacquart, D. (2008). Islamic pharmacology in the Middle Ages: Theories and substances. *European Review, 16*(2), 219–227.

Judd, L. L. (1997). The clinical course of unipolar major depressive disorders. *Archives of General Psychiatry, 54*(11), 989–991.

Judd, L. L., Akiskal, H. S., Maser, J. D., Zeller, P. J., Endicott, J., Coryell, W., et al. (1998). A prospective 12-year study of subsyndromal and syndromal depressive symptoms in unipolar major depressive disorders. *Archives of General Psychiatry, 55*(8),694–700.

Kaltenboeck, A., & Harmer, C. (2018). The neuroscience of depressive disorders: A brief review of the past and some considerations about the future. *Brain and Neuroscience Advances, 2*(8), 2398212818799269.

Kapur, S., Phillips, A. G., & Insel, T. R. (2012). Why has it taken so long for biological psychiatry to develop clinical tests and what to do about it? *Molecular Psychiatry, 17,* 1174–1179.

Kessing, L. V., Willer, I., Andersen, P. K., & Bukh, J. D. (2017). Rate and predictors of conversion from unipolar to bipolar disorder: A systematic review and meta-analysis. *Bipolar Disorders, 19*(5), 324–335.

Kessler, R. C., Berglund, P., Demler, O., Jin, R., Koretz, D., Merikangas, K. R., et al. (2003). The epidemiology of major depressive disorder: Results from the National Comorbidity Survey Replication (NCS-R). *Journal of the American Medical Association, 289*(23), 3095–3105.

Khodaei, M. A., Noorbala, A. A., Parsian, Z., Targhi, S. T., Emadi, F., Alijaniha, F., et al. (2017). Avicenna (980–1032 C.E.): The pioneer in treatment of depression. *Transylvanian Review, 25*(17), 4377–4389.

Kraepelin, E. (1903). *Psychiatrie: Ein Lehrbuch fur Studierende und Aerzte.* Leipzig, Germany: Barth.

Kraepelin, E. (1915). Clinical psychiatry: A text-book for students and physicians. In A. Ross Diefendorf (Ed. & Trans.), *The seventh German edition of Kraepelin's Lehrbuch der Psychiatrie* (2nd ed.). New York: Macmillan.

Kraepelin, E. (1917). *Lectures on clinical psychi*atry (3rd English ed.; T. Johnstone, Ed. &Trans.). New York: Wood.

Kraepelin, E. (1921). *Manic-depressive insanity and paranoia* (8th ed.; R. M. Barclay, Trans.). Edinburgh, UK: E & S Livingstone.

Lagay, F. (2002). The legacy of humoral medicine. *Virtual Mentor, 4*(7), virtualmentor.2002.4.7.mhst1-0207.

Liddell, H., & Robert, S. (1980). *A Greek-English Lexicon* (abridged ed.). Oxford, UK: Oxford University Press

Lupien, S. J., Sasseville, M., François, N., Giguère, C. E., Boissonneault, J., Plusquellec, P., et al. (2017). The DSM5/RDoC debate on the future of mental health research: Implication for studies on human stress and presentation of the signature bank. *Stress, 20*(1), 2–18.

Meyer, A. (1922). Interrelations of the domain of neuropsychiatry. *Archives of Neurology and Psychiatry, 8*, 111–121.

Musliner, K. L., & Østergaard, S. D. (2018). Patterns and predictors of conversion to bipolar disorder in 91,587 individuals diagnosed with unipolar depression. *Acta Psychiatrica Scandinavica, 137*(5),422–432.

Pizzagalli, D. A. (2020). Introduction. *Harvard Review of Psychiatry, 28*(1), 1–3.

Radden, J. (2003). Is this dame melancholy?: Equating today's depression and past melancholia. *Philosophy, Psychiatry, and Psychology, 10*(1), 37–52.

Rao, U. (2014). DSM-5: Disruptive mood dysregulation disorder. *Asian Journal of Psychiatry, 11*, 119–123.

Reed, G. M., First, M. B., Kogan, C. S., Hyman, S. E., Gureje, O., Gaebel, W., et al. (2019). Innovations and changes in the ICD-11 classification of mental, behavioural and neurodevelopmental disorders. *World Psychiatry, 18*(1), 3–19.

Reed, G. M., Mendonça Correia, J., Esparza, P., Saxena, S., & Maj, M. (2011). The WPA-WHO Global survey of psychiatrists' attitudes towards mental disorders classification. *World Psychiatry, 10*(2), 118–131.

Rogler, L. H. (1997). Making sense of historical changes in the Diagnostic and Statistical Manual of Mental Disorders: Five propositions. *Journal of Health and Social Behavior, 38*(1), 9–20.

Rush, A. J., Fava, M., Wisniewski, S. R., Lavori, P. W., Trivedi, M. H., Sackeim, H. A., et al. (2004). Sequenced treatment alternatives to relieve depression (STAR*D): Rationale and design. *Controlled Clinical Trials, 25*(1),119–142.

Sadock, V. A., Sadock, B. J., & Kaplan, H. I. (2003). *Kaplan & Sadock's synopsis of psychiatry: behavioral sciences/clinical psychiatry.* Philadelphia: Lippincott Williams & Wilkins.

Safavi-Abbasi, S., Brasiliense, L. B. C, & Workman, R. K. (2007). The fate of medical knowledge and the neurosciences during the time of Genghis Khan and the Mongolian Empire. *Neurosurgical Focus, 23*(1), E13.

Shakeri, A., Sahebkar, A., & Javadi, B. (2016). *Melissa officinalis L.*—A review of its traditional uses, phytochemistry and pharmacology. *Journal of Ethnopharmacology, 188*, 204–224.

Sibille, E., & French, B. (2013). Biological substrates underpinning diagnosis of major depression. *International Journal of Neuropsychopharmacology, 16*(8), 1893–1909.

Solomon, D. A., Keller, M. B., Leon, A. C., Mueller, T. I., Lavori, P. W., Shea, M. T., et al. (2000). Multiple recurrences of major depressive disorder. *American Journal of Psychiatry, 157*, 229–233.

Spitzer, R. L., Endicott, J., & Robins, E. (1978). Research diagnostic criteria: Rationale and reliability. *Archives of General Psychiatry, 35*(6), 773–782.

Stegenga, B. T., Kamphuis, M. H., King, M., Nazareth, I., & Geerlings, M. I. (2010). The natural course and outcome of major depressive disorder in primary care: The PREDICT-NL study. *Social Psychiatry and Psychiatric Epidemiology, 47*(1), 87–95.

Stuart-Parrigon, K., & Stuart, S. (2014). Perinatal depression: An update and overview. *Current Psychiatry Reports, 16*(9), 468.

Wolpert, L. (1999). *Malignant sadness: The anatomy of depression.* London: Faber & Faber.

World Health Organization. (1948a). *International classification of diseases: Manual of the international statistical classification of diseases, injuries and causes of death, 6th revision.* Geneva: Author.

World Health Organization. (1948b) *Manual of the international classification of diseases, injuries, and causes of death.* Geneva: Author.

World Health Organization. (1975). *International classification of diseases, 9th revision.* Geneva: Author.

World Health Organization. (2019). *International classification of diseases, 11th revision.* Retrieved from *https://icd.who.int.*

CHAPTER 2

Neuroanatomy and Neural Networks in Depression

Michelle Thai
Kathryn Cullen
Bonnie Klimes-Dougan

Some of the earliest etiological theories of depression emphasized the physical, presumably rooted in an imbalance of humors of body fluids (Horwitz, Wakefield, & Lorenzo-Luaces, 2017). The prominent, 21st-century integrative, biopsychosocial etiological model of depression has also placed an importance on underlying biological processes. Indeed, some of the most rapid advances in the field are due to tools that have been developed and refined to noninvasively peer under the skull. These efforts to understand brain structure and function in those who suffer from depression have promoted important new insights into this disorder.

This chapter provides foundational knowledge for critical neural structures and networks implicated in depression. We start by presenting a brief overview of the broader range of methods and describing the primary noninvasive magnetic resonance imaging (MRI) techniques used to examine brain structure and functioning. We then review abnormalities in some of the key networks implicated in depression, briefly considering structural evidence but highlighting evidence related to activation and connectivity during tasks and at rest. This work is highly relevant to examining the pathophysiology of depression and identifying targets and mechanisms of treatments. As we will see, each technique provides an important but narrow glimpse into the brain. Research in the coming decades will likely be enhanced by a more integrative picture within and across these networks as we develop a better understanding of the mind–body connections in depression and treatments for depression.

FOUNDATIONAL KNOWLEDGE

Numerous approaches have been used to examine the morphology and cytoarchitecture of the brain within the context of depression. Early efforts involved a range of techniques, many of which continue to be used today. It is only in the last two decades that scientists have emphasized the anomalies in the structure and function of key brain circuits (Baumann et al., 1999). The scant research on depression that existed was often based on using depression as a psychiatric control for schizophrenia, a disorder in which neurodevelopmental anomalies were more clearly evident (Jeste, Lohr, & Goodwin, 1988).

Some of the long-standing methods for studying the brain have provided critical foundational knowledge. Postmortem evaluation showed that depressed patients had changes in monoamine receptors, transports, and other secondary messenger systems in the brainstem nuclei (Rajkowska, 2003). This evaluation helped support the noradrenergic hypothesis of the pathophysiology of depression (Ordway & Klimek, 2001). More recent postmortem evaluations of the brain have shown that specific quantitative and qualitative cellular characteristics of the brain (e.g., density, shape, size of glial cells) can play a role in mood disorders (reviewed by Price & Drevets, 2010).

Invasive technologies have advanced our understanding of adult depression by examining brain function *in vivo*. Invasive functional imaging methods include positron emission tomography and single-photon emission computed tomography. These procedures are considered invasive because they involve injecting radioactive substances to generate contrasts that assess blood flow, blood perfusion, and glucose metabolism in the brain as an indirect measure of neural activity. These studies have reported altered brain function at the neuromolecular level, including dysfunctional interaction between specific neurotransmitters and their corresponding receptor sites (Dougherty et al., 2006) and increased or decreased (relative to healthy controls [HC]) cerebral blood flow with respect to specific brain regions (Kowatch et al., 1999).

Some noninvasive technologies have a lengthy history for examining brain structure and function with regard to depression. For example, the use of computerized tomography (CT) scans more broadly helped to advance the understanding of ventricular enlargement (Shima et al., 1984). Electroencephalography (EEG) is another noninvasive technology used to examine depressed patients as early as 1936 (Lemere, 1936) and continues to provide essential information. EEG provides direct measurements of the time course of electrical activity, allowing for the isolation of different cortical frequency bands (delta, theta, alpha, and beta). Some of the important contributions of EEG research involve evidence of alpha asymmetry and connectivity dysfunction in depressed populations. More specifically, depressed individuals exhibited higher left alpha band activity (associated with approach motivation) and lower right alpha band activity (associated with withdrawal motivation) when compared with healthy controls (Stewart, Coan, Towers, & Allen, 2014). In addition, EEG connectivity has revealed lower overall functional connectivity between the subgenual anterior cingulate cortex (sgACC) and lateral and medial regions of the prefrontal cortex (Iseger et al., 2017). While best suited to measure peripheral brain functioning, these methods have provided a wealth of information to date and are beginning to be paired with other technologies.

While assessing brain structure and functioning is critically important, neuropsychological testing can provide a behavioral metric for examining brain functioning and provides complementary information to brain imaging technologies (see Cullum, Denney, & Bailey, Chapter 11, this volume, for more information on neuropsychological assessment in depression). Impairments in verbal memory, information-processing speed, and executive functioning have been identified, most consistently in adult patients with late-onset depression (Koenig, Bhalla, & Butters, 2014; Snyder, 2013), implicating the hippocampus and prefrontal cortex. Undoubtedly, many of these established techniques will continue to critically inform our understanding of the pathophysiology of depression, but the focus of this chapter is on some key advances brain imaging technology has provided to advance the understanding of depression.

Magnetic Resonance Imaging Methods to Evaluate Brain Structure and Function

While many types of neuroimaging methodologies have been established and utilized in psychiatric research, this review will focus on structural and functional MRI, a noninvasive neuroimaging technique that has made continual advances in increasing the quality of primarily spatial but, to some extent, temporal resolution.

Neuroimaging to Assess Brain Structure

Morphometric estimates include volume, thickness, and surface area. Voxel-based morphology is based on the estimates of three-dimensional voxels for the whole brain or for individual structures. Based to some extent on the level of gyrification, surface-based techniques can allow for an estimate of both the white and pial surfaces combined. These indices of cortical thickness and surface area can also be used to examine anatomical detail across the whole brain or localized brain regions to identify brain pathology. Structural connectivity between brain regions can also be estimated using diffusion tensor imaging. Some research on depression has focused on indices of white matter integrity, although the issue of whether anomalies are associated with depression remains largely unresolved (e.g., Cullen et al., 2020). Subtle differences in white matter integrity have been found across a number of different tracts in adults but not in adolescents with depression (van Velzen et al., 2020). Although structural and functional connectivities are correlated, in this chapter, we focus on functional instead of structural connectivity because functional connectivity also encompasses indirect connections between brain regions (Batista-García-Ramó & Fernández-Verdecia, 2018; Damoiseaux & Greicius, 2009).

Neuroimaging to Assess Brain Functioning: Activity and Connectivity

Functional MRI (fMRI) is a technique that provides useful temporal information about brain function by measuring changes in the hemodynamic response, or blood flow. fMRI typically relies on the blood-oxygen-level-dependent (BOLD) contrast. As a brain region becomes more active, it requires more resources, or glucose and oxygen, and blood flow increases to the brain region. When blood releases oxygen to a brain region, the blood becomes deoxygenated. Oxygenated and deoxygenated blood have different magnetic properties, and fMRI records these differences in magnetization over time as an index of brain activity.

fMRI can be used to record brain activity while an individual is completing a task or while an individual is at rest. Task-based activation utilizes experimental paradigms to look at relative activation or deactivation to certain types of stimuli or conditions. To understand brain functioning in depression, researchers commonly compare activation to negative conditions relative to positive or neutral conditions (e.g., sad vs. happy faces, reward vs. punishment conditions). Neural activation during cognitive tasks (e.g., working memory, executive functioning) is also examined.

Functional connectivity is the degree to which neural activity in one brain region is associated with the pattern of responding in another brain region(s). Since functionally connected regions have synchronized resting-state BOLD signals (Biswal, Yetkin, Haughton, & Hyde, 1995), this approach can estimate brain connectivity within neural networks of interest at rest (resting-state functional connectivity [RSFC]). Brain connectivity can also be examined while an individual is completing a task.

Neural Networks in Depression

Depression symptoms can be largely attributed to biased processing and interpretation of external and internal events (De Raedt & Koster, 2010). These biases result in maladaptive thought processes and behaviors. Processing of external events is driven by bottom-up brain structures that draw attention to salient stimuli in the environment that signal threat or reward (Menon & Uddin, 2010). Once these salient stimuli are detected, top-down structures must synthesize this information to shape ideas about the external world and make decisions about behavior (Miller & D'Esposito, 2005). Individuals must decide whether to approach or avoid environmental stimuli, such as who to associate with, what food to consume, or which places to avoid. In the short term, successful avoidance of threat promotes survival, and successful approach may optimize opportunities to obtain rewards (Elliot & Covington, 2001). Excessive avoidance and insufficient approach characterize depression and may lead to missed opportunities for maximizing one's potential and deriving pleasure, accounting for symptoms of depression, like anhedonia (Trew, 2011).

Beyond processing stimuli immediately in one's present environment, an individual must also integrate information from one's past and formulate ideas about the future. Although some brain regions activate and support behavior for a task at hand, there are other brain regions that are active at rest and direct attention inward toward self-reflection and autobiographical memories (Whitfield-Gabrieli & Ford, 2012). While thoughts centered on oneself and one's experience may help with planning and guiding behavior, excessive self-referential thinking may result in perseverative patterns of thinking that interfere with adaptive behavior and goal pursuit. In depression, these perseverative patterns of thinking are inherently negative and are termed rumination (Nolen-Hoeksema, Wisco, & Lyubomirsky, 2008).

The brain regions that are thought to drive these processes include four neural networks, or groups of brain regions that tend to activate and deactivate together. The prefrontal cortex (PFC), which is part of the cognitive control network (CCN), is the first network. The CCN drives top-down processing and is responsible for regulating bottom-up processing of critical brain regions to facilitate adaptive behavior (Miller & D'Esposito, 2005). Dysfunction of the CCN may underlie impaired attention, concentration, and executive functioning in depression (Corbetta & Shulman, 2002; Disner, Beevers, Haigh, & Beck, 2011). The CCN may be particularly impaired when the affective load is substantial.

Two networks are involved in detecting salient motivational features of the environment (sometimes when combined referred to as the salience network): the threat network is the avoidance system involved in the salience of threat to safety, and the reward network is the approach system involved in the salience of reward. Impaired threat network functioning may underlie negative affect, poor affect regulation, and autonomic dysfunction (Mayberg et al., 1999; Phillips, Drevets, Rauch, & Lane, 2003). Impaired reward network functioning may underlie deficits in reward processing and experiences of pleasure (Admon & Pizzagalli, 2015). The fourth network of interest is the default mode network (DMN), which works in opposition to task-positive prefrontal regions. Excessive DMN functioning in depression may underlie perseverative negative thoughts and self-reflection (Fox & Raichle, 2007; Gusnard & Raichle, 2001; Ochsner & Gross, 2005; Raichle et al., 2001).

In this chapter, we focus on the most compelling evidence from MRI research in populations with depression of brain structural and functional abnormalities in these four different networks: the CCN, threat network, reward network, and the DMN (see Plate 2.1 in the color insert). Although we focus on case-control studies with adults, for indeed, most research has centered on adults diagnosed with major depressive disorder (MDD), this chapter includes recent advancements in developmental psychopathology and neurophysiology. We consider briefly normal developmental patterns of change over time as well as what may go awry in the context of depression. Importantly, treatment tends to normalize the functioning of these four networks (Li et al., 2018). As this literature shows, we are beginning to understand how these brain networks are involved in the pathophysiology of depression, setting the stage for the development of treatments that directly target these aberrant neural circuits.

THE CCN/PFC

A student with depression had planned to start writing a paper this morning. Instead, it is noon and he is still in bed. He is staring at the ceiling thinking, "I can't do this. I'm never going to understand Shakespeare. What's the point? I'll get an F anyways." It's 5:00 P.M. by the time he has his laptop open, but he finds he cannot focus on his paper. Instead, he finds himself thinking about how he will disappoint his teachers and his family. This student had started out the school year well and had been receiving A's. His teacher had even nominated one of his papers for an award. However, a few months into the year, his class attendance dropped, missing assignments accumulated, and his grades started dropping to C's and D's. This student is catastrophizing and fortune-telling, two cognitive distortions commonly associated with depression. He is also struggling to regulate these negative thoughts and feelings in order to complete an important task. He finds it difficult to break out of the negative spiral. This inadequate regulation of negative processes can be due to impaired CCN functioning.

The CCN underlies regulatory abilities, including top-down control of cognitive processes and the regulation of negative emotions, two processes that often go awry in depression. Based on task-based neuroimaging across different executive function domains, the CCN includes the dorsolateral prefrontal cortex (dlPFC), the dorsal anterior cingulate cortex (dACC), the posterior parietal cortex (PPC), and the orbitofrontal cortex (OFC; Cole &

Schneider, 2007; Niendam et al., 2012). Recruitment of the CCN increases across development in accordance with the development of executive functioning abilities (Rubia, 2013), and regions of the CCN, like the anterior cingulate cortex (ACC), develop more extensive connections across development (Kelly et al., 2009).

Abnormal functioning of the PFC and cingulate cortex are theorized to underlie cognitive mechanisms of depression, including deficits in both "hot" and "cold" cognitive processing. The dACC and more lateral areas of the PFC tend to be implicated in cold cognition, whereas the ventral ACC, OFC, and more ventral and medial regions of the PFC tend to be implicated in hot cognition (Pessoa, 2008; Stevens, 2016). Cold cognition encompasses general executive control processes such as response inhibition, set shifting, and sustained attention. In contrast, hot cognition, or affective cognition, is the intersection between emotion processing and executive functioning and also involves the ability to use cognitive processes to regulate emotion (e.g., cognitive reappraisal). For example, the lateral PFC subserves active emotion regulation, such as when individuals try reappraising negative situations while the medial PFC (mPFC) subserves automatic emotion regulation (Groenewold et al., 2013). Additionally, the OFC is implicated in valuation and plays a critical role in the reward network (Pujara & Koenigs, 2014).

The CCN in general shows abnormalities in depression that contribute to global deficits in executive abilities, including impaired concentration, which is a common symptom of depression (Disner et al., 2011). These executive deficits interfere with regulation of emotional processing through prefrontal connections with the other neural networks implicated in depression. Some of the most effective treatments for depression, including cognitive-behavioral therapy (CBT), focus on cognitive regulation as a key process (Kerestes, Davey, Stephanou, Whittle, & Harrison, 2014; see Milanovic, McNeely, Qureshi, McKinnon, & Holshausen, Chapter 17, this volume, and Bowie, Best, Tran, & Boyd, Chapter 18, also this volume, for information on CBT for depression).

Brain Structure of the CCN

Depression, particularly early onset depression, consistently shows subtle volumetric abnormalities localized to structures of the CCN. Some of the most prominent gray matter reductions in volume in MDD have been noted in the sgACC, as well as OFC and the ventral lateral PFC (vlPFC) (Drevets, Price, & Furey, 2008), implicating regions involved in emotion regulation. Patterns of surface area and cortical thickness in depression have recently been examined by the Enhancing Neuroimaging Genetics through Meta-Analyses (ENIGMA; Schmaal et al., 2017) work group, which analyzed the largest compilation of data to date, including scans of over 10,000 patients with MDD or HC from 20 sites. They found no differences in surface area for adults. However, adolescents with MDD had lower total surface area in frontal regions (medial OFC and superior frontal gyrus). By contrast, there is now considerable evidence of cortical thinning in key areas of the frontal lobe associated with MDD in adults. Adults with MDD, but not adolescents with MDD, had thinner cortical gray matter in the OFC and ACC compared to healthy controls. Adults with MDD also had thinner cortical gray matter than controls in the cingulate cortex (Schmaal et al., 2017). Additional evidence is provided by a recent systematic literature review of 36 studies and meta-analysis of 24 studies that included about 2,000 participants (Suh et al., 2019). Cortical thinning was observed in the MDD group in the bilateral OFC (Brodmann's area 11). The mechanisms and dynamic processes relevant to cortical thinning are not well understood, though some researchers have suggested that the initial thickening may be due to maturational delays in the thinning process or a compensatory process that takes place to regulate limbic functioning (van Eijndhoven et al., 2013).

Resting-State Functional Connectivity of the CCN

In general, the CCN shows reduced within-network connectivity in depression (Mulders, van Eijndhoven, Schene, Beckmann, & Tendolkar, 2015). The dlPFC is hypoconnected to regions within the CCN, including the PPC (Kaiser, Andrews-Hanna, Wager, & Pizzagalli, 2015; Mulders et al., 2015). Decreased functional connectivity within the CCN (dACC and dlPFC seeds) is associated with poorer treatment response, apathy, and executive dysfunction (Dichter, Gibbs, & Smoski, 2015). Lower intrinsic connectivity within the CCN may interfere with coordination among the regions of the CCN, which may make engaging regulatory processes more difficult. The CCN also shows abnormal between-network RSFC with the threat network, reward network, and DMN, which will be reviewed in later sections.

Task-Based Activation of the CCN

Abnormal prefrontal activation in individuals suffering from depression is shown on both "cold" and "hot" cognitive tasks (Song et al., 2018). Cold cognitive tasks use neutral stimuli (e.g., arrows) whereas hot cognitive tasks use emotional stimuli (e.g., threatening faces) to examine preferential processing or the degree of distraction. Cognitive appraisal tasks are another type of hot cognitive task that involves regulating one's response to emotional stimuli. For example, a common task used to look at cognitive regulation is Ochsner's emotion regulation task in which participants are asked to respond normally or to try to decrease their negative feelings in response to negative pictures (Moran, Jendrusina, & Moser, 2013).

Behaviorally, populations with depression tend to show subtle deficits in executive functioning. For example, on the flanker task, a commonly used task to assess executive functioning, one must indicate the direction of a central arrow flanked by two arrows on each side that can either be pointing in the same direction (congruent) or in the opposite direction (incongruent) as the central arrow. Patients with depression tend to show greater interference (i.e., longer response times) on the incongruent trials, indicating difficulty resolving conflict (Sommerfeldt et al., 2016). Individuals with depression also have deficits in hot cognition, showing a bias toward negativity, evidenced by quicker response times to negative stimuli and greater distractibility by negative stimuli (Roiser & Sahakian, 2013).

Adults and youth with depression tend to show hypoactivation of the prefrontal cortex across hot and cold cognitive tasks (Fitzgerald, Laird, Maller, & Daskalakis, 2008; Hamilton et al., 2012; Kerestes et al., 2014; Miller, Hamilton, Sacchet, & Gotlib, 2015; Song et al., 2018). Prefrontal regions, including the dlPFC, vlPFC, and dACC, are underactive when downregulating negative emotions, processing positive stimuli, and engaging in executive functioning, like working memory, response inhibition, and verbal fluency (Groenewold et al., 2013; Kerestes et al., 2014; Klumpp & Deldin, 2010; Nord et al., 2020; Zilverstand, Parvaz, & Goldstein, 2017). Although the dlPFC, particularly the left dlPFC, shows lower activation to negative stimuli in adults with depression, some regions of the right dlPFC show increased activation to negative and positive stimuli (Fitzgerald et al., 2008). Differences in the right and left dlPFC to emotional stimuli are in line with a laterality effect that proposes hypoactivity in the "positive" left hemisphere and hyperactivity in the "negative" right hemisphere in populations with depression (Gadea, Espert, Salvador, & Martí-Bonmatí, 2011; Rutherford & Lindell, 2011). Hypoactivation of the CCN indicates that populations with depression are not engaging the CCN to actively direct attention away from irrelevant or negative stimuli and are failing to direct attention toward potential rewarding aspects of the environment.

Patients with depression have also exhibited hyperactivation of the CCN. Greater PFC activity has been found in response to negative stimuli (dACC; Groenewold et al., 2013; Hamilton et al., 2012), to positive stimuli (OFC; Groenewold et al., 2013), and during reward processing and reward anticipation (bilateral dlPFC; Zhang, Chang, Guo, Zhang, & Wang, 2013). When adults with MDD perform comparably to healthy controls on cold cognitive tasks, they tend to show greater prefrontal activation (Kerestes et al., 2014; Pizzagalli, 2011). Likewise, during cognitive reappraisal compared to passive viewing of negative stimuli, adults with MDD show greater lateral and medial PFC activation compared to healthy controls (Kerestes et al., 2014). Over-recruitment of CCN regions during cold and hot processing suggests that when populations with depression do engage the CCN, they are not efficiently recruiting the CCN and may be compensating for deficits by utilizing more resources. Notably, this compensation is not shown in adolescents, who do not exhibit PFC hyperactivation during cold cognitive tasks (Kerestes et al., 2014). Because the prefrontal cortex undergoes development into early adulthood, children and adolescents with depression may be less able to engage in these compensatory efforts.

Summary of CCN Findings

In summary, patients with depression demonstrate inadequate and/or inefficient CCN recruitment. Structural abnormalities of CCN regions are not consistent across development but may circumscribe the ability of patients with depression to draw on the CCN. Lower RSFC within the CCN may signal a lack of synchrony within the CCN that may interfere with coordinated functioning. Reduced prefrontal activation and connectivity may underlie difficulties regulating responses to negativity; depressed individuals may not be activating their CCN to downregulate hyperactive limbic regions that direct attention to negative stimuli, leading to a persistent negative mood. Overrecruitment, on the other hand, suggests that individuals with depression have to work harder to regulate their processing, which may result in feelings of fatigue and interfere with the ability to continually regulate mood given that cognitive resources are limited. The fact that the CCN is also underactive during cold cognitive tasks and shows reduced within-network RSFC may indicate general deficits in executive control and account for symptoms of poor concentration.

THE THREAT NETWORK/CORTICOLIMBIC NETWORK

Imagine an individual with depression is giving a presentation in front of a large audience. Most of the audience members may be smiling and nodding, but one audience member in the back is frowning. The speaker quickly detects this displeased audience member, and she begins to notice that he is rolling his eyes and starting to look at his phone. The speaker finds it hard to ignore the displeased audience member and starts thinking that she is inadequate and a failure. She leaves feeling discouraged and disappointed and starts thinking about how her speech must have been perceived poorly and about other past presentations that were unsuccessful, setting off a negative spiral of depressed mood and thoughts. On the way home, she notices the sharp tone of voice of the taxi driver and feels worse. An overactive threat network can lead to this pattern of quick detection and in-depth processing of negative features of the environment.

The threat network or corticolimbic network is involved in emotion activation and regulation. The threat network includes the limbic regions that emphasize bottom-up emotion processing, including the amygdala, hippocampus, insula, and the hypothalamus (Lindquist, Satpute, Wager, Weber, & Barrett, 2016; Vytal & Hamann, 2010). The threat network is also widely connected to the top-down regions of the CCN. Prefrontal regions like the lateral PFC, mPFC, ACC, and OFC contribute to the top-down regulation of these negative emotions (Seminowicz et al., 2004). Positive RSFC between limbic regions and the PFC, which may set the stage for recruiting top-down regulation, develops at age 10 and increases into adulthood (Alarcón, Cservenka, Rudolph, Fair, & Nagel, 2015). In response to negative stimuli, however, prefrontal to amygdala functional connectivity changes from positive to negative during puberty (Gee et al., 2013), a switch representing more successful top-down regulation of negative emotions in adolescence and adulthood.

The amygdala rapidly processes sensory information about the environment received from the thalamus and transmits this information to cortical regions for higher processing. The amygdala is well known for the quick detection of threat, but the amygdala also includes projections to the striatum to in turn influence both behavioral approach and avoidance (Janak & Tye, 2015). The hippocampus is critical for memory and stress responding (Lupien & Lepage, 2001). Importantly, these limbic regions have a large number of glucocorticoid receptors and are involved in hypothalamic–pituitary–adrenal (HPA) axis functioning and responses to stress (Liu et al., 2017). The insula and the cingulate cortex are involved in the communication between bottom-up and top-down structures, showing extensive connections with prefrontal regions and limbic structures. The insula is involved in regulating autonomic responses to threat and has connections to the motor system to initiate a behavioral response (Menon & Uddin, 2010). Like the insula, the ACC is an intermediary structure within the threat network and may serve to support affect regulation. The sgACC in particular is strongly implicated in the experience of negative emotions and is connected with brain regions that subserve emotion, regulate autonomic functioning, and underlie reward processing (Stevens, 2016).

In depression, limbic regions are commonly highly reactive. A growing body of evidence shows that hypoactive prefrontal regions fail to effectively downregulate over-activity in limbic regions, leading to persistent negative mood (Disner et al., 2011). As previously noted, however, the opposite pattern of prefrontal hyperactivity is also common and may indicate inefficiency, such that those with depression must work harder or recruit more resources than healthy individuals to downregulate limbic activity (Diener et al., 2012). Likewise, frontal regions have been shown to be both over- and underconnected to limbic regions (Heller, 2016). On the one hand, hyperconnectivity is usually interpreted as evidence of excessive feedforward information from limbic regions to frontal regions, such that negative stimuli are readily brought to conscious awareness. Hypoconnectivity, on the other hand, is taken as evidence of insufficient feedback from frontal regions to downregulate limbic regions.

Brain Structure of the Threat Network

Some of the most consistent findings for those suffering from depression involves the link between depression and hippocampal volume. Preclinical studies have provided a basis for a causal link between stress and hippocampal atrophy (Lupien & Lepage, 2001). Considered in the family of stress regulatory diseases, MDD is associated with decrements in hippocampal volume. For example, in the ENIGMA study (Schmaal et al., 2016), significantly lower hippocampal volume was measured in MDD than HC. Importantly, this result was driven by patients with recurrent MDD, and there were no group differences for depressed adults who only had one major depressive episode. Additionally, patients with early-onset MDD had smaller hippocampal volumes. Fortunately, the hippocampus continues to undergo neurogenesis throughout adulthood (Lupien & Lepage, 2001), and there is some evidence that when recovery takes place, the hippocampus may regain some of the previously lost brain volume (Mateus-Pinheiro et al., 2013). These volumetric differences in the hippocampus are common to a number of severe types of psychopathology and are not unique to MDD (Haukvik, Tamnes, Söderman, & Agartz, 2018).

Volumetric findings for the amygdala are more mixed (Schmaal et al., 2016). Enhanced dendritic arborization and increased spine density in the amygdala could translate into larger volumes (Mitra, Jadhav, McEwen, Vyas, & Chattarji, 2005; Vyas, Mitra, Rao, & Chattarji, 2002). However, in the previously described ENIGMA study on subcortical volumes, no overall group differences in amygdala volume were found. However, the developmental progression requires continued examination given that early-onset MDD had marginally lower amygdala volumes than late-onset MDD. Other subcortical regions did not differ across MDD and HC groups based on standard volumetric analyses, but when considering cortical thickness, adults with MDD have been shown to have thinner cortical gray matter than HC in some brain structures, including the insula (Schmaal et al., 2016, 2017).

Resting-State Functional Connectivity of the Threat Network

In depression, the threat network tends to show greater within-network connectivity among limbic regions, reduced connectivity between limbic and prefrontal regions (i.e., frontolimbic connectivity), and abnormal connectivity with the DMN (see section on the DMN). There is evidence of increased connectivity among the limbic structures. The amygdala and insula are hyperconnected (Li et al., 2018). Likewise, the sgACC shows increased connectivity with other limbic regions (e.g., insula, amygdala, superior temporal gyrus; Connolly et al., 2013). Greater amygdala and sgACC connectivity is associated with higher levels of negative affect and tends to increase at the onset of depression (Li et al., 2018). Greater connectivity among limbic regions may predispose patients with depression to more readily detect negative information, and greater synchrony among these regions may increase the likelihood that this information is passed along to be processed by higher-level brain regions and brought into conscious awareness.

Abnormal frontolimbic connectivity in depression may represent heightened feedforward activity from limbic regions, resulting in excessive processing of negative information as well as reduced feedback from frontal regions to downregulate limbic overactivity. Respectively, both greater and lower frontolimbic connectivity has been found in support of both of these theories. The ACC shows reduced connectivity with the thalamus and the amygdala (Wang, Hermens, Hickie, & Lagopoulos, 2012). The OFC also shows reduced connectivity with the amygdala (Cheng et al., 2018). The sgACC shows reduced RSFC with the left dlPFC (greater negative) but greater positive RSFC with the right dlPFC (Connolly et al., 2013). This laterality effect is consistent with hemispheric laterality research in depression that shows the left PFC is hypoactive while the right PFC is hyperactive. The left PFC may play a particularly critical role in inhibiting limbic activity to regulate negative emotions, whereas the right PFC may be involved in processing negative information from limbic regions. Accordingly, reduced negative RSFC between the sgACC and left dlPFC is related to lower levels of depression (Connolly et al., 2013). Greater negative frontolimbic connectivity may suggest a lack of coordination between frontal and limbic regions, such that heightened limbic activity is not triggering a regulatory response from frontal regions. Critically, treatment has shown to reverse abnormal threat network RSFC. Treatment increases frontolimbic connectivity (hypothalamus with dlPFC, OFC, and ACC; ACC with thalamus, amygdala, and pallidostriatum; Dichter et al., 2015; Wang et al., 2012).

Task-Based Activation of the Threat Network

Given the threat network's involvement in the experience of negative emotion, researchers commonly look at threat network activation during emotion processing. Common emotion processing tasks compare activation to negative emotional faces (e.g., sad or angry), to positive or neutral faces, or to non-face stimuli (e.g., shapes). Participants can be asked to respond to certain stimuli or to passively view the stimuli. One of the most commonly used emotion processing tasks that elicits amygdala activity requires participants to match either faces (e.g., angry, fearful, or happy) or shapes (Hariri, Tessitore, Mattay, Fera, & Weinberger, 2002). Typically, these tasks capture quick, bottom-up processing of limbic structures. In depression, limbic regions tend to be hyperactive in response to negative stimuli. Behaviorally, individuals with depression tend to show a negativity bias, responding faster to negative stimuli, having better recall for negative stimuli, or being more distracted by negative stimuli.

Adult and adolescent patients suffering from depression tend to show overactivity of threat network regions to negativity. Regions like the amygdala, dACC, sgACC, and the insula are hyperactive in response to threatening and nonthreatening negative stimuli, in anticipation of negative stimuli, and when downregulating or maintaining negative emotion (Hamilton et al., 2012; Joormann & Stanton, 2016; Kerestes et al., 2014; Miller et al., 2015; Zilverstand et al., 2017). Adolescents at risk for developing MDD also show amygdala hyperactivity (Kerestes et al., 2014). Hyperactivation of threat network regions in response to negative emotional stimuli support behavioral findings of a negativity bias in depression (Gotlib, Krasnoperova, Yue, & Joormann, 2004). Limbic hyperactivity drives this fast, automatic detection of negative features of the environment and greater processing of these negative features in depression.

Regions of the threat network also play a prominent role in the salient detection of positive features of the environment. In response to positive stimuli and to reward, populations with depression tend to show reduced threat network activation in regions like the amygdala, insula, ACC, and hippocampus (Groenewold et al., 2013; Miller et al., 2015; Zhang et al., 2013). Decreased activation of threat network regions to positive stimuli may indicate that individuals with depression may not detect and process positive stimuli as thoroughly, which may reduce opportunities for pleasure and enjoyment that may help break one out of a chronic low mood.

The threat network continues to show evidence of abnormal functioning even on cold cognitive tasks. Some regions of the threat network tend to be hypoactive during executive functioning tasks, like the dACC and the dorsal anterior insula, in depressed youth (Miller et al., 2015). Other regions of the threat network, like the sgACC, show evidence of hyperactivity during cold cognitive tasks in adolescents (Kerestes et al., 2014). Hypoactivity of threat network regions during executive functioning tasks may indicate that individuals with depression may not be thoroughly processing critical signals, like a stop signal, so they can override automatic tendencies when necessary. On the other hand, hyperactivity of other threat network regions during these cognitive tasks may suggest excessive processing of negative aspects of the tasks, like errors, and negative features outside of the task, like self-reflective thoughts, which detracts attention away from the task at hand. In conjunction, both underactivity and overactivity of the threat network during cold cognitive tasks suggest that patients with depression are not efficiently utilizing their neural resources to focus on the task at hand. They may fail to thoroughly process relevant features of the task and to disengage from negative feedback or irrelevant thoughts or feelings in order to perform the task successfully, which may contribute to the impaired concentration commonly found in depression.

Treatment has been shown to reduce hyperactivation of the threat network (Kerestes et al., 2014). This suggests that an important component of treating depression is reducing detection and processing of negative stimuli. In accordance, treatments like CBT train patients with depression to notice and challenge automatic negative thoughts. Interestingly, greater baseline levels of amygdala activation and lower pregenual ACC activation predict better CBT treatment response (Kerestes et al., 2014). These patients with greater threat network activation at baseline may have more room to improve and can receive greater benefit from treatments targeting automatic negative processing.

Task-Based Connectivity of the Threat Network

Threat network connectivity also shows abnormalities during hot and cold tasks. There is evidence of increased task-based connectivity within the threat network. For example, on an emotional face-matching task, patients with depression show increased connectivity between the bilateral extended amygdala and the sgACC (Kerestes et al., 2014). Excessive within-network connectivity of the threat network during tasks complements RSFC findings. The threat network is predisposed to rapid transmission between different regions that detect negative stimuli, and greater coherence between these regions is exhibited in response to threat. Greater coherence within the threat network in response to negativity may increase the likelihood that negative stimuli detected by bottom-up structures are processed by higher-order regions.

Moreover, patients with depression show reduced frontolimbic connectivity during both hot and cold tasks. Amygdala and prefrontal connectivity is reduced during emotion processing in depression (Dannlowski et al., 2009). Effective connectivity methods demonstrate lower top-down and bottom-up amygdala-OFC connectivity during the processing of emotional faces (Carballedo et al., 2011; de Almeida et al., 2009). During an emotion regulation task, adolescents with depression show reduced amygdala connectivity with the mPFC and the insula while maintaining their normal responses (Perlman et al., 2012) and greater mPFC and sgACC connectivity when asked to decrease their negative emotions. Adults (dlPFC-amygdala: Song et al., 2018) and adolescents (sgACC-vmPFC: Kerestes et al., 2014) suffering from depression also show lower threat network-PFC connectivity during cold cognitive tasks. Reduced frontolimbic connectivity likely contributes to difficulties in regulating negative emotions in depression. The PFC is less able to turn down excessive limbic reactivity and focus attention on the task at hand. Limbic regions, on the other hand, may fail to or inefficiently recruit top-down regions. Critically, attenuated left amygdala and ACC connectivity normalizes following antidepressant treatment in adults (Kerestes et al., 2014), suggesting that an important component of treatment may be increasing frontal regulatory control over regions of the threat network.

Summary of Threat Network Findings

In depression, limbic regions of the threat network tend to be overactive and overconnected, which may facilitate rapid detection and transmission of negative information. In contrast, frontal regulatory regions are underactive and less connected with limbic regions, which may interfere with downregulation of limbic regions and therefore, the ability to regulate negative emotions. A predisposition to notice and process negative stimuli may maintain the chronic, pervasive negative mood characteristic of depression and contribute to other symptoms, such as low self-esteem and rumination.

THE REWARD NETWORK/CORTICOSTRIATAL NETWORK

A pre-med student with depression takes his first biology exam. He receives an A but dismisses it as due to luck. He begins to assume he will fail the next exam and never become a doctor. He then struggles with motivation to do homework, gives up on studying altogether, and stops attending class. Ultimately, he may end up doing poorly in the class and feeling hopeless about the future. This pattern of behavior is driven by dysfunction in the reward network. Reduced processing of rewarding features of the environment interferes with goal-pursuit and may result in a negative, reinforcing spiral of isolation as well as lack of motivation and interest.

The reward network or the corticostriatal network is centrally implicated in reward processing, but different loops within these circuits are also implicated in executive control, emotional behavior, and motor control. Dysfunction in reward network functioning is related to anhedonia, rumination, and psychomotor retardation (Treadway & Zald, 2011). Task-based neuroimaging of pleasure and reward processing shows that the reward network includes frontal regions (vmPFC, dlPFC, ACC, and OFC), the thalamus, and striatal regions (nucleus accumbens, caudate, and putamen; Berridge & Kringelbach, 2008; Haber & Knutson, 2010; Liu, Hairston, Schrier, & Fan, 2011; Sescousse, Caldú, Segura, & Dreher, 2013). Striatal regions of the reward network undergo significant development during adolescence (Kerestes et al., 2014), and connectivity between striatal and frontal regions increases across development (Stevens, 2016).

The striatum is responsible for reward processing, activating to both reward (e.g., winning money) and loss or punishment (e.g., losing money or receiving an electric shock) (Admon & Pizzagalli, 2015). In particular, the nucleus accumbens (NAcc), part of the ventral striatum, is a key dopamine receptor and a neurotransmitter central for reward-related signaling, and is involved in all three stages of reward processing: anticipation, evaluation, and outcome (Pizzagalli, 2014). The dorsal striatum, composed of the caudate and putamen, activates to reward learning, adapting behavior to achieve rewards. The striatum sends information about reward outcomes to the OFC and vmPFC, closely connected structures that then use this information for valuation and guiding future decisions, including making determinations about risk, probability, reward, and loss as well as delaying gratification for later, larger rewards (Pujara & Koenigs, 2014). Healthy individuals show high levels of vmPFC/OFC-ventral striatum connectivity at rest and during reward-related tasks (Pujara & Koenigs, 2014).

Individuals suffering from depression commonly have difficulty deriving pleasure from activities they once enjoyed and motivating themselves in pursuit of a goal. An underactive reward network may underlie these key symptoms of anhedonia and avolition in depression, which are perhaps the most distinct features of depression (Clark & Watson, 1991; Treadway & Zald, 2011). In depression, reward-related regions fail to activate to pleasurable events and aspects of the environment as well as to anticipated reward. This hypoactivation of the reward network likely reduces the experience of joy and interferes with motivation, diminishing the inclination to get oneself out of bed and going about day-to-day activities (e.g., Pizzagalli, 2014).

Brain Structure of the Reward Network

There is limited evidence of volumetric differences in the striatal structures. In a series of meta-analyses, smaller caudate and putamen volumes were found (Bora, Harrison, Davey, Yücel, & Pantelis, 2012). However, the largest compilation of data to date (Schmaal et al., 2016) found no group differences in the caudate, putamen, pallidum, accumbens, or thalamus.

Resting-State Functional Connectivity of the Reward Network

In depression, the reward network shows abnormal connectivity with widespread brain regions that are part of the CCN, threat network, and DMN. There is some evidence of increased RSFC between the reward network and the CCN. The dorsal caudate shows greater RSFC with the dlPFC (Furman, Hamilton, & Gotlib, 2011; Mulders et al., 2015), which is related to depression severity and rumination (Furman et al., 2011). Greater connectivity between the reward network and the CCN may represent excessive dampening down of reward-related activity and positive emotions, predisposing individuals with depression to feelings of hopelessness.

On the other hand, the reward network tends to show reduced connectivity with regions of the threat network. The ventral striatum shows reduced RSFC with the sgACC in adult and adolescent patients with depression (Heller, 2016; Mulders et al., 2015). The ventral and dorsal putamen show reduced RSFC with the superior temporal gyrus and the posterior insula (Furman et al., 2011). Reduced connectivity may suggest that the reward network is not coordinated with the threat network in depression. Because the reward and threat networks typically work together to detect salient stimuli, reduced communication between these two systems may result in imbalanced decision making in favor of avoiding any threat over pursuing any reward. Importantly, treatment increases reward network connectivity with the threat network (hypothalamus with putamen and caudate; Dichter et al., 2015; Wang et al., 2012).

In terms of the DMN, regions of the reward network tend to show lower connectivity with anterior regions (mPFC) and mixed connectivity with posterior regions (precuneus, PCC). The ventral striatum, dorsal caudate, and ventral putamen all show reduced positive RSFC with the mPFC in adult and adolescent patients with depression (Furman et al., 2011; Heller, 2016; Mulders et al., 2015). Reduced dorsal caudate-mPFC RSFC specifically has been linked with psychomotor retardation (Furman et al., 2011). On the other hand, posterior regions of the DMN, like the precuneus and the PCC, show increased RSFC with the ventral striatum (Furman et al., 2011) but decreased connectivity with the caudate bilaterally (Bluhm et al., 2009). However, both increased positive connectivity and lower connectivity provide evidence of a lack of anticorrelation between the reward network and the DMN (Bluhm et al., 2009; Furman et al., 2011; Heller, 2016; Mulders et al., 2015). Reduced anticorrelation between the reward network and the DMN in depression may account for difficulty shifting out of perseverative, self-directed negative thinking and focusing on positive events that may be occurring externally. Approach-related brain centers may have deficits in communicating reward to frontal regions that regulate focus, such that positive stimuli may not undergo further processing. Instead, focus is predisposed to get stuck on negative self-reflection, even in the face of reward.

Task-Based Activation of the Reward Network

Processing the positive aspects of the environment is typically impaired in depression. Simple tasks to examine the processing of pleasant stimuli involve looking at or listening to positive stimuli, including pictures and music. To look at reward processing, tasks commonly rely on monetary rewards, although other rewarding stimuli, such as social feedback, have also been used. Reward network activation can be examined across three different stages of reward processing: reward selection, anticipation, and outcome. The Iowa Gambling Task (IGT) is commonly used to look at reward-related decision making. During the IGT, one chooses a card from one of four different decks that vary in the probability of winning and in the magnitude of the reward or loss. Researchers can examine the extent of learning on this task, risk aversion, and reward processing. Those with depression struggle with probabilistic learning or learning the probability of different outcomes, underestimating the likelihood of or undervaluing positive outcomes. Behaviorally, depressed individuals demonstrate low reward sensitivity and tend to experience lower levels and shorter duration of positive affect following rewards (Admon & Pizzagalli, 2015; Li et al., 2018).

In response to positive stimuli, regions of the reward network, such as the ventral striatum, NAcc, caudate, thalamus, and the OFC, show blunted activation. This pattern is also observed in children at risk for developing depression and individuals with remitted depression (Jenkins et al., 2018; Pizzagalli, 2014; Zhang et al., 2013). Individuals with depression are also less able to upregulate positive affect and show reduced NAcc activation over time (Heller et al., 2009). Reduced ventral striatum activation to positive stimuli is related to greater levels of anhedonia (Pizzagalli, 2014) and to lower levels of positive affect (Kerestes et al., 2014).

During reward-processing tasks, depressed individuals similarly show reduced activation in the reward network (Kerestes et al., 2014; Pujara & Koenigs, 2014; Zhang et al., 2013) across all three stages of reward processing, particularly patients with more severe depression (Hall, Milne, & MacQueen, 2014). Hypoactivity of the NAcc is found in response to reward (Pizzagalli, 2014), especially to larger rewards (Hall et al., 2014), and is associated with decreased pleasure (Admon & Pizzagalli, 2015). Reduced activation of the caudate is found during reward anticipation and reward outcome (Zhang et al., 2013) and is associated with deficits in reward learning (Admon & Pizzagalli, 2015; Pizzagalli, 2014). Hypoactivity of the putamen is found in response to reward cues and is associated with impaired reward prediction (Admon & Pizzagalli, 2015; Pizzagalli, 2014). Children and adolescents with depression show the same pattern of hypoactivation of reward regions during reward anticipation and outcome (Kerestes et al., 2014; Pizzagalli, 2014). Depression is also associated with a decreased ability to sustain reward-related activation and with greater declines in activity in reward-related regions (e.g., NAcc) over time (Carl et al., 2016; Jenkins et al., 2018). This pattern of reward network hypoactivation suggests that patients with depression are not detecting and processing positive and rewarding stimuli, which may account for the diminished experience of pleasure. Notably, antidepressant treatment upregulates reward network activity in regions like the ventral striatum, caudate, putamen, and vmPFC during reward-processing tasks and in response to positive stimuli (Kerestes et al., 2014; Pizzagalli, 2014; Pujara & Koenigs, 2014).

Study of the frontal regions of the reward network during reward-related tasks produces mixed findings, with both hypo- and hyperactivity found (Pujara & Koenigs, 2014). Mixed findings may be related to differences in reward and loss magnitudes. In response to and in anticipation of large losses and large rewards, patients with depression show reduced activation in the vmPFC, ACC, and inferior OFC (Hall et al., 2014; Kerestes et al., 2014). In contrast, hyperactivation of the bilateral middle and superior OFC is found during reward anticipation of small rewards (Kerestes et al., 2014). This may indicate that depression interferes particularly with incorporating larger rewards to shape behavior. In day-to-day life, this may manifest as difficulty imagining the future and long-term goals, resulting in feelings of hopelessness.

In terms of connectivity between frontal and striatal regions, individuals with depression tend to show reduced connectivity between frontal and bottom-up reward regions, although increased frontostriatal connectivity has been found in response to loss (Admon et al., 2015; Walsh et al., 2017). Depressed individuals tend to show greater bottom-up connectivity during reward anticipation, whereas healthy individuals tend to show top-down frontostriatal connectivity (Li et al., 2018). This suggests that depressed individuals may make decisions based more on the salience of wins or losses that is processed by striatal regions rather than on the synthesis of different sources of information across trials. In conjunction with a negativity bias and a preferential focus on penalties, depressed individuals may be strongly driven toward avoidance rather than approach.

Summary of Reward Network Findings

In individuals with depression, bottom-up striatal regions of the reward network tend to be underactive in response to positive stimuli and throughout different stages of reward processing in depression. These reward-related regions also tend to show abnormal connectivity with top-down prefrontal regions. Reward-processing signals go awry in early stages of the reward process, so individuals with depression may not allocate the attentional resources to detect the positive stimuli. Bottom-up regions may then fail to send reward-related information to prefrontal regions for further processing. In turn, prefrontal control regions may excessively quiet reward signaling, such that valid reward signals do not factor into decision making. Failure to process positive stimuli reinforces chronic depressed mood and prevents experiences that can challenge depressive concepts about one's self, others, and the world. Likewise, reduced processing of reward likely underlies symptoms of avolition and may result in negatively biased decisions that maintain depressive symptoms, like the decision to stay in bed all day. Patients with depression may struggle with motivation because reward network dysfunction fails to keep potential gains in mind, undermining goal pursuit, which may reinforce depressive symptoms.

THE DEFAULT MODE NETWORK

A patient with depression receives a text message from a friend with whom she had been planning to have dinner. The message reads, "Hey, something came up. I can't meet up tonight. Sorry." Her first thoughts may be "She doesn't want to hang out with me because she doesn't like me. I must have done something wrong. She must be mad." These thoughts quickly spiral into negative self-perceptions. "I'm boring. I'm not a good friend. No one will ever want to be my friend." These thoughts may escalate into a negative cascade of similar negative experiences. "My ex-boyfriend canceled a lot too right before we broke up. Dad did the same thing to mom before they got divorced. No one will ever love me.

I'm going to be alone forever." Individuals with depression tend to perseverate on negative self-reflections, and the DMN is associated with these ruminative thoughts.

The DMN is a task-negative network, meaning these brain regions are typically more active at rest and less active when engaged in a demanding or goal-directed task. Processes subserved by the DMN include self-referential processing, social cognition, and autobiographical memory. Importantly, in healthy individuals, the DMN is associated with mind-wandering and creativity (Whitfield-Gabrieli & Ford, 2012). Notably, the DMN is anticorrelated with task-positive networks, like the CCN, that are more active when engaged in a task. In healthy individuals, the anterior insula cortex and the ACC are involved in switching between the DMN and CCN, and thus are critical for directing the focus of conscious awareness (Craig & Craig, 2009). Using resting-state neuroimaging and tasks of introspection, social cognition, and autobiographical memory, the DMN can be divided into anterior and posterior subnetworks with the anterior subnetwork centered on the mPFC and the posterior subnetwork centered on the precuneus and posterior cingulate cortex (PCC) (Andrews-Hanna, Reidler, Sepulcre, Poulin, & Buckner, 2010; Buckner, Andrews-Hanna, & Schacter, 2008; Li et al., 2018; Raichle, 2015; Spreng, Mar, & Kim, 2009). Other regions of the DMN include the parietal cortex (medial, lateral, and inferior), angular gyrus, and medial temporal lobe.

Functional connectivity within the DMN is generally similar in children and adults, and posterior regions of the DMN show strong connectivity in infants (Supekar et al., 2010; Whitfield-Gabrieli & Ford, 2012). DMN structural connectivity and anterior to posterior DMN (e.g., mPFC to PCC) functional connectivity, however, are weak in childhood. Anterior to posterior connectivity strengthens into adulthood but decreases after age 60. The DMN and the CCN anticorrelation also increases into adulthood (Stevens, 2016).

There are regional differences in DMN activity during self-referential and memory processing. Anterior regions of the DMN tend to subserve self-referential processing and social cognition. Posterior regions are involved in retrieving autobiographical memories. The medial temporal lobe and associated structures are critical for episodic memory and prospection. The anterior mPFC and a region encompassing the precuneus and PCC make up a midline core of the DMN that is strongly connected with all regions within the DMN (Andrews-Hanna et al., 2010; Buckner et al., 2008; Whitfield-Gabrieli & Ford, 2012).

In depression, the DMN tends to show excessive within-network connectivity and greater connectivity with more affective nodes, like the sgACC (Hamilton, Farmer, Fogelman, & Gotlib, 2015). Patients with depression also have difficulty turning off DMN activation and engaging other networks, like the CCN, to focus on a task at hand. The tendency for individuals with depression to get "stuck" in a negative spiral of perseverative, self-reflective thoughts of failure, worthlessness, and guilt is attributed to abnormalities in the DMN. In addition, the negative valence of these ruminative thoughts is attributed to excessive connectivity between the DMN and limbic regions, leading to low self-esteem and self-blame.

Brain Structure of the DMN

There is no consistent evidence of structural differences between depressed and well participants, including no evidence of surface area differences in brain regions implicated in the DMN. While there is some preliminary evidence of less cortical thickness in regions of the DMN, including the PCC and the right precuneus in early-onset compared to late-onset MDD (Truong et al., 2013), it is possible that these regions are particularly influenced by disturbances in sleep that are common accompaniments of MDD (Yu et al., 2018). A meta-analysis of social phobia, a common precursor of depression, shows evidence of greater volume of the left precuneus (Wang et al., 2018). Other indices of structure for the DMN have not typically been assessed for relevance to depression. However, in the previously discussed ENIGMA study (Schmaal et al., 2017), adults (but not adolescents) with MDD had thinner cortical gray matter (but not cortical surface areas) than HC in related structures, including the temporal lobes.

Resting-State Functional Connectivity of the DMN

In MDD, there is evidence of hyperconnectivity both within and between the DMN and other networks implicated in depression (Whitfield-Gabrieli & Ford, 2012). Patients with depression exhibit increased RSFC in both the anterior and posterior regions of the DMN (Dichter et al., 2015). In terms of the anterior subnetwork, functional connectivity in the ventral and dorsal mPFC (vmPFC and dmPFC) and the ventral ACC is increased in adults and adolescents with MDD (Kerestes et al., 2014; Zhu et al., 2011). Higher functional connectivity of the vmPFC and vACC is related to rumination (Zhu et al., 2011). Posterior regions of the DMN also show greater within-network connectivity. Greater connectivity has been found between the PCC with the precuneus, bilateral lateral parietal lobes, and dmPFC (Dichter et al., 2015; Mulders et al., 2015). Greater functional connectivity within the DMN is associated with symptoms of pessimism (Dichter et al., 2015). DMN hyperconnectivity tends to persist into remission (Li et al., 2018), particularly in the anterior DMN (Dichter et al., 2015). Reduced within-DMN RSFC has also been found, particularly in posterior regions of the DMN, including the PCC, precuneus, and angular gyrus. Reduced posterior DMN RSFC is related to over-general memory (Zhu et al., 2011). The midline core also shows decreased connectivity with the dmPFC (anterior medial PFC–dmPFC, PCC-dmPFC, precuneus-dmPFC; Mulders et al., 2015; Zhu et al., 2011). Treatment-resistant depression is particularly associated with reduced functional connectivity within the DMN (Dichter et al., 2015). These differences in within-DMN connectivity may be accounted for by different symptom profiles and depression severity.

The DMN also shows abnormal patterns of connectivity with the CCN and the threat network. The DMN shows predominance over the CCN in depression in contrast to the typical anticorrelated DMN-CCN connectivity found in healthy populations. Instead, populations with depression evidence greater positive RSFC and reduced negative RSFC between the DMN and the dlPFC (Kaiser et al., 2015). This predominance of the DMN over the CCN is associated with rumination (Whitfield-Gabrieli & Ford, 2012). DMN dominance over frontal executive regions may indicate that individuals with depression may struggle to disengage the DMN and engage the CCN, resulting in a spiral of negative perseverative thoughts. Critically, treatment increases DMN-CCN anticorrelation (Mulders et al., 2015).

The DMN is hyperconnected to the threat network in depression. DMN RSFC is increased with regions like the sgACC in adults and adolescents (Hamilton et al., 2015;

Kerestes et al., 2014; Li et al., 2018; Mulders et al., 2015; Whitfield-Gabrieli & Ford, 2012). There is also greater positive amygdala and precuneus RSFC in adolescents with depression (Cullen et al., 2014). Greater sgACC and DMN RSFC is positively associated with depression severity (Kerestes et al., 2014) and with rumination symptoms (Li et al., 2018). Excessive threat network and DMN connectivity may contribute to the negative content of rumination in depression by making it easy for negative external stimuli to elicit perseverative, self-referential thoughts. However, greater negative connectivity between the threat network and DMN has also been found (amygdala-mPFC: Kaiser et al., 2015; sgACC-precuneus: Connolly et al., 2013), which has been associated with greater depression symptoms. Because the threat network is involved in saliency detection, greater negative connectivity may indicate that external stimuli may be ineffective in interrupting ruminative cascades to redirect focus in populations with depression. Notably, treatment reduces functional connectivity between limbic regions and the DMN (medial frontal gyrus, precuneus; Dichter et al., 2015; Wang et al., 2012).

There is also increased DMN connectivity with temporal regions, like the temporal pole, the temporal parietal junction/lateral temporal cortex, and the hippocampus (Kaiser et al., 2015; Zhu, Zhu, Shen, Liao, & Yuan, 2017). Temporal regions are involved in short-term and working memory. Greater DMN connectivity with temporal regions is positively correlated with rumination symptoms (Zhu et al., 2017). Greater connectivity between the DMN and temporal regions may contribute to the perseverative nature of rumination. The temporal lobe may maintain negative thoughts in conscious awareness and also elicit other recent negative events in short-term memory, which may lead to a cascade of negative thinking.

Task-Based Activation of the DMN

Overall, the DMN tends to be overactive across a variety of tasks in patients with depression. When healthy individuals engage in a task, the DMN tends to deactivate, and this phenomenon is known as DMN suppression. In depression, there is reduced DMN suppression. Instead, individuals with depression show greater anterior and posterior DMN activity during both hot and cold tasks (Whitfield-Gabrieli & Ford, 2012). Tasks that have shown increased DMN activity in depression include affective processing tasks, reward processing tasks, and cold cognitive tasks. The PCC shows increased activation to positive and negative stimuli in depressed individuals (Fitzgerald et al., 2008), and anterior regions of the DMN fail to deactivate during emotion judgment (Grimm et al., 2011). The cuneus and the mPFC are hyperactive during reward-processing tasks (Kerestes et al., 2014; Zhang et al., 2013). Patients with depression also fail to suppress activation in the medial temporal lobe and precuneus during word-generation tasks (Backes et al., 2014; Takamura et al., 2016). While listening to music, greater anhedonia is associated with greater activity in DMN regions like the PCC, mPFC, and precuneus (Jenkins et al., 2018) and with greater CCN activity in the inferior frontal gyrus. This may suggest that the CCN is ineffectively downregulating DMN activity (Jenkins et al., 2018). The DMN is also hyperconnected and fails to show anticorrelation with the CCN during working memory, self-referential thinking, and emotion processing (Li et al., 2018; Rayner, Jackson, & Wilson, 2016). DMN hyperactivity during tasks is associated with greater depression severity and feelings of hopelessness in depressed patients (Whitfield-Gabrieli & Ford, 2012). DMN hyperactivity has been shown to normalize following successful depression treatment (Takamura et al., 2016). DMN hyperactivity suggests that individuals with depression may attend less to features of the task and instead are stuck on negative, task-unrelated thoughts (i.e., ruminate).

Studies that have directly examined neural activity during rumination have also shown DMN hyperactivity. Rumination is most commonly assessed by self-report measures. Rumination induction tasks have been developed in which individuals are asked to think about different statements designed to elicit either ruminative or neutral thoughts (e.g., "the degree of helplessness you feel" vs. "the shape of a cello"; Nolen-Hoeksema & Morrow, 1991, 1993). While ruminating, depressed individuals show greater activation in prefrontal (dlPFC, OFC, dACC and rACC), limbic (amygdala, sgACC), and DMN regions (PCC, mPFC). They show reduced activation in reward-related regions (caudate) and other DMN regions (precuneus, cuneus) (Cooney, Joormann, Eugène, Dennis, & Gotlib, 2010). Adolescents with remitted depression also show greater DMN (precuneus, inferior parietal lobule, medial temporal gyrus) and limbic (amygdala, thalamus, insula) activation during rumination (Burkhouse et al., 2017). These rumination paradigms provide direct evidence of DMN involvement in rumination.

Summary of DMN Findings

In summary, the DMN tends to dominate over other networks in depression. The DMN shows excessive within- and between-network connectivity and is hyperactive when ruminating and on a range of tasks. Self-report questions and rumination tasks have linked the DMN with ruminative thinking in depressed populations, and hyperactivity of DMN regions on other tasks suggests that patients with depression struggle to shut down this task-negative network. Predominance of the DMN may result in a trade-off such that other networks are not adequately recruited as needed (e.g., reward network regions for reward processing or the CCN for regulatory controls). Depression, then, may impair day-to-day functioning because attention is directed inward toward unrelated, perseverative negative thoughts and away from the present situation.

DISCUSSION

As noted in this chapter, key structural and functional anomalies associated with depression are evident in control, threat, reward, and default mode networks. Overall, the studies show evidence of disruption in these four networks, but there is variability across methods of evaluation. The most convincing evidence comes from connectivity analyses, more variable results from across activation paradigms, and the most tentative evidence from examination of brain structure. In some cases, the evidence is consistent across different imaging parameters of structure and function. Structural brain differences are not consistently evident, but overall the data shows some evidence of subtle differences between depressed and healthy controls. By contrast, techniques that employ brain-functioning indices show some relatively robust patterns of atypical brain connectivity and activation.

The most research and the strongest evidence are evident in the threat and reward networks, but overall all four networks show evidence of functional anomalies in populations with depression.

In other cases, considerable variation is noted, sometimes due to inadequately powered studies. Several key features about populations with depression likely contribute to this variation. One issue pertains to differences in types of depression and the tremendous variation in symptom presentation within and across samples. A second issue pertains to considering depressive problems within the broader context of psychopathology. The emphasis on transdiagnostic approaches is currently getting some traction. Indeed, most of the literature fails to fully consider patterns of comorbidities and to embed depressive problems within the broader context of psychopathology. A recent review of imaging evidence for transdiagnostic approaches provides some evidence for differences in bipolar and unipolar depression, but notes that more research is needed to determine if we will be able to transcend the use of current nosological systems using these strategies (Mitelman, 2019). A third issue of note is developmental context. Indeed, we are just beginning to more fully understand differences among age of onset, chronicity (including treatment-resistant depression), the developmental context in which symptoms are assessed (e.g., samples of adolescents vs. elderly populations), and severity (e.g., those with mild, moderate, or severe impairment). Emerging evidence suggests that biotypes of depression may help inform treatment responses. Given these notable variations, perhaps it is surprising that any evidence of consensus is emerging. However, these brain networks are likely to be critically important when considering targets of treatments across types of depression, but these four networks may show differences in the degree or even directionality of abnormalities in different subsets of depression.

The technology involved in precise measurement of key networks is continually evolving. For example, in a recent study using a 7 Tesla MRI whole-brain analysis, Schmidt and colleagues (2017) were able to measure habenula volumes. The habenula is a paired epithalamic structure involved in the pathogenesis of MDD, specifically with an impact on the regulation of serotonergic and dopaminergic neurons. While absolute and relative total habenula volumes did not differ significantly, correlations were found between bilateral habenula volumes and depressive symptom severity. These increasingly more clearly focused and precise brain measurements will likely provide critical information about how to pair specific pharmacological agents. Similarly, computational advancements will be critically important. Recently, machine learning was used to identify networks that distinguish between MDD and HC adults with a classification accuracy of 97% (Guo, Qin, Chen, Xu, & Xiang, 2017). The regions of most significance were generally consistent with previous studies (e.g., bilateral temporal pole, left superior frontal gyrus, right lateral dorsolateral frontal gyrus, left thalamus, left pallidum, right putamen, left lingual gyrus, right cuneus, and left PCC). Advances in measurement and analysis of these brain networks will likely clarify variability in the current literature.

Precision is one issue, but integration is another. Even if these networks prove to be those primarily implicated in depression, we have little knowledge about whether or not all four are commonly disrupted. Do most individuals show anomalies across the cognitive, threat, reward, and default mode networks? Are there specific types of depression that correspond to specific brain regions?

A related issue is that much of our current work on neurobiological mechanisms of depression falls short by providing an account of individual indices at play. With increasing attention being given to neurobiological correlates of psychopathology, research has begun to consider the use of multiple levels of analysis of a system and how they interact with one another. The Research Domain Criteria project approach calls for increased focus on multilevel analyses, but this objective remains largely aspirational as integrative pictures of biological functioning are sparse. Depressive problems are well suited for the application of this approach as they may be considered within a dimension that is relevant to core biological processes. These concepts are foundational to the organizational perspective of development (Toth & Cicchetti, 2010), with early maladaptation probabilistically setting the individual up for later derailments in functioning. Additionally, vulnerability to developing psychopathology is associated with incoherence within and across various biological and psychological systems, potentially allowing for a more holistic understanding of the various sequelae that may occur following aberrant development of neurobiological indices. One line of work that has an emerging literature is threat system functioning at the neural and physiological levels. For example, our group published the first paper on the interplay between brain structure and activation and HPA axis functioning within the context of a stressor with depressed adolescents (Klimes-Dougan et al., 2014). We have also considered the correspondence of activation and connectivity within the context of self-harming adolescents (Westlund Schreiner, Klimes-Dougan, Parenteau, Hill, & Cullen, 2019). Multilevel analytical frameworks will help advance the understanding of more cross-talk across systems and remains a largely unexplored frontier.

In closing, the focus of this review has been on the pathological processes and corresponding brain anomalies in depression, but even these changes may be examples of largely adaptive mechanisms. Cameron and Schoenfeld (2018) provide an exceptional example of possible adaptive mechanisms of the affective system. Rapid learning is important in aversive environments by the use of fear generalization, setting the stage for how the individual can respond to or avoid threats and increase their survival. Importantly, they argue that the failure to rapidly adjust perceptions of fear may be adaptive in some contexts. Importantly, targets of intervention must consider adaptive capacities of the individual and disentangle when a neural anomaly is impairing and when it is beneficial. The hope is that this review of the central neural systems involved in depression may provide a platform for examining possible treatments.

REFERENCES

Admon, R., Nickerson, L. D., Dillon, D. G., Holmes, A. J., Bogdan, R., Kumar, P., et al. (2015). Dissociable cortico-striatal connectivity abnormalities in major depression in response to monetary gains and penalties. *Psychological Medicine, 45*(1), 121–131.

Admon, R., & Pizzagalli, D. A. (2015). Dysfunctional reward processing in depression. *Current Opinion in Psychology, 4*, 114–118.

Alarcón, G., Cservenka, A., Rudolph, M. D., Fair, D. A., & Nagel, B. J. (2015). Developmental sex differences in resting state functional connectivity of amygdala sub-regions. *NeuroImage, 115*, 235–244.

Andrews-Hanna, J. R., Reidler, J. S., Sepulcre, J., Poulin, R., & Buckner, R. L. (2010). Functional-anatomic fractionation of the brain's default network. *Neuron, 65*(4), 550–562.

Backes, H., Dietsche, B., Nagels, A., Stratmann, M., Konrad, C., Kircher, T., et al. (2014). Increased neural activity during overt and continuous semantic verbal fluency in major depression: Mainly a failure to deactivate. *European Archives of Psychiatry and Clinical Neuroscience, 264*(7), 631–645.

Batista-García-Ramó, K., & Fernández-Verdecia, C. I. (2018). What we know about the brain structure–function relationship. *Behavioral Sciences, 8*(4), 39.

Baumann, B., Danos, P., Krell, D., Diekmann, S., Wurthmann, C., Bielau, H., et al. (1999). Unipolar–bipolar dichotomy of mood disorders is supported by noradrenergic brainstem system morphology. *Journal of Affective Disorders, 54*(1), 217–224.

Berridge, K. C., & Kringelbach, M. L. (2008). Affective neuroscience of pleasure: Reward in humans and animals. *Psychopharmacology, 199*(3), 457–480.

Biswal, B., Yetkin, F. Z., Haughton, V. M., & Hyde, J. S. (1995). Functional connectivity in the motor cortex of resting human brain using echo-planar MRI. *Magnetic Resonance in Medicine, 34*(4), 537–541.

Bluhm, R., Williamson, P., Lanius, R., Théberge, J., Densmore, M., Bartha, R., et al. (2009). Resting state default-mode network connectivity in early depression using a seed region-of-interest analysis: Decreased connectivity with caudate nucleus. *Psychiatry and Clinical Neurosciences, 63*(6), 754–761.

Bora, E., Harrison, B. J., Davey, C. G., Yücel, M., & Pantelis, C. (2012). Meta-analysis of volumetric abnormalities in cortico-striatal-pallidal-thalamic circuits in major depressive disorder. *Psychological Medicine, 42*(4), 671–681.

Buckner, R. L., Andrews-Hanna, J. R., & Schacter, D. L. (2008). The brain's default network: Anatomy, function, and relevance to disease. *Annals of the New York Academy of Sciences, 1124*(1), 1–38.

Burkhouse, K. L., Jacobs, R. H., Peters, A. T., Ajilore, O., Watkins, E. R., & Langenecker, S. A. (2017). Neural correlates of rumination in adolescents with remitted major depressive disorder and healthy controls. *Cognitive, Affective, and Behavioral Neuroscience, 17*(2), 394–405.

Cameron, H. A., & Schoenfeld, T. J. (2018). Behavioral and structural adaptations to stress. *Frontiers in Neuroendocrinology, 49*, 106–113.

Carballedo, A., Scheuerecker, J., Meisenzahl, E., Schoepf, V., Bokde, A., Möller, H.-J., et al. (2011). Functional connectivity of emotional processing in depression. *Journal of Affective Disorders, 134*(1–3), 272–279.

Carl, H., Walsh, E., Eisenlohr-Moul, T., Minkel, J., Crowther, A., Moore, T., et al. (2016). Sustained anterior cingulate cortex activation during reward processing predicts response to psychotherapy in major depressive disorder. *Journal of Affective Disorders, 203*, 204–212.

Cheng, W., Rolls, E. T., Qiu, J., Xie, X., Lyu, W., Li, Y., et al. (2018). Functional connectivity of the human amygdala in health and in depression. *Social Cognitive and Affective Neuroscience, 13*(6), 557–568.

Clark, L. A., & Watson, D. (1991). Tripartite model of anxiety and depression: psychometric evidence and taxonomic implications. *Journal of Abnormal Psychology, 100*(3), 316–336.

Cole, M. W., & Schneider, W. (2007). The cognitive control network: Integrated cortical regions with dissociable functions. *NeuroImage, 37*(1), 343–360.

Connolly, C. G., Wu, J., Ho, T. C., Hoeft, F., Wolkowitz, O., Eisendrath, S., et al. (2013). Resting-state functional connectivity of subgenual anterior cingulate cortex in depressed adolescents. *Biological Psychiatry, 74*(12), 898–907.

Cooney, R. E., Joormann, J., Eugène, F., Dennis, E. L., & Gotlib, I. H. (2010). Neural correlates of rumination in depression. *Cognitive, Affective, and Behavioral Neuroscience, 10*(4), 470–478.

Corbetta, M., & Shulman, G. L. (2002). Control of goal-directed and stimulus-driven attention in the brain. *Nature Reviews Neuroscience, 3*(3), 201.

Craig, A. D., & Craig, A. D. B. (2009). How do you feel—now?: The anterior insula and human awareness. *Nature Reviews Neuroscience, 10*(1), 59–70.

Cullen, K. R., Brown, R., Schreiner, M. W., Eberly, L. E., Klimes-Dougan, B., Reigstad, K., et al. (2020). White matter microstructure relates to lassitude but not diagnosis in adolescents with depression. *Brain Imaging and Behavior, 14*(5), 1507–1520.

Cullen, K. R., Westlund, M. K., Klimes-Dougan, B., Mueller, B. A., Houri, A., Eberly, L. E., et al. O.

(2014). Abnormal amygdala resting-state functional connectivity in adolescent depression. *JAMA Psychiatry, 71*(10), 1138–1147.

Damoiseaux, J. S., & Greicius, M. D. (2009). Greater than the sum of its parts: A review of studies combining structural connectivity and resting-state functional connectivity. *Brain Structure and Function, 213*(6), 525–533.

Dannlowski, U., Ohrmann, P., Konrad, C., Domschke, K., Bauer, J., Kugel, H., et al. (2009). Reduced amygdala–prefrontal coupling in major depression: Association with MAOA genotype and illness severity. *International Journal of Neuropsychopharmacology, 12*(1), 11.

de Almeida, J. R. C., Versace, A., Mechelli, A., Hassel, S., Quevedo, K., Kupfer, D. J., et al. (2009). Abnormal amygdala-prefrontal effective connectivity to happy faces differentiates bipolar from major depression. *Biological Psychiatry, 66*(5), 451–459.

De Raedt, R., & Koster, E. H. W. (2010). Understanding vulnerability for depression from a cognitive neuroscience perspective: A reappraisal of attentional factors and a new conceptual framework. *Cognitive, Affective and Behavioral Neuroscience, 10*(1), 50–70.

Dichter, G. S., Gibbs, D., & Smoski, M. J. (2015). A systematic review of relations between resting-state functional-MRI and treatment response in major depressive disorder. *Journal of Affective Disorders, 172*, 8–17.

Diener, C., Kuehner, C., Brusniak, W., Ubl, B., Wessa, M., & Flor, H. (2012). A meta-analysis of neurofunctional imaging studies of emotion and cognition in major depression. *NeuroImage, 61*(3), 677–685.

Disner, S. G., Beevers, C. G., Haigh, E. A. P., & Beck, A. T. (2011). Neural mechanisms of the cognitive model of depression. *Nature Reviews Neuroscience, 12*(8), 467–477.

Dougherty, D. D., Bonab, A. A., Ottowitz, W. E., Livni, E., Alpert, N. M., Rauch, S. L., et al. (2006). Decreased striatal D1 binding as measured using PET and [11C]SCH 23,390 in patients with major depression with anger attacks. *Depression and Anxiety, 23*(3), 175–177.

Drevets, W. C., Price, J. L., & Furey, M. L. (2008). Brain structural and functional abnormalities in mood disorders: Implications for neurocircuitry models of depression. *Brain Structure and Function, 213*(1), 93–118.

Elliot, A. J., & Covington, M. V. (2001). Approach and avoidance motivation. *Educational Psychology Review, 20*, 73–92.

Fitzgerald, P. B., Laird, A. R., Maller, J., & Daskalakis, Z. J. (2008). A meta-analytic study of changes in brain activation in depression. *Human Brain Mapping, 29*(6), 683–695.

Fox, M. D., & Raichle, M. E. (2007). Spontaneous fluctuations in brain activity observed with functional magnetic resonance imaging. *Nature Reviews Neuroscience, 8*(9), 700–711.

Furman, D. J., Hamilton, J. P., & Gotlib, I. H. (2011). Frontostriatal functional connectivity in major depressive disorder. *Biology of Mood and Anxiety Disorders, 1*(1), 11.

Gadea, M., Espert, R., Salvador, A., & Martí-Bonmatí, L. (2011). The sad, the angry, and the asymmetrical brain: Dichotic listening studies of negative affect and depression. *Brain and Cognition, 76*(2), 294–299.

Gee, D. G., Humphreys, K. L., Flannery, J., Goff, B., Telzer, E. H., Shapiro, M., et al. (2013). A developmental shift from positive to negative connectivity in human amygdala-prefrontal circuitry. *Journal of Neuroscience, 33*(10), 4584–4593.

Gotlib, I. H., Krasnoperova, E., Yue, D. N., & Joormann, J. (2004). Attentional biases for negative interpersonal stimuli in clinical depression. *Journal of Abnormal Psychology, 113*(1), 127–135.

Grimm, S., Ernst, J., Boesiger, P., Schuepbach, D., Boeker, H., & Northoff, G. (2011). Reduced negative BOLD responses in the default-mode network and increased self-focus in depression. *World Journal of Biological Psychiatry, 12*(8), 627–637.

Groenewold, N. A., Opmeer, E. M., de Jonge, P., Aleman, A., & Costafreda, S. G. (2013). Emotional valence modulates brain functional abnormalities in depression: Evidence from a meta-analysis of fMRI studies. *Neuroscience and Biobehavioral Reviews, 37*(2), 152–163.

Guo, H., Qin, M., Chen, J., Xu, Y., & Xiang, J. (2017). Machine-learning classifier for patients with major depressive disorder: Multifeature approach based on a high-order minimum spanning tree functional brain network. *Computational and Mathematical Methods in Medicine, 2017*, 4820935.

Gusnard, D. A., & Raichle, M. E. (2001). Searching for a baseline: Functional imaging and the resting human brain. *Nature Reviews Neuroscience, 2*(10), 685–694.

Haber, S. N., & Knutson, B. (2010). The reward circuit: Linking primate anatomy and human imaging. *Neuropsychopharmacology, 35*(1), 4–26.

Hall, G. B. C., Milne, A. M. B., & MacQueen, G. M. (2014). An fMRI study of reward circuitry in patients with minimal or extensive history of major depression. *European Archives of Psychiatry and Clinical Neuroscience, 264*(3), 187–198.

Hamilton, J. P., Etkin, A., Furman, D. J., Lemus, M. G., Johnson, R. F., & Gotlib, I. H. (2012). Functional neuroimaging of major depressive disorder: A meta-analysis and new integration of baseline activation and neural response data. *American Journal of Psychiatry, 169*(7), 693–703.

Hamilton, J. P., Farmer, M., Fogelman, P., & Gotlib, I. H. (2015). Depressive rumination, the default-mode network, and the dark matter of clinical neuroscience. *Biological Psychiatry, 78*(4), 224–230.

Hariri, A. R., Tessitore, A., Mattay, V. S., Fera, F., & Weinberger, D. R. (2002). The amygdala response to emotional stimuli: A comparison of faces and scenes. *NeuroImage, 17*(1), 317–323.

Haukvik, U. K., Tamnes, C. K., Söderman, E., & Agartz, I. (2018). Neuroimaging hippocampal subfields in schizophrenia and bipolar disorder: A systematic review and meta-analysis. *Journal of Psychiatric Research, 104,* 217–226.

Heller, A. S. (2016). Cortical-subcortical interactions in depression: From animal models to human psychopathology. *Frontiers in Systems Neuroscience, 10,* 1–10.

Heller, A. S., Johnstone, T., Shackman, A. J., Light, S. N., Peterson, M. J., Kolden, G. G., et al. (2009). Reduced capacity to sustain positive emotion in major depression reflects diminished maintenance of fronto-striatal brain activation. *Proceedings of the National Academy of Sciences, 106*(52), 22445–22450.

Horwitz, A. V., Wakefield, J. C., & Lorenzo-Luaces, L. (2017). History of depression. In R. J. DeRubeis & D. R. Strunk (Eds.), *Oxford handbook of mood disorders* (Vol. 1, pp. 11–23). New York: Oxford University Press.

Iseger, T. A., Korgaonkar, M. S., Kenemans, J. L., Grieve, S. M., Baeken, C., Fitzgerald, P. B., et al. (2017). EEG connectivity between the subgenual anterior cingulate and prefrontal cortices in response to antidepressant medication. *European Neuropsychopharmacology, 27*(4), 301–312.

Janak, P. H., & Tye, K. M. (2015). From circuits to behaviour in the amygdala. *Nature, 517,* 284–292.

Jenkins, L. M., Skerrett, K. A., DelDonno, S. R., Patrón, V. G., Meyers, K. K., Peltier, S., et al. (2018). Individuals with more severe depression fail to sustain nucleus accumbens activity to preferred music over time. *Psychiatry Research: Neuroimaging, 275,* 21–27.

Jeste, D. V., Lohr, J. B., & Goodwin, F. K. (1988). Neuroanatomical studies of major affective disorders: A review and suggestions for further research. *British Journal of Psychiatry, 153*(4), 444–459.

Joormann, J., & Stanton, C. H. (2016). Examining emotion regulation in depression: A review and future directions. *Behaviour Research and Therapy, 86,* 35–49.

Kaiser, R. H., Andrews-Hanna, J. R., Wager, T. D., & Pizzagalli, D. A. (2015). Large-scale network dysfunction in major depressive disorder: A meta-analysis of resting-state functional connectivity. *JAMA Psychiatry, 72*(6), 603–611.

Kelly, C., de Zubicaray, G., Di Martino, A., Copland, D. A., Reiss, P. T., Klein, D. F., et al. (2009). L-dopa modulates functional connectivity in striatal cognitive and motor networks: A double-blind placebo-controlled study. *Journal of Neuroscience, 29*(22), 7364–7378.

Kerestes, R., Davey, C. G., Stephanou, K., Whittle, S., & Harrison, B. J. (2014). Functional brain imaging studies of youth depression: A systematic review. *NeuroImage: Clinical, 4,* 209–231.

Klimes-Dougan, B., Eberly, L. E., Westlund Schreiner, M., Kurkiewicz, P., Houri, A., Schlesinger, A., et al. (2014). Multilevel assessment of the neurobiological threat system in depressed adolescents: Interplay between the limbic system and hypothalamic–pituitary–adrenal axis. *Development and Psychopathology, 26*(4, Pt. 2), 1321–1335.

Klumpp, H., & Deldin, P. (2010). Review of brain functioning in depression for semantic processing and verbal fluency. *International Journal of Psychophysiology, 75*(2), 77–85.

Koenig, A. M., Bhalla, R. K., & Butters, M. A. (2014). Cognitive functioning and late-life depression. *Journal of the International Neuropsychological Society, 20*(5), 461–467.

Kowatch, R. A., Devous, M. D., Harvey, D. C., Mayes, T. L., Trivedi, M. H., Emslie, G. J., et al. (1999). A SPECT HMPAO study of regional cerebral blood flow in depressed adolescents and normal controls. *Progress in Neuro-Psychopharmacology and Biological Psychiatry, 23*(4), 643–656.

Lemere, F. (1936). The significance of individual differences in the Berger rhythm. *Brain: A Journal of Neurology, 59,* 366–375

Li, B.-J., Friston, K., Mody, M., Wang, H.-N., Lu, H.-B., & Hu, D.-W. (2018). A brain network model for depression: From symptom understanding to disease intervention. *CNS Neuroscience and Therapeutics, 24*(11), 1004–1019.

Lindquist, K. A., Satpute, A. B., Wager, T. D., Weber, J., & Barrett, L. F. (2016). The brain basis of positive and negative affect: Evidence from a meta-analysis of the human neuroimaging literature. *Cerebral Cortex, 26*(5), 1910–1922.

Liu, W., Ge, T., Leng, Y., Pan, Z., Fan, J., Yang, W., et al. (2017). The role of neural plasticity in depression: From hippocampus to prefrontal cortex. *Neural Plasticity, 2017,* 1–11.

Liu, X., Hairston, J., Schrier, M., & Fan, J. (2011). Common and distinct networks underlying reward valence and processing stages: A meta-analysis of functional neuroimaging studies. *Neuroscience and Biobehavioral Reviews, 35*(5), 1219–1236.

Lupien, S. J., & Lepage, M. (2001). Stress, memory, and the hippocampus: Can't live with it, can't live without it. *Behavioural Brain Research, 127*(1–2), 137–158.

Mateus-Pinheiro, A., Pinto, L., Bessa, J. M., Morais, M., Alves, N. D., Monteiro, S., et al. (2013). Sustained remission from depressive-like behavior depends on hippocampal neurogenesis. *Translational Psychiatry, 3*(1), e210.

Mayberg, H. S., Liotti, M., Brannan, S. K., McGinnis, S., Mahurin, R. K., Jerabek, P. K., et al. (1999). Reciprocal limbic-cortical function and negative mood: Converging PET findings in depression and normal sadness. *American Journal of Psychiatry, 156,* 675–682.

Menon, V., & Uddin, L. Q. (2010). Saliency, switching, attention and control: A network model of insula function. *Brain Structure and Function, 214*(5–6), 655–667.

Miller, B. T., & D'Esposito, M. (2005). Searching for "the top" in top-down control. *Neuron, 48*(4), 535–538.

Miller, C. H., Hamilton, J. P., Sacchet, M. D., & Gotlib, I. H. (2015). Meta-analysis of functional neuroimaging of major depressive disorder in youth. *JAMA Psychiatry, 72*(10), 1045–1053.

Mitelman, S. A. (2019). Transdiagnostic neuroimaging in psychiatry: A review. *Psychiatry Research, 277,* 23–38.

Mitra, R., Jadhav, S., McEwen, B. S., Vyas, A., & Chattarji, S. (2005). Stress duration modulates the spatiotemporal patterns of spine formation in the basolateral amygdala. *Proceedings of the National Academy of Sciences, 102*(26), 9371–9376.

Moran, T. P., Jendrusina, A. A., & Moser, J. S. (2013). The psychometric properties of the late positive potential during emotion processing and regulation. *Brain Research, 1516,* 66–75.

Mulders, P. C., van Eijndhoven, P. F., Schene, A. H., Beckmann, C. F., & Tendolkar, I. (2015). Resting-state functional connectivity in major depressive disorder: A review. *Neuroscience and Biobehavioral Reviews, 56,* 330–344.

Niendam, T. A., Laird, A. R., Ray, K. L., Dean, Y. M., Glahn, D. C., & Carter, C. S. (2012). Meta-analytic evidence for a superordinate cognitive control network subserving diverse executive functions. *Cognitive, Affective, and Behavioral Neuroscience, 12*(2), 241–268.

Nolen-Hoeksema, S., & Morrow, J. (1991). A prospective study of depression and posttraumatic stress symptoms after a natural disaster: The 1989 Loma Prieta earthquake. *Journal of Personality and Social Psychology, 61*(1), 115.

Nolen-Hoeksema, S., & Morrow, J. (1993). Effects of rumination and distraction on naturally occurring depressed mood. *Cognition and Emotion, 7*(6), 561–570.

Nolen-Hoeksema, S., Wisco, B. E., & Lyubomirsky, S. (2008). Rethinking rumination. *Perspectives on Psychological Science, 3*(5), 400–424.

Nord, C. L., Halahakoon, D. C., Lally, N., Limbachya, T., Pilling, S., & Roiser, J. P. (2020). The neural basis of hot and cold cognition in depressed patients, unaffected relatives, and low-risk healthy controls: An fMRI investigation. *Journal of Affective Disorders, 274,* 389–398.

Ochsner, K. N., & Gross, J. J. (2005). The cognitive control of emotion. *Trends in Cognitive Sciences,* 9(5), 242–249.

Ordway, G. A., & Klimek, V. (2001). Noradrenergic pathology in psychiatric disorders: postmortem studies. *CNS Spectrums,* 6(8), 697–703.

Perlman, G., Simmons, A. N., Wu, J., Hahn, K. S., Tapert, S. F., Max, J. E., et al. (2012). Amygdala response and functional connectivity during emotion regulation: A study of 14 depressed adolescents. *Journal of Affective Disorders,* 139(1), 75–84.

Pessoa, L. (2008). On the relationship between emotion and cognition. *Nature Reviews Neuroscience,* 9(2), 148–158.

Phillips, M. L., Drevets, W. C., Rauch, S. L., & Lane, R. (2003). Neurobiology of emotion perception I: The neural basis of normal emotion perception. *Biological Psychiatry,* 54(5), 504–514.

Pizzagalli, D. A. (2011). Frontocingulate dysfunction in depression: Toward biomarkers of treatment response. *Neuropsychopharmacology,* 36(1), 183–206.

Pizzagalli, D. A. (2014). Depression, stress, and anhedonia: Toward a synthesis and integrated model. *Annual Review of Clinical Psychology,* 10(1), 393–423.

Price, J. L., & Drevets, W. C. (2010). Neurocircuitry of mood disorders. *Neuropsychopharmacology,* 35(1), 192–216.

Pujara, M., & Koenigs, M. (2014). Mechanisms of reward circuit dysfunction in psychiatric illness: Prefrontal–striatal interactions. *The Neuroscientist,* 20(1), 82–95.

Raichle, M. E. (2015). The brain's default mode network. *Annual Review of Neuroscience,* 38(1), 433–447.

Raichle, M. E., MacLeod, A. M., Snyder, A. Z., Powers, W. J., Gusnard, D. A., & Shulman, G. L. (2001). A default mode of brain function. *Proceedings of the National Academy of Sciences,* 98(2), 676.

Rajkowska, G. (2003). Depression: What we can learn from postmortem studies. *The Neuroscientist,* 9(4), 273–284.

Rayner, G., Jackson, G., & Wilson, S. (2016). Cognition-related brain networks underpin the symptoms of unipolar depression: Evidence from a systematic review. *Neuroscience and Biobehavioral Reviews,* 61, 53–65.

Roiser, J. P., & Sahakian, B. J. (2013). Hot and cold cognition in depression. *CNS Spectrums,* 18(03), 139–149.

Rubia, K. (2013). Functional brain imaging across development. *European Child and Adolescent Psychiatry,* 22(12), 719–731.

Rutherford, H. J. V., & Lindell, A. K. (2011). Thriving and surviving: Approach and avoidance motivation and lateralization. *Emotion Review,* 3(3), 333–343.

Schmaal, L., Hibar, D. P., Sämann, P. G., Hall, G. B., Baune, B. T., Jahanshad, N., et al. (2017). Cortical abnormalities in adults and adolescents with major depression based on brain scans from 20 cohorts worldwide in the ENIGMA Major Depressive Disorder Working Group. *Molecular Psychiatry,* 22(6), 900–909.

Schmaal, L., Veltman, D. J., van Erp, T. G. M., Sämann, P. G., Frodl, T., Jahanshad, N., et al. (2016). Subcortical brain alterations in major depressive disorder: Findings from the ENIGMA major depressive disorder working group. *Molecular Psychiatry,* 21(6), 806–812.

Schmidt, F. M., Schindler, S., Adamidis, M., Strauß, M., Tränkner, A., Trampel, R., et al. (2017). Habenula volume increases with disease severity in unmedicated major depressive disorder as revealed by 7T MRI. *European Archives of Psychiatry and Clinical Neuroscience,* 267(2), 107–115.

Seminowicz, D. A., Mayberg, H. S., McIntosh, A. R., Goldapple, K., Kennedy, S., Segal, Z., et al. (2004). Limbic–frontal circuitry in major depression: A path modeling metanalysis. *NeuroImage,* 22(1), 409–418.

Sescousse, G., Caldú, X., Segura, B., & Dreher, J.-C. (2013). Processing of primary and secondary rewards: A quantitative meta-analysis and review of human functional neuroimaging studies. *Neuroscience and Biobehavioral Reviews,* 37(4), 681–696.

Shima, S., Shikano, T., Kitamura, T., Masuda, Y., Tsukumo, T., Kanba, S., & Asai, M. (1984). Depression and ventricular enlargement. *Acta Psychiatrica Scandinavica,* 70(3), 275–277.

Snyder, H. R. (2013). Major depressive disorder is associated with broad impairments on neuropsychological measures of executive function: A meta-analysis and review. *Psychological Bulletin, 139*(1), 81–132.

Sommerfeldt, S. L., Cullen, K. R., Han, G., Fryza, B. J., Houri, A. K., & Klimes-Dougan, B. (2016). Executive attention impairment in adolescents with major depressive disorder. *Journal of Clinical Child and Adolescent Psychology, 45*(1), 69–83.

Song, T., Han, X., Du, L., Che, J., Liu, J., Shi, S., et al. (2018). The role of neuroimaging in the diagnosis and treatment of depressive disorder: A recent review. *Current Pharmaceutical Design, 24*(22), 2515–2523.

Spreng, R. N., Mar, R. A., & Kim, A. S. N. (2009). The common neural basis of autobiographical memory, prospection, navigation, theory of mind, and the default mode: A quantitative meta-analysis. *Journal of Cognitive Neuroscience, 21*(3), 489–510.

Stevens, M. C. (2016). The contributions of resting state and task-based functional connectivity studies to our understanding of adolescent brain network maturation. *Neuroscience and Biobehavioral Reviews, 70*, 13–32.

Stewart, J. L., Coan, J. A., Towers, D. N., & Allen, J. J. B. (2014). Resting and task-elicited prefrontal EEG alpha asymmetry in depression: Support for the capability model. *Psychophysiology, 51*(5), 446–455.

Suh, J. S., Schneider, M. A., Minuzzi, L., MacQueen, G. M., Strother, S. C., Kennedy, S. H., et al. (2019). Cortical thickness in major depressive disorder: A systematic review and meta-analysis. *Progress in Neuro-Psychopharmacology and Biological Psychiatry, 88*, 287–302.

Supekar, K., Uddin, L. Q., Prater, K., Amin, H., Greicius, M. D., & Menon, V. (2010). Development of functional and structural connectivity within the default mode network in young children. *NeuroImage, 52*(1), 290–301.

Takamura, M., Okamoto, Y., Okada, G., Toki, S., Yamamoto, T., Yamamoto, O., et al. (2016). Disrupted brain activation and deactivation pattern during semantic verbal fluency task in patients with major depression. *Neuropsychobiology, 74*(2), 69–77.

Toth, S. L., & Cicchetti, D. (2010). The historical origins and developmental pathways of the discipline of developmental psychopathology. *Israel Journal of Psychiatry and Related Sciences, 47*(2), 95–104.

Treadway, M. T., & Zald, D. H. (2011). Reconsidering anhedonia in depression: Lessons from translational neuroscience. *Neuroscience and Biobehavioral Reviews, 35*(3), 537–555.

Trew, J. L. (2011). Exploring the roles of approach and avoidance in depression: An integrative model. *Clinical Psychology Review, 31*(7), 1156–1168.

Truong, W., Minuzzi, L., Soares, C. N., Frey, B. N., Evans, A. C., MacQueen, G. M., et al. (2013). Changes in cortical thickness across the lifespan in major depressive disorder. *Psychiatry Research, 214*(3), 204–211.

van Eijndhoven, P., Wingen, G. van, Katzenbauer, M., Groen, W., Tepest, R., Fernández, G., et al. (2013). Paralimbic cortical thickness in first-episode depression: Evidence for trait-related differences in mood regulation. *American Journal of Psychiatry, 170*(12), 1477–1486.

van Velzen, L. S., Kelly, S., Isaev, D., Aleman, A., Aftanas, L. I., Bauer, J., et al. (2020). White matter disturbances in major depressive disorder: A coordinated analysis across 20 international cohorts in the ENIGMA MDD working group. *Molecular Psychiatry, 25*(7), 1511–1525.

Vyas, A., Mitra, R., Rao, B. S. S., & Chattarji, S. (2002). Chronic stress induces contrasting patterns of dendritic remodeling in hippocampal and amygdaloid neurons. *Journal of Neuroscience, 22*(15), 6810–6818.

Vytal, K., & Hamann, S. (2010). Neuroimaging support for discrete neural correlates of basic emotions: A voxel-based meta-analysis. *Journal of Cognitive Neuroscience, 22*(12), 2864–2885.

Walsh, E., Carl, H., Eisenlohr-Moul, T., Minkel, J., Crowther, A., Moore, T., et al. (2017). Attenuation of frontostriatal connectivity during reward processing predicts response to psychotherapy in major depressive disorder. *Neuropsychopharmacology, 42*(4), 831–843.

Wang, L., Hermens, D. F., Hickie, I. B., & Lagopoulos, J. (2012). A systematic review of resting-state functional-MRI studies in major depression. *Journal of Affective Disorders, 142*(1), 6–12.

Wang, Y., Chen, G., Zhong, S., Jia, Y., Xia, L., Lai, S., et al. (2018). Association between resting-state brain functional connectivity and cortisol levels in unmedicated major depressive disorder. *Journal of Psychiatric Research, 105*, 55–62.

Westlund Schreiner, M., Klimes-Dougan, B., Parenteau, A., Hill, D., & Cullen, K. R. (2019). A framework for identifying neurobiologically based intervention targets for NSSI. *Current Behavioral Neuroscience Reports, 6*(4), 177–187.

Whitfield-Gabrieli, S., & Ford, J. M. (2012). Default mode network activity and connectivity in psychopathology. *Annual Review of Clinical Psychology, 8*(1), 49–76.

Yu, S., Shen, Z., Lai, R., Feng, F., Guo, B., Wang, Z., et al. (2018). The orbitofrontal cortex gray matter is associated with the interaction between insomnia and depression. *Frontiers in Psychiatry, 9*, 651.

Zhang, W.-N., Chang, S.-H., Guo, L.-Y., Zhang, K.-L., & Wang, J. (2013). The neural correlates of reward-related processing in major depressive disorder: A meta-analysis of functional magnetic resonance imaging studies. *Journal of Affective Disorders, 151*(2), 531–539.

Zhu, X., Wang, X., Xiao, J., Zhong, M., Liao, J., & Yao, S. (2011). Altered white matter integrity in first-episode, treatment-naive young adults with major depressive disorder: A tract-based spatial statistics study. *Brain Research, 1369*, 223–229.

Zhu, X., Zhu, Q., Shen, H., Liao, W., & Yuan, F. (2017). Rumination and default mode network subsystems connectivity in first-episode, drug-naive young patients with major depressive disorder. *Scientific Reports, 7*(1), 1–10.

Zilverstand, A., Parvaz, M. A., & Goldstein, R. Z. (2017). Neuroimaging cognitive reappraisal in clinical populations to define neural targets for enhancing emotion regulation. A systematic review. *NeuroImage, 151*, 105–116.

CHAPTER 3

Depression across the Adult Lifespan

Vonetta M. Dotson
Shellie-Anne Levy
Hannah R. Bogoian
Andrew M. Gradone

PREVALENCE AND RISK FACTORS ACROSS THE ADULT LIFESPAN

Prevalence

The lifetime prevalence of major depressive disorder (MDD), as measured by the U.S. National Comorbidity Survey Replication (NCS-R), is estimated to be 19.2% (Kessler et al., 2010); however, the numbers vary significantly across age groups. Both lifetime and 12-month prevalence rates are lower in older adults (ages ≥65 years; 9.8% and 2.6%, respectively) relative to younger groups (ages 18–64 years; 19.4–22.7% and 7.7–10.4%, respectively; Kessler et al., 2010). Many studies estimate that as many as a third of older adults experience clinically significant subthreshold depressive symptoms (Djernes, 2006; Judd & Kunovac, 1998). Across the adult lifespan, women reliably have higher rates of MDD (female lifetime prevalence: 22.9%; male lifetime prevalence: 15.1%; Kessler et al., 2010). Data from the National Institute of Mental Health's Collaborative Psychiatric Epidemiology Surveys, which included the NCS-R, showed that the prevalence of MDD in U.S.-born ethnic groups was nearly double that of foreign-born ethnic groups, but not in older adults (González, Tarraf, Whitfield, & Vega, 2010). Healthy immigrant effects do not appear to hold into old age, and prevalence rates for foreign-born ethnic groups tend to exceed rates for U.S.-born groups in later life.

Risk Factors

Multiple risk factors are associated with MDD across the lifespan, generally falling within the biopsychosocial framework. Being female, poor, unmarried, disabled, or unemployed places an individual at the greatest risk for MDD (Kessler et al., 2010). With the exception of employment status, all of these sociodemographic factors are greater predictors of MDD in late life.

Recurrent, early-onset MDD (defined as two or more major depressive episodes [MDEs] before the age of 25) is associated with a stronger family history of mood disorders. It is more likely to reoccur and less likely to respond to treatment (Zubenko, Zubenko, Spiker, Giles, & Kaplan, 2001). People with a high genetic vulnerability for mood disorders relative to those with a low vulnerability are more likely to experience depression after stressful life events (Kendler & Karkowski-Shuman, 1997). Additionally, people with MDD are more likely to self-generate stressful events, which in turn could be interpreted as more negative if they have a high genetic vulnerability for depression along with neurotic personality traits (Smith & Blackwood, 2004). On one hand, life events and changes rated as negative and uncontrollable, particularly those that occur in the social context of family, work, educational settings, and living conditions, are significantly more closely associated with the development of MDD (Friis, Wittchen, Pfister, & Lieb, 2002). On the other hand, the occurrence of more positive events has been associated with a decreased chance of developing MDD. This finding suggested that the occurrence of positive events would be a protective factor (Friis et al., 2002).

Biological risk factors for developing MDD in late life include chronic disease, vascular factors (such as cardiac and cerebrovascular conditions), health status (including sleep disturbance and low exercise), disability, and poor health habits such as severe alcohol and tobacco use (Vink, Aartsen, & Schoevers, 2008). Poor self-perceived health is also a risk factor for late-life depression. Psychological risk factors include personality traits (e.g., high neuroticism, external locus of control), poor coping strategies, negative self-image, and psychopathology such as more psychiatric symptoms at baseline or a chronic history of psychiatric illness (Vink et al., 2008). Social risk factors include smaller network size, single marital status, qualitative aspects of the social network (e.g., lack of satisfaction with friends, marital problems), and stressful life events (Vink et al., 2008).

DEPRESSION MORBIDITY AND MORTALITY

Epidemiological studies have consistently found that MDD is strongly comorbid with anxiety disorders and is comorbid with substance use and impulse control disorders (Andrade et al., 2003; Kessler et al., 2003). About three-fourths (72.1%) of those surveyed in the NCS-R study who met diagnostic criteria for lifetime MDD also met criteria for another disorder in the fourth edition of the *Diagnostic and Statistical Manual of Mental Disorders* (DSM-IV; American Psychiatric Association, 1994) that was measured in the survey (Kessler et al., 2003). Approximately 59.2% of the sample with MDD additionally had an anxiety disorder, 24% had a substance use disorder, and 30% had an impulse control disorder.

Across all age groups, MDD is associated with numerous negative consequences, including insomnia, extreme fatigue, weight fluctuations, greater sensitivity to pain, more incidents of physical illness, poorer social functioning, increased risk for suicide, and cognitive deficits in processing speed, attention, memory, and executive functioning (American Psychiatric Association, 2013; Lee, Hermens, Porter, & Redoblado-Hodge, 2012). Chronic recurrent depression, in particular, is associated with changes in neural functioning (Greden, 2001). Specifically, individuals with chronic depression often have volumetric reductions in hippocampal and prefrontal areas, which contribute to the observed cognitive deficits (Greden, 2001).

Morbidity and Mortality in Young Adults

Unipolar depression often develops into bipolar disorder in younger adults (Smith & Blackwood, 2004), and comorbidity rates of MDD and bipolar disorder range from 16.0 to 20.0% (Angst et al., 2011; Kessler et al., 2010). Some researchers have argued that this comorbidity rate vastly underestimates the true comorbidity of these disorders. For example, using validated bipolarity specifier criteria that are more sensitive than the text revision of DSM-IV (DSM-IV-TR; American Psychiatric Association, 2000) criteria in identifying patients with bipolar features, Angst and colleagues (2011) showed that nearly half (47%) of adults with MDD met the bipolarity specifier criteria.

Morbidity and Mortality in Older Adults

Morbidity in older adults can be complicated because many physical disorders become more prevalent as one ages, which can lead to underdiagnosis, or in some cases, misdiagnosis of MDD due to confusion with symptoms of physical disorders (Kessler et al., 2010). That being said, MDD in older adults is commonly comorbid with medical and neurological disorders in addition to the previously discussed psychiatric disorders (Alexopoulos, Buckwalter, et al., 2002). Older adults with depression relative to those without depression have significantly more vascular comorbidities, including hypertension, cardiovascular disease, artherosclerosis, and gastrointestinal ulcers (Taylor, McQuoid, & Krishnan, 2004). Neurological disorders, such as dementia, are also comorbid with MDD and often lead to functional impairment due to cognitive deficits (Alexopoulos, Buckwalter, et al., 2002; Bennett & Thomas, 2014). Many of these comorbidities have a bidirectional effect on each other.

In older adults, depression may lead to self-neglect and impairment in instrumental activities of daily living, increased mortality because of physical illness, as well as risk of suicide (Abrams, Lachs, McAvay, Keohane, & Bruce, 2002; Penninx et al., 2001). Even after controlling for illness severity and disability in hospitalized patients, depression still independently predicts mortality (Covinsky et al., 1998). In a study of completed suicides among older adults, recurrent MDD was the disorder most strongly associated with suicide (Wærn et al., 2002). Among people who commit suicide, approximately 90% had a psychiatric diagnosis at the time of death (Cavanagh, Carson, Sharpe, & Lawrie, 2003). Of these people, the most common diagnosis was MDD (consistent with the findings in late life), which occurs in approximately half to two-thirds of the cases (Conwell et al., 1996). A meta-analysis of risk factors that increase one's chances of committing suicide found that male gender, family history of psychiatric disease, severe depression, hopelessness, comorbid anxiety disorders, substance misuse, and previous suicide attempts increase suicide risk (Hawton, Casanas, Haw, & Saunders, 2013).

DEPRESSIVE SYMPTOM PRESENTATION

Depression across the adult lifespan tends to follow a U-shaped pattern by age, such that depressive symptoms are highest in early adulthood, decrease in middle adulthood, and increase again in late life (Sutin et al., 2013). This trajectory as well as depressive symptom presentation is likely influenced by a complex interplay of biopsychosocial factors. The fifth edition of DSM (DSM-5) describes seven depressive disorders (see Salem, Soares,

& Selvaraj, Chapter 1, this volume, for comprehensive details of the depressive disorders) that can be diagnosed in adulthood, which include MDD, persistent depressive disorder (dysthymia), premenstrual dysphoric disorder, substance/medication-induced depressive disorder, depressive disorder due to another medical condition, other specified depressive disorder, and unspecified depressive disorder (American Psychiatric Association, 2013). Although there are differences in etiology, duration, time of onset, and symptom presentation among all these depressive disorders, all their core symptoms include sad, empty, or irritable mood that can manifest as somatic and cognitive changes and significantly interfere with day-to-day functioning (American Psychiatric Association, 2013). This section details the differences in depressive symptom presentation across the adult lifespan.

Depression in Early and Middle Adulthood

Young adults exhibit greater depressive symptoms relative to middle-aged and older adults, with depressed affect being the most prominent symptom, followed by interpersonal problems and somatic complaints (Sutin et al., 2013). Early-onset depression (EOD), operationalized as symptoms that occur before age 40, tends have a more chronic illness course with persistent depressive symptoms (Korten, Comijs, Lamers, & Penninx, 2012). Individuals with EOD have a higher genetic load (i.e., positive family history), tend to have a history of childhood trauma and suicide attempts, and exhibit neuroticism personality traits (Korten et al., 2012).

Research is mixed regarding the differences in depressive symptom profiles among middle-aged individuals relative to younger and older adults. Not only is there variability in the age ranges used to operationalize middle age, but middle-aged individuals are often grouped together with younger adults in study samples. While there is a tendency to report symptoms of sad mood (Hybels, Landerman, & Blazer, 2012), variability in depressive symptom reports limits the ability across studies to identify distinct symptom profiles in middle-aged individuals with depression compared to their younger or older peers. For example, relative to early and late adulthood, onset of major depression in middle age (30–50 years) was marked by less endorsement of suicidal thoughts and insomnia (Charlton, Lamar, Ajilore, & Kumar, 2013). In contrast, Hybels and colleagues (2012) found that younger/middle-aged individuals (18–50) reported greater crying spells, feeling of dislike by others, and suicidal ideation, but no differences in sleep disturbance in comparison to older adults. These two examples highlight methodological differences between studies of young and middle age adults that has produced more questions than provided answers with regard to specific depressive symptom profiles for that age band.

Late-Life Depression

Depression in older adults is typically classified as recurrent from early life, new or late onset (60–65 years of age), secondary to a general medical illness, or secondary to medication or substance use (Aziz & Steffens, 2013). Depression in older relative to younger individuals has been found to have a more chronic course, poorer prognosis, and higher relapse rate (Mitchell & Subramaniam, 2005). Also, the etiology is more heterogeneous in older than younger age groups (Aziz & Steffens, 2013; Gottfries, 1998).

Older relative to younger individuals may be more hesitant to report sad mood and may minimize reports of guilt and loss of sexual interest (Hegeman, Kok, van der Mast, & Giltay, 2012; Shahpesandy, 2005). Moreover, older individuals may be more likely to report psychomotor retardation, less time spent in work or activities, hypochondriasis, insomnia, and somatic symptoms (e.g., fatigue, loss of energy, pain, and gastrointestinal disturbance) (Alexopoulos, Kiosses, Klimstra, Kalayam, & Bruce, 2002; Hegeman et al., 2012; Shahpesandy, 2005). Of note, increased prevalence of somatic depressive symptoms in older adults is not always supported in research (Hybels et al., 2012). Nonetheless, age differences in clinical presentation can adversely affect detection and appropriate diagnosis of MDD in older adults.

The term *vascular depression* was coined in 1997 to describe the symptom presentation and cognitive pattern in late-onset individuals with MDD with vascular disease and vascular risk factors, such as diabetes, hypertension, and coronary artery disease (Alexopoulos, Meyers, Young, Campbell, et al., 1997). Individuals with vascular depression compared to those with nonvascular depression show greater psychomotor slowing, less agitation, less guilt, poorer insight, and less depressive ideation (Alexopoulos, Meyers, Young, Kakuma, et al., 1997). Alexopoulos, Kiosses, and colleagues (2002) proposed a late-life "depression–executive dysfunction syndrome," which is similar in behavioral presentation to vascular depression. This syndrome manifests as loss of interest/pleasure in activities, psychomotor retardation, paranoia, reduced verbal fluency, and impaired visual confrontation naming. Also, a mild vegetative state is associated with this syndrome. Frontostriatal disruption is the putative etiology and has been supported by converging neuroimaging, neuropathological, and clinical evidence (Alexopoulos, Kiosses, et al., 2002).

The tendency for older adults to report a different symptom presentation than younger individuals can likely be attributed to a combination of age-related changes (e.g., decreased libido, lack of a living partner), comorbid physical illness/cognitive impairment, and/or cohort and personality effects (Alexopoulos, Meyers, Young, Kakuma, et al., 1997; Aziz & Steffens, 2013; Bouwman, 2008; Gottfries, 1998; Naarding et al., 2005; Wetherell et al., 2009). A recent narrative review (Haigh, Bogucki, Sigmon, & Blazer, 2018) concluded that despite evidence that depression in late life differs in symptomatic presentation from depression in young adults, particularly in regards to higher somatic symptoms, there is insufficient evidence to separate the impact of medical comorbidity on these differences.

Gender and Depressive Symptoms

According to the "gendered responding" framework, depressive symptomology differs in men and women due to differences in their conditioned experience of and response to negative affect and life events (Addis, 2008). This framework posits that individuals who adhere to a masculine gender role are more prone to exhibit externalizing depressive symptoms (e.g., anger, irritability, somatic symptoms, and substance use; Addis, 2008), and are less likely to endorse symptoms like crying or sad mood (Addis, 2008; Rodgers et al., 2014).

Within this "gendered responding" framework, gender differences in depressive symptoms can also manifest differently in younger and older age groups. Older adults are often stereotyped to assume traditional gender roles. Cohort effects (i.e., coming of age in the same historical and sociopolitical context) can influence adherence to gender roles and "masculine or feminine" traits (Strough, Leszczynski, Neely, Flinn, & Margrett, 2007). Data from systematic clinic interviews have indicated that older men relative to women have the tendency to report less psychological or depressive symptoms but may report more sleep, cognitive, and pain symptoms (Hinton, Zweifach, Oishi, Tang, & Unutzer, 2006). As adherence to traditional masculine values or identity may partially account for this gender difference (Hinton et al., 2006), older men may be less likely to seek help or report typical depressive symptoms when their masculinity is threatened by increasing age (e.g., reduced physical stamina, loss of powerful role in work or at home; Calasanti, 2004). Price, Gregg, Smith, and Fiske (2018) found that younger and older women who endorsed masculine traits reported fewer typical depressive symptoms (e.g., sad mood, crying) and greater atypical symptoms (e.g., somatic symptoms, anger, hostility). This pattern was better defined in women than in men and suggested that differences in depressive symptom presentation may be related to identification with masculine traits rather than sex (Price et al., 2018). Overall, continued investigation of the "gendered responding" framework is warranted to help elucidate age and gender differences in depressive symptom manifestation and assessment.

RACIAL/ETHNIC AND CULTURAL CONSIDERATIONS

From a sociocultural perspective, the expression of depressive symptoms is often shaped by an individual's cultural values and norms (for additional information, see Tureson, Gold, & Thames, Chapter 13, this volume) that influence the perception, interpretation, and meaning of life experiences and stressors (Kleinman, Eisenberg, & Good, 1978). When examining mental illness in culturally diverse populations, researchers may need to take an emic (i.e., culture-specific) approach to fully understand differences in racial/ethnic presentations, as Western or majority group conceptualizations and normative standards can be insufficient. Past research supports racial/ethnic differences in clinical presentation and symptom profiles of depression relative to White reference groups (Ballenger et al., 2001; Mitchell, Watkins, Shires, Chapman, & Burnett, 2017; Myers et al., 2002; Weissman et al., 1996). However, investigations of racial/ethnic differences in trajectory or symptom presentation with aging is sparse (Bracken & Reintjes, 2010; Fiske, Wetherell, & Gatz, 2009; Mitchell et al., 2017). We present a brief review of the literature regarding racial/ethnic and cultural presentations of depressive symptoms in U.S. minority populations as well as differences from an adult lifespan perspective if available, with the caveat that symptom generalizations may not fully capture the heterogeneity within ethnic and cultural groups.

African Americans

African Americans may present with somatic and vegetative depressive symptoms (e.g., weight loss, sleep disturbance, fatigue, and appetite changes) rather than low mood, guilt, or suicidal thoughts (Carter, 1974; Fabrega, Mezzich, & Ulrich, 1988). These findings however, have been inconsistent across studies (Blazer, Landerman, Hays, Simonsick, & Saunders, 1998; Gallo, Cooper-Patrick, & Lesikar, 1998; Hamilton, 1960; Rhoades & Overall, 1983; Wohl, Lesser, & Smith, 1997). Through a qualitative analysis of clinical interviews, Baker (2001) found that African Americans with MDD either denied feeling sad, blue, or helpless ("the stoic believer"); showed increased anger/hostility or irritability ("the angry, 'evil' one"); or continued to take on additional responsibilities despite exhaustion ("the John Henry doer").

In predominantly White samples, older relative to younger adults tend to report less affective depressive symptoms (Baker, Espino, Robinson, & Stewart, 1994; Gallo, Anthony, & Muthen, 1994; Hegeman et al., 2012). There is some evidence to suggest that older African Americans relative to Whites are less likely to report dysphoria and are more likely to report thoughts of death ideation despite less frequent endorsement of thoughts of suicide (Gallo et al., 1998). Despite the likelihood of reporting less dysphoria and even when accounting for socioeconomic status and health factors, a recent 10-year longitudinal study indicated that older African Americans relative to their White counterparts were more likely to experience the onset of depression during the study period and those aged 70–79 were significantly more likely to have depression (Barry et al., 2014). Overall, age and race appear to uniquely intersect to influence the risk for depression onset among African American elders.

Hispanic Americans

Current research is mixed regarding the predominance of somatic depressive symptoms in Hispanic Americans in comparison to Whites, but there are widely accepted cultural and linguistic differences in somatic symptom expression. Many Hispanics express their somatization through cultural idioms of distress (Guarnaccia, Lewis-Fernandez, & Marano, 2003; Lewis-Fernandez, Guarnaccia, Patel, Lizardi, & Diaz, 2005). Latinx in the United States may describe their symptoms as *nervios* (nerves), which may include headaches, *dolor de cerebro* ("brain ache"), irritability, stomach problems, sleep problems, and/or *mareos* (dizziness). Additionally, given the cultural stigma associated with psychiatric disease, Hispanic Americans may explain their depressive symptoms as *sufrimiento* or chronic worry or suffering related to life stressors (Jenkins & Cofresi, 1998).

Older Hispanic Americans and Latinx relative to Whites and African Americans have greater rates of depression (Blazer, 2003; Gonzalez, Haan, & Hinton, 2001; Mui, 1993). Additionally, older immigrant and low-acculturated Latinx are at greater risk for depression relative to younger immigrant Latinx and U.S.-born Latinx (Gonzalez et al., 2001). In addition to age and low acculturation, other factors associated with increased depression rates in older Latinx include low income, low social support, high stress, financial stress, and functional decline (Liang, Xu, Quinones, Bennett, & Ye, 2011).

Asian Americans

Asian Americans are heterogeneous, with more than 28 Asian groups across the United States with distinct cultures, languages, and migration histories. Regardless of depression prevalence rates among Asian Americans, which is beyond the scope of this chapter, research supports the ideas that once diagnosed, depression tends to be more chronic and that Asian Americans relative to Whites are less likely to seek antidepressant treatment (Le Meyer, Zane, Cho, & Takeuchi, 2009; Leong, 1986). Research on mental health and

MDD in Asian Americans is significantly limited even without addressing within-group diversity, but the long-standing view is that Asian Americans may somatically present distress (e.g., with more predominant body aches, fatigue, or changes in appetite or sleep; Kleinman, 1996; Lin & Cheung, 1999; Lu, Bond, Friedman, & Chan, 2010). However, when directly queried, Asian Americans do describe and endorse psychological and affective depressive symptoms on symptom questionnaires (Lin & Cheung, 1999; Ryder et al., 2008; Yeung, Chang, Gresham, Nierenberg, & Fava, 2004). Therefore, Asian Americans' spontaneous report of somatic complaints do not necessarily serve as a denial of affective symptoms (Yang & WonPat-Borja, 2007).

From a Western cultural perspective, individuality and self-sufficiency are valued, and lack thereof is often associated with depressive symptoms of perceived helplessness and loss of power/poor self-esteem. In contrast, in some Eastern Asian cultures, collectivism and an undifferentiated self-structure are valued. Therefore, we have a different depressive manifestation with the presence of helplessness, but without loss of power/poor self-esteem (Marsella, 2003). In older Asian Americans who may be less acculturated, loneliness and perceived family disharmony can be likely manifestations of depression (Pang, 1995).

American Indians and Alaska Natives

American Indians and Alaska Natives (AI/AN) have 561 federally recognized tribes in the United States and speak over 200 indigenous languages (Fleming, 1992). AI/AN conceptualize mental health differently than mainstream Western culture (Beals et al., 2005; Hodge, Limb, & Cross, 2009). Traditionally, the concept of mental illness tends to be perceived as a supernatural possession, disharmony between inner and outer natural forces of the earth, expression of a special gift, or terminal phase of a physical/medical illness (Kunitz, 1983; Thompson, Walker, & Silk-Walker, 1993). The term *depressed* does not exist in some American Indian and Alaska native languages, but two prominent culture-bound syndromes, "ghost sickness" and "heart break syndrome," are recognized (Manson, Shore, & Bloom, 1985). Individuals with "ghost sickness" are believed to be possessed by the deceased and may have depressive symptoms of fatigue, loss of appetite, dizziness, and nightmares. "Heart break syndrome" is a sudden, temporary weakening of the muscle of the heart brought on by emotional distress, often by the death of a loved one. There is a dearth of research on the symptom presentation of mood disorders in this minority group. However, screening of mood in two studies that used the Center for Epidemiologic Studies Depression Scale (CES-D) found no differential experience of somatic versus psychological depressive symptoms (Manson, Ackerson, Dick, Baron, & Fleming, 1990; Somervell et al., 1992).

RELATIONSHIP TO UNDERLYING NEUROMECHANISMS

There are both similarities and differences in the neurobiological contributors to depression across the adult lifespan. Overall, evidence points to the disruption of frontolimbic brain networks as important in the etiology of depression (Mayberg, 1997; Phillips, Ladouceur, & Drevets, 2008; Price & Drevets, 2012). Comprehensive details regarding the neurobiology of MDD in adults are provided by Thai, Cullen, & Klimes-Dougan (Chapter 2, this volume). Here, we highlight important age differences in neurobiological mechanisms related to MDD.

Neuroimaging studies that include a lifespan sample are limited and remain an important area for future research. Nonetheless, there is some evidence that the neurobiological contributors to depression differ across the lifespan. A meta-analysis (Arnone, McIntosh, Ebmeier, Munafo, & Anderson, 2012) of studies that examined brain volume reduction in depression in samples that ranged from 12 to 74 years of age showed that later age of MDD onset was associated with greater volume reductions in the left amygdala but smaller volume reductions in the left anterior cingulate. In addition, older age was associated with greater white matter lesions. Another meta-analysis (Bora, Harrison, Davey, Yucel, & Pantelis, 2012) of magnetic resonance imaging (MRI) studies with mean ages that ranged from 14 to 76 years showed that volumetric reductions tended to be more pronounced in late-life depression (onset after ages 50–65) compared to early-onset depression in the prefrontal cortex, orbitofrontal cortex, putamen, caudate, and thalamus, although the difference only reached statistical significance for the thalamus. In contrast, in individuals ages 18–61 years who were either high or low risk for the development of depression, Peterson and colleagues (2009) found that participants in the high-risk group showed cortical thinning in the subgenual, anterior, and posterior cingulate and medial orbitofrontal cortex, though the effect was similar across ages. In general, later onset of depression has been associated with more severe cognitive deficits and structural MRI abnormalities (Disabato et al., 2014; Herrmann, Goodwin, & Ebmeier, 2007), although some studies have shown the opposite pattern (e.g., Sachs-Ericsson et al., 2018).

In addition to structural and functional brain changes, there is evidence of age differences in other neuromechanisms of depression. For example, a recent meta-analysis (Cao et al., 2018) found that in the overall analysis, leptin changes were not found in MDD. However, subgroup analyses showed that leptin levels were increased in participants with MDD and with body mass index (BMI) ≥ 25 or age ≥ 40. Leptin is an anti-obesity hormone and a major anorexigenic factor, which is secreted proportionally to the volume of body fat (Zeman et al., 2009) and BMI (Gecici et al., 2005). Leptin decreases food intake and increases energy expenditure (Yang & WonPat-Borja, 2007). Leptin may be an underlying neuromechanism of depression in the subsample of depressed individuals age 40 years and over with high BMI.

Increasingly, research suggests that many of the neurobiological mechanisms associated with depression are also associated with the aging process, even in nondepressed older adults. For example, both aging and depression are associated with decreases in brain-derived neurotrophic factor, metabolic dysregulation, mitochondrial dysfunction, and reduction in prefrontal cortex volumes (Sibille, 2013). Thus, depression may lead to "accelerated aging" (Wolkowitz, Reus, & Mellon, 2011), and in at least some cases, late-life rather than earlier-life depression might represent a different disease entity with distinct etiologies and unique clinical presentation (Fiske et al., 2009). A recent review

(Rutherford, Taylor, Brown, Sneed, & Roose, 2017) delineated three late-life depressive subtypes that were distinguishable by underlying biomarkers: (1) cerebrovascular aging, (2) inflammation and dopamine depletion, and (3) oxidative stress and mitochondrial aging. Each of these subtypes and pathways to late-life depression is supported by numerous studies that have documented not only that aging is associated with changes in each mechanism, but also that these neurobiological mechanisms are similarly altered in depression. Notably, these neurobiological mechanisms have inconsistently been associated with depression in earlier adulthood, which supports the idea of distinct etiologies of depression in late life.

EVALUATION AND TREATMENT ISSUES ACROSS THE ADULT LIFESPAN

Not all diagnostic and treatment tools are made equal in regards to their ability to appropriately assess and treat depression across the adult lifespan. This section reviews the major diagnostic tools for depression in adults and discusses issues regarding treatment.

Diagnostic and Evaluation Tools

Structured and Semistructured Interviews

Structured and semistructured interviews remain the *gold standard* of MDD assessment (for additional information, see Pace & Husain, Chapter 10, this volume). Given that the presence of depression in older adults is often complicated by the presence of medical issues (Alexopoulos et al., 2001), interview-style assessment of depression allows clinicians to more thoroughly assess psychiatric symptoms that might otherwise be masked by co-occurring health conditions. The Mini-International Neuropsychiatric Interview (MINI; Sheehan et al., 1998) is a short, structured diagnostic interview that can be administered in approximately 15 minutes. The MINI has acceptable psychometric properties and is reported to have greater than 80% sensitivity (Amorim, Lecrubier, Weiller, Hergueta, & Sheehan, 1998). Given its straightforward format of yes/no questions (Pettersson, Bostrom, Gustavsson, & Ekselius, 2015), research has found that adult patients of all ages and general practitioners in primary care settings endorsed it as a comprehensive and easy-to-use psychiatric diagnostic screening tool. This is an important finding, especially given that 80% of older American adults with MDD are treated through primary care settings (Kessler et al., 2010).

Another important tool in the assessment of MDD is the Structured Clinical Interview for DSM-5 (SCID-5; First, Williams, Karg, & Spitzer, 2016). The SCID-5 is a semistructured clinical interview designed to assess clinically significant psychiatric disorders as noted in DSM-5. The SCID-5 takes approximately 45–90 minutes to administer (though the mood module can be given as a stand-alone measure in less time) and has excellent psychometric properties for both current and lifetime psychiatric illness (Shankman et al., 2018).

Depression Symptom Severity Questionnaires

Beck Depression Inventory, 2nd Edition

The Beck Depression Inventory, 2nd Edition (BDI-II; Beck, Steer, & Brown, 1996) was designed to assess depressive symptoms as described in DSM-IV-TR (American Psychiatric Association, 2000) over the course of the previous 2 weeks via a 21-item, self-report format. While originally demonstrating high internal consistency ($\alpha = 0.91$) and high test–retest reliability ($r = .93$) among a sample of mostly college-aged adults (Beck et al., 1996), the BDI-II's utility has been supported for use among community-dwelling older adults (Segal, Coolidge, Cahill, & O'Riley, 2008).

Center for Epidemiologic Studies Depression Scale

The CES-D is a commonly used 20-item self-report measure of depressive symptoms with high internal consistency among the general population (Cronbach's $\alpha = 0.85$). This scale has well-supported validity in both general adults and older adult populations (Gellis, 2010; Gomez & McLaren, 2015; Lewinsohn, Seeley, Roberts, & Allen, 1997). It has additional utility given its well-replicated four-factor structure across adult lifespan samples, which include depressed mood, somatic symptoms, lack of positive affect, and interpersonal difficulties (Cosco, Prina, Stubbs, & Wu, 2017; Radloff, 1977; Ros et al., 2011).

Geriatric Depression Scale

The Geriatric Depression Scale (GDS) is a 30-item, self-report measure developed specifically to identify depressive symptoms in older adults over the course of the previous week (Yesavage et al., 1983). The yes/no format it utilizes has a Flesch–Kincaid reading level of grade 4.8, which makes it easily accessible to older adults of varying educational backgrounds and current cognitive status (Guerin, Copersino, & Schretlen, 2018; Yesavage et al., 1983). A short form of the GDS, the GDS-15, which further reduced the cognitive demands of the scale, has also been validated for use with older adults (Cullum, Tucker, Todd, & Brayne, 2006; Friedman, Heisel, & Delavan, 2005; Sheikh & Yesavage, 1986). While developed specifically for older adults, this scale also has strong specificity and sensitivity among younger and middle-aged adults (Guerin et al., 2018).

Patient Health Questionnaire–9

The Patient Health Questionnaire–9 (PHQ-9) is a nine-item scale taken from the larger Patient Health Questionnaire (used to assess a range of common mental illnesses) that uses a self-report, 4-point response scale format that asks individuals to identify depressive symptoms they have experienced in the prior 2 weeks (Bradley, Backus, & Gray, 2016; Kroenke, Spitzer, & Williams, 2001). Across studies, the PHQ-9 has demonstrated sound psychometric properties in the assessment of depression in adults of all ages (Kroenke et al., 2001; Pettersson et al., 2015; Santos et al., 2014); it has specificity and sensitivity comparable to that of both the MINI and SCID (Pettersson et al., 2015).

The American Geriatric Society guidelines recommend administering the PHQ-2 (i.e., frequency of depressed mood and anhedonia over the past 2 weeks) to screen older adults for depression, then following up positive screens with the PHQ-9 or GDS (Bradley et al., 2016). Given the somewhat complex format of the BDI-II and CES-D, the simpler format of the GDS or PHQ-9 is recommended for use with older adults.

Antidepressant Treatment Issues across the Adult Lifespan

Older adults often delay seeking out formal help for depression due to stigma (Polacsek, Boardman, & McCann, 2019) and ageism in treatment settings (Lyons et al., 2017), which consequently leads to poorer health outcomes (Atkins, Naismith, Luscombe, & Hickie, 2015; Connor, McKinnon, Roker, Ward, & Brown, 2016). This result was illustrated through a large cohort study (Sanglier, Saragoussi, Milea, & Tournier, 2015) that found that more than half of adults age 65 and older, relative to a third of younger adults (aged 25–64 years), received no antidepressant treatment or the initiation of such treatment was delayed for a significant period of time.

Medical Complications of Antidepressant Treatment

Antidepressant treatment (see Rosenblat, Chapter 15, this volume, for additional information) in older adults is complicated by the fact that older compared with younger adults tend to present with more co-occurring medical conditions (Ho et al., 2014). While the same antidepressant medication doses are as effective as those prescribed to younger adults, it is necessary to titrate them more slowly (Kok & Reynolds, 2017) due to potential medical complications that may make antidepressants less tolerable for this population (Mitchell & Subramaniam, 2005). For instance, older relative to younger adults tend to have increased sensitivity to antidepressant-induced anticholinergic effects (Bradley et al., 2016). In fact, most, if not all, antidepressants are on the *potentially inappropriate medications* list from the Beers Criteria (American Geriatrics Society Beers Criteria Update Expert Panel, 2015), and antidepressant medication use has been associated with the presence of Alzheimer's disease (Moraros, Nwankwo, Patten, & Mousseau, 2017). An increased risk of falls, hyponatremia (Filippatos, Makri, Elisaf, & Liamis, 2017), gastrointestinal upset, and drug–drug iatrogenic interactions are some potential consequences associated with antidepressant medication use in older adults (Bradley et al., 2016) that necessitates a more cautious approach to psychotropic treatment.

Psychotherapy

Antidepressant medication treatment alone will fail to be beneficial for approximately two-thirds of older adults with MDD (Kok, Nolen, & Heeren, 2012). Thus, it is important for health care providers to explore nonpharmacological treatment options with this population. Meta-analyses have revealed that psychotherapy (see Milanovic, McNeely, Qureshi, McKinnon, & Holshausen, Chapter 17, this volume, for additional information) designed to specifically target MDD has a moderate to high beneficial effect on depressive symptoms and that these effects remained stable for up to 6 months (Cuijpers, Karyotaki,

TABLE 3.1. Summary of Depression across the Lifespan

Prevalence

The estimated lifetime prevalence of major depressive disorder (MDD) is 19.2%, but estimates are lower in older adults (9.8%). As many as a third of older adults experience clinically significant subthreshold depressive symptoms.

Risk factors

Risk factors for MDD include being female, poor, unmarried, and disabled or unemployed. Stressful life events and changes seen as negative and uncontrollable increase the risk for a depressive episode, especially in people with high genetic vulnerability. Biological risk factors include chronic disease, vascular factors, and poor health status/habits. Psychological risk factors include high neuroticism, an external locus of control, poor coping strategies, negative self-image, and psychopathology. Social risk factors include having a small or unsatisfying social network and being unmarried.

Morbidity and mortality

MDD is often comorbid with anxiety disorders, substance use, and impulse control disorders. MDD is associated with numerous negative consequences, including poor physical health, cognitive impairment, and changes in brain structure and function. Vascular comorbidities and neurological disorders, such as dementia, are common in late-life depression. Depression is associated with functional disability in older adults.

Depressive symptom presentation

Depression across the adult lifespan tends to follow a U-shaped pattern by age (symptoms are highest in early adulthood, decrease in middle adulthood, and increase again in late life). Depression in older adults tends to have a more chronic course, poorer prognosis, and higher relapse rate compared to young adults. There is mixed evidence regarding age differences in the clinical presentation of depression, with some suggestion that young adults exhibit more prominent depressed affect and interpersonal problems, while older adults exhibit less sad mood and more somatic symptoms.

Gender, racial/ethnic, and cultural considerations

According to the "gendered responding" framework, depressive symptomology differs in men and women due to differences in their conditioned experience of and response to negative affect and life events. From a sociocultural perspective, the expression of depressive symptoms is often shaped by an individual's cultural values and norms that influence the perception, interpretation, and meaning of life experiences and stressors.

Relationship to underlying neuromechanisms

There is evidence that the neurobiological contributors to depression differ across the lifespan, with older adults often having more severe changes to brain structure and function. However, neuroimaging studies that include a lifespan sample are limited and remain an important area for future research.

Evaluation and treatment issues

Structured and semistructured interviews are the gold standard for diagnosing depression. Symptom severity questionnaires can be used as an alternative or complementary tool. Caution should be taken when prescribing antidepressant medications for older adults due to their increased risk for falls and other adverse side effects. Psychotherapy is an effective and safe alternative.

Pot, & Al, 2014). Success with psychotherapeutic antidepressant treatment approaches of acute depression in older adults has shown similar success rates as that found in younger adults; randomized controlled trials of evidenced-based cognitive-behavioral therapy and problem-solving therapy, for example, have demonstrated moderate to large effect sizes (Fiske et al., 2009). Importantly, a treatment goal of psychotherapy should be the maintenance of acute antidepressant gains given that older adults are more prone to relapse and recurrence of depressive symptoms (Haigh et al., 2018).

CONCLUSION

Overall, the literature to date has suggested that age is an important and critical factor in both clinical research and practice related to depression. Across stages of the adult lifespan, prevalence rates, risk factors, clinical correlates, etiology, and outcomes of depression can vary (see Table 3.1). Moreover, special considerations must be made for the assessment and treatment of depression across the lifespan in order to maximize safety, tolerability, and antidepressant efficacy. The limited studies that have focused on depression in different ethnic and racial groups highlight significant gaps that warrant research, such as the importance of intersections of diversity (e.g., unique issues in depressed older adults from ethnic minority groups). As the population ages and becomes more diverse across the globe, there is a clear need for depression studies that include diverse samples from across the entire adult lifespan.

REFERENCES

Abrams, R. C., Lachs, M., McAvay, G., Keohane, D. J., & Bruce, M. L. (2002). Predictors of self-neglect in community-dwelling elders. *American Journal of Psychiatry, 159*(10), 1724–1730.

Addis, M. E. (2008). Gender and depression in men. *Clinical Psychology: Science and Practice, 15*(3), 153–168.

Alexopoulos, G. S., Buckwalter, K., Olin, J., Martinez, R., Wainscott, C., & Krishnan, K. R. (2002). Comorbidity of late life depression: An opportunity for research on mechanisms and treatment. *Biological Psychiatry, 52*(6), 543–558.

Alexopoulos, G. S., Kiosses, D. N., Klimstra, S., Kalayam, B., & Bruce, M. L. (2002). Clinical presentation of the "depression-executive dysfunction syndrome" of late life. *American Journal of Geriatric Psychiatry, 10*(1), 98–106.

Alexopoulos, G. S., Meyers, B. S., Young, R. C., Campbell, S., Silbersweig, D., & Charlson, M. (1997). "Vascular depression" hypothesis. *Archives of General Psychiatry, 54*(10), 915–922.

Alexopoulos, G. S., Meyers, B. S., Young, R. C., Kakuma, T., Silbersweig, D., & Charlson, M. (1997). Clinically defined vascular depression. *American Journal of Psychiatry, 154*(4), 562–565.

American Geriatrics Society Beers Criteria Update Expert Panel. (2015). American Geriatrics Society 2015 Beers Criteria. *Journal of American Geriatric Society, 63*(11), 2227–2246.

American Psychiatric Association. (1994). *Diagnostic and statistical manual of mental disorders* (4th ed.). Washington, DC: Author.

American Psychiatric Association. (2000). *Diagnostic and statistical manual of mental disorders* (4th ed., text rev.). Washington, DC: Author.

American Psychiatric Association. (2013). *Diagnostic and statistical manual of mental disorders* (5th ed.). Arlington, VA: Author.

Amorim, P., Lecrubier, Y., Weiller, E., Hergueta, T., & Sheehan, D. (1998). DSM-IH-R Psychotic Disorders: Procedural validity of the Mini International Neuropsychiatric Interview (MINI). Concordance and causes for discordance with the CIDI. *European Psychiatry, 13*(1), 26–34.

Andrade, L., Caraveo-Anduaga, J. J., Berglund, P., Bijl, R. V., De Graaf, R., Vollebergh, W., et al. (2003). The epidemiology of major depressive episodes: Results from the International Consortium of Psychiatric Epidemiology (ICPE) surveys. *International Journal of Methods in Psychiatric Research, 12*(1), 3–21.

Angst, J., Azorin, J. M., Bowden, C. L., Perugi, G., Vieta, E., Gamma, A., et al. (2011). Prevalence and characteristics of undiagnosed bipolar disorders in patients with a major depressive episode: The BRIDGE study. *Archives of General Psychiatry, 68*(8), 791–799.

Arnone, D., McIntosh, A. M., Ebmeier, K. P., Munafo, M. R., & Anderson, I. M. (2012). Magnetic resonance imaging studies in unipolar depression: Systematic review and meta-regression analyses. *European Neuropsychopharmacology, 22*(1), 1–16.

Atkins, J., Naismith, S. L., Luscombe, G. M., & Hickie, I. B. (2015). Elderly care recipients' perceptions of treatment helpfulness for depression and the relationship with helpseeking. *Clinical Interventions in Aging, 10,* 287–295.

Aziz, R., & Steffens, D. C. (2013). What are the causes of late-life depression? *The Psychiatric Clinics of North America, 36*(4), 497–-516.

Baker, F. M. (2001). Diagnosing depression in African Americans. *Community Mental Health Journal, 37*(1), 31–38.

Baker, F. M., Espino, D. V., Robinson, B. H., & Stewart, B. (1994). Assessing depressive symptoms in African American and Mexican American elders. *Clinical Gerontologist, 14*(1), 15–29.

Ballenger, J. C., Davidson, J. R., Lecrubier, Y., Nutt, D. J., Kirmayer, L. J., Lépine, J., et al. (2001). Consensus statement on transcultural issues in depression and anxiety from the International Consensus Group on Depression and Anxiety. *Journal of Clinical Psychiatry, 13,* 47–55.

Barry, L. C., Thorpe, R. J., Jr., Penninx, B. W., Yaffe, K., Wakefield, D., Ayonayon, H. N., et al. (2014). Race-related differences in depression onset and recovery in older persons over time: The health, aging, and body composition study. *American Journal of Geriatric Psychiatry, 22*(7), 682–691.

Beals, J., Manson, S. M., Whitesell, N. R., Spicer, P, Novins, D. K., & Mitchell, C. M. (2005). Prevalence of DSM-IV disorders and attendant help-seeking in 2 American Indian reservation populations. *Archives of General Psychiatry, 62*(1), 99–108.

Beck, A. T., Steer, R. A., & Brown, G. K. (1996). *Manual for the Beck Depression Inventory–II.* San Antonio, TX: Psychological Corporation.

Bennett, S., & Thomas, A. J. (2014). Depression and dementia: Cause, consequence or coincidence? *Maturitas, 79*(2), 184–190.

Blazer, D. G. (2003). Depression in late life: review and commentary. *Journals of Gerontology Series A: Biological Sciences and Medical Sciences, 58*(3), 249–265.

Blazer, D. G., Landerman, L. R., Hays, J. C., Simonsick, E. M., & Saunders, W. B. (1998). Symptoms of depression among community-dwelling elderly African-American and white older adults. *Psychological Medicine, 28*(6), 1311–1320.

Bora, E., Harrison, B. J., Davey, C. G., Yucel, M., & Pantelis, C. (2012). Meta-analysis of volumetric abnormalities in cortico-striatal-pallidal-thalamic circuits in major depressive disorder. *Psychological Medicine, 42*(4), 671–681.

Bouwman, W. P. (2008). Sexual, ethics and medico-legal issues. In R. O. Jacoby, C. Oppenheimer, T. Dening, & A. Thomas (Eds.), *Oxford textbook of old age psychiatry.* Oxford, UK: Oxford University Press.

Bracken, B. A., & Reintjes, C. (2010). Age, race, and gender differences in depressive symptoms: A lifespan developmental investigation. *Journal of Psychoeducational Assessment, 28*(1), 40–53.

Bradley, B., Backus, D., & Gray, E. (2016). Depression in the older adult: What should be considered? *Mental Health Clinician, 6*(5), 222–228.

Calasanti, T. (2004). Feminist gerontology and old men. *Journal of Gerontology, Series B: Psychological Sciences and Social Sciences, 59*(6), S305–314.

Cao, B., Chen, Y., Brietzke, E., Cha, D., Shaukat, A., Pan, Z., et al. (2018). Leptin and adiponectin levels in major depressive disorder: A systematic review and meta-analysis. *Journal of Affective Disorders, 238*, 101–110.

Carter, J. H. (1974). Recognizing psychiatric symptoms in black Americans. *Geriatrics, 29*(11), 95–99.

Cavanagh, J. T. O., Carson, A. J., Sharpe, M., & Lawrie, S. M. (2003). Psychological autopsy studies of suicide: A systematic review. *Psychological Medicine, 33*(3), 395–405.

Charlton, R. A., Lamar, M., Ajilore, O., & Kumar, A. (2013). Preliminary analysis of age of illness onset effects on symptom profiles in major depressive disorder. *International Journal of Geriatric Psychiatry, 28*(11), 1166–1174.

Connor, K. O., McKinnon, S. A., Roker, R., Ward, C. J., & Brown, C. (2016). Mitigating the stigma of mental illness among older adults living with depression: The benefit of contact with a peer educator. *Stigma and Health, 3*(2), 93–101.

Conwell, Y., Duberstein, P. R., Cox, C., Herrmann, J. H., Forbes, N. T., & Caine, E. (1996). Relationships of age and axis I diagnoses in victims of completed suicide: A psychological autopsy study. *American Journal of Psychiatry, 153*(8), 1001–1008.

Cosco, T. D., Prina, M., Stubbs, B., & Wu, Y. T. (2017). Reliability and validity of the Center for Epidemiologic Studies Depression Scale in a population-based cohort of middle-aged U.S. adults. *Journal of Nursing Measurement, 25*(3), 476–485.

Covinsky, K. E., Palmer, R. M., Kresevic, D. M., Kahana, E., Counsell, S. R., Fortinsky, R. H., et al. (1998). Improving functional outcomes in older patients: Lessons from an acute care for elders unit. *Joint Commission Journal on Quality Improvement, 24*(2), 63–76.

Cuijpers, P., Karyotaki, E., Pot, A. M., & Al, E. (2014). Managing depression in older age: Psychological interventions. *Maturitas, 79*, 160–169.

Cullum, S., Tucker, S., Todd, C., & Brayne, C. (2006). Screening for depression in older medical inpatients. *International Journal of Geriatric Psychiatry, 21*(5), 469–476.

Disabato, B. M., Morris, C., Hranilovich, J., D'Angelo, G. M., Zhou, G, Wu, N., et al. (2014). Comparison of brain structural variables, neuropsychological factors, and treatment outcome in early-onset versus late-onset late-life depression. *American Journal of Geriatric Psychiatry, 22*(10), 1039–1046.

Djernes, J. K. (2006). Prevalence and predictors of depression in populations of elderly: A review. *Acta Psychiatrica Scandinavica, 113*(5), 372–387.

Fabrega, H., Jr., Mezzich, J., & Ulrich, R. F. (1988). Black-white differences in psychopathology in an urban psychiatric population. *Comprehensive Psychiatry, 29*(3), 285–297.

Filippatos, T. D., Makri, A., Elisaf, M. S., & Liamis, G. (2017). Hyponatremia in the elderly: challenges and solutions. *Clinical Interventions in Aging, 12*, 1957–1965.

First, M. B., Williams, J. B. W., Karg, R. S., & Spitzer, R. L. (2016). *Structured Clinical Interview for DSM-5 disorders. Clinician version (SCID-5-CV)*. Arlington, VA: American Psychiatric Association.

Fiske, A., Wetherell, J. L., & Gatz, M. (2009). Depression in older adults. *Annual Review of Clinical Psychology, 5*, 363–389.

Fleming, C. M. (1992). American Indians and Alaska Natives: Changing societies past and present. In M. A. Orlandi, R. Weston, & L. G. Epstein (Eds.), *Cultural competence for evaluators: A guide for alcohol and other drug abuse prevention practitioners working with ethnic/racial communities* (pp. 147–171). Rockville, MD: U.S. Department of Health and Human Services.

Friedman, B., Heisel, M. J., & Delavan, R. L. (2005). Psychometric properties of the 15-item geriatric depression scale in functionally impaired, cognitively intact, community-dwelling elderly primary care patients. *Journal of the American Geriatrics Society, 53*(9), 1570–1576.

Friis, R. H., Wittchen, H.-U., Pfister, H., & Lieb, R. (2002). Life events and changes in the course of depression in young adults. *European Psychiatry, 17*(5), 241–253.

Gallo, J. J., Anthony, J. C., & Muthen, B. O. (1994). Age differences in the symptoms of depression: A latent trait analysis. *Journal of Gerontology, 49*(6), 251–264.

Gallo, J. J., Cooper-Patrick, L., & Lesikar, S. (1998). Depressive symptoms of Whites and African Americans aged 60 years and older. *Journals of Gerontology Series B: Psychological Sciences and Social Sciences, 53*(5), 277–286.

Gecici, O., Kuloglu, M., Atmaca, M., Tezcan, A. E., Tunckol, H., Emül, H. M., et al. (2005). High serum leptin levels in depressive disorders with atypical features. *Psychiatry and Clinical Neurosciences, 59*(6), 736–738.

Gellis, Z. D. (2010). Assessment of a brief CES-D measure for depression in homebound medically ill older adults. *Journal of Gerontological Social Work, 53*(4), 289–303.

Gomez, R., & McLaren, S. (2015). The Center for Epidemiological Studies Depression Scale: Measurement and structural invariance across ratings of older adult men and women. *Personality and Individual Differences, 75,* 130–134.

Gonzalez, H. M., Haan, M. N., & Hinton, L. (2001). Acculturation and the prevalence of depression in older Mexican Americans: Baseline results of the Sacramento Area Latino Study on Aging. *Journal of the American Geriatrics Society, 49*(7), 948–953.

González, H. M., Tarraf, W., Whitfield, K. E., & Vega, W. A. (2010). The epidemiology of major depression and ethnicity in the United States. *Journal of Psychiatric Research, 44*(15), 1043–1051.

Gottfries, C. G. (1998). Is there a difference between elderly and younger patients with regard to the symptomatology and aetiology of depression? *International Clinical Psychopharmacology, 13*(Suppl. 5), S13–S18.

Greden, J. F. (2001). The burden of recurrent depression: causes, consequences, and future prospects. *Journal of Clinical Psychiatry, 62,* 5–9.

Guarnaccia, P. J., Lewis-Fernandez, R., & Marano, M. R. (2003). Toward a Puerto Rican popular nosology: Nervios and ataque de nervios. *Culture, Medicine and Psychiatry, 27*(3), 339–366.

Guerin, J. M., Copersino, M. L., & Schretlen, D. J. (2018). Clinical utility of the 15-item Geriatric Depression Scale (GDS-15) for use with young and middle-aged adults. *Journal of Affective Disorders, 241,* 59–62.

Haigh, E. A. P., Bogucki, O. E., Sigmon, S. T., & Blazer, D. G. (2018). Depression among older adults: A 20-year update on five common myths and misconceptions. *American Journal of Geriatric Psychiatry, 26*(1), 107–122.

Hamilton, M. (1960). A rating scale for depression. *Journal of Neurology, Neurosurgery, and Psychiatry, 23,* 56–62.

Hawton, K., Casanas, I. C. C., Haw, C., & Saunders, K. (2013). Risk factors for suicide in individuals with depression: A systematic review. *Journal of Affective Disorders, 147*(1–3), 17–28.

Hegeman, J. M., Kok, R. M., van der Mast, R. C., & Giltay, E. J. (2012). Phenomenology of depression in older compared with younger adults: meta-analysis. *British Journal of Psychiatry, 200*(4), 275–281.

Herrmann, L. L., Goodwin, G. M., & Ebmeier, K. P. (2007). The cognitive neuropsychology of depression in the elderly. *Psychological Medicine, 37*(12), 1693–1702.

Hinton, L., Zweifach, M., Oishi, S., Tang, L., & Unutzer, J. (2006). Gender disparities in the treatment of late-life depression: Qualitative and quantitative findings from the IMPACT trial. *American Journal of Geriatric Psychiatry, 14*(10), 884–892.

Ho, C. S., Feng, L., Fam, J., Mahendran, R., Kua, E. H., & Ng, T. (2014). Coexisting medical comorbidity and depression: Multiplicative effects on health outcomes in older adults. *International Psychogeriatrics, 26*(7), 1221–1229.

Hodge, D. R., Limb, G. E., & Cross, T. L. (2009). Moving from colonization toward balance and harmony: A Native American perspective on wellness. *Social Work, 54*(3), 211–219.

Hybels, C. F., Landerman, L. R., & Blazer, D. G. (2012). Age differences in symptom expression in patients with major depression. *International Journal of Geriatric Psychiatry, 27*(6), 601–611.

Jenkins, J. H., & Cofresi, N. (1998). The sociosomatic course of depression and trauma: A cultural analysis of suffering and resilience in the life of a Puerto Rican woman [see comment]. *Psychosomatic Medicine, 60*(4), 439–447.

Judd, L. L., & Kunovac, J. L. (1998). Bipolar and unipolar depressive disorders in geriatric patients. In N. Brunello, S. Z. Langer, & G. Racagni (Eds.), *Mental disorders in the elderly: New therapeutic approaches* (Vol. 13, pp. 1–10). Basel, Switzerland: Karger.

Kendler, K. S., & Karkowski-Shuman, L. (1997). Stressful life events and genetic liability to major depression: Genetic control of exposure to the environment? *Psychological Medicine, 27*(3), 539–547.

Kessler, R. C., Berglund, P., Demler, O., Jin, R., Koretz, D., Merikangas, K. R., et al. (2003). The epidemiology of major depressive disorder: Results from the National Comorbidity Survey Replication (NCS-R). *Journal of the American Medical Association, 289*(23), 3095–3105.

Kessler, R. C., Birnbaum, H., Bromet, E., Hwang, I., Sampson, N., & Shahly, V. (2010). Age differences in major depression: Results from the National Comorbidity Survey Replication (NCS-R). *Psychological Medicine, 40*(2), 225–237.

Kleinman, A. (1996). How is culture important for DSM-IV. In J. E. Mezzich, A. Kleinman, H. Fabrega, & D. L. Parron (Eds.), *Culture and psychiartric diagnosis: A DSM-IV perspective* (pp. 15–26). Washington, DC: American Psychiatric Press.

Kleinman, A., Eisenberg, L., & Good, B. (1978). Culture, illness, and care: Clinical lessons from anthropologic and cross-cultural research. *Annals of Internal Medicine, 88*(2), 251–258.

Kok, R. M., Nolen, W. A., & Heeren, T. J. (2012). Efficacy of treatment in older depressed patients: A systematic review and meta-analysis of double-blind randomized controlled trials with antidepressants. *Journal of Affective Disorders, 141*(2–3), 103–115.

Kok, R. M., & Reynolds, C. F. (2017). Management of depression in older adults: A review. *Journal of the American Medical Association, 317*(20), 2114–2122.

Korten, N. C. M., Comijs, H. C., Lamers, F., & Penninx, B. W. J. H. (2012). Early and late onset depression in young and middle aged adults: Differential symptomatology, characteristics and risk factors? *Journal of Affective Disorders, 138*(3), 259–267.

Kroenke, K., Spitzer, R. L., & Williams, J. B. W. (2001). The PHQ-9: Validity of a brief depression severity measure. *Journal of General Internal Medicine, 16*(9), 606–613.

Kunitz, S. J. (1983). *Disease change and the role of medicine: The Navajo experience.* Berkeley, CA: University of California Press.

Le Meyer, O., Zane, N., Cho, Y. I., & Takeuchi, D. T. (2009). Use of specialty mental health services by Asian Americans with psychiatric disorders. *Journal of Consulting and Clinical Psycholology, 77*(5), 1000–1005.

Lee, R. S. C., Hermens, D. F., Porter, M. A., & Redoblado-Hodge, M. A. (2012). A meta-analysis of cognitive deficits in first-episode major depressive disorder. *Journal of Affective Disorders, 140*(2), 113–124.

Leong, F. T. (1986). Counseling and psychotherapy with Asian-Americans: Review of the literature. *Journal of Counseling Psychology, 33*(2), 196–206.

Lewinsohn, P. M., Seeley, J. R., Roberts, R. E., & Allen, N. B. (1997). Center for epidemiologic studies depression scale (CES-D) as a screening instrument for depression among community-residing older adults. *Psychology and Aging, 12*(2), 277–287.

Lewis-Fernandez, R., Guarnaccia, P. J., Patel, S., Lizardi, D., & Diaz, N. (2005). Ataque de nervios: Anthropological, epidemiological, and clinical dimensions of a cultural syndrome. In A. M. Georgiopoulos & J. F. Rosenbaum (Eds.), *Perspectives in cross cultural psychiatry* (pp. 63–85). Philadelphia: Lippincott Williams & Wilkins.

Liang, J., Xu, X., Quinones, A. R., Bennett, J. M., & Ye, W. (2011). Multiple trajectories of depressive symptoms in middle and late life: racial/ethnic variations. *Psychology and Aging, 26*(4), 761–777.

Lin, K. M., & Cheung, F. (1999). Mental health issues for Asian Americans. *Psychiatric Services, 50*(6), 774–780.

Lu, A., Bond, M. H., Friedman, M., & Chan, C. (2010). Understanding cultural influences on depression by analyzing a measure of its constituent symptoms *International Journal of Psychological Studies, 2*(1), 55–70.

Lyons, A., Alba, B., Heywood, W., Fileborn, B., Minichiello, V., Barrett, C., et al. (2017). Experiences of ageism and the mental health of older adults. *Aging and Mental Health, 7863,* 1–9.

Manson, S. M., Ackerson, L. M., Dick, R. W., Baron, A. E., & Fleming, C. M. (1990). Depressive symptoms among American Indian adolescents: Psychometric characteristics of the Center for Epidemiologic Studies Depression Scale (CES-D). *Psychological Assessment, 2*(3), 231–237.

Manson, S. M., Shore, J. H., & Bloom, J. D. (1985). The depressive experience in American Indian communities: A challenge for psychiatric theory and diagnosis. In A. Kleinman & B. Good (Eds.), *Culture and Depression* (pp. 331–368). Berkeley, CA: University of California Press.

Marsella, A. J. (2003). Cultural aspects of depressive experience and disorders. In W. J. Lonner, D. L. Dinnel, S. A. Hayes, & D. N. Sattler (Eds.), *Online Readings in Psychology and Culture* (Vol. 9). Bellingham, WA: Center for Cross-Cultural Research, Western Washington University

Mayberg, H. S. (1997). Limbic-cortical dysregulation: A proposed model of depression. *Journal of Neuropsychiatry and Clinical Neurosciences, 9*(3), 471–481.

Mitchell, A. J., & Subramaniam, H. (2005). Prognosis of depression in old age compared to middle age: A systematic review of comparative studies. *American Journal of Psychiatry, 162*(9), 1588–1601.

Mitchell, J. A., Watkins, D. C., Shires, D., Chapman, R. A., & Burnett, J. (2017). Clues to the blues: Predictors of self-reported mental and emotional health among older African American men. *American Journal of Men's Health, 11*(5), 1366–1375.

Moraros, J., Nwankwo, C., Patten, S. B., & Mousseau, D. D. (2017). The association of antidepressant drug usage with cognitive impairment or dementia, including Alzheimer disease: A systematic review and meta-analysis. *Depression and Anxiety, 34*(3), 217–226.

Mui, A. C. (1993). Self-reported depressive symptoms among Black and Hispanic frail elders: A sociocultural perspective. *Journal of Applied Gerontology, 12*(2), 170–187.

Myers, H. F. Lesser, I., Rodriguez, N., Mira, C. B., Hwang, W. C., Camp, C., et al. (2002). Ethnic differences in clinical presentation of depression in adult women. *Cultural Diversity and Ethnic Minority Psychology, 8*(2), 138–156.

Naarding, P., Schoevers, R. A., Janzing, J. G., Jonker, C., Koudstaal, P. J., & Beekman, A. T. (2005). A study on symptom profiles of late-life depression: The influence of vascular, degenerative and inflammatory risk-indicators. *Journal of Affective Disorders, 88*(2), 155–162.

Pang, K. Y. (1995). A cross-cultural understanding of depression among elderly Korean immigrants. *Clinical Gerontologist, 15*(4), 3–20.

Penninx, B. W., Beekman A. T., Honig A., Deeg D. J., Schoevers R. A., van Eijk J. T., et al. (2001). Depression and cardiac mortality: Results from a community-based longitudinal study. *Archives of General Psychiatry, 58*(3), 221–227.

Peterson, B. S., Warner, V., Bansal, R., Zhu, H., Hao, X., Liu, J, et al. (2009). Cortical thinning in persons at increased familial risk for major depression. *Proceedings of the National Academy of Sciences of the United States of America, 106*(15), 6273–6278.

Pettersson, A., Bostrom, K. B., Gustavsson, P., & Ekselius, L. (2015). Which instruments to support diagnosis of depression have sufficient accuracy?: A systematic review. *Nordic Journal of Psychiatry, 69*(7), 497–508.

Phillips, M. L., Ladouceur, C. D., & Drevets, W. C. (2008). A neural model of voluntary and automatic emotion regulation: implications for understanding the pathophysiology and neurodevelopment of bipolar disorder. *Molecular Psychiatry, 13*(9), 829, 833–857.

Polacsek, M., Boardman, G. H., & McCann, T. V. (2019). Help-seeking experiences of older adults with a diagnosis of moderate depression. *International Journal of Mental Health Nursing, 28*(1), 278–287.

Price, E. C., Gregg, J. J., Smith, M. D., & Fiske, A. (2018). Masculine traits and depressive symptoms in older and younger men and women. *American Journal of Men's Health, 12*(1), 19–29.

Price, J. L., & Drevets, W. C. (2012). Neural circuits underlying the pathophysiology of mood disorders. *Trends in Cognitive Sciences, 16*(1), 61–71.

Radloff, L. S. (1977). The CES-D scale: A self-report depression scale for research in the general population. *Applied Psychological Measurement, 1,* 385–401.

Rhoades, H., & Overall, J. (1983). The Hamilton Depression Scale: Factor scoring and profile classification. *Psychopharmacology Bulletin, 19*(91–96).

Rodgers, S., Grosse Holtforth, M., Müller, M., Hengartner, M. P., Rössler, W., & Ajdacic-Gross, V. (2014). Symptom-based subtypes of depression and their psychosocial correlates: A person-centered approach focusing on the influence of sex. *Journal of Affective Disorders, 156,* 92–103.

Ros, L., Latorre, J. M., Aguilar, M. J., Serrano, J. P., Navarro, B., & Ricarte, J. J. (2011). Factor structure and psychometric properties of the Center for Epidemiologic Studies Depression Scale (CES-D) in older populations with and without cognitive impairment. *International Journal of Aging and Human Development, 72*(2), 83–110.

Rutherford, B. R., Taylor, W. D., Brown, P. J., Sneed, J. R., & Roose, S. P. (2017). Biological aging and the future of geriatric psychiatry. *Journals of Gerontology Series A: Biological and Medical Sciences, 72*(3), 343–352.

Ryder, A. G., Yang, J., Zhu, X., Yao, S., Yi, J., Heine, S. J., & Bagby, R. M. (2008). The cultural shaping of depression: Somatic symptoms in China, psychological symptoms in North America? *Journal of Abnormal Psychology, 117*(2), 300–313.

Sachs-Ericsson, N. J., Hajcak, G., Sheffler, J. L., Stanley, I. H., Selby, E. A., Potter, G. G., et al. (2018). Putamen volume differences among older adults: Depression status, melancholia, and age. *Journal of Geriatric Psychiatry and Neurology, 31*(1), 39–49.

Sanglier, T., Saragoussi, D., Milea, D., & Tournier, M. (2015). Depressed older adults may be less cared for than depressed younger ones. *Psychiatry Research, 229*(3), 905–912.

Santos, N. C., Costa, P. S., Cunha, P., Portugal-Nunes, C., Amorim, L., Cotter, J., et al. (2014). Clinical, physical and lifestyle variables and relationship with cognition and mood in aging: A cross-sectional analysis of distinct educational groups. *Frontiers in Aging Neuroscience, 6*, 21.

Segal, D. L., Coolidge, F. L., Cahill, B. S., & O'Riley, A. A. (2008). Psychometric properties of the Beck Depression Inventory II (BDI-II) among community-dwelling older adults. *Behavior Modification, 32*(1), 3–20.

Shahpesandy, H. (2005). Different manifestation of depressive disorder in the elderly. *Neuroendocrinology Letters, 26*(6), 691–695.

Shankman, S. A., Funkhouser, C. J., Klein, D. N., Davila, J., Lerner, D., & Hee, D. (2018). Reliability and validity of severity dimensions of psychopathology assessed using the Structured Clinical Interview for DSM-5 (SCID). *International Journal of Methods in Psychiatric Research, 27*(1), e1590.

Sheehan, D. V., Lecrubier, Y., Sheehan, K. H., Amorim, P., Janavs, J., Weiller, E., et al. (1998). The Mini-International Neuropsychiatric Interview (M.I.N.I.): The development and validation of a structured diagnostic psychiatric interview for DSM-IV and ICD-10. *Journal of Clinical Psychiatry, 59*(Suppl. 20), 22–33; quiz 34–57.

Sheikh, J. I., & Yesavage, J. A. (1986). Geriatric Depression Scale (GDS): Recent evidence and development of a shorter version. *Journal of Aging and Mental Health, 5*(1–2), 165–173.

Sibille, E. (2013). Molecular aging of the brain, neuroplasticity, and vulnerability to depression and other brain-related disorders. *Dialogues in Clinical Neuroscience, 15*(1), 53–65.

Smith, D. J., & Blackwood, D. H. R. (2004). Depression in young adults. *Advances in Psychiatric Treatment, 10*(1), 4–12.

Somervell, P. D., Beals, J., Kinzie, J. D., Boehnlein, J., Leung, P., & Manson, S. M. (1992). Use of the CES-D in an American Indian village. *Culture, Medicine, and Psychiatry, 16*(4), 503–517.

Strough, J., Leszczynski, J. P., Neely, T. L., Flinn, J. A., & Margrett, J. (2007). From adolescence to later adulthood: Femininity, masculinity, and androgyny in six age groups. *Sex Roles, 57*(5), 385–396.

Sutin, A. R., Terracciano, A., Milaneschi, Y., An, Y., Ferrucci, L., & Zonderman, A. B. (2013). The trajectory of depressive symptoms across the adult life span. *JAMA Psychiatry, 70*(8), 803–811.

Taylor, W. D., McQuoid, D. R., & Krishnan, K. R. R. (2004). Medical comorbidity in late-life depression. *International Journal of Geriatric Psychiatry, 19*(10), 935–943.

Thompson, J. W., Walker, R. D., & Silk-Walker, P. (1993). Psychiatric care of American Indians and Alaska Natives. In A. C. Gaw (Ed.), *Culture, ethnicity and mental illness* (pp. 189–243). Washington, DC: American Psychiatric Press.

Vink, D., Aartsen, M. J., & Schoevers, R. A. (2008). Risk factors for anxiety and depression in the elderly: A review. *Journal of Affective Disorders, 106*(1), 29–44.

Wærn, M., Runeson, B. S., Allebeck, P., Beskow, J., Rubenowitz, E., Skoog, I., et al. (2002). Mental disorder in elderly suicides: A case-control study. *American Journal of Psychiatry, 159*(3), 450–455.

Weissman, M. M., Bland, R. C., Canino, G. J., Faravelli, C., Greenwald, S., Hwu H. G., et al. (1996). Cross-national epidemiology of major depression and bipolar disorder. *Journal of the American Medical Association, 276*(4), 293–299.

Wetherell, J. L., Petkus, A. J., McChesney, K., Stein, M. B., Judd, P. H., Rockwell, E., et al. (2009). Older adults are less accurate than younger adults at identifying symptoms of anxiety and depression. *Journal of Nervous and Mental Disease, 197*(8), 623–626.

Wohl, M., Lesser, I., & Smith, M. (1997). Clinical presentations of depression in African American and white outpatients. *Cultural Diversity and Mental Health, 3*(4), 279–284.

Wolkowitz, O. M., Reus, V. I., & Mellon, S. H. (2011). Of sound mind and body: depression, disease, and accelerated aging. *Dialogues in Clinical Neuroscience, 13*(1), 25–39.

Yang, L. H., & WonPat-Borja, A. J. (2007). Psychopathology among Asian Americans. In F. T. L. Leong, A. Ebreo, L. Kinoshita, A. G. Inman, & L. H. Yang (Eds.), *Handbook of Asian American osychology* (2nd ed., pp. 379–405). Thousand Oaks, CA: Sage.

Yesavage, J. A., Brink, T. L., Rose, T. L., Lum, O., Huang, V., Adey, M., et al. (1983). Development and validation of a geriatric depression screening scale: A preliminary report. *Journal of Psychiatric Research, 17*(1), 37–49.

Yeung, A., Chang, D., Gresham, R. L., Jr., Nierenberg, A. A., & Fava, M. (2004). Illness beliefs of depressed Chinese American patients in primary care. *Journal of Nervous and Mental Disease, 192*(4), 324–327.

Zeman, M., Jirak, R., Jachymova, M., Vecka, M., Tvrzicka, E., & Zak, A. (2009). Leptin, adiponectin, leptin to adiponectin ratio and insulin resistance in depressive women. *Neuroendocrinology Letters, 30*(3), 387–395.

Zubenko, G. S., Zubenko, W. N., Spiker, D. G., Giles, D. E., & Kaplan, B. B. (2001). Malignancy of recurrent, early-onset major depression: A family study. *American Journal of Medical Genetics, 105*(8), 690–699.

CHAPTER 4

Depression and Comorbid Neuropsychiatric Disorders

Sara Kashani
Olusola Ajilore

In the latest version of the *Diagnostic and Statistical Manual of Mental Disorders* (DSM-5; American Psychiatric Association, 2013), a criterion for the diagnosis of major depressive disorder (MDD) includes the "diminished ability to think or concentrate, or indecisiveness, nearly every day" (see Salem, Soares, & Selvaraj, Chapter 1, this volume, for additional information). Concentration problems and inattention may be especially salient in patients with MDD who have comorbid neuropsychiatric disorders. These cognitive difficulties fall under the domain of the neurovegetative symptoms of depression. The neurocognitive dysfunction seen in mood disorders, such as MDD, is thought to be related to the dysfunction of information processing in the central nervous system at the cortical level (Sadock, Sadock, & Ruiz, 2017). The latest data for the prevalence of cognitive dysfunction in depression, based on an inpatient sample, estimated that up to 37.5% had impairment in two or more cognitive domains (Douglas et al., 2018). This chapter explores depression and common comorbid neuropsychiatric disorders such as Alzheimer's disease (AD), vascular dementia, frontotemporal dementia (FTD), multiple sclerosis (MS), epilepsy, and traumatic brain injury (TBI) (see Table 4.1).

EPIDEMIOLOGY OF DEPRESSION AND COMORBIDITIES

The lifetime prevalence of MDD in high-income, developed nations such as the United States may range from 12 to 18%. Specific estimates include a lifetime prevalence of 16.6% and a projected lifetime risk of 23.3% by age 75 years. Although the diagnosis of psychiatric disorders often occurs earlier in life, the development of depression later in life may be secondary to comorbid conditions that often occur in parallel with age-related decline (Kessler et al., 2005).

TABLE 4.1. Summary of Comorbid Neuropsychiatric Disorders

Comorbidity	Epidemiology	Clinical presentation	Treatment
Alzheimer's disease	Approximately 33%	Depression, agitation, aggression, irritability, social withdrawal, suicidality	Cholinesterase inhibitors, antipsychotics (with caution)
Vascular dementia	Approximately 19%, ranges from 6 to 45%	Psychomotor retardation, apathy, abulia, poor executive functioning, impaired concentration, limited processing speed, abnormal brain lesions on magnetic resonance imaging	Antidepressants, psychotherapy
Frontotemporal dementia	Ranges from 33 to 40%	Earlier age of onset, mood lability, extreme apathy, atrophy of frontotemporal lobes	Antidepressants such as selective serotonin reuptake inhibitors (SSRIs), trazodone, psychotherapy
Multiple sclerosis	Approximately 50%	Sleep changes, fatigue, suicidality, changes in attention or memory, poor executive functioning, white matter disease on brain imaging	Antidepressants, psychotherapy, exercise training
Epilepsy	Ranges from 6 to 34%	Depression or anxiety ictally, postictally, or interictally; mania	Antidepressants such as SSRIs and serotonin–norepinephrine reuptake inhibitors, psychotherapies such as cognitive-behavioral therapy or acceptance and commitment therapy
Traumatic brain injury	Ranges from 6 to 77%	Changes in cognition such as in attention, concentration and memory; mood symptoms such as depression; anxiety	Antidepressants, specific psychotherapies such as problem-solving therapy or cognitive-behavioral therapy

Depression is thought to affect approximately one-third of patients with AD (Sadock et al., 2017), but estimates of prevalence have varied across studies. Indeed, estimates have ranged from as low as 13% to as high as 87% (Chi et al., 2015; Winter, Korchounov, Zhukova, & Bertschi, 2011). The variability in reported estimate rates may depend on the diagnostic criteria that are applied, as well as the confounding nature of depressive symptoms in the context of neurological illness, especially changes in cognitive function. In some studies, depression may be related to a prognosis of dementia later in life, though this risk may depend on whether the onset of depression occurs in early, mid-, or late life (Barnes et al., 2012; Byers & Yaffe, 2011; Korczyn & Halperin, 2009).

Cerebrovascular disease may also herald the later development of depression (Kumar, Selim, & Caplan, 2010; Robinson, 2003). The prevalence of depression in vascular dementia is estimated at 19%, with a wide range that varies from 6 to 45% (Ballard et al., 2000). Heightened recognition of depressive symptoms in patients with vascular disease has led to description of a clinical entity known as "vascular depression," which speaks to the recently increased interest in inflammatory processes that may underlie both depression and cerebrovascular disease (Baldwin, 2005).

Relative to other neuropsychiatric comorbidities, studies of depression in FTD have been limited. The prevalence rate has been estimated to range from 33 to 40% but may depend on the assessment method and could vary by the subtype of FTD (Blass & Rabins, 2009; Chakrabarty, Sepehry, Jacova, & Hsiung, 2015). As in other neuropsychiatric disorders, the diagnosis of depression in FTD with stringent DSM-5 diagnostic criteria has been challenging due to the overlap in the neurovegetative symptoms of depression with FTD-induced neurological symptoms (Chakrabarty et al., 2015). Some studies have used more lax criteria to define the presence or absence of depression such as a focus on the presence of sad mood as the sole indicator of depression. These between-study methodological differences reflect the heterogeneity of psychiatric nosology in the diagnosis of depression in patients with neuropsychiatric disorders.

Depression is a well-known comorbidity of multiple sclerosis. The lifetime prevalence is estimated at 50%, with an annual rate of 20% (Marrie et al., 2015; Siegert & Abernethy, 2005). The prevalence of depression in patients with epilepsy has been reported to range from 6 to 34% and may be as high as 50% in those seen in tertiary care centers (Kanner, 2003; Sadock et al., 2017). While medications used to treat epilepsy may have adverse effects on mood, similar studies on agents such as interferon (used to treat multiple sclerosis) have not confirmed an association of iatrogenic-induced depression with medication (Patten & Metz, 2002). In fact, future research directions may study the role of biological agents in the treatment of depression as interest in the inflammatory theories underlying depression pathophysiology continues to grow (Syed et al., 2018).

Greater awareness of the occurrence of TBI in athletes and military personnel has led to the increased study of adverse postconcussive outcomes such as depression. The rates of depression after TBI range from 6 to 77% (Sadock et al., 2017). In the first year after injury, depression may occur in approximately 25 to 50% of cases, with a lifetime prevalence that has been found to range from 26 to 64% (Sadock et al., 2017). The risk of depression may remain elevated years or even decades after the original injury. The presence of depression appears to be directly related to the TBI, as patients with similar traumatic injuries that had no brain impact had lower rates of depression (Jorge et al., 2004).

CLINICAL PRESENTATION

The DSM-5 diagnosis of MDD requires at minimum the presence of either sad mood or anhedonia. Anhedonia is defined as the loss of interest in activities that one previously enjoyed. Other presenting depressive symptoms include changes in appetite or weight, insomnia or hypersomnia, psychomotor agitation or retardation, fatigue or decreased energy, feelings of worthlessness or guilt, concentration difficulties, and suicidality. In addition to sad mood or anhedonia, at least five of these symptoms must be present for at minimum 2 weeks. These criteria, based on DSM-5, help guide clinical judgment and should not be used as a rote checklist to make a diagnosis (Sadock et al., 2017).

As mentioned earlier, the diagnosis of depression within an existing neuropsychiatric disorder can pose a challenge due to overlap of symptoms. However, depending on the specific neuropsychiatric disorder under consideration, the presentation may differ slightly.

Patients ultimately diagnosed with AD may in fact first present with depression as a chief complaint (Sadock et al., 2017). The American Association for Geriatric Psychiatry (AAGP) has proposed an alternative set of diagnostic criteria for depression in this patient population. Specifically, the AAGP has recommended the inclusion of behavioral symptoms for diagnostic criteria such as aggression or agitation that may be related to underlying irritability (Sepehry et al., 2017). Also, social withdrawal may be a prominent feature (Olin et al., 2002). Importantly, while this population may endorse less suicidality in part due to less verbalization, they nonetheless may experience increased passive death wishes (Sepehry at al., 2017). Thus, it is critical to assess the DSM-5 MDD symptoms as well as the symptoms recommended by the AAGP to help ensure diagnostic accuracy.

Depression in vascular dementia may include psychomotor retardation and changes in motivation such as apathy and abulia. A patient may appear sad, that is, their general display of emotion—or affect—appears sad, whereas apathy refers to a lack of emotion or interest, and abulia represents a more extreme form of apathy, such as a complete absence of will or initiative altogether. Cognitive abnormalities are common in vascular dementia and include worsened executive functioning, impaired concentration, and poor processing speed. The entity described earlier with the nomenclature of "vascular depression" depends specifically on the concurrent presence of abnormal brain lesions as documented with magnetic resonance imaging (Aizenstein et al., 2016).

Depression in FTD may involve mood lability as a prominent feature. Lability refers to quick and sudden changes in expressed emotionality, such that the emotion appears unexpectedly and out of proportion or may even be inappropriate to the situation at hand. At the same time, extreme apathy may be a common manifestation of a depressive syndrome in this population (Blass & Rabins, 2009). Relative to other neurodegenerative illnesses, FTD has an earlier age of onset, and those around the affected individual may suspect a "midlife crisis" or depressive episode. The diagnosis of FTD is confirmed by structural or even functional brain imaging that documents atrophy of the frontotemporal lobes (Sadock et al., 2017).

The most prominent symptoms overlapping with depression in those with MS may be sleep changes and fatigue. Fatigue in this situation, however, may be directly attributed to the demyelinating disorder, thus potentially leading to overdiagnosis of depression.

Suicidality has been found to be increased in patients with MS (Brønnum-Hansen, Stenager, Stenager, & Kock-Henriksen, 2005). Cognitive difficulties experienced by patients with MS may include changes in attention, working memory, and executive function, which some researchers believe may be directly related to the severity of white matter disease as documented on brain imaging (Rao, 1995). The pathophysiology, and thus the specific presentation, of depression in MS remains unclear. Indeed, depression in this population may be reactive, and the cognitive changes may be more related to the underlying neurological disease than to depression (Sadock et al., 2017; Siegert & Abernethy, 2005). Other theories about MS have postulated that depression may be a prodrome or an independent condition, may share the same etiology as MS, or as mentioned previously, may result from the medications used to treat MS (Galeazzi et al., 2005, as cited in Sadock et al., 2017).

In epilepsy, neurologists describe the clinical presentation of a given patient's seizures as its "semiology." Unsurprisingly, depression or anxiety may compose the ictal or postictal semiology in a given patient, or may even occur as part of the aura (Kanner, 2003). In some clinical scenarios, the mood symptoms might be the only manifestation of the seizure episode. Specific depressive symptoms in epilepsy include anhedonia or suicidal ideation (Kanner, 2003). The depressive symptoms may present interictally, that is, outside the context of the seizure episode. Once thought to be rare, mania is now increasingly recognized as also being a manifestation of epilepsy (Kanner, 2003).

Major depressive episodes following TBI are common and are often comorbid with anxiety disorders. These patients often have a personal history of MDD prior to the occurrence of the brain injury (Jorge et al., 2004). Patients with a history of TBI and concurrent depression relative to those with TBI without a history of MDD show poorer performance on cognitive tests. However, some research has suggested that patients with TBI with history of depression relative to those without a psychiatric history may show similar performance on psychological evaluation metrics (Jorge et al., 2004).

Increasing media attention to the clinical sequelae of concussions, for example, in professional athletes, has led to research of an entity known as chronic traumatic encephalopathy (CTE), for which depression is a major presenting symptom (McKee et al., 2009). Early manifestations of CTE include changes in cognitive domains such as attention, concentration, and memory, but mood symptoms such as depression have also been found to be common (McKee et al., 2009). As CTE is a relatively new diagnosis, additional research is warranted to clarify and confirm diagnostic symptomatology.

TREATMENT CONSIDERATIONS

Across all of the aforementioned neurological disorders, comorbid depression poses a significant treatment challenge compared to either a neurological illness or MDD alone. Treatment must take into account the nuances of both the neuropsychiatric disorder and the depressive disorder, while optimizing benefit to the patient and minimizing harm. For treatment of MDD, patients have myriad options, including pharmacological agents, psychotherapy, or neuromodulation treatments either alone or in combination. Deciding on the optimal therapy of choice will involve input from the integrated health care team to ensure optimal antidepressant efficacy and safety.

In AD, data supporting the use of antidepressants is variable and depends on the pharmacological properties of the specific agent in question. For example, due to their anticholinergic properties, medications such as tricyclic antidepressants are not recommended as they can worsen mental status in these patients. However, cholinesterase inhibitor medications may have modest efficacy for the treatment of apathy (Sadock et al., 2017). Second-generation antipsychotics for the treatment of behavioral disturbances seen in AD and other dementias have been given an FDA "black-box" warning against their use in the geriatric population. The warning specifically advises that the mortality risk increases in patients who have dementia and also take these medications. On the other hand, the agitation seen in these patients poses a treatment challenge. Thus, there is a possible short-term benefit for use of an atypical antipsychotic agent to treat acute agitation, but potential harm with long-term use of this medication class.

Antidepressants have been explored as a mainstay of treatment for depressive as well as behavioral symptoms of FTD; these antidepressants include selective serotonin reuptake inhibitors (SSRIs), such as paroxetine, and medications traditionally used for insomnia, such as trazodone (Lebert, Stekke, Hasenbroekx, & Pasquier, 2004; Moretti, Torre, Antonello, Cazzato, & Bava, 2003; Swartz, Miller, Lesser, & Darby, 1997). Antidepressants, as well as psychotherapy, also constitute the cornerstone of treatment for depression in MS (Mohr & Goodkin, 1999). Given that a broad range of antidepressants is available, clinicians may choose to select an agent based on the presence of other symptoms that could be addressed or assuaged by that same agent (Fiest et al., 2016). As a non-pharmacological treatment option, exercise training—such as water aerobics or resistance training—offers potential benefit for patients with both MS and depression, particularly for their symptoms of fatigue (Feinstein, Rector, & Motl, 2013).

SSRIs and selective serotonin–norepinephrine reuptake inhibitors also have utility in the treatment of epilepsy with comorbid depression (Maguire, Weston, Singh, & Marson, 2014). Treatment considerations for depression in patients with epilepsy include assessing if medications could potentially alter the seizure threshold or have effects on the metabolism of antiepileptic drugs, which these patients may be taking concurrently. Psychotherapy, such as cognitive-behavioral therapy (CBT) or acceptance and commitment therapy, offers an alternative but comparable treatment option for patients with both epilepsy and depression who cannot tolerate medications or wish to forego medications based on their personal preferences (Hoppe & Elger, 2011).

Online and group problem-solving therapy has helped to improve executive functioning deficits in pediatric, adolescent, and adult patients with TBI (Rath, Simon, Langenbahn, Sherr, & Diller, 2003; Wade, Wolfe, Brown, & Pestian, 2005; Wade et al., 2010). This type of therapy may help utilize compensatory mechanisms in patients with other deficits due to the TBI, which allows them to better live their day-to-day lives (Rath et al., 2003). Other reviews have demonstrated the efficacy of serotonin-based antidepressant agents and CBT for the treatment of post-TBI-induced depression (Fann, Hart, & Schomer, 2009).

Clinical guidelines for the treatment of depression or other mood or behavioral disturbances in neuropsychiatric disorders remain both underdeveloped and underutilized.

For example, recommendations for the treatment of depression in MS may depend on the clinical experience of the treatment team rather than results from studies or recommendations from the literature. Further research is needed to elucidate the specific pharmacology or type of antidepressant therapies that may best benefit patients with depression and a specific neuropsychiatric disorder.

AREAS FOR FUTURE RESEARCH

Research in the past several decades has helped to characterize the characteristics of depression in comorbid neuropsychiatric disorders. Areas for further research include treatment considerations, which have high clinical utility, and pathophysiology, which can help develop new antidepressant treatment options. In either case, the question that remains is how to best address the clinical symptoms of these patients in order to help them remain depression free and lead a higher quality of life. Exciting new therapies convey new hope and optimism for the treatment of depression in patients with comorbid neuropsychiatric disorders. For example, on the basis of neuroinflammatory theories of MDD, renewed interest in the use of statins as an adjunctive medication has shown some benefits for improvement in mood (Köhler et al., 2016; Salagre, Fernandes, Dodd, Brownstein, & Berk, 2016).

Given that depression in comorbid neuropsychiatric disorders may be especially difficult to treat, non-first-line therapies such as electroconvulsive therapy (ECT; see Finnegan & McLoughlin, Chapter 20, this volume) or transcranial magnetic stimulation (TMS; see Kavanaugh & Croarkin, Chapter 23, this volume) could play a role. ECT may confer remission of depression in just a few treatments with effective results. Geriatric depression, especially, may remit well with ECT, as these patients often have refractory or severe depression and may be unable to tolerate the side effects of the serotonergic agents traditionally used to treat depression (Kelly & Zisselman, 2000).

TMS, a relatively newer antidepressant therapy, continues to be studied in patients with neurological illness and comorbid MDD. Research continues to identify new brain targets for treatment delivery, which can allow for more precise medical treatment on the basis of the specific neuropsychiatric disorder in question. For example, localization of lesions or deficits and lesion-based network analysis could allow for the targeting of specific brain regions or circuits that contribute to mood pathology in neurological conditions (Fox, 2018). Typically, TMS is targeted to the brain region known as the dorsolateral prefrontal cortex. Current research has found that targeting this region specifically allows patients to better engage in cognitive reappraisal, which is a reframing technique often utilized in CBT to help patients view their experiences and situation in a more positive light (Golkar et al., 2012).

Theta burst transcranial magnetic stimulation allows for delivery of this treatment at higher frequencies, which could lead to potentially more rapid effects (Huang, Edwards, Rounis, Bhatia, & Rothwell, 2005). This modification of the protocol for TMS has been touted as a "rapid-acting antidepressant" and may help treat even treatment-refractory cases of depression in patients with neurological illnesses (Chung, Hoy, & Fitzgerald, 2015; Williams et al., 2018).

CONCLUSION

In comorbid neuropsychiatric disorders, depression may present in varying degrees with a diverse spectrum of clinical manifestations that can include affective, behavioral, and neurocognitive symptoms. This highlights the complex interplay of emotional processing and cognitive processing at the level of the neuron to the level of specific brain regions, and even the cortex as a whole. In more modern studies, this suggests that clinicians and scientists will need to look at the level of specific brain circuits and networks in order to develop and implement antidepressant therapies for this unique patient population with neuropsychiatric illnesses. Sophisticated techniques in neuroimaging, alongside complex network analyses, have been combined with computational biology and psychiatry to help uncover the neurological basis for depression in these neuropsychiatric illnesses. Further research is warranted to inform how depression manifests in comorbid neuropsychiatric disorders, which can then lead to exciting new discoveries and treatments and help develop our current understanding of the human brain.

REFERENCES

Aizenstein, H. J., Baskys, A., Boldrini, M., Butters, M. A., Diniz, B. S., Jaiswal, M. K., et al. (2016). Vascular depression consensus report—a critical update. *BMC Medicine, 14*(1), 161.

American Psychiatric Association. (2013). *Diagnostic and statistical manual of mental disorders* (5th ed.). Arlington, VA: Author.

Baldwin, R. C. (2005). Is vascular depression a distinct sub-type of depressive disorder?: A review of causal evidence. *International Journal of Geriatric Psychiatry, 20*(1), 1–11.

Ballard, C., Neill, D., O'Brien, J., McKeith, I. G., Ince, P., & Perry, R. (2000). Anxiety, depression and psychosis in vascular dementia: prevalence and associations. *Journal of Affective Disorders, 59*(2), 97–106.

Barnes, D. E., Yaffe, K., Byers, A. L., McCormick, M., Schaefer, C., & Whitmer, R. A. (2012). Midlife vs. late-life depressive symptoms and risk of dementia: Differential effects for Alzheimer disease and vascular dementia. *Archives of General Psychiatry, 69*(5), 493–498.

Blass, D. M., & Rabins, P. V. (2009). Depression in frontotemporal dementia. *Psychosomatics, 50*(3), 239–247.

Brønnum-Hansen, H., Stenager, E., Stenager, E. N., & Koch-Henriksen, N. (2005). Suicide among Danes with multiple sclerosis. *Journal of Neurology, Neurosurgery and Psychiatry, 76*(10), 1457–1459.

Byers, A. L., & Yaffe, K. (2011). Depression and risk of developing dementia. *Nature Reviews Neurology, 7*(6), 323.

Chakrabarty, T., Sepehry, A. A., Jacova, C., & Hsiung, G. Y. R. (2015). The prevalence of depressive symptoms in frontotemporal dementia: a meta-analysis. *Dementia and Geriatric Cognitive Disorders, 39*(5–6), 257–271.

Chi, S., Wang, C., Jiang, T., Zhu, X. C., Yu, J. T., & Tan, L. (2015). The prevalence of depression in Alzheimer's disease: a systematic review and meta-analysis. *Current Alzheimer Research, 12*(2), 189–198.

Chung, S. W., Hoy, K. E., & Fitzgerald, P. B. (2015). Theta-burst stimulation: a new form of TMS treatment for depression? *Depression and Anxiety, 32*(3), 182–192.

Douglas, K. M., Gallagher, P., Robinson, L. J., Carter, J. D., McIntosh, V. V., Frampton, C. M., et al. (2018). Prevalence of cognitive impairment in major depression and bipolar disorder. *Bipolar disorders, 20*(3), 260–274.

Fann, J. R., Hart, T., & Schomer, K. G. (2009). Treatment for depression after traumatic brain injury: A systematic review. *Journal of Neurotrauma, 26*(12), 2383–2402.

Feinstein, A., Rector, N., & Motl, R. (2013). Exercising away the blues: Can it help multiple sclerosis-related depression? *Multiple Sclerosis Journal, 19*(14), 1815–1819.

Fiest, K. M., Walker, J. R., Bernstein, C. N., Graff, L. A., Zarychanski, R., Abou-Setta, A. M., et al. (2016). Systematic review and meta-analysis of interventions for depression and anxiety in persons with multiple sclerosis. *Multiple Sclerosis and Related Disorders, 5*, 12–26.

Fox, M. D. (2018). Mapping symptoms to brain networks with the human connectome. *New England Journal of Medicine, 379*(23), 2237–2245.

Galeazzi, G. M., Ferrari, S., Giaroli, G., Mackinnon, A., Merelli, E., Motti, L., et al. (2005). Psychiatric disorders and depression in multiple sclerosis outpatients: Impact of disability and interferon beta therapy. *Neurological Sciences, 26*(4), 255–262.

Golkar, A., Lonsdorf, T. B., Olsson, A., Lindstrom, K. M., Berrebi, J., Fransson, P., et al. (2012). Distinct contributions of the dorsolateral prefrontal and orbitofrontal cortex during emotion regulation. *PloS One, 7*(11), e48107.

Hoppe, C., & Elger, C. E. (2011). Depression in epilepsy: A critical review from a clinical perspective. *Nature Reviews Neurology, 7*(8), 462–472.

Huang, Y. Z., Edwards, M. J., Rounis, E., Bhatia, K. P., & Rothwell, J. C. (2005). Theta burst stimulation of the human motor cortex. *Neuron, 45*(2), 201–206.

Jorge, R. E., Robinson, R. G., Moser, D., Tateno, A., Crespo-Facorro, B., & Arndt, S. (2004). Major depression following traumatic brain injury. *Archives of General Psychiatry, 61*(1), 42–50.

Kanner, A. M. (2003). Depression in epilepsy: Prevalence, clinical semiology, pathogenic mechanisms, and treatment. *Biological Psychiatry, 54*(3), 388–398.

Kelly, K. G., & Zisselman, M. (2000). Update on electroconvulsive therapy (ECT) in older adult. *Journal of the American Geriatrics Society, 48*(5), 560–566.

Kessler, R. C., Berglund, P., Demler, O., Jin, R., Merikangas, K. R., & Walters, E. E. (2005). Lifetime prevalence and age-of-onset distributions of DSM-IV disorders in the National Comorbidity Survey Replication. *Archives of General Psychiatry, 62*(6), 593–602.

Köhler, O., Gasse, C., Petersen, L., Ingstrup, K. G., Nierenberg, A. A., Mors, O., et al. (2016). The effect of concomitant treatment with SSRIs and statins: A population-based study. *American Journal of Psychiatry, 173*(8), 807–815.

Korczyn, A. D., & Halperin, I. (2009). Depression and dementia. *Journal of the Neurological Sciences, 283*(1–2), 139–142.

Kumar, S., Selim, M. H., & Caplan, L. R. (2010). Medical complications after stroke. *The Lancet Neurology, 9*(1), 105–118.

Lebert, F., Stekke, W., Hasenbroekx, C., & Pasquier, F. (2004). Frontotemporal dementia: A randomised, controlled trial with trazodone. *Dementia and Geriatric Cognitive Disorders, 17*(4), 355–359.

Maguire, M. J., Weston, J., Singh, J., & Marson, A. G. (2014). Antidepressants for people with epilepsy and depression. *Cochrane Database of Systematic Reviews*, Issue 12, CD010682.

Marrie, R. A., Reingold, S., Cohen, J., Stuve, O., Trojano, M., Sorensen, P. S., et al. (2015). The incidence and prevalence of psychiatric disorders in multiple sclerosis: A systematic review. *Multiple Sclerosis Journal, 21*(3), 305–317.

McKee, A. C., Cantu, R. C., Nowinski, C. J., Hedley-Whyte, E. T., Gavett, B. E., Budson, A. E., et al. (2009). Chronic traumatic encephalopathy in athletes: Progressive tauopathy after repetitive head injury. *Journal of Neuropathology and Experimental Neurology, 68*(7), 709–735.

Mohr, D. C., & Goodkin, D. E. (1999). Treatment of depression in multiple sclerosis: Review and meta-analysis. *Clinical Psychology: Science and Practice, 6*(1), 1–9.

Moretti, R., Torre, P., Antonello, R. M., Cazzato, G., & Bava, A. (2003). Frontotemporal dementia: Paroxetine as a possible treatment of behavior symptoms. *European Neurology, 49*(1), 13–19.

Olin, J. T., Schneider, L. S., Katz, I. R., Meyers, B. S., Alexopoulos, G. S., Breitner, J. C., et al. (2002). Provisional diagnostic criteria for depression of Alzheimer disease. *American Journal of Geriatric Psychiatry, 10*(2), 125–128.

Patten, S. B., & Metz, L. M. (2002). Interferon β1a and depression in secondary progressive MS: Data from the SPECTRIMS Trial. *Neurology, 59*(5), 744–746.

Rao, S. M. (1995). Neuropsychology of multiple sclerosis. *Current Opinion in Neurology, 8*(3), 216–220.

Rath, J. F., Simon, D., Langenbahn, D. M., Sherr, R. L., & Diller, L. (2003). Group treatment of problem-solving deficits in outpatients with traumatic brain injury: a randomised outcome study. *Neuropsychological Rehabilitation, 13*(4), 461–488.

Robinson, R. G. (2003). Poststroke depression: Prevalence, diagnosis, treatment, and disease progression. *Biological Psychiatry, 54*(3), 376–387.

Sadock, B. J., Sadock, V. A., & Ruiz, P. (2017). *Kaplan and Sadock's comprehensive textbook of psychiatry* (10th ed.). Philadelphia: Lippincott Williams & Wilkins.

Salagre, E., Fernandes, B. S., Dodd, S., Brownstein, D. J., & Berk, M. (2016). Statins for the treatment of depression: A meta-analysis of randomized, double-blind, placebo-controlled trials. *Journal of Affective Disorders, 200*, 235–242.

Sepehry, A. A., Lee, P. E., Hsiung, G. Y. R., Beattie, B. L., Feldman, H. H., & Jacova, C. (2017). The 2002 NIMH Provisional Diagnostic Criteria for depression of Alzheimer's disease (PDC-dAD): Gauging their validity over a decade later. *Journal of Alzheimer's Disease, 58*(2), 449–462.

Siegert, R. J., & Abernethy, D. A. (2005). Depression in multiple sclerosis: A review. *Journal of Neurology, Neurosurgery and Psychiatry, 76*(4), 469–475.

Swartz, J. R., Miller, B. L., Lesser, I. M., & Darby, A. L. (1997). Frontotemporal dementia: treatment response to serotonin selective reuptake inhibitors. *Journal of Clinical Psychiatry, 58*(5), 212–216.

Syed, S. A., Beurel, E., Loewenstein, D. A., Lowell, J. A., Craighead, W. E., Dunlop, B. W., et al. (2018). Defective inflammatory pathways in never-treated depressed patients are associated with poor treatment response. *Neuron, 99*(5), 914–924.

Wade, S. L., Walz, N. C., Carey, J., Williams, K. M., Cass, J., Herren, L., et al. (2010). A randomized trial of teen online problem solving for improving executive function deficits following pediatric traumatic brain injury. *Journal of Head Trauma Rehabilitation, 25*(6), 409–415.

Wade, S. L., Wolfe, C. R., Brown, T. M., & Pestian, J. P. (2005). Can a web-based family problem-solving intervention work for children with traumatic brain injury? *Rehabilitation Psychology, 50*(4), 337.

Williams, N. R., Sudheimer, K. D., Bentzley, B. S., Pannu, J., Stimpson, K. H., Duvio, D., et al. (2018). High-dose spaced theta-burst TMS as a rapid-acting antidepressant in highly refractory depression. *Brain, 141*(3), e18.

Winter, Y., Korchounov, A., Zhukova, T. V., & Bertschi, N. E. (2011). Depression in elderly patients with Alzheimer dementia or vascular dementia and its influence on their quality of life. *Journal of Neurosciences in Rural Practice, 2*(1), 27.

CHAPTER 5

Depression and Comorbid Medical Illness

Laura Howe-Martin
Tori Knox-Rice
Deanna Denman
E. Sherwood Brown

D epression is commonly comorbid with other chronic medical illnesses, and emerging research has continued to evaluate a potential common pathway for both. We are hopeful that 20 years from now, much of the information in this chapter regarding the complex, likely bidirectional, relationship between depression and medical common illnesses will be obsolete and replaced with a better understanding of shared causal mechanisms. Until that time, we will highlight the areas that complicate the relationship between medical illnesses and depression, including the rate of common overlap, difficulties associated with differential diagnosis, and the impact of depression on medical illness (as well the impact of medical illness on depression). In addition, research and theories on potential common pathways for certain medical illnesses and depression will be briefly reviewed, using type 2 diabetes as one common pathway example.

THE IMPORTANCE OF CAREFUL DIFFERENTIAL DIAGNOSIS

Many different types of depressive disorders share several symptoms. Each disorder, however, has a unique set of symptoms, and therefore, careful differentiation among disorders is imperative to determine the correct diagnosis and to facilitate appropriate treatment. The risk of inadequate diagnosis is that untreated or undertreated depression may result in disability, exacerbation of physical symptoms, and increased mortality.

Differentiating Depression from Other Major Psychiatric Disorders

All depressive disorders are characterized by a sad/irritable mood or lack of interest in previously enjoyed activities (i.e., anhedonia), in addition to cognitive and physical symptoms. However, these disorders differ in etiology, number of symptoms present, and timing (American Psychiatric Association, 2013). Major depressive disorder (MDD) is the most commonly diagnosed form of depression (American Psychiatric Association, 2013) and is characterized by discrete episodes of depressed or irritable mood most of the day, every day, or a loss of interest or pleasure in activities (anhedonia) lasting at least 2 weeks. To meet the criteria for a major depressive episode (MDE), an individual must experience at least five of the diagnostic symptoms, including depressed mood or anhedonia. The other diagnostic symptoms include changes in appetite, sleep patterns, and psychomotor activity, as well as fatigue, challenges concentrating, feelings of worthlessness or guilt, and thoughts of death or suicide (American Psychiatric Association, 2013). MDEs are typically recurrent, but a single episode may occur.

Bipolar and related disorders are often misdiagnosed as MDD (Angst et al., 2011; Hirschfeld, 2014; Hirschfeld, Lewis, & Vornik, 2003). Bipolar I disorder is characterized by discrete periods of elevated or irritable mood and increased energy lasting most of the day every day for at least a week (mania); in the case of bipolar II, there is a period of at least 4 days (hypomania). During a manic or hypomanic episode, an individual must also show evidence of at least three of the following diagnostic symptoms: inflated self-esteem or grandiosity, decreased need for sleep, pressured speech, flight of ideas or racing thoughts, distractibility, increase in goal-directed activity, and engagement in high-risk activities (American Psychiatric Association, 2013). For a bipolar I disorder diagnosis, a manic episode is sufficient for a diagnosis; for a bipolar II disorder diagnosis, however, there must also be a history of past or current major depressive episode(s). Cyclothymic disorder is diagnosed when adults experience 2 years (one year for children and adolescents) of hypomanic and depressive episodes that do not meet the criteria for (hypo)manic or major depressive episodes (American Psychiatric Association, 2013). Misdiagnosis of bipolar disorders as major depression may occur when a patient presents for treatment during a depressive phase; depressive episodes are typically more frequent and distressing than hypomanic episodes, and thus, patients are more likely to seek treatment (Angst et al., 2011). Additionally, patients may experience irritability and agitation during major depressive *or* manic or hypomanic episodes, further complicating diagnosis. Bipolar disorder cannot be effectively managed through psychotherapy or antidepressants (the latter may aggravate or trigger manic symptoms) alone and is more appropriately treated initially with mood stabilizers or atypical antipsychotics (Cruz et al., 2010). It is therefore critical to obtain a full, thorough history to assess for past episodes of mania or hypomania. MDD may present with a handful of hypomanic symptoms (particularly irritability). Therefore, it is important to distinguish between bipolar disorders and MDD, during which criteria will not be met for a true hypomanic episode due to shortened duration of symptoms or fewer symptoms. Thus, unless clinicians are vigilant about assessing past history of manic and hypomanic episodes or phases, misdiagnosis of bipolar and cyclothymic disorders as unipolar depression is likely (Smith & Ghaemi, 2006; Van Meter, Youngstrom, & Findling, 2012).

Adjustment disorders constitute the "development of emotional or behavioral symptoms in response to a stressor or multiple stressors" (American Psychiatric Association, 2013, p. 287). Adjustment disorders with depressed mood can develop within medically ill or injured populations, due to the stress of a new diagnosis, unexpected or prolonged hospitalization, or the stress of dealing with chronic disease. An important exclusion criterion for adjustment disorder is that the symptoms *may not* meet the criteria for MDD. If, in response to a stressor, an individual develops symptoms that meet the full criteria for a major depressive episode, diagnosis of MDD is more appropriate than an adjustment disorder. In addition, the symptom profile of an adjustment disorder with depressed mood differs from MDD and includes low mood, tearfulness, and feelings of hopelessness. Thus, symptoms of an adjustment disorder do not include the time criterion, anhedonia, or neurovegetative symptoms of MDD. Among individuals who develop low mood and marked distress in response to a medical condition, it is also important to differentiate symptoms of the condition (e.g., fatigue and weight loss due to cancer) from neurovegetative symptoms of depression to arrive at an appropriate diagnosis.

Differentiating Depression from Another Medical Condition

MDD must also be distinguished from a depressive disorder due to another medical condition (AMC). Clinical and research evidence points to clear associations between several neurological and neuroendocrine disorders. For example, depressive symptoms and presentation may be *directly caused by* stroke, Parkinson's disease, several forms of dementia, Cushing's disease, or hypothyroidism. Care should be taken to avoid both under- and overdiagnosis of depression in the context of such conditions. Inappropriately attributing symptoms of depression to the direct cause of a physical illness (when other mood symptoms are present) would lead to underdiagnosis and treatment of MDD, while failing to consider that the symptoms of physical illness could lead to overdiagnosis. While the prominent feature of depression due to AMC is a persistent period of depressed mood or anhedonia (Criterion A), there *must be* evidence that the symptoms are a *direct* pathophysiological response to a medical condition (Criterion B) and not merely an emotional reaction to the idea of having a difficult diagnosis or disease. Thus, depression due to AMC must be distinguished from MDD, as well as an adjustment disorder, when a medical condition is the identified stressor.

To determine whether depression is due to AMC, it must be established that the etiology of the change in mood is the medical condition (i.e., that an established physiological mechanism is causing the depression). This determination may be based on the timeline of the onset of mood symptoms and the medical condition, coupled with a review of the patient's medical information. Thus, determining whether the patient experienced depressive episodes prior to onset of the medical condition is critical, as is determining how the depressive symptoms may have progressed following the identification and treatment of the causative medical condition and treatment. Literature supporting a direct link between the medical condition and mood disorder is also helpful to review when considering this differential diagnosis. Prior research describes differential features specific to depression due to another medical condition such as increased likelihood of vegetative symptoms, social withdrawal, and irritability (Ehrt et al., 2006; Olin et al., 2002; Paradiso, Vaidya, Tranel, Kosier, & Robinson, 2008; Park et al., 2007).

Differentiating Depression
from Substance- or Medication-Induced Depression

Substance- or medication-induced depressive disorder has the same clinical features of MDD; however, the depressive symptoms are directly related to the use of a substance or medication. Thus, the patient's clinical and medical history shows that the onset of depressive symptoms directly follows the use of (or withdrawal from) a substance that may produce depressive symptoms. The symptoms *may not* be explained by another depressive disorder (i.e., the symptoms may not precede the use of, or withdrawal from, the substance). Differential diagnosis of substance/medication-induced depressive disorder versus a primary depressive disorder may be made by considering the timeline of symptom onset and course. Individuals with substance/medication-induced depressive disorder will have a history of medication/substance use, or withdrawal, that precedes development of the depressive symptoms. Several forms of substance use are associated with depressive symptoms, including alcohol, phencyclidine, opioids, anxiolytics, and amphetamines. Depressive symptoms may also result from the withdrawal from substances (e.g., cocaine).

Commonly prescribed medication such as beta blockers, central nervous system (CNS) medications, calcium channel blockers, corticosteroids, hormones and hormone blockers, anti-Parkinson drugs, benzodiazepines, cytokine interferon alpha, and many others may also cause depressive symptoms (Alexopoulous, 2005; Blazer, 2003; Djernes, 2006). Of note, providers should take care to clearly differentiate between substance/medication-induced depressive disorder and depression due to AMC. It is always possible that, rather than being a result of the medication, the depressive symptoms are direct sequelae of the medical condition. In such instances, the provider must examine the history carefully and consider whether the medication, or the underlying medical condition, is the cause.

Finally, a pitfall that results in underdiagnosis and undertreatment of depressive symptoms is the "understandable" trap. In clinical settings, this refers to underdiagnosis of a psychiatric disorder (typically MDD) due to the patient experiencing an understandable reaction to a chronic or recent stressor, such as the diagnosis of an illness or the impact of significant psychosocial stressors. Once psychosocial risk factors are better understood, it becomes quite reasonable that the person may develop symptoms of sadness, anhedonia, and even guilt, sleep disturbance, or suicidal ideation. However, this increases a risk of underdiagnosing comorbid depression.

THE IMPACT OF SOCIAL AND CULTURAL FACTORS

Psychosocial variables impact both risk for and experiences of depression and comorbid medical illnesses. A multitude of psychosocial risk factors have been studied as predisposing individuals to developing depression and/or medical illnesses (e.g., poor prenatal care), precipitating symptoms of both (e.g., an incident trauma), and perpetuating the problems (e.g., lack of access to care). The bidirectional interaction between psychosocial risk factors, depression and chronic medical disorders has been outlined by Katon (2003, 2011; Katon & Ciechanowski, 2002), and others (see reviews by Chen & Miller, 2013; Druss & Walker, 2011; Matthews & Gallo, 2011; see Figure 5.1).

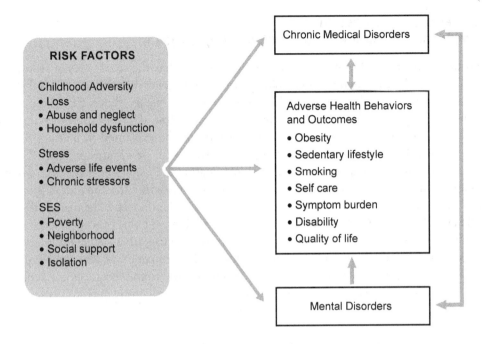

FIGURE 5.1. Model of the interaction between mental disorders and medical illness. From Druss and Walker (2011). Copyright © 2011 Robert Wood Johnson Foundation. Reprinted by permission.

These and other models highlight the importance of predisposing risk factors such as childhood adversity (e.g., early loss, abuse/neglect) and low socioeconomic status (SES; e.g., poverty, neighborhood characteristics, isolation). Stress—in the form of adverse life events and/or additional chronic stressors—is also a notable risk factor. However, the challenge in highlighting adversity and stress alongside SES is that these factors are intertwined and may influence the same underlying biological pathway(s) that give rise to both chronic medical illnesses and depression. Therefore, it is difficult to assess the unique, individual impact each factor has on the development of depression and chronic medical illnesses.

In addition, the scope of all individual and combined psychosocial risk factors (and the related risk models) is far beyond what can be covered in this chapter. Instead, we will specifically highlight the impact of three areas on depression and comorbid medical illness: (1) the impact of childhood adversity and trauma, (2) SES, (3) health disparities, and (4) chronic ongoing stressors, such as discrimination.

Childhood Adversity and Trauma

Early childhood adversity is a clear risk factor for later development of both depression and chronic medical illnesses (e.g., Chapman et al., 2004; Felitti et al., 1998; Poole, Dobson, & Pusch, 2017; Youssef et al., 2017). The most prominent findings regarding this relationship have emerged from the Adverse Childhood Experiences study (see Feletti et al., 1998, and subsequent related publications and replications). Although the participants in the original study were primarily White and middle- to upper-middle-class insured patients, findings from this study provided further empirical insight into the relationship between childhood abuse and household dysfunction on mental health problems later in life, as well as adult medical disease rates, health care utilization, and mortality. The initial and subsequent replication studies from this data note a graded relationship between the total number of categories of reported adverse childhood experiences and later adult health risk behaviors. For example, individuals who reported four or more categories of adverse childhood experiences were significantly more likely than those without any reported adverse experiences to also have myriad poor health conditions, including severe obesity, diabetes, liver disease, cancer, ischemic heart disease, stroke, and/or chronic bronchitis or emphysema (Dong, Dube, Velitti, Giles, & Anda, 2003; Felitti et al., 1998; Ramiro, Madrid, & Brown, 2010; Springer, Sheridan, Kuo, & Carnes, 2003; Wade et al., 2016). The original study (Felitti et al., 1998) also reflected an even greater risk for history of depressed mood within the past year (adjusted odds ratio [OR] = 4.6) and/or history of suicide attempt (adjusted OR = 12.2), alongside an increased risk for problematic substance use and risky sexual behaviors, for those who reported four or more categories of adverse childhood experiences (Chapman et al., 2004; Felitti et al., 1998).

Socioeconomic Status

Socioeconomic status is composed of a multitude of factors that go beyond income, education, and job status to involve specific neighborhood factors (e.g., toxin exposure, violence, access to social capital) and that have an impact on family characteristics (such as level of conflict and parental disciplinary style). There is strong, consistent evidence for the relationship between SES and health, in that lower SES consistently places individuals at higher risk for an array of health problems than their higher-SES counterparts (Lantz, House, Mero, & Williams, 2005; Ribeiro, Fraga, Costa, McCroy, & Barros, 2018; Smith, 2004; Williams, Priest, & Anderson, 2016). This array of health problems ranges from headaches to osteoarthritis to hypertension and coronary artery disease to cervical cancer. SES is also strongly associated with the development of depression. In addition, research on the relationship between low SES and risk for depression and chronic illnesses shows that SES is both a predisposing and perpetuating risk factor (Everson, Maty, Lynch, & Kaplan, 2002).

Lack of insurance and resulting differential access to health care only partially explain poor health outcomes among low-SES individuals (see review by Chen & Miller, 2013). Worse living conditions, increased engagement in health-compromising behaviors (e.g., smoking), and individual psychological characteristics (e.g., depression and anxiety resulting from family conflict; hostility and pessimism) also play a role. Not surprisingly, Lynch, Kaplan, Cohen, Tuomilehto, and Salonen (1996) found that the relationship between low SES and poor health outcomes such as cardiovascular mortality was significantly reduced when psychological risk factors (e.g., depression, hopelessness) were statistically controlled. Although negative emotions do not fully mediate this relationship, this ongoing relationship between negative health outcomes and depression requires ongoing examination.

Low-SES environments also perpetuate negative health outcomes due to exposure to chronic and perceived stress, increased risk of traumatic life events, and daily hassles (Gallo, Bogart, Vranceanu, & Matthews, 2005; Hatch & Dohrenwend, 2007). Other models posit that psychosocial resources (e.g., social support, self-esteem, optimism) are an important link between SES and health problems, with limited amounts of these resources reported by individuals with lower SES (Gallo & Matthews, 2003). However, these resources may have a role as helpful mediators between SES and health outcome (Bosma et al., 2005; Matthews, Gallo, & Taylor, 2010). Chen and Miller (2013) propose a "shift-and-persist" model of adaptation that may protect low-SES individuals from poorer health outcomes. Specifically, "shifting" (cognitive reappraisal and emotion regulation) and "persisting" (finding meaning and retaining optimism) may ameliorate the impact of underlying biological risk factors that lead to worsen chronic conditions such as cardiovascular disease and asthma (Chen & Miller, 2013). However, it is the specific nature of chronic depression and its symptoms that clearly impede this level of cognitive/emotional flexibility and hopefulness, therefore limiting coping and increasing the risk of chronic disease impact.

Health Disparities

Health disparities due to SES, gender, race/ethnicity, and other important areas of identity are clearly documented in the literature (for more information, see Tureson, Gold, & Thames, Chapter 13, this volume, on inclusion and diversity), with significantly poorer outcomes for depression and chronic medical illnesses seen across various marginalized groups (Adler et al., 1994; Braveman, Cubbin, Egerter, Williams, & Pamuk, 2010; Egede, 2006; Matthews & Gallo, 2011). Ethnic/racial minorities, sexual and gender minorities, individuals with disabilities, and individuals living in poverty are all considered to be at a higher risk of disparate care within the health care system (Braveman et al., 2010; Fiscella & Williams, 2004). In addition, although not traditionally viewed as marginalized, white men are also at heightened risk for poorer depression-related and disease-related outcomes, such as increased risk for suicide completion (Curtin, Warner, & Hedegaard, 2016). lower rates of psychological help-seeking behaviors (Yousaf, Grunfeld, & Hunter, 2015), and overall decreased lifespan expectancy (Kochanek, Murphy, Xu, & Arias, 2014).

When lack of access to care is coupled with lack of care utilization, mental health disorders and chronic medical diseases are often underdiagnosed and therefore undertreated. This results in increased health care costs, cumulative symptom burden, and premature mortality, particularly when these diseases co-occur. Approaches such as integrating mental health providers into primary care settings or using a collaborative care approach have been encouraged to address health disparities among individuals with comorbid chronic diseases and depression.

Chronic Discrimination as Chronic Stress

One underappreciated form of chronic stress is the role of systematic discrimination. For example, there is a significant relationship between experienced racial discrimination and a host of difficulties across the lifespan, including hypertension, birthweight, respiratory illness, body mass index (BMI), insulin resistance, and perceived health, as well as anxiety, depression, and psychosis (Brody, Yu, Chen, Ehrlich, & Miller, 2018; Collins et al., 2000; Janssen et al., 2003; Karlsen & Nazroo, 2002).

Cultural trauma (also referred to as *historical trauma*) reflects another form of chronic stress and refers to "when members of a collectivity feel they have been subjected to a horrendous event that leaves indelible marks upon group consciousness, marking their memories forever and changing their identity in fundamental and irreversible ways" (Alexander, Eyerman, Giesen, Smelser, & Sztompka, 2004, p. 1). This concept may be salient to the diagnosis and treatment of depression in that experiences of vicarious violence, loss, and historical discrimination may present as symptoms of depression, particularly when current events trigger the recall of historical ones. When specific social incidents occur to trigger culturally traumatic memories (e.g., denial of Holocaust events, police shootings of unarmed African Americans, appropriation of land owned by indigenous people), acute symptoms of distress may become more apparent. Symptoms of cultural trauma can include feelings of helplessness, hopelessness, and internalized guilt (Alexander et al., 2004; Mohatt, Thompson, Thai, & Tebes, 2014). Cultural trauma has also been used to conceptualize the development of significant depression, self-destructive behaviors, substance use, chronic health disparities, and earlier mortality rates among indigenous populations (Evans-Campbell, 2008; Gone, 2013; Hill, Lau, & Wing Sue, 2010; Kirmayer, Gone, & Moses, 2014). As there have been limited studies on the relationship between cultural trauma, depression, and comorbid medical illness, evaluation of cultural trauma as one form of chronic stressor that could give rise to both depression and comorbid chronic illnesses is needed.

PREVALENCE RATES OF DEPRESSION AND COMORBID MEDICAL ILLNESS

Within the literature, depressive disorders have been identified as a significant public health issue due to their rising prevalence and chronicity (Cassano & Fava, 2002). Some researchers have cited a higher prevalence of MDD in medically ill populations when compared to the "healthy" population (Fava, 2005). Various studies have investigated ties between medical illness and co-occurring depression. Depression has been shown to significantly impact medical outcomes in numerous comorbid conditions such as cardiovascular disease, HIV, diabetes, and chronic obstructive pulmonary disease (Albrecht et al., 2016; Gross & Malaspina, 2015; Hare, Toukhsati, Johansson, & Jaarsma, 2014; Nanni, Caruso, Mitchell, Meggiolaro, & Grassi, 2015; see Table 5.1).

Cardiovascular disease in particular has shown a high prevalence of comorbid depression (Larsen, 2013; Lichtman et al., 2008). Higher rates (24–42%) have also been found in those with congestive heart failure (Guck, Elsasser, Kavan, & Eugene, 2003). A wealth of research on diabetes, type 1 and type 2, highlights the association between the diagnosis and depression. Studies have looked not only at the mere presence of depression, but the bidirectional relationship of both diagnoses (Pan et al., 2010). Some studies have asserted that individuals with type 1 or 2 diabetes mellitus have a 20–30% prevalence of MDD (Nouwen et al., 2010), two to three times more than that of the general population.

TABLE 5.1. Ten Medical Illnesses Commonly Comorbid with Depression

Cardiovascular disease	Depressive disorders have been associated with risk factors for cardiovascular disease. This association extends to health behaviors that impact illness, such as smoking and physical inactivity (Hayward, 1995; Larsen, 2013; Nemeroff, Musselman, & Evans, 1998).
Type 2 diabetes	Elevated rates of depression have consistently been associated with diabetes (Talbot, Nouwen, Gingras, Bélanger, & Audet, 1999). It has been proposed that depressive symptoms may be a risk factor for the development of diabetes (Gross & Malaspina, 2015; Yu, Zhang, Lu, & Fang, 2015).
Substance use disorder	Depression and substance use disorders are highly prevalent in the general population and can co-occur (Lai, Cleary, Sitharthan, & Hunt, 2015; Wu & Blazer, 2014).
Stroke	Depression following stroke is highly prevalent, with estimates ranging around 31% (Hackett & Pickles, 2014).
Chronic obstructive pulmonary disease (COPD)	A diagnosis of COPD is associated with a higher risk for the development of depression (van den Bemt et al., 2009). Depression in COPD can impact compliance with medical treatment and smoking cessation (Albrecht et al., 2016).
HIV	Depressive disorders among individuals with HIV may approach nearly 50% (Forstein et al., 2006; Nanni, Caruso, Mitchell, Meggiolaro, & Grassi, 2015). The presence of depression in HIV has been associated with negative disease outcomes such as accelerated disease progression, nonadherence to antiretrovirals, and mortality (Carrico et al., 2011; Gonzalez, Batchelder, Psaros, & Safren, 2011).
Multiple sclerosis	Research has shown that up to 50% of patients with multiple sclerosis have comorbid depression (Marrie, 2016). The occurrence of this comorbidity is estimated to be three times the rate of major depression in community-based samples and greater than the rate of depression among patients with other neurological disorders (Siegert & Abernethy, 2005).
Epilepsy	Depression is the most common comorbid psychiatric disorder in patients with epilepsy (Fiest et al., 2013; Kanner, 2003). Depression has a profound negative impact on the quality of life in individuals with epilepsy (Jehi, Tesar, Obuchowski, Novak, & Najm, 2011).
Asthma	Symptoms such as dyspnea and disruptive nighttime sleep cycles are associated with a higher risk for major depression (Goldney, Ruffin, Fisher, & Wilson, 2003). Depressive symptoms have been associated with poor asthma-related outcomes (Eisner, Katz, Lactao, & Iribarren, 2005).
Arthritis	Individuals diagnosed with arthritis or those experiencing arthritis-related debility/arthritic symptoms have been found to report greater incidence of depression (Dickens, McGowan, Clark-Carter, & Creed, 2002; Matcham, Rayner, Steer, & Hotopf, 2013). Functional status has been correlated with depression, with greater depressive symptoms reported in those experiencing severe symptoms (Kwiatkowska, Kłak, Maślińska, Mańczak, & Raciborski, 2018).

Although it is estimated that a significant proportion of individuals with HIV have clinically significant depressive symptoms, depression remains underdiagnosed within this population (Forstein et al., 2006; Pence, O'Donnell, & Gaynes, 2012). Treatment of HIV includes not only the initial awareness of the illness, but consistent engagement in medical care that adheres to an antiretroviral therapy regimen. Depression can impact this process by contributing to nonadherence (Gonzalez, Batchelder, Psaros, & Safren, 2011).

Chronic obstructive pulmonary disease (COPD) is a prevalent lung disease and often co-occurs with depression (Pumar et al., 2014). This high rate of comorbidity exists among those diagnosed with COPD when compared to both smoker and nonsmokers without the diagnosis (Hanania et al., 2011).

HOW DEPRESSION COMPLICATES MEDICAL ILLNESSES

Pathways associated with comorbidity among medical and mental disorders are likely bidirectional. Medical conditions can result in mental disorders, and mental disorders can increase the risk for medical conditions (Katon, 2003). Some prior epidemiological studies investigated the bidirectional nature of this phenomenon, with results showing the significant impact that can easily flow both ways (Patten et al., 2008). Chronic illness may increase the risk of depression or the duration of depressive episodes; either effect could lead to an increased prevalence. Alternatively, MDD may predispose individuals to certain chronic illnesses (Druss & Walker, 2011; Evans et al., 2005).

When depression co-occurs with a chronic medical condition, an individual's functional impairment and symptoms burden increases significantly (Katon, Lin, & Kroenke, 2007). Some researchers have found an association with notably reduced quality of life and length of life, not to mention a higher cost burden of treatment (Egede, 2007; Katon, 2003). According to some estimates, the risk of premature mortality stands at two to four times that of the general population for those with mental disorders (Colton & Manderscheid, 2006). In such studies, death was found to be due to "natural" causes such as cardiovascular disease rather than accidents and suicides (Druss & Walker, 2011). In a multistate mortality study based on public mental health agencies from 1997 to 2000, clients were found to die, on average, 25 years earlier than the average life expectancy for the general population (Colton & Manderscheid, 2006). These studies further highlight the association between mental health and general health outcomes.

When examining comorbid medical illness and depression, lifestyle factors should be strongly considered. Mental illness can have a significant impact on health behaviors, putting those affected at a higher risk of developing or exacerbating medical conditions (DiMatteo, Lepper, & Croghan, 2000). Many behaviors, such as tobacco use, alcohol consumption, drug use, dietary habits, and physical activity, can be viewed as modifiable (Spring, Moller, & Coons, 2012). These health behaviors become much more complicated when considering a key component of depressive disorder—anhedonia or reduced motivation or ability to experience pleasure. Positive self-care, which may include consistent medication adherence, exercise, diet, or stress relief, is often essential in managing chronic medical conditions. These self-care behaviors can be negatively impacted by anhedonia or mental conditions that decrease or reduce motivation to actively engage in aspects of day-to-day life (Druss & Walker, 2011; Katon, 2003). The likelihood of treatment nonadherence with medical treatment regimens are three times greater for depressed patients compared with nondepressed patients (DiMatteo et al., 2000; Sawada et al., 2009). Nonadherence is highly associated with poorer medical outcomes as a whole and should be considered when discussing treatment in those affected by comorbid affective conditions.

HOW MEDICAL ILLNESSES COMPLICATE DEPRESSION TREATMENT

As previously noted, depression rates are highly comorbid among those with other medical conditions. Chronic illness is associated with increased prevalence of both depressive symptoms and disorders. As previously discussed, illness can cause and contribute to depression in various ways, as it may be the stressor leading to depressive symptomatology (i.e., MDD or adjustment disorder) or directly cause depression through pathophysiological mechanisms (i.e., depression due to AMC or depression due to substance/medication use). For others, however, biological risk factors or changes associated with illness may interact with psychosocial factors contributing to depression. Thus, the experience of having a medical condition—changes in functional limitations, pain due to cancer and disease—can contribute to depression (Bair, Robinson, Katon, & Kroenke, 2003; Egede, 2007). Some chronic conditions may also contribute to depression through behavioral mechanisms (e.g., chronic pain leading to a lack of activity and withdrawal from enjoyable activities; Fiske, Wetherell, & Gatz, 2009). Consequently, understanding the complex ways medical illness may contribute to depressive disorders is paramount to successful treatment.

The biopsychosocial model is currently one of the best ways to understand the relationship between medical illness and depression (Engel, 1980). It views chronic conditions through a multifaceted framework that integrates physical, psychological, and social factors that can impact the development and maintenance of an individual's clinical presentation. The interplay between physical (medical illness), psychological (mood and cognition), behavioral, and social influences helps to explain how medical illness may complicate depression treatment.

Illness is influenced by personal experience and how a person responds to a disease. The relationship between chronic illness and depression is well suited to conceptualization in a biopsychosocial framework that can help account for varying psychosocial aspects of experience that can contribute to differing clinical presentations. Thus, when considering how medical conditions may impact depression, one must consider how changes in the physical experience may be related to psychological and social factors.

The experience of chronic illness gives people many reasons to change their behavior and cognitions. For example, individuals are likely to reduce their activities in response to symptoms such as pain and fatigue. Negative self-talk is also likely as individuals are prone to worry about their condition and potentially feel hopeless about their prognosis or the management of a chronic illness. Those managing chronic illness are likely to experience temporary or permanent changes in functional limitations (e.g., muscle weakness, physical disability, nausea), which is related to increased incidence of depression (Egede, 2007; Fiske et al., 2009). These negative cognitions and behavioral changes can lead to depressive symptoms such as low mood, anhedonia, and feelings of hopelessness. Such changes may also contribute to the maintenance of depression. For example, a person struggling with pain and fatigue is likely to decrease their participation in activities and stay in bed more. This could lead the person to experience negative emotions and further withdraw from social support and enjoyable activities, ultimately leading to further deconditioning, increased pain and fatigue, and greater distress and depressive symptomatology.

Medical illness may also impact the process of psychotherapy. While patients may be willing to participate in therapy, challenges inherent to the treatment of their medical condition may impede psychotherapy. For example, for hospitalized patients engaging in psychotherapy, the length of their hospitalization limits the number of sessions they can have with a hospital psychotherapist. Other challenges may include unpredictable schedules, interruptions to therapy sessions by other providers, or procedures or symptoms rendering a patient unavailable/incapable of participation. The experience of illness can impede one's ability to participate in psychotherapy. For example, a person may feel too unwell to attend, and participate, in psychotherapy sessions. Medications could render a person too somnolent to participate in, or recall, sessions. Impaired functioning (e.g. extreme nausea or impaired mobility) may also limit individuals' ability to participate in elements of treatment such as scheduling of positive activity for behavioral activation.

Physical illness also represents a change in biological risk factors for depression. Studies exploring the links between illness and depressive disorders have considered genetic influences, poor treatment adherence and lifestyle factors, and changes in the endocrine system, inflammation and immune functioning, cardiovascular functioning, and neuroanatomy as factors increasing risk for, or causing, depression (Fiske et al., 2009; Krishnan, 2002; Whooley et al., 2007). These associations are highest among individuals with cardiovascular disease (Carney & Freedland, 2003) and neurological disorders (e.g., stroke; Park et al., 2007).

Treatment of medical illness may also complicate treatment of depression through medication effects and interactions. Individuals coping with chronic illness typically take several medications that may cause fatigue, sedation, and other challenges to participation. As noted previously, certain medications (e.g., beta blockers, CNS medications, corticosteroids, hormone blockers) may cause depressive symptoms (Alexopoulous, 2005; Blazer, 2003; Celano, Freudenrich, Fernandez-Robles, Stern, & Huffman, 2011; Djernes, 2006). Additionally, some medications that are used to treat medical conditions may preclude the use of antidepressant medications due to the potential for interactions (e.g., citalopram and paroxetine may increase the serum levels of metoprolol and cause bradycardia; see Kurdyak, Manno, Gomes, Mamadani, & Juurlink, 2012).

In summary, chronic illness may impact treatment of depressive disorders through multiple avenues. In addition to the ways that medical conditions and their treatments may cause depressive symptoms, medical conditions can impact and impede treatment of depressive disorders through the burden of illness, biological changes, and maintenance of symptoms. Recognizing the unique challenges that medical illnesses can contribute to depression is key to successful treatment.

COMMON-PATHWAYS MODELS AND AREAS FOR FURTHER RESEARCH

An exciting area of research involves searching for common pathways for all chronic diseases, including chronic depression. Much of this research can be quite translational, as it has emerged from both bench scientists and clinicians who are observing similar phenomena in different settings. Why does chronic depression coexist with chronic medical diseases at such a high rate? Does depression as a disease prompt sedentary and other unhealthy behaviors that lead to increased risk for chronic diseases such as type 2 diabetes? Do specific underlying diseases, such as coronary artery disease, prompt the development of depressive symptoms in certain individuals? Or, as this section reviews, is there evidence for common underlying pathways for all chronic diseases?

One issue that hampers research in this area is the variety of methodologies used to assess depression. For example, some studies utilize self-report assessment of depressive symptoms, whereas others assess for MDD and other nuances of diagnosable depression using structured clinical interviews. Furthermore, many studies rely on cross-sectional designs, therefore limiting the conclusions that can be drawn.

In addition, the complicated nature of the brain as an organ significantly hampers clear findings in this field of research. Advances in neuroimaging have helped research in this area tremendously, although much of the common pathways research continues to build on animal models (inasmuch as they can inform interpretation of human behaviors). Areas of common pathway research for depression and chronic diseases include investigating the role(s) of metabolism, chronic inflammation, abnormalities in the hypothalamic–pituitary–adrenal axis (HPA), cortisol changes, homeostatic changes between the sympathetic and parasympathetic nervous systems, and the "gut microbiome" (microbiota–gut–brain axis), to name a few (Foster & Neufeld, 2013; Gragnoli, 2014; Heijtz et al., 2011; Katon, 2011; Moulton, Pickup, & Ismail, 2015; Wang & Kasper, 2014).

Type 2 Diabetes as One Example

One example of the complex relationship between chronic depression and medical illness is type 2 diabetes (T2DM). Most individuals with depression do not develop this medical disease, nor do most individuals with T2DM develop chronic depression. However, T2DM is associated with an approximately 20% increased risk of incident depression (Nouwen et al., 2010), while depression is associated with a 60% increased risk of incident T2DM (Mezuk, Eaton, Albrecht, & Golden, 2008; Nouwen et al., 2010). Furthermore, there is a genetic correlation of $r = .19$ (Scherrer et al., 2011, although with a broad confidence interval [CI] cited of 0 to 0.46), and both MDD and T2DM have similar heritability rates (40% for MDD vs. 35% for T2DM, per Krishnan & Nestler, 2008). A 10-year longitudinal study by Pan and colleagues (2010) reported women with depression have an increased risk of developing T2DM (odds ratios [OR] 1.17; 95% CI 1.05–1.30), while women with T2DM exhibited an increased relative risk of clinical depression (OR 1.29; 95% CI 1.18–1.40). Both disorders are associated with significant morbidity, mortality, and increased health care costs (Egede & Ellis, 2010). In fact, the American Diabetes Association (ADA; 2019) recommends assessment of depression, among other psychological issues, in those with diabetes, particularly T2DM, as this form of diabetes comprises 90% of diabetes cases.

A wealth of issues impact the prevalence data and research examining the relationship between depression and T2DM, including depression assessment instrumentation (e.g., structured diagnostic interview vs. self-report rating scales), depressive symptoms that are typical of diabetes as well (e.g., fatigue, weight changes), heavy reliance on cross-sectional study design, and not controlling for important variables such as gender, age, SES, lifestyle factors, and BMI. For example, as described by Roy and Lloyd (2012), women with T2DM have significantly higher rates of depression than men with T2DM, which mirrors the pattern of depression in the general nondiabetic population. In addition, there is an emphasis on European American medical models and participants in most studies on the overlap between diabetes and depression.

Methodological variability and diagnostic error are not the only proposed explanations for this consistently reported overlap. As noted previously in this chapter, T2DM shares many underlying risk factors with chronic depression, including early childhood adversity, ongoing social system adversity, and deprivation related to poverty and/or low SES (Matthews & Gallo, 2011). There are also poorer health behaviors among individuals with both diseases, including increased rates of smoking and lower rates of physical activity (Manson et al., 1991; Mathew, Hogarth, Leventhal, Cook, & Hitsman, 2017; Nefs, Pop, Denollet, & Pouwer, 2016; Schuch et al., 2017). In addition, several biological common pathways between T2DM and depression have been identified (see Katon, 2011; Moulton et al., 2015) and are highlighted next.

Chronic inflammation has been implicated in the increased risk for both depression and T2DM. One example includes the role of inflammatory cytokines, albeit not clearly and not without the impact of specific moderators (e.g., BMI). For example, it has been a long-standing clinical standard of care that patients awaiting treatment with cytokine interferon alpha should also undergo careful pretreatment psychological evaluation to assess for a history of depression and/or suicidal behaviors. For example, a significant number of patients (almost 35% per meta-analysis by Machado et al., 2017) with hepatitis C develop a major depressive episode during interferon treatment. Increased production of proinflammatory cytokines has been demonstrated to contribute directly to the development of depressive symptoms through inducing stress-related neuroendocrine and central neurotransmitter changes similar to those found in depression (Anisman & Merali, 2003; Dowlati et al., 2010). Furthermore, levels of proinflammatory cytokines in plasma and cerebrospinal fluid can influence how depressive disorders are exhibited, as well as the associated severity of symptoms (Young, Bruno, & Pomara, 2014).

Diabetes-associated inflammation has also been implicated in the development and exhibition of sickness behavior and diabetes treatment nonadherence (see review by Rustad, Musselman, & Nemeroff, 2011). Furthermore, chronic inflammation has been implicated in the relationship between chronic life stressors, including adverse childhood experiences, and the later development of both T2DM risk and depression in adulthood (Moulton et al., 2015). As such, modification of inflammation may prove to be a common treatment pathway for patients with both T2DM and depression. For example, anti-inflammatory treatments as an adjuvant to selective serotonin reuptake inhibitors may increase the antidepressant effect for patients affected by both diseases (Akhondzadeh et al., 2009; Müller, 2013).

HPA axis dysregulation is related to chronic inflammation and has also been implicated in these two diseases, specifically with regard to chronic stress, chronically elevated and/or excess cortisol levels, glycemic control, and specific brain structure development (i.e., hippocampus and amygdala; Barden, 2004; Krishnan & Nestler, 2008). It has been proposed that hyperactivation of the neuroendocrine cortisol pathway gives rise to T2DM, metabolic syndrome, and depression via corticotropin-releasing hormone, adrenocorticotropic hormone, and glucocorticoid receptor dysfunction (Hoyo-Becerra, Schlaak, & Hermann, 2014; Loftis & Hauser, 2004; Machado et al., 2017). In addition, a host of candidate genes have been proposed as playing a role in depression, antidepressant response, obesity, and T2DM (Gragnoli, 2014). However, while the relationship between elevated cortisol levels and metabolic syndrome (and later T2DM) has been established, the relationship to depression is less clear, although abnormalities in the HPA axis have been implicated in depression (Gold, 2015). For example, overactivation of the HPA axis may impair neuroplasticity in brain areas related to emotion and mood regulation (Duman, 2004; Gold, 2015), although this condition may be more prominent in only certain types of depression, such as in the more severe or melancholic types of depression. Further research is needed to evaluate this relationship prior to pursuing treatments that alter HPA axis regulation to target both depression and T2DM.

Circadian rhythm disruption has also been implicated in the overlap between depression and diabetes. Sleep disruption and fatigue are common symptoms of depression, particularly insomnia (although hypersomnia is present for some). Clinically, sleep architecture among individuals with depression and those with T2DM display commonalities, including increased rapid-eye-movement density and decreased slow-wave sleep (Kudlow, Cha, Lam, & McIntyre, 2016; Moulton et al., 2015). In addition, clock genes (which are involved in circadian rhythm regulation) have been implicated in fasting glucose concentrations (Jha, Challet, & Kalsbeek, 2015; Laermans & Depoortere, 2016) and are posited to play a significant role in mood disorders such as depression and bipolar disorder (Bunney et al., 2015; Zaki et al., 2018). It has long been posited that antidepressant therapy works at a clock gene level to regulate the sleep cycle as a necessary part of overall depressive symptom management. For example, low-dose ketamine therapy for depression is thought to restore circadian rhythms due to impact on clock genes (Bunney et al., 2015).

The *gut microbiome* or the *gut–brain axis* has been implicated in diseases such as depression and T2DM. Dysbiosis (the opposite of symbiosis) in gut microbiota have been implicated in several health conditions, including asthma, autism, obesity, diabetes, inflammation, and stress (see reviews by Rieder, Wisniewski, Alderman, & Campbell, 2017; Wang & Kasper, 2014). In addition, gut microbiota are demonstrably important to CNS functioning (Foster & Neufeld, 2013; Heijtz et al., 2011; Wang & Kasper, 2014). Specifically, it has been found that bacteria can activate neural pathways and CNS signaling systems, therefore shifting aspects of neuroplasticity, serotonergic, and GABA-ergic systems. This opens up potential treatments for underlying microbiota dysbiosis that may give rise to both diabetes and depression. For example, probiotic treatment has demonstrated suppression of depression in animal models in specific cases, such as maternal separation-induced depression (Gareau, Jury, MacQueen, Sherman, & Perdue, 2007). Given the importance of these symptoms for mental health and mental illness, emerging research beyond animal models will provide further information on the impact of altered microbiota profiles in chronic disorders such as autism and depression.

Taken together, these proposed common pathways suggest that upstream biomarker identification and modification could prevent the development of both disorders, or at least promote common medical treatment approaches (Moulton, Pickup, & Ismail, 2015). However, it should be noted that nonpharmacological treatments for comorbid depression and T2DM are already in place. For example, a meta-analysis of multiple randomized controlled trials demonstrated that cognitive-behavioral therapy produces long-term improvements in depressive symptoms for patients with both disorders through improving adherence and targeting underlying negative thoughts (Li et al., 2017). In fact, the ADA and the American Psychological Association have recently partnered to promote the Mental Health Provider Diabetes Education Program (ADA, n.d.) as a way of promoting treatment of comorbid depression and anxiety in the diabetes population. Interventions that ameliorate chronic stress, target traumatic experiences, and/or decrease the impact of chronic adverse experiences (e.g., poverty, cultural trauma) could also be posited to decrease the impact of both of these diseases.

CONCLUSION

This chapter has reviewed the very broad and complex relationship between depression and comorbid medical illnesses, beginning with the significant challenges to differential diagnosis and prevalence rates regarding comorbidity. Early childhood, social, and cultural factors were introduced as important risk factors for the development of both depression and medical diseases. Furthermore, clinical complications when both diseases are present were highlighted. Finally, some of the common research pathways were introduced. The latter represents a significant and hopeful path toward understanding depression as a chronic disease, and the value of integrated models of care within medicine.

REFERENCES

Adler, N. E., Boyce, T., Chesney, M. A., Cohen, S., Folkman, S., Kahn, R. L., et al. (1994). Socioeconomic status and health: The challenge of the gradient. *American Psychologist, 49*(1), 15.

Akhondzadeh, S., Jafari, S., Raisi, F., Nasehi, A. A., Ghoreishi, A., Salehi, B., et al. (2009). Clinical trial of adjunctive celecoxib treatment in patients with major depression: A double blind and placebo controlled trial. *Depression and Anxiety, 26*(7), 607–611.

Albrecht, J. S., Park, Y., Hur, P., Huang, T. Y., Harris, I., Netzer, G., et al. (2016). Adherence to maintenance medications among older adults with chronic obstructive pulmonary disease. The role of depression. *Annals of the American Thoracic Society, 13*(9), 1497–1504.

Alexander, J., Eyerman, R., Giesen, B., Smelser, N., & Sztompka, P. (2004). *Cultural trauma and collective identity.* Berkeley: University of California Press.

Alexopoulos, G. S. (2005). Depression in the elderly. *Lancet, 365,* 1961–1970.

American Diabetes Association. (2019). Standards of medical care in diabetes. *Diabetes Care, 42*(Suppl. 1), S34–S45.

American Diabetes Association. (n.d.). Mental Health Provider Diabetes Education Program. Retrieved May 8, 2020, from *https://professional.diabetes.org/meeting/other/mental-health-provider-diabetes-education-program.*

American Psychiatric Association. (2013). *Diagnostic and statistical manual of mental disorders* (5th ed.). Arlington, VA: Author.

Angst, J. (2011). Prevalence and characteristics of undiagnosed bipolar disorders in patients with a major depressive episode: The BRIDGE study. *Archives of General Psychiatry, 68*(8), 791.

Anisman, H., & Merali, Z. (2003). Cytokines, stress and depressive illness: Brain-immune interactions. *Annals of Medicine, 35*(1), 2–11.

Bair, M. J., Robinson, R. L., Katon, W., & Kroenke, K. (2003). Depression and pain comorbidity: A literature review. *Archives of Internal Medicine, 163*(20), 2433.

Barden, N. (2004). Implication of the hypothalamic–pituitary–adrenal axis in the physiopathology of depression. *Journal of Psychiatry and Neuroscience, 29*(3), 185.

Blazer, D. G. (2003). Depression in late life: Review and commentary. *The Journals of Gerontology, Series A: Biological Sciences and Medical Sciences, 58,* 249–265.

Bosma, H., Van Jaarsveld, C. H. M., Tuinstra, J., Sanderman, R., Ranchor, A. V., Van Eijk, J. T. M., et al. (2005). Low control beliefs, classical coronary risk factors, and socio-economic differences in heart disease in older persons. *Social Science and Medicine, 60*(4), 737–745.

Braveman, P. A., Cubbin, C., Egerter, S., Williams, D. R., & Pamuk, E. (2010). Socioeconomic disparities in health in the United States: What the patterns tell us. *American Journal of Public Health, 100*(Suppl. 1), S186–S196.

Brody, G. H., Yu, T., Chen, E., Ehrlich, K. B., & Miller, G. E. (2018). Racial discrimination, body mass index, and insulin resistance: A longitudinal analysis. *Health Psychology, 37*(12), 1107.

Bunney, B. G., Li, J. Z., Walsh, D. M., Stein, R., Vawter, M. P., Cartagena, P., et al. (2015). Circadian dysregulation of clock genes: Clues to rapid treatments in major depressive disorder. *Molecular Psychiatry, 20*(1), 48.

Carney, R. M., & Freedland, K. E. (2003). Depression, mortality, and medical morbidity in patients with coronary heart disease. *Biological Psychiatry, 54*(3), 241–247.

Carrico, A. W., Riley, E. D., Johnson, M. O., Charlebois, E. D., Neilands, T. B., Remien, R. H., et al. (2011). Psychiatric risk factors for HIV disease progression: The role of inconsistent patterns of anti-retroviral therapy utilization. *Journal of Acquired Immune Deficiency Syndromes, 56*(2), 146.

Cassano, P., & Fava, M. (2002). Depression and public health: An overview. *Journal of Psychosomatic Research, 53*(4), 849–857.

Celano, C. M., Freudenrich, O., Fernandez-Robles, C., Stern, T. A., & Huffman, J. C. (2011). Depressogenic effects of medications: A review. *Dialogues in Clinical Neuroscience, 13*(1), 17.

Chapman, D. P., Whitfield, C. L., Felitti, V. J., Dube, S. R., Edwards, V. J., & Anda, R. F. (2004). Adverse childhood experiences and the risk of depressive disorders in adulthood. *Journal of Affective Disorders, 82*(2), 217–225.

Chen, E., & Miller, G. E. (2013). Socioeconomic status and health: Mediating and moderating factors. *Annual Review of Clinical Psychology, 9,* 723–749.

Collins, J. W., Jr., David, R. J., Symons, R., Handler, A., Wall, S. N., & Dwyer, L. (2000). Low-income African-American mothers' perception of exposure to racial discrimination and infant birth weight. *Epidemiology, 11*(3), 337–339.

Colton, C. W., & Manderscheid, R. W. (2006). Congruencies in increased mortality rates, years of potential life lost, and causes of death among public mental health clients in eight states. *Preventing Chronic Disease, 3*(2), A42.

Cruz, N., Sanchez-Moreno, J., Torres, F., Goikolea, J. M., Valentí, M., & Vieta, E. (2010). Efficacy of modern antipsychotics in placebo-controlled trials in bipolar depression: A meta-analysis. *International Journal of Neuropsychopharmacology, 13*(1), 5.

Curtin, S. C., Warner, M., & Hedegaard, H. (2016). Suicide rates for females and males by race and ethnicity: United States, 1999 and 2014. *NCHS Health E-stat.*

Dickens C., McGowan L., Clark-Carter D., Creed F. (2002). Depression in rheumatoid arthritis: A systematic review of the literature with meta-analysis. *Psychosomatic Medicine, 64*(1):52–60.

DiMatteo, M. R., Lepper, H. S., & Croghan, T. W. (2000). Depression is a risk factor for noncompliance with medical treatment: Meta-analysis of the effects of anxiety and depression on patient adherence. *Archives of Internal Medicine, 160*(14), 2101–2107.

Djernes, J. K. (2006). Prevalence and predictors of depression in populations of elderly: A review. *Acta Psychiatrica Scandinavica, 113,* 372–387.

Dong, M., Dube, S. R., Felitti, V. J., Giles, W. H., & Anda, R. F. (2003). Adverse childhood experiences and self-reported liver disease: New insights into the causal pathway. *Archives of Internal Medicine, 163*(16), 1949–1956.

Dowlati, Y., Herrmann, N., Swardfager, W., Liu, H., Sham, L., Reim, E. K., & Lanctôt, K. L. (2010). A meta-analysis of cytokines in major depression. *Biological Psychiatry, 67*(5), 446–457.

Druss, B. G., & Walker, E. R. (2011). Mental disorders and medical comorbidity. *Robert Wood Johnson Foundation Synthesis Project: Research Synthesis Report* (21), 1–26.

Duman, R. S. (2004). Depression: a case of neuronal life and death? *Biological Psychiatry, 56*(3), 140–145.

Egede, L. E. (2006). Race, ethnicity, culture, and disparities in health care. *Journal of General Internal Medicine, 21*(6), 667–669.

Egede, L. E. (2007). Major depression in individuals with chronic medical disorders: Prevalence, correlates and association with health resource utilization, lost productivity and functional disability. *General Hospital Psychiatry, 29*(5), 409–416.

Egede, L. E., & Ellis, C. (2010). Diabetes and depression: Global perspectives. *Diabetes Research and Clinical Practice, 87*(3), 302–312.

Ehrt, U., Brønnick, K., Leentjens, A. F. G., Larsen, J. P., & Aarsland, D. (2006). Depressive symptom profile in Parkinson's disease: A comparison with depression in elderly patients without Parkinson's disease. *International Journal of Geriatric Psychiatry, 21*(3), 252–258.

Eisner, M. D., Katz, P. P., Lactao, G., & Iribarren, C. (2005). Impact of depressive symptoms on adult asthma outcomes. *Annals of Allergy, Asthma and Immunology, 94*(5), 566–574.

Engel, G. L. (1980). The clinical application of the biopsychosocial model. *American Journal of Psychiatry, 137*(5), 535–544.

Evans, D. L., Charney, D. S., Lewis, L., Golden, R. N., Gorman, J. M., Krishnan, K. R. R., et al. (2005). Mood disorders in the medically ill: Scientific review and recommendations. *Biological Psychiatry, 58*(3), 175–189.

Evans-Campbell, T. (2008). Historical trauma in American Indian/Native Alaska communities: A multilevel framework for exploring impacts on individuals, families, and communities. *Journal of Interpersonal Violence, 23*(3), 316–338.

Everson, S. A., Maty, S. C., Lynch, J. W., Kaplan, G. A. (2002). Epidemiologic evidence for the relation between socioeconomic status and depression, obesity, and diabetes. *Journal of Psychosomatic Research, 53* (4), 891–895.

Fava, M. (2005). Identifying and managing depression in the medical patient. *Primary Care Companion to the Journal of Clinical Psychiatry, 7*(6), 282–295.

Felitti, V. J., Anda, R. F., Nordenberg, D., Williamson, D. F., Spitz, A. M., Edwards, V., et al. (1998). Relationship of childhood abuse and household dysfunction to many of the leading causes of death in adults: The Adverse Childhood Experiences (ACE) Study. *American Journal of Preventive Medicine, 14*(4), 245–258.

Fiest, K. M., Dykeman, J., Patten, S. B., Wiebe, S., Kaplan, G. G., Maxwell, C. J., et al. (2013). Depression in epilepsy a systematic review and meta-analysis. *Neurology, 80*(6), 590–599.

Fiscella, K., & Williams, D. R. (2004). Health disparities based on socioeconomic inequities: Implications for urban health care. *Academic Medicine, 79*(12), 1139–1147.

Fiske, A., Wetherell, J. L., & Gatz, M. (2009). Depression in older adults. *Annual Review of Clinical Psychology, 5*(1), 363–389.

Forstein, M., Cournos, F., Douaihy, A., Goodkin, K., Wainberg, M., & Wapenyi, K. (2006). *Guideline Watch: Practice guideline for the treatment of patients with HIV/AIDS.* Washington, DC: American Psychiatric Association.

Foster, J. A., & Neufeld, K. A. M. (2013). Gut–brain axis: How the microbiome influences anxiety and depression. *Trends in Neurosciences, 36*(5), 305–312.

Gallo, L. C., Bogart, L. M., Vranceanu, A. M., & Matthews, K. A. (2005). Socioeconomic status, resources, psychological experiences, and emotional responses: A test of the reserve capacity model. *Journal of Personality and Social Psychology, 88*(2), 386.

Gallo, L. C., & Matthews, K. A. (2003). Understanding the association between socioeconomic status and physical health: Do negative emotions play a role? *Psychological Bulletin, 129*(1), 10–51.

Gareau, M. G., Jury, J., MacQueen, G., Sherman, P. M., Perdue, M. H. (2007). Probiotic treatment of rat pups normalises corticosterone release and ameliorates colonic dysfunction induced by maternal separation. *Gut, 56,* 1522–1528.

Gold, P. W. (2015). The organization of the stress system and its dysregulation in depressive illness. *Molecular Psychiatry, 20*(1), 32.

Goldney, R. D., Ruffin R., Fisher, L. J., & Wilson, D. H. (2003). Asthma symptoms associated with depression and lower quality of life: A population survey. *Medical Journal of Australia, 178*(9):437–441.

Gone, J. P. (2013). Redressing First Nations historical trauma: Theorizing mechanisms for indigenous culture as mental health treatment. *Transcultural Psychiatry, 50*(5), 683–706.

Gonzalez, J. S., Batchelder, A. W., Psaros, C., & Safren, S. A. (2011). Depression and HIV/AIDS treatment nonadherence: A review and meta-analysis. *Journal of Acquired Immune Deficiency Syndromes, 58*(2), 181–187.

Gragnoli, C. (2014). Hypothesis of the neuroendocrine cortisol pathway gene role in the comorbidity of depression, type 2 diabetes, and metabolic syndrome. *Application of Clinical Genetics, 7,* 43–53.

Gross, R., & Malaspina, D. (2015). Differential associations between depression, risk factors for insulin resistance and diabetes incidence in a large US sample. *Israel Journal of Psychiatry and Related Sciences, 52*(2), 85.

Guck, T. P., Elsasser, G. N., Kavan, M. G., & Eugene, J. E. J. (2003). Depression and congestive heart failure. *Congestive Heart Failure, 9*(3), 163–169.

Hackett, M. L., & Pickles, K. (2014). Part I: Frequency of depression after stroke: An updated systematic review and meta-analysis of observational studies. *International Journal of Stroke, 9*(8), 1017–1025.

Hanania, N. A., Müllerova, H., Locantore, N. W., Vestbo, J., Watkins, M. L., Wouters, E. F., et al. (2011). Determinants of depression in the ECLIPSE chronic obstructive pulmonary disease cohort. *American Journal of Respiratory and Critical Care Medicine, 183*(5), 604–611.

Hare, D. L., Toukhsati, S. R., Johansson, P., & Jaarsma, T. (2014). Depression and cardiovascular disease: A clinical review. *European Heart Journal, 35,* 1365–1372.

Hatch, S. L., & Dohrenwend, B. P. (2007). Distribution of traumatic and other stressful life events by race/ethnicity, gender, SES and age: A review of the research. *American Journal of Community Psychology, 40*(3–4), 313–332.

Hayward, C. (1995). Psychiatric illness and cardiovascular risk. *Epidemiological Reviews, 17*(1), 129–138.

Heijtz, R. D., Wang, S., Anuar, F., Qian, Y., Björkholm, B., Samuelsson, A., et al. (2011). Normal gut microbiota modulates brain development and behavior. *Proceedings of the National Academy of Sciences, 108*(7), 3047–3052.

Hill, J. S., Lau, M. Y., & Wing Sue, D. (2010). Integrating trauma psychology and cultural psychology: Indigenous perspectives on theory, research, and practice. *Traumatology, 16*(4), 39–47.

Hirschfeld, R. M. (2014). Differential diagnosis of bipolar disorder and major depressive disorder. *Journal of Affective Disorders, 169,* S12–S16.

Hirschfeld, R. M., Lewis, L., & Vornik, L. A. (2003). Perceptions and impact of bipolar disorder: How far have we really come?: Results of the National Depressive and Manic-Depressive Association 2000 survey of individuals with bipolar disorder. *Journal of Clinical Psychiatry, 64*(2), 161–174.

Hoyo-Becerra, C., Schlaak, J. F., & Hermann, D. M. (2014). Insights from interferon-?-related depression for the pathogenesis of depression associated with inflammation. *Brain, Behavior, and Immunity, 42,* 222–231.

Janssen, I., Hanssen, M., Bak, M. L. F. J., Bijl, R. V., De Graaf, R., Vollebergh, W., et al. (2003). Discrimination and delusional ideation. *British Journal of Psychiatry, 182*(1), 71–76.

Jehi, L., Tesar, G., Obuchowski, N., Novak, E., & Najm, I. (2011). Quality of life in 1931 adult patients with epilepsy: Seizures do not tell the whole story. *Epilepsy and Behavior, 22*(4), 723–727.

Jha, P. K., Challet, E., & Kalsbeek, A. (2015). Circadian rhythms in glucose and lipid metabolism in nocturnal and diurnal mammals. *Molecular and Cellular Endocrinology, 418,* 74–88.

Kanner, A. M. (2003). Depression in epilepsy: Prevalence, clinical semiology, pathogenic mechanisms, and treatment. *Biological Psychiatry, 54*(3), 388–398.

Karlsen, S., & Nazroo, J. Y. (2002). Relation between racial discrimination, social class, and health among ethnic minority groups. *American Journal of Public Health, 92*(4), 624–631.

Katon, W. J. (2003). Clinical and health services relationships between major depression, depressive symptoms, and general medical illness. *Biological Psychiatry, 54*(3), 216–226.

Katon, W. J. (2011). Epidemiology and treatment of depression in patients with chronic medical illness. *Dialogues in Clinical Neuroscience, 13*. Retrieved from *www.dialogues-cns.org.*

Katon, W. J., & Ciechanowski, P. (2002). Impact of major depression on chronic medical illness. *Journal of Psychosomatic Research, 53*(4), 859–863.

Katon, W., Lin, E. H., & Kroenke, K. (2007). The association of depression and anxiety with medical symptom burden in patients with chronic medical illness. *General Hospital Psychiatry, 29*(2), 147–155.

Kirmayer, L. J., Gone, J. P., & Moses, J. (2014). Rethinking historical trauma. *Transcultural Psychiatry, 51*(3), 299–319.

Kochanek, K. D., Murphy, S. L., Xu, J., & Arias, E. (2014). Mortality in the United States, 2013. *NCHS Data Brief, 178,* 1–8.

Krishnan, K. R. R. (2002). Biological risk factors in late life depression. *Biological Psychiatry, 52*(3), 185–192.

Krishnan, V., & Nestler, E. J. (2008). The molecular neurobiology of depression. *Nature, 455,* 894–902.

Kudlow, P. A., Cha, D. S., Lam, R. W., & McIntyre, R. S. (2013). Sleep architecture variation: A mediator of metabolic disturbance in individuals with major depressive disorder. *Sleep Medicine, 14*(10), 943–949.

Kurdyak, P. A., Manno, M., Gomes, T., Mamdani, M. M., & Juurlink, D. N. (2012). Antidepressants, metoprolol and the risk of bradycardia. *Therapeutic Advances in Psychopharmacology, 2*(2), 43–49.

Kwiatkowska, B., Kłak, A., Maślińska, M., Mańczak, M., & Raciborski, F. (2018). Factors of depression among patients with rheumatoid arthritis. *Reumatologia, 56*(4), 219–227.

Laermans, J., & Depoortere, I. (2016). Chronobesity: Role of the circadian system in the obesity epidemic. *Obesity Reviews, 17*(2), 108–125.

Lai, H. M. X., Cleary, M., Sitharthan, T., & Hunt, G. E. (2015). Prevalence of comorbid substance use, anxiety and mood disorders in epidemiological surveys, 1990–2014: A systematic review and meta-analysis. *Drug and Alcohol Dependence, 154,* 1–13.

Lantz, P. M., House, J. S., Mero, R. P., Williams, D. R. (2005). Stress, life events, and socioeconomic disparities in health: Results from the Americans' Changing Lives Study. *Journal of Health and Social Behavior, 46,* 274–288.

Larsen, K. K. (2013). Depression following myocardial infarction. *Danish Medical Journal, 60*(7), B4689.

Li, C., Xu, D., Hu, M., Tan, Y., Zhang, P., Li, G., & Chen, L. (2017). A systematic review and meta-analysis of randomized controlled trials of cognitive behavior therapy for patients with diabetes and depression. *Journal of Psychosomatic Research, 95,* 44–54.

Lichtman, J. H., Bigger, J. T., Blumenthal, J. A., Frasure-Smith, N., Kaufmann, P. G., Lespérance, F., et al. (2008). Depression and coronary heart disease: Recommendations for screening, referral, and treatment. *Circulation, 118*(17), 1768–1775.

Loftis, J. M., & Hauser, P. (2004). The phenomenology and treatment of interferon-induced depression. *Journal of Affective Disorders, 82*(2), 175–190.

Lynch, J. W., Kaplan, G. A., Cohen, R. D., Tuomilehto, J., & Salonen, J. T. (1996). Do cardiovascular risk factors explain the relation between socioeconomic status, risk of all-cause mortality, cardiovascular mortality, and acute myocardial infarction? *American Journal of Epidemiology, 144*(10), 934–942.

Machado, M. O., Oriolo, G., Bortolato, B., Köhler, C. A., Maes, M., Solmi, M., et al. (2017). Biological mechanisms of depression following treatment with interferon for chronic hepatitis C: A critical systematic review. *Journal of Affective Disorders, 209,* 235–245.

Manson, J. E., Stampfer, M. J., Colditz, G. A., Willett, W. C., Rosner, B., Hennekens, C. H., et al. (1991). Physical activity and incidence of non-insulin-dependent diabetes mellitus in women. *Lancet, 338*(8770), 774–778.

Marrie, R. A. (2016). Comorbidity in multiple sclerosis: Some answers, more questions. *International Journal of MS Care, 18*(6), 271–272.

Matcham, F., Rayner, L., Steer, S., & Hotopf, M. (2013). The prevalence of depression in rheumatoid arthritis: A systematic review and meta-analysis. *Rheumatology (Oxford, England), 52*(12), 2136–2148

Mathew, A. R., Hogarth, L., Leventhal, A. M., Cook, J. W., & Hitsman, B. (2017). Cigarette smoking and depression comorbidity: Systematic review and proposed theoretical model. *Addiction, 112*(3), 401–412.

Matthews, K. A., & Gallo, L. C. (2011). Psychological perspectives on pathways linking socioeconomic status and physical health. *Annual Review of Psychology, 62,* 501–530.

Matthews, K. A., Gallo L. C., & Taylor S. E. (2010). Are psychosocial factors mediators of socioeconomic status and health connections?: A progress report and blueprint for the future. *Annals of the New York Academy of Sciences, 1186,* 146–173.

Mezuk, B., Eaton, W. W., Albrecht, S., & Golden, S. H. (2008). Depression and type 2 diabetes over the lifespan: A meta-analysis. *Diabetes Care, 31*(12), 2383–2390.

Mohatt, N. V., Thompson, A. B., Thai, N. D., & Tebes, J. K. (2014). Historical trauma as public narrative: A conceptual review of how history impacts present-day health. *Social Science and Medicine, 106,* 128–136.

Moulton, C. D., Pickup, J. C., & Ismail, K. (2015). The link between depression and diabetes: The search for shared mechanisms. *Lancet: Diabetes and Endocrinology, 3*(6), 461–471.

Müller, N. (2013). The role of anti-inflammatory treatment in psychiatric disorders. *Psychiatria Danubina, 25*(3), 292–298.

Nanni, M. G., Caruso, R., Mitchell, A. J., Meggiolaro, E., & Grassi, L. (2015). Depression in HIV infected patients: A review. *Current Psychiatry Reports, 17*(1), 530.

Nefs, G., Pop, V. J., Denollet, J., & Pouwer, F. (2016). Depressive symptoms and all-cause mortality in people with type 2 diabetes: A focus on potential mechanisms. *British Journal of Psychiatry, 209*(2), 142–149.

Nemeroff, C. B., Musselman, D. L., & Evans, D. L. (1998). Depression and cardiac disease. *Depression and Anxiety, 8,* 71–79.

Nouwen, A., Winkley, K., Twisk, J. et al. (2010). Type 2 diabetes mellitus as a risk factor for the onset of depression: A systematic review and meta-analysis. *Diabetologia, 53,* 2480.

Olin, J. T., Schneider, L. S., Katz, I. R., Meyers, B. S., Alexopoulos, G. S., Breitner, J. C., et al. (2002). Provisional diagnostic criteria for depression of Alzheimer disease. *American Journal of Geriatric Psychiatry, 10*(2), 125–128.

Pan, A., Lucas, M., Sun, Q., van Dam, R. M., Franco, O. H., Manson, J. E., et al. (2010). Bidirectional association between depression and type 2 diabetes mellitus in women. *Archives of Internal Medicine, 170*(21), 1884–1891.

Paradiso, S., Vaidya, J., Tranel, D., Kosier, T., & Robinson, R. (2008). Nondysphoric depression following stroke. *Journal of Neuropsychiatry and Clinical Neurosciences, 20*(1), 52–61.

Park, J. H., Lee, S. B., Lee, T. J., Lee, D. Y., Jhoo, J. H., Youn, J. C., et al. (2007). Depression in vascular dementia is quantitatively and qualitatively different from depression in Alzheimer's disease. *Dementia and Geriatric Cognitive Disorders, 23*(2), 67–73.

Patten, S. B., Williams, J. V. A., Lavorato, D. H., Modgill, G., Jetté, N., & Eliasziw, M. (2008). Major depression as a risk factor for chronic disease incidence: Longitudinal analyses in a general population cohort. *General Hospital Psychiatry, 30*(5), 407–413.

Pence, B. W., O'Donnell, J. K., & Gaynes, B. N. (2012). Falling through the cracks: The gaps between depression prevalence, diagnosis, treatment, and response in HIV care. *AIDS, 26*(5), 656–658.

Poole, J. C., Dobson, K. S., & Pusch, D. (2017). Childhood adversity and adult depression: The protective role of psychological resilience. *Child Abuse and Neglect, 64,* 89–100.

Pumar, M. I., Gray, C. R., Walsh, J. R., Yang, I. A., Rolls, T. A., & Ward, D. L. (2014). Anxiety and depression—Important psychological comorbidities of COPD. *Journal of Thoracic Disease, 6*(11), 1615–1631.

Ramiro, L. S., Madrid, B. J., & Brown, D. W. (2010). Adverse childhood experiences (ACE) and health-risk behaviors among adults in a developing country setting. *Child Abuse and Neglect, 34*(11), 842–855.

Ribeiro, A. I., Fraga, S., Costa, L., McCroy, C., & Barros, H. (2018). Socioeconomic inequalities in health during early childhood: Evidence from a birth cohort. *Journal of Epidemiology and Community Health, 66,* 354–355.

Rieder, R., Wisniewski, P. J., Alderman, B. L., & Campbell, S. C. (2017). Microbes and mental health: A review. *Brain, Behavior, and Immunity, 66,* 9–17.

Roy, T., & Lloyd, C. E. (2012). Epidemiology of depression and diabetes: A systematic review. *Journal of Affective Disorders, 142,* S8–S21.

Rustad, J. K., Musselman, D. L., & Nemeroff, C. B. (2011). The relationship of depression and diabetes: Pathophysiological and treatment implications. *Psychoneuroendocrinology, 36*(9), 1276–1286.

Sawada, N., Uchida, H., Suzuki, T., Watanabe, K., Kikuchi, T., Handa, T., et al. (2009). Persistence and compliance to antidepressant treatment in patients with depression: A chart review. *BMC Psychiatry, 9*(1), 38.

Scherrer, J. F., Xian, H., Lustman, P. J., Franz, C. E., McCaffery, J., Lyons, M. J., et al. (2011). A test for common genetic and environmental vulnerability to depression and diabetes. *Twin Research and Human Genetics, 14*(2), 169–172.

Schuch, F., Vancampfort, D., Firth, J., Rosenbaum, S., Ward, P., Reichert, T., et al. (2017). Physical activity and sedentary behavior in people with major depressive disorder: A systematic review and meta-analysis. *Journal of Affective Disorders, 210,* 139–150.

Siegert, R. J., & Abernethy, D. A. (2005). Depression in multiple sclerosis: A review. *Journal of Neurology, Neurosurgery and Psychiatry, 76*(4), 469–475.

Smith, D., & Ghaemi, S. (2006). Hypomania in clinical practice. *Advances in Psychiatric Treatment, 12*(2). 110–120.

Smith, J. P. (2004). Unraveling the SES: health connection. *Population and Development Review, 30,* 108–132.

Spring, B., Moller, A. C., & Coons, M. J. (2012). Multiple health behaviours: Overview and implications. *Journal of Public Health, 34,* i3–i10.

Springer, K. W., Sheridan, J., Kuo, D., & Carnes, M. (2003). The long-term health outcomes of childhood abuse. *Journal of General Internal Medicine, 18*(10), 864–870.

Talbot, F., Nouwen, A., Gingras, J., Bélanger, A., & Audet, J. (1999). Relations of diabetes intrusiveness and personal control to symptoms of depression among adults with diabetes. *Health Psychology, 18*(5), 537–542.

van den Bemt, L., Schermer, T., Bor, H., Smink, R., van Weel-Baumgarten, E., Lucassen, P., et al. (2009). The risk for depression comorbidity in patients with COPD. *Chest, 135*(1), 108–114.

Van Meter, A. R., Youngstrom, E. A., & Findling, R. L. (2012). Cyclothymic disorder: A critical review. *Clinical Psychology Review, 32,* 229–243.

Wade, R., Jr., Cronholm, P. F., Fein, J. A., Forke, C. M., Davis, M. B., Harkins-Schwarz, M., et al. (2016). Household and community-level adverse childhood experiences and adult health outcomes in a diverse urban population. *Child Abuse and Neglect, 52,* 135–145.

Wang, Y., & Kasper, L. H. (2014). The role of microbiome in central nervous system disorders. *Brain, Behavior, and Immunity, 38,* 1–12.

Whooley, M. A., Caska, C. M., Hendrickson, B. E., Rourke, M. A., Ho, J., & Ali, S. (2007). Depression and inflammation in patients with coronary heart disease: Findings from the Heart and Soul Study. *Biological Psychiatry, 62*(4), 314–320.

Williams, D. R., Priest, N., & Anderson, N. B. (2016). Understanding associations among race, socioeconomic status, and health: Patterns and prospects. *Health Psychology, 35*(4), 407–411.

Wu, L., & Blazer, D. (2014). Substance use disorders and psychiatric comorbidity in mid- and later life: A review. *International Journal of Epidemiology, 43*(2), 304–317.

Young, J. J., Bruno, D., & Pomara, N. (2014). A review of the relationship between proinflammatory cytokines and major depressive disorder. *Journal of Affective Disorders, 169,* 15–20.

Yousaf, O., Grunfeld, E. A., & Hunter, M. S. (2015). A systematic review of the factors associated with delays in medical and psychological help-seeking among men. *Health Psychology Review, 9*(2), 264–276.

Youssef, N. A., Belew, D., Hao, G., Wang, X., Treiber, F. A., Stefanek, M., et al. (2017). Racial/ethnic differences in the association of childhood adversities with depression and the role of resilience. *Journal of Affective Disorders, 208,* 577–581.

Yu, M., Zhang, X., Lu, F., & Fang, L. (2015). Depression and risk for diabetes: A meta-analysis. *Canadian Journal of Diabetes, 39*(4), 266–272.

Zaki, N. F., Spence, D. W., BaHammam, A. S., Pandi-Perumal, S. R., Cardinali, D. P., & Brown, G. M. (2018). Chronobiological theories of mood disorder. *European Archives of Psychiatry and Clinical Neuroscience, 268*(2), 107–118.

PART II

NEUROPSYCHOLOGICAL DOMAINS

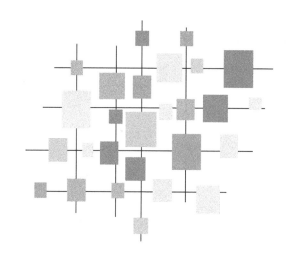

CHAPTER 6

The Role of Cognitive Reserve in Depression

Sonya Dhillon
Konstantine K. Zakzanis

Patients with major depressive disorder (MDD) can demonstrate cognitive impairments that vary in severity and resultant impediment or disablement in terms of instrumental activities of daily living (Gomez et al., 2006; Landro, Stiles, & Sletvold, 2001; Schatzberg, 2002; Shenal, Harrison, & Demaree, 2003; Zakzanis, Leach, & Kaplan, 1998). Cognitive impairments that characterize the disorder can include reduced component aspects of executive functions (Harvey et al., 2004), slowed processing speed (Nebes et al., 2000), reduced verbal fluency (Zakzanis et al., 1998), inattention (Kampf-Sherf et al., 2004), and difficulties in component memory processes such as learning and retrieval (Iverson, Brooks, Langenecker, & Young, 2011).

While neuropsychological testing can elucidate the cognitive profile of any given individual with MDD, there currently exists no MDD-specific neuropsychological signature. Indeed, the published literature is inconsistent regarding what cognitive domains are reliably impacted by the illness (see McClintock, Husain, Greer, & Cullum, 2010). One explanation for this inconsistency might relate to the heterogeneity of research methods employed across studies. For example, there is considerable variability regarding between- and within-sample characteristics across studies. Such variability can include whether patients are acutely depressed or are in remission, are medicated or not medicated, or have comorbid illnesses. Moreover, depressive symptom presentation in patients meeting formal DSM-5 diagnostic criteria (see Salem, Soares, & Selvaraj, Chapter 1, this volume, regarding DSM-5 criteria for MDD) can present with complete nonoverlap in depressive symptoms, while the severity of same can also vary considerably (Chen, Eaton, Gallo, & Nestadt, 2000; Merikangas, Wicki, & Angst, 1994). Also, the moderating roles of motivation, effort (Cohen, Weingartner, Smallberg, Pickar, & Murphy, 1982), and response bias (see Boone, 2007) are important to underscore in the neuropsychology of depression, as patients are prone to present with motivational difficulties coupled with cognitive bias that inherently may contribute to neuropsychological test score variability. Indeed, the relationship between cognitive bias and neuropsychological presentation is itself an area of important study but is beyond the scope of this chapter (see Dhillon, Videla-Nash, Foussias, Segal, & Zakzanis, 2020).

While various candidate factors beyond those described above have been understood to drive cognitive inefficiency and impairment in the context of MDD, a relatively unexplored and potentially contributing factor is that of cognitive reserve. In this chapter, we examine the cognitive reserve hypothesis and identify how this construct may relate to, and operate in relation to, depression and related disorders and their neuropsychological presentation.

THE COGNITIVE RESERVE HYPOTHESIS

Cognitive reserve was first described by Stern, Alexander, Prohovnik, and Mayeux (1992) and later operationalized (Stern, 2002) in the context of Alzheimer's disease (AD). Stern (2002) explained that there were individual differences in the information-processing speed of cognitive and/or functional tasks. Here, we describe the active model of non-orgranic brain reserve. Individuals with higher or a larger cognitive reserve have been found to experience fewer consequences as a result of brain injury or disease (Colangeli et al., 2016). While "brain reserve" relates to the actual physical differences in neurological structure or function, or "hardware," cognitive reserve can be regarded as the "software" (see Figure 6.1).

To this end, rather than suggesting that there are anatomical differences in the brain that contribute to differences in functional abilities that follow neurological disease or injury, the cognitive reserve hypothesis posits that the processing of cognitive tasks can vary in terms of efficiency from one individual to another (Stern, 2002). Baseline or rather, "innate" long-standing intellectual ability (IQ), and life experiences may serve as a protective and/or compensatory mechanism for brain injury or disease.

Accordingly, the cognitive reserve hypothesis has helped to explain the contributory role that higher intelligence, education, and occupational attainment play in terms of functional preservation in the context of neuropathological alterations. That is, patients may have the same brain reserve (e.g., cerebral volume) but experience different functional outcomes based on their cognitive reserve. As such, a reduced cognitive reserve can result

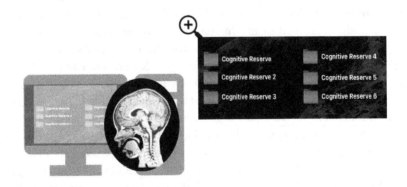

FIGURE 6.1. Conceptual representation of brain reserve and cognitive reserve.

in greater functional decline; although it is noteworthy that emerging research has identified the contribution of "functional reserve" in this context as a construct that may delay and/or slow functional decline and maintain functional independence in the context of cognitive impairment.

The concept of cognitive reserve has been examined in the extant literature with an emphasis on clinical populations with neurological pathologies and presentations. For example, the cognitive reserve hypothesis in the context of AD and AD-related pathology has been extensively studied (Querbes et al., 2009; Scarmeas & Stern, 2004; Stern, 2012). AD pathology affords researchers the opportunity to study neurodegenerative disease progression over time in the context of reliable pathology and expected cortical and subcortical atrophy (e.g., temporal–parietal atrophy). The observed effects of age, education, and occupational attainment on functional outcomes have been reliably replicated in AD (Paradise, Cooper, & Livingston, 2009; Roe, Xiong, Miller, & Morris, 2007; Stern, 2012; Tucker & Stern, 2011). Moreover, cognitive reserve has been shown to serve as a protective and compensatory factor in this illness.

The cognitive reserve hypothesis has also been examined in a host of other conditions such as HIV (Foley et al., 2012; Shapiro, Mahoney, Peyser, Zingman, & Verghese, 2014; Stern, Silva, Chaisson, & Evans, 1996), multiple sclerosis (Booth et al., 2013; Schwartz, Snook, Quaranto, Benedict, & Vollmer, 2013; Sumowski & Leavitt, 2013), stroke (Nunnari, Bramanti, & Marino, 2014; Willis & Hakim, 2013), and traumatic brain injury (TBI; Levi, Rassovsky, Agranov, Sela-Kaufman, & Vakil, 2013) as well as normal aging (Solé-Padullés et al., 2009; Tucker & Stern, 2011). Collectively, such research has supported the concept of cognitive reserve. For example, a study that examined cognitive and brain reserve in a sample with TBI found that IQ, years of education, and brain volume were related to cognitive deficits regardless of injury severity (Kesler, Adams, Blasey, & Bigler, 2003). The study used the American College Testing (ACT) scores (or equivalent) as their preinjury IQ estimate and as a purportedly more valid estimate of the IQ cognitive domain relative to years of education alone. The brain volume metrics that were used were generally resistant to atrophy (e.g., total intracranial value). The results illustrated that both cognitive and brain reserve were associated with the magnitude of cognitive deficits.

In other studies, cognitive reserve has been found to be a moderating factor in postconcussive syndrome in children, regardless of injury severity (Fey et al., 2010); it has been found to be a robust and independent predictor of disability-free recovery one year postmoderate and severe TBI (Schneider et al., 2014). Collectively, evidence strongly supports the cognitive reserve hypothesis in various neuropsychiatric conditions, and it may serve as a protective, compensatory, or combined protective and compensatory factor.

THE PROBLEM WITH EDUCATION AS AN INDEX OF COGNITIVE RESERVE

In general, most studies have indirectly examined cognitive reserve through assessment of proxies such as years of education. Fewer studies have used purportedly more valid indicators of cognitive reserve in combination, such as premorbid IQ (e.g., vocabulary tests, word reading tests). Using educational attainment as a proxy measure of cognitive reserve may underrepresent the construct of reserve and may only be a subcomponent of a larger construct. For instance, studies have demonstrated that years of education are associated with help-seeking behaviors, health promotion behaviors, and so on, and may moderate recovery by way of these pro-cognitive health behaviors rather than reserve per se (Jackson-Triche et al., 2000). In the case of depression, this can lead to proactive behaviors that include seeking psychological services, access to pharmaceutical treatment, increased exercise and nutrition, and availability of information that may not be available to those with lower education.

Educational attainment is influenced by numerous factors (e.g., socioeconomic status, financial status, parental education) that do not necessarily converge on an individual's innate 'intelligence' or cognitive ability. It may very well be that IQ estimates, by way of standardized tests, are more useful metrics for documenting cognitive reserve rather than only the use of educational attainment (see Satz et al., 1993). Ideally, cognitive reserve can be defined as a latent construct with indicator variables that include IQ (Koenen et al., 2009), educational and occupational attainment (Murray et al., 2011), and engagement in recreational activities (Scarmeas & Stern, 2004; see Fratiglioni & Wang, 2007, for a review). Moreover, less attention has been paid to the examination of cognitive reserve as the ability to adapt one's performance for task demands, a potentially valid index of cognitive reserve (Yang, Krampe, & Baltes, 2006) that is in line with Stern's (2002) original cognitive reserve hypothesis.

CAN THE HETEROGENEITY OF COGNITIVE INEFFICIENCY AND IMPAIRMENT IN DEPRESSION BE ASCRIBED TO COGNITIVE RESERVE?

Stern (2002) described cognitive reserve as consisting of two main components. The first component infers that cognitive functioning can be robust and resilient against brain pathology; that is a protective factor. In the context of depression, neurological pathology has yet to be reliably determined in terms of a candidate marker, and as such, depression is not an obvious candidate for the cognitive reserve hypothesis. On the other hand, psychopathology can be identified based on constellations of depressive symptoms and diagnostic reliability and validity, as is the case with MDD diagnostic criteria in the fifth edition of the *Diagnostic and Statistical Manual of Mental Disorders* (DSM-5; American Psychiatric Association, 2013). Functional neuroanatomical regions are implicated in depression, the most consistently involved regions being the anterior cingulate cortex and the dorsolateral prefrontal cortex. These prefrontal brain regions are associated with various cognitive domains, including executive functions and social cognition (for a review, see Rogers et al., 2004). As such, cognitive reserve may be applicable to depression and serve to protect against depression-induced pathology.

Stern's second component of the cognitive reserve hypothesis is related to one's ability to use alternative functions when another function is compromised (i.e., make use of compensatory mechanisms and strategies); that is a compensatory factor. Cognitive reserve is distinguishable from compensation of the brain and one's behavior observed in response to brain damage (Tucker & Stern, 2012). Cognitive reserve has also been shown to be involved in the preservation of functioning and cognition in normal aging as well as a variation that is observed in normal aging. As such, it may apply to conditions that have no confirmed organicity such as depression and related psychiatric disorders. Here, the rationale and application of cognitive reserve to depression are plausible, as the functional impairments observed in depression exist on a spectrum that ranges from intact instrumental activities of daily living to profound disability (see American Psychiatric Association, 2013). Accordingly, the cognitive reserve hypothesis may help explain the prevalence of cognitive impairment, and varied functional impairment that is observed across depressive disorders. Furthermore, engaging in compensatory strategies in response to inefficiency and impairment in one (or more) cognitive domains may also be a product of motivation and effort, which are cognitive processes that can be profoundly impacted by depression and related pathologies.

While clinical research efforts to understand cognitive reserve have focused on neurological conditions, the cognitive reserve hypothesis may also be applicable to psychiatric conditions. Collectively, functional neuroanatomical evidence and the markedly variable presentation of cognitive impairments and functional outcome in depression demonstrate that investigating the cognitive reserve hypothesis in depression is warranted (Dhillon et al., 2020; Ebmeier, Rose, & Steele, 2006)

DEPRESSION AND THE COGNITIVE RESERVE HYPOTHESIS

To date, no systematic reviews or meta-analyses have examined the cognitive reserve hypothesis in the context of depression. However, a few empirical studies do exist. In particular, as with many psychiatric conditions, there are challenges in elucidating the cause-and-effect relationship between cognitive impairments and depression. While DSM-5 deleniates diagnostic criteria for the disorder that includes both psychological symptoms and cognitive disturbance (e.g., decreased concentration, unable to make decisions), it is unclear whether the cognitive disturbance is a precursor, vulnerability factor, or consequence of the disorder itself. For example, although scientists have collected significant and replicable evidence of neuropsychological dysfunction related to schizophrenia (American Psychiatric Association, 2013; Heinrichs & Zakzanis, 1998), the cause and effect of this relationship has yet to be elucidated (see Bilder et al., 2000), which poses a challenge for both clinicians and researchers. Without longitudinal, population-based studies with baseline examinations of cognitive functioning before the onset of a major depressive episode, the temporal relationship of cognitive impairment cannot be determined at this time.

What can be addressed is the degree of influence that factors related to cognitive reserve (i.e., education, IQ, occupational achievement) have on individuals with depression and how such factors impact activities of daily living (i.e., functional outcomes). As of 2018, only three studies had specifically addressed depression and the cognitive reserve hypothesis. Across studies, it appeared evident there existed no equivocal estimate or proxy of cognitive reserve, nor had a specific metric been identified as the most appropriate for depression. Some studies utilized crude metrics of cognitive reserve, such as occupation and years of education, whereas other studies investigated latent constructs of cognitive reserve with indicators that included IQ, recreational activities, and performance on cognitive flexibility measures (see Stern, 2009). While no consensus has been reached as to what is the best metric or what the incremental utility of these variables is in the context of depression, researchers have investigated different proxies of cognitive reserve in depression. To help elucidate the properties of depression-related cognitive reserve, these studies are reviewed in the following sections.

EDUCATION, SUBCLINICAL DEPRESSION, AND COGNITIVE OUTCOMES

McLaren, Szymkowicz, Kirton, and Dotson (2015) examined the effect of education on memory in a sample of participants with subclinical depression. Notably, studies have shown that cognitive deficits are observed in populations with subthreshold depression (see, e.g., in older adults, Dotson, Resnick & Zondermon, 2008; Elderkin-Thomson et al., 2003)—that is, in populations that experience depressive symptoms without meeting diagnostic criteria for MDD. Here, higher depressive symptom severity was associated with poorer neuropsychological test performance for individuals with less years of education. In contrast, cognitive performance was preserved for individuals with higher years of education and higher depressive symptom severity. Specifically, this interaction effect of depression severity and level of education was significant for performance on tests of verbal memory (e.g., Hopkins Verbal Learning Test—Revised; Brandt, 1991) but not for tests of executive functions (e.g., Stroop Color and Word Test [Golden, 1978]; Trail Making Test Part B [Reitan, 1958]) and processing speed (Trail Making Test Part A [Reitan, 1958]). These results are consistent with previous studies reviewed in that proxies of cognitive reserve may serve as protective factors in depression, attenuating the influence of the disorder on cognitive abilities, and in turn buffer against functional consequences.

PREMORBID IQ, MAJOR DEPRESSIVE DISORDER, AND COGNITIVE OUTCOMES

In 2018, researchers sought to tackle the confounds in studying cognitive impairment in depression,and proposed that cognitive reserve may mitigate variable cognitive impairments. Venezia and colleagues (2018) share our position that the heterogeneity of study samples with regard to diagnostic thresholds, medications, and comorbidities may account for the variance observed in cognitive impairments. Yet, cognitive reserve may be a factor that accounts for this variance that has yet to be empirically investigated. In the study by Venezia and colleages, psychiatric diagnosis was confirmed with the Structured Clinical Interview for DSM-IV (First & Gibbon, 2004), and comparisons across measures were made to a healthy volunteer sample. All participants completed a neuropsychological test battery that examined domains commonly implicated in depression (processing speed, interference processing, memory, and executive functions; McClintock et al., 2010; Zakzanis et al., 1998). Estimates of premorbid IQ were derived from the Wechsler Adult Intelligence Scale—3rd Edition (WAIS-III; Wechsler, 1997) vocabulary subtest. The participants self-reported their years of education.

The results indicated that WAIS-III vocabulary scores moderated differences in processing speed and executive functions between the MDD and healthy groups.

Furthermore, the expression of these differences was attenuated with higher estimates of intellectual ability, or cognitive reserve. These results were consistent with previous work (McClaren et al., 2015) that demonstrated the protective effects of cognitive reserve in the context of neuropsychological inefficiency and impairment in depression. Furthermore, Venezia and colleagues (2018) found that years of education was not a significant factor when WAIS-III vocabulary scores were accounted for. This finding suggested that education level may measure some aspects of cognitive reserve but may be a weaker estimate of cognitive reserve than standardized tests of premorbid intellectual abilities.

PROXIES OF COGNITIVE RESERVE IN DEPRESSION

In another study, Coloma Andrews and Zihl (2014) evaluated cognitive reserve in depression in a different manner. Cognitive reserve was operationalized via testing the limits procedure whereby cognitive reserve was measured as an index of performance improvement on the Digit Symbol Substitution Task (DSST). Here, maximal performance improvement across testing timepoints was used as an estimate of the magnitude of cognitive reserve as based on the following formula: $CR_i = [1 + (1 + x_1/x_{\text{maxgroup}})] * [(x_i - x_1) / x_{\text{maxgroup}}]$ (Coloma Andrews & Zihl, 2014, p. 17). While most studies have used estimates of crystallized intelligence or years of education, here the authors posited that this formula was a metric of the size of an individual's cognitive reserve, as it measured a construct related to adaptation of performance (i.e., compensatory cognitive reserve). In this study, participants completed a cognitive screen (Mini-Mental Status Examination; Strub & Black 1985); 10 administrations of the German version of the DSST (Neubauer & Horn, 2006), in order to derive a metric of performance improvement and cognitive reserve; a cognitive test battery, including measures of attention, memory, and executive functions; self-report inventories that measured the "Big Five" personality traits (see McCrae & Costa, 1987, 1989); and depression symptom severity (Montgomery–Åsberg Depression Rating Scale; Davidson, Turnbull, Strickland, Miller, & Graves, 1986).

Overall, after controlling for age and years of education, the results suggested that cognitive reserve was significantly associated with attention, openness to experience, and depression severity. Interestingly, the relationship between years of education and cognitive reserve was insignificant. There were no significant differences on cognitive reserve between healthy controls and patients with depression overall. However, differences in cognitive reserve were found between controls and patients with depression with or without cognitive impairments. Here, the researchers examined differences among groups with depression with intact cognitive function, depression with cognitive impairments, and healthy controls. Relative to the healthy controls and depression with intact cognitive functions groups, the depression with cognitive impairments group had smaller cognitive reserve and poorer performance on attention measures. However, like many other studies that have examined cognitive impairments in depression, inefficiency and impairment were observed across all cognitive domains (i.e., attention, memory, executive functions) in half of the patient sample. This finding suggested that there was no pathognomic cognitive signature of depression.

Collectively, these results illustrate that a reduced cognitive reserve is associated with poorer attention and memory performance for individuals with MDD and cognitive impairments. It does not, however, support the notion that cognitive reserve is a predictive protective factor for depression.

COGNITIVE RESERVE AND DEPRESSION IN OLDER ADULTS

A further area of focus of the cognitive reserve hypothesis has been older adults (e.g., 65 years or older) with depression. In a cross-sectional study of healthy older adults, Murphy and O'Leary (2010) found that education and depressive symptoms were associated with verbal memory (e.g., word list recall). In particular, education level was positively associated with delayed recall performance, while depressive symptoms were associated with immediate recall performance. These results suggested that depression and education level had differential effects on verbal memory but did not address how education and other factors related to cognitive reserve may have impacted depression related outcomes.

Lara and colleagues (2017) published a large-scale population-based study that examined the influence of cognitive reserve on quality of life and the role that depression and disability played in that relationship. Data were collected from 1973 participants greater than 50 years of age, cross sectionally, using self-report measures of cognitive reserve (Cognitive Reserve Questionnaire; Rami et al., 2011), quality of life (WHOQOL-AGE; Caballero et al., 2013), disability (WHODAS 2.0; Üstün, Kostanjsek, Chatterji, & Rehm, 2010), and depression severity. Participants also completed a battery of cognitive tests that assessed multiple cognitive domains, including attention, verbal fluency, verbal memory, and working memory. Cross-sectional analyses were performed, and results illustrated that there was an association between cognitive reserve and quality of life and that this association was mediated by depression, cognitive function, and disability. Disability status had the strongest mediating effect in the total sample and in subgroups ages 50–64 and 65+ (β = −.45, −.43 and −.45, respectively). Specifically, the direct mediation effects of depression were insignificant in a 50- to 64-year-old age group but were significant in the 65+ group. The effects of cognitive functions and disability were significant for both groups. While this study was cross-sectional, which limited the predictability of the reported effects (see Maxwell & Cole, 2007), it suggested that cognitive reserve may have indirect quality-of-life persevering properties, particularly in older adults with presumably more cognitive deficits (Balota, Dolan, & Duchek, 2000).

COGNITIVE RESERVE AND OTHER PSYCHIATRIC DISORDERS

Broadly speaking, the cognitive reserve hypothesis has been examined, to some degree, in other psychiatric disorders. In a large-scale longitudinal study, Koenen and colleagues (2009) examined this hypothesis in a cohort study of patients with various psychiatric disorders. Here, IQ and diagnostic status were assessed across multiple timepoints and ages (up to age 32). IQ was averaged over three ages (7, 9, and 11) and examined as a potential predictive factor in developing one or more psychiatric condition(s). Overall, higher childhood IQ was associated with a 42% reduction in the odds of developing a lifetime schizophrenia disorder, a 26% reduction of an adult anxiety disorder, and 23% reduction for adult depressive disorder. On the contrary, lower childhood IQ was associated with a higher risk of psychiatric comorbidity and greater duration of major depression (i.e., recurrent or longer lasting depressive episodes). The results also suggested that higher IQ increased the risk for the development of mania, though this finding should be interpreted with caution as the sample size was small ($n = 8$). Overall, the results illustrated that childhood IQ was a protective factor against the development of depression later in life.

In a sample of patients with schizophrenia, Munro, Russell, Murray, Kerwin, and Jones (2002) found that children with higher scores on IQ scales had better functional outcomes at a 21-year follow-up. IQ scores; however, were not predictive of clinical symptoms in general. It has also been shown that patients with schizophrenia who have a higher premorbid or childhood IQ have better functional outcomes (Aylward, Walker, & Bettes, 1984). More broadly, in the schizophrenia-spectrum literature, studies have shown that those with better cognitive abilities (e.g., higher performance on neuropsychological tests) have better functional outcomes as based on return to work and work-related rehabilitation success (Bell & Bryson, 2001; Bryson et al., 1998; Gold, Goldberg, McNary, Dixon, & Lehman, 2002). Cognitive abilities have also been found to be predictive of social cognition and executive function (e.g., social decision making and problem solving; Addington & Addington, 2000). While these studies were not a direct indication of cognitive reserve per se, they underscore the importance of cognitive abilities independent of psychiatric symptoms in activities of daily living in the context of psychiatric disorder,.

Barnett, Salmond, Jones, and Sahakian (2006) suggested that cognitive reserve was a protective and diagnostic factor in psychiatric disorders and outcomes. With respect to psychiatric disorders, cognitive reserve may moderate the impact of the illness on daily social and occupational functioning, as has been the case in the AD and normal aging literature (see Stern, 2012). That is, higher education and IQ, regardless of psychiatric symptom severity, produce better outcomes for individuals. As such, there is a theoretical and empirical basis for examining the cognitive reserve hypothesis in the context of depression and related disorder.

COGNITIVE RESERVE AND DEPRESSIVE SYMPTOMS IN OTHER DISORDERS: BORROWING INSIGHTS FROM CLINICAL SAMPLES

While there are inconsistencies in research, some evidence does support the cognitive reserve hypothesis relationship with depression when insights from the TBI literature are considered (Salmond, Menon, Chatfeld, Pickard, & Sahakian, 2006). When reviewing studies of individuals with TBI, some studies have found no significant differences between patients with TBI with and without depression (Gomez-Hernandez, Max, Kosier, Paradiso, & Robinson, 1997; Groom, Shaw O'Connor, Howard, & Pickens, 1998; Hibbard et al., 2004; Holsinger et al., 2002), while other studies have found differences (Deb, Lyons, Koutzoukis, Ali, & McCarthy, 1999). Deb and colleagues (1999) found that education level was predictive of depressive symptoms postinjury, but scores on the National Adult

Reading Test (Nelson & Willison, 1991), which is a widely used measure to estimate premorbid IQ, did not find this. Although education was a significant factor associated with depressive symptoms, it is also well known that low education itself is a risk for psychiatric disorder in the general population (Lishman, 2008). Therefore, it is difficult to ascertain if cognitive reserve is implicated in all psychiatric illnesses, and if the proxy measures of cognitive reserve (such as years of education) are producing statistical artifacts.

Recently, Cadden, Guty, and Arnett (2019) examined whether two related, but different cognitive reserve proxies mediated the relationship between depression and disability in a sample of patients with multiple sclerosis (MS). The authors operationalized two types of cognitive reserve: malleable (e.g., leisure time) and fixed (e.g., years of education). The two subtypes of cognitive reserve were highly correlated but conceptually different. Although a limitation of this study was the cross-sectional design, the results nonetheless suggested that the type of reserve was unimportant in the relationship, but that higher rates of disability predicted depression only in individuals who were lower on either malleable or fixed cognitive reserve. On the other hand, the relationship between depression and disability was insignificant for individuals who had either high malleable or fixed reserve. These results suggested the presence of a protective effect of cognitive reserve, such that higher reserve buffers the effects of depression resulting from disability in patients with MS.

Collectively, findings from these studies are congruent with the previous hypotheses that cognitive reserve may be an explanatory variable in the risk and functional outcomes related to psychiatric symptoms in adults, such that those with higher cognitive reserve may have better instrumental activities of daily living and quality of life, regardless of symptoms in that these factors are likely related to functional outcomes (e.g., disability). Of course, these results are also influenced by age, neurological differences, and potential neurodegenerative disease processes. As such, they may not be generalizable to other populations with depression and related disorders in isolation. Furthermore, the literature reviewed is relatively recent, and while it has shown promise, it is limited by cross-sectional rather than longitudinal studies and use of crude rather than useful measures of cognitive reserve. A summary table, Table 6.1, outlines the appropriateness of proxies for cognitive reserve for interested researchers and/or clinicians.

TABLE 6.1. Proxies of Cognitive Reserve and Means of Data Collection

Self-report/interview	Standardized testing
Educational attainment	IQ
Occupational attainment	Vocabulary tests
Recreational activity involvement[a]	Reading tests
	Adaptation to task demands[a]
	Executive functioning[a]
	Processing speed[a]
	Brain volume

[a]Recommended for populations with depression.

CONCLUSION

Evidence generated from multiple studies has suggested that a relationship exists between measures of cognitive reserve and neuropsychological inefficiencies and impairments and that cognitive reserve may protect or compensate for neuropsychological inefficiencies impairments in neuropsychiatric illnesses.

In addition to previously conducted cross-sectional studies, longitudinal research is warranted that can examine cognitive reserve as a moderator of neuropsychological and psychiatric sequelae of depression and can offer a better understanding of the relationship. First, causality could be inferred. Second, predictions could be made for the course and progression of disease burden for the afflicted individual. Third, early interventions could be developed that could target neuropsychological abilities in a more personalized manner as based on one's specific ability levels. For instance, individuals with greater and less cognitive reserve could be taught to make use of compensatory strategies that would attenuate the influence of cognitive impairments in day-to-day living.

Rather than using only one crude cognitive reserve proxy such as years of education, researchers may consider using multiple proxies of cognitive reserve (e.g., executive functioning, adaptation to task demands), particularly in the context of depression. Numerous psychosocial factors contribute to one's ability to attain lower or higher levels of education. Such factors are likely magnified with the diagnosis of a psychiatric illness (e.g., depression) and simply produce more error in analyses that limits both internal and external study validity. Utilizing age- and education-normed general intellectual functioning measures, as well as proxies of reserve that measure information processing and flexibility such as testing limits and adaptation, can help elucidate the relationship between cognitive reserve, neuropsychological inefficiency and impairment, and depression. In an era when depression is the leading cause of global disability, and much of this disability can be attributed to neuropsychological impairment, it is critical to investigate the possible influence of cognitive reserve on functional outcomes in order to promote population health and improve overall functional outcomes.

REFERENCES

Addington, J., & Addington, D. (2000). Neurocognitive and social functioning in schizophrenia: A 2.5 year follow-up study. *Schizophrenia Research, 44*(1), 47–56.

American Psychiatric Association. (2013). *Diagnostic and statistical manual of mental disorders* (5th ed.). Arlington, VA: Author.

Aylward, E., Walker, E., & Bettes, B. (1984). Intelligence in schizophrenia: Meta-analysis of the research. *Schizophrenia Bulletin, 10*(3), 430–459.

Balota, D. A., Dolan, P. O., & Duchek, J. M. (2000). Memory changes in healthy older adults. In E. Tulving & F. I. M. Craik (Eds.), *The Oxford handbook of memory* (pp. 395–409). New York: Oxford University Press.

Barnett, J. H., Salmond, C. H., Jones, P. B., & Sahakian, B. J. (2006). Cognitive reserve in neuropsychiatry. *Psychological Medicine, 36*(8), 1053–1064.

Bell, M. D., & Bryson, G. (2001). Work rehabilitation in schizophrenia: Does cognitive impairment limit improvement? *Schizophrenia Bulletin, 27*(2), 269–279.

Bilder, R. M., Goldman, R. S., Robinson, D., Reiter, G., Bell, L., Bates, J. A., et al. (2000). Neuropsychology of first-episode schizophrenia: Initial characterization and clinical correlates. *American Journal of Psychiatry, 157*(4), 549–559.

Boone, K. B. (Ed.). (2007). *Assessment of feigned cognitive impairment: A neuropsychological perspective.* New York: Guilford Press.

Booth, A. J., Rodgers, J. D., Schwartz, C. E., Quaranto, B. R., Weinstock-Guttman, B., Zivadinov, R., & Benedict, R. H. (2013). Active cognitive reserve influences the regional atrophy to cognition link in multiple sclerosis. *Journal of the International Neuropsychological Society, 19*(10), 1128–1133.

Brandt, J. (1991). The Hopkins Verbal Learning Test: Development of a new memory test with six equivalent forms. *The Clinical Neuropsychologist, 5*(2), 125–142.

Caballero, F. F., Miret, M., Power, M., Chatterji, S., Tobiasz-Adamczyk, B., Koskinen, S., et al. (2013). Validation of an instrument to evaluate quality of life in the aging population: WHOQOL-AGE. *Health and Quality of Life Outcomes, 11,* 177.

Cadden, M. H., Guty, E. T., & Arnett, P. A. (2019). Cognitive reserve attenuates the effect of disability on depression in multiple sclerosis. *Archives of Clinical Neuropsychology, 34*(4), 495–502.

Chen, L. S., Eaton, W. W., Gallo, J. J., & Nestadt, G. (2000). Understanding the heterogeneity of depression through the triad of symptoms, course and risk factors: A longitudinal, population-based study. *Journal of Affective Disorders, 59*(1), 1–11.

Cohen, R. M., Weingartner, H., Smallberg, S. A., Pickar, D., & Murphy, D. L. (1982). Effort and cognition in depression. *Archives of General Psychiatry, 39*(5), 593–597.

Colangeli, S., Boccia, M., Verde, P., Guariglia, P., Bianchini, F., & Piccardi, L. (2016). Cognitive reserve in healthy aging and Alzheimer's disease: A meta-analysis of fMRI studies. *American Journal of Alzheimer's Disease and Other Dementias, 31*(5), 443–449.

Coloma Andrews, L. C., & Zihl, J. (2014). Cognitive reserve in major depression–Associations with cognitive status, age, education, personality, and depression severity. *Austin Journal of Psychiatry and Behavioral Sciences, 1*(3), 1015–1025.

Davidson, J., Turnbull, C. D., Strickland, R., Miller, R., & Graves, K. (1986). The Montgomery–Åsberg Depression Scale: Reliability and validity. *Acta Psychiatrica Scandinavica, 73*(5), 544–548.

Deb, S., Lyons, I., Koutzoukis, C., Ali, I., & McCarthy, G. (1999). Rate of psychiatric illness 1 year after traumatic brain injury. *American Journal of Psychiatry, 156*(3), 374–378.

Dhillon, S., Videla-Nash, G., Foussias, G., Segal, Z. V., & Zakzanis, K. K. (2020). On the nature of objective and perceived cognitive impairments in depressive symptoms and real-world functioning in young adults. *Psychiatry Research, 287,* 112932.

Dotson, V. M., Resnick, S. M., & Zonderman, A. B. (2008). Differential association of concurrent, baseline, and average depressive symptoms with cognitive decline in older adults. *American Journal of Geriatric Psychiatry, 16*(4), 318–330.

Ebmeier, K., Rose, E., & Steele, D. (2006). Cognitive impairment and fMRI in major depression. *Neurotoxicity Research, 10*(2), 87–92.

Elderkin-Thompson, V., Kumar, A., Bilker, W. B., Dunkin, J. J., Mintz, J., Moberg, P. J., et al. (2003). Neuropsychological deficits among patients with late-onset minor and major depression. *Archives of Clinical Neuropsychology, 18*(5), 529–549.

Fay, T. B., Yeates, K. O., Taylor, H. G., Bangert, B., Dietrich, A. N. N., Nuss, K. E., et al. (2010). Cognitive reserve as a moderator of postconcussive symptoms in children with complicated and uncomplicated mild traumatic brain injury. *Journal of the International Neuropsychological Society, 16*(1), 94–105.

First, M. B., & Gibbon, M. (2004). The Structured Clinical Interview for DSM-IV Axis I Disorders (SCID-I) and the Structured Clinical Interview for DSM-IV Axis II Disorders (SCID-II). In M. J. Hilsenroth & D. L. Segal (Eds.), *Comprehensive handbook of psychological assessment: Vol. 2. Personality assessment* (pp. 134–143). Hoboken, NJ: Wiley.

Foley, J. M., Ettenhofer, M. L., Kim, M. S., Behdin, N., Castellon, S. A., & Hinkin, C. H. (2012). Cognitive reserve as a protective factor in older HIV-positive patients at risk for cognitive decline. *Applied Neuropsychology. Adult, 19*(1), 16–25.

Fratiglioni, L., & Wang, H. X. (2007). Brain reserve hypothesis in dementia. *Journal of Alzheimer's Disease, 12*(1), 11–22.

Gold, J. M., Goldberg, R. W., McNary, S. W., Dixon, L. B., & Lehman, A. F. (2002). Cognitive correlates of job tenure among patients with severe mental illness. *American Journal of Psychiatry, 159*(8), 1395–1402.

Golden, C. J. (1978). *Stroop Color and Word Test: A manual for clinical and experimental uses.* Chicago: Stoelting.

Gomez, R. G., Fleming, S. H., Keller, J., Flores, B., Kenna, H., DeBattista, C., et al. (2006). The neuropsychological profile of psychotic major depression and its relation to cortisol. *Biological Psychiatry, 60*(5), 472–478.

Gomez-Hernandez, R., Max, J. E., Kosier, T., Paradiso, S., & Robinson, R. G. (1997). Social impairment and depression after traumatic brain injury. *Archives of Physical Medicine and Rehabilitation, 78*(12), 1321–1326.

Groom, K. N., Shaw, T. G., O'Connor, M. E., Howard, N. I., & Pickens, A. (1998). Neurobehavioral symptoms and family functioning in traumatically brain-injured adults. *Archives of Clinical Neuropsychology, 13*(8), 695–711.

Harvey, P. O., Le Bastard, G., Pochon, J. B., Levy, R., Allilaire, J. F., Dubois, B. E. E. A., et al. (2004). Executive functions and updating of the contents of working memory in unipolar depression. *Journal of Psychiatric Research, 38*(6), 567–576.

Heinrichs, R. W., & Zakzanis, K. K. (1998). Neurocognitive deficit in schizophrenia: A quantitative review of the evidence. *Neuropsychology, 12*(3), 426–445.

Hibbard, M. R., Ashman, T. A., Spielman, L. A., Chun, D., Charatz, H. J., & Melvin, S. (2004). Relationship between depression and psychosocial functioning after traumatic brain injury1. *Archives of Physical Medicine and Rehabilitation, 85*, 43–53.

Holsinger, T., Steffens, D. C., Phillips, C., Helms, M. J., Havlik, R. J., Breitner, J. C., et al. (2002). Head injury in early adulthood and the lifetime risk of depression. *Archives of General Psychiatry, 59*(1), 17–22.

Iverson, G. L., Brooks, B. L., Langenecker, S. A., & Young, A. H. (2011). Identifying a cognitive impairment subgroup in adults with mood disorders. *Journal of Affective Disorders, 132*, 360–367.

Jackson-Triche, M. E., Sullivan, J. G., Wells, K. B., Rogers, W., Camp, P., & Mazel, R. (2000). Depression and health-related quality of life in ethnic minorities seeking care in general medical settings. *Journal of Affective Disorders, 58*(2), 89–97.

Kampf-Sherf, O., Zlotogorski, Z., Gilboa, A., Speedie, L., Lereya, J., Rosca, P., et al. (2004). Neuropsychological functioning in major depression and responsiveness to selective serotonin reuptake inhibitors antidepressants. *Journal of Affective Disorders, 82*(3), 453–459.

Kesler, S. R., Adams, H. F., Blasey, C. M., & Bigler, E. D. (2003). Premorbid intellectual functioning, education, and brain size in traumatic brain injury: An investigation of the cognitive reserve hypothesis. *Applied Neuropsychology, 10*(3), 153–162.

Koenen, K. C., Moffitt, T. E., Roberts, A. L., Martin, L. T., Kubzansky, L., Harrington, H., et al. (2009). Childhood IQ and adult mental disorders: A test of the cognitive reserve hypothesis. *American Journal of Psychiatry, 166*(1), 50–57.

Landrø, N. I., Stiles, T. C., & Sletvold, H. (2001). Neuropsychological function in nonpsychotic unipolar major depression. *Cognitive and Behavioral Neurology, 14*(4), 233–240.

Lara, E., Koyanagi, A., Caballero, F., Domènech-Abella, J., Miret, M., Olaya, B., et al. (2017). Cognitive reserve is associated with quality of life: A population-based study. *Experimental Gerontology, 87*, 67–73.

Levi, Y., Rassovsky, Y., Agranov, E., Sela-Kaufman, M., & Vakil, E. (2013). Cognitive reserve components as expressed in traumatic brain injury. *Journal of the Internatinal Neuropsychological Society, 19*, 664–671.

Lishman, W. A. (2008). *Organic psychiatry: The psychological consequences of cerebral disorder* (3rd ed.). Oxford, UK: Blackwell Science.

Maxwell, S. E., & Cole, D. A. (2007). Bias in cross-sectional analyses of longitudinal mediation. *Psychological Methods, 12*(1), 23–44.

McClintock, S. M., Husain, M. M., Greer, T. L., Cullum, C. M. (2010). Association between depression severity and neurocognitive function in major depressive disorder: A review and synthesis. *Neuropsychology, 24*(1), 9–34.

McCrae, R. R., & Costa, P. T. (1987). Validation of the five-factor model of personality across instruments and observers. *Journal of Personality and Social Psychology, 52*(1), 81–90.

McCrae, R. R., & Costa, P. T., Jr. (1989). More reasons to adopt the five-factor model. *American Psychologist, 44*(2), 451–452.

McLaren, M. E., Szymkowicz, S. M., Kirton, J. W., & Dotson, V. M. (2015). Impact of education on memory deficits in subclinical depression. *Archives of Clinical Neuropsychology, 30*(5), 387–393.

Merikangas, K. R., Wicki, W., & Angst, J. (1994). Heterogeneity of depression: Classification of depressive subtypes by longitudinal course. *British Journal of Psychiatry, 164*(3), 342–348.

Munro, J. C., Russell, A. J., Murray, R. M., Kerwin, R. W., & Jones, P. B. (2002). IQ in childhood psychiatric attendees predicts outcome of later schizophrenia at 21 year follow-up. *Acta Psychiatrica Scandinavica, 106*(2), 139–142.

Murphy, M., & O'Lleary, E. (2010). Depression, cognitive reserve and memory performance in older adults. *International Journal of Geriatric Psychiatry, 25*(7), 665–671.

Murray, A. D., Staff, R. T., McNeil, C. J., Salarirad, S., Ahearn, T. S., Mustafa, N., et al. (2011). The balance between cognitive reserve and brain imaging biomarkers of cerebrovascular and Alzheimer's diseases. *Brain, 134*(12), 3687–3696.

Nebes, R. D., Butters, M. A., Mulsant, B. H., Pollock, B. G., Zmuda, M. D., Houck, P. R., et al. (2000). Decreased working memory and processing speed mediate cognitive impairment in geriatric depression. *Psychological Medicine, 30*(3), 679–691.

Nelson, H. E., & Willison, J. (1991). *National Adult Reading Test (NART)*. Windsor: NFER-Nelson.

Neubauer, A., & Horn, R. V. (2006). *Wechsler Intelligenztest für Erwachsene: WIE; Übersetzung und Adaption der WAIS-III*. M. San Antonio, TX: Harcourt Test Services.

Nunnari, D., Bramanti, P., & Marino, S. (2014). Cognitive reserve in stroke and traumatic brain injury patients. *Neurological Sciences, 35*(10), 1513–1518.

Paradise, M., Cooper, C., & Livingston, G. (2009). Systematic review of the effect of education on survival in Alzheimer's disease. *International Psychogeriatrics, 21*(1), 25–32.

Querbes, O., Aubry, F., Pariente, J., Lotterie, J. A., Démonet, J. F., Duret, V., et al. (2009). Early diagnosis of Alzheimer's disease using cortical thickness: Impact of cognitive reserve. *Brain, 132*(8), 2036–2047.

Rami, L., Valls-Pedret, C., Bartrés-Faz, D., Caprile, C., Solé-Padullés, C., Castellvi, M., et al. (2011). Cognitive reserve questionnaire. Scores obtained in a healthy elderly population and in one with Alzheimer's disease. *Revista de Neurologia, 52*(4), 195–201.

Reitan, R. M. (1958). Validity of the Trail Making Test as an indicator of organic brain damage. *Perceptual and Motor Skills, 8*(3), 271–276.

Roe, C. M., Xiong, C., Miller, J. P., & Morris, J. C. (2007). Education and Alzheimer disease without dementia support for the cognitive reserve hypothesis. *Neurology, 68*(3), 223–228.

Rogers, M. A., Kasai, K., Koji, M., Fukuda, R., Iwanami, A., Nakagome, K., et al. (2004). Executive and prefrontal dysfunction in unipolar depression: A review of neuropsychological and imaging evidence. *Neuroscience Research, 50*(1), 1–11.

Salmond, C. H., Menon, D. K., Chatfield, D. A., Pickard, J. D., & Sahakian, B. J. (2006). Cognitive reserve as a resilience factor against depression after moderate/severe head injury. *Journal of Neurotrauma, 23*(7), 1049–1058.

Satz, P., Morgenstern, H., Miller, E. N., Selnes, O. A., McArthur, J. C., Cohen, B. A., et al. (1993). Low education as a possible risk factor for cognitive abnormalities in HIV-1: Findings from the multicenter AIDS Cohort Study (MACS). *Journal of Acquired Immune Deficiency Syndromes, 6*(5), 503–511.

Scarmeas, N., & Stern, Y. (2004). Cognitive reserve: Implications for diagnosis and prevention of Alzheimer's disease. *Current Neurology and Neuroscience Reports, 4*(5), 374–380.

Schatzberg, A. F. (2002). Major depression: Causes or effects. *American Journal of Psychiatry, 159.* 1077–1079.

Schneider, E. B., Sur, S., Raymont, V., Duckworth, J., Kowalski, R. G., Efron, D. T., et al. (2014). Functional recovery after moderate/severe traumatic brain injury: A role for cognitive reserve? *Neurology, 82*(18), 1636–1642.

Schwartz, C. E., Snook, E., Quaranto, B., Benedict, R. H., & Vollmer, T. (2013). Cognitive reserve and patient-reported outcomes in multiple sclerosis. *Multiple Sclerosis, 19*(1), 87–105.

Shapiro, M. E., Mahoney, J. R., Peyser, D., Zingman, B. S., & Verghese, J. (2014). Cognitive reserve protects against apathy in individuals with human immunodeficiency virus. *Archives of Clinical Neuropsychology, 29*(1), 110–120.

Shenal, B. V., Harrison, D. W., & Demaree, H. A. (2003). The neuropsychology of depression: A literature review and preliminary model. *Neuropsychology Review, 13*(1), 33–42.

Solé-Padullés, C., Bartrés-Faz, D., Junqué, C., Vendrell, P., Rami, L., Clemente, I. C., et al. (2009). Brain structure and function related to cognitive reserve variables in normal aging, mild cognitive impairment and Alzheimer's disease. *Neurobiology of Aging, 30*(7), 1114–1124.

Stern, R. A., Silva, S. G., Chaisson, N., & Evans, D. L. (1996). Influence of cognitive reserve on neuropsychological functioning in asymptomatic human immunodeficiency virus-1 infection. *Archives of Neurology, 53*(2), 148–153.

Stern, Y. (2002). What is cognitive reserve?: Theory and research application of the reserve concept. *Journal of the International Neuropsychological Society, 8*(3), 448–460.

Stern, Y. (2009). Cognitive reserve. *Neuropsychologia, 47*(10), 2015–2028.

Stern, Y. (2012). Cognitive reserve in ageing and Alzheimer's disease. *The Lancet Neurology, 11*(11), 1006–1012.

Stern, Y., Alexander, G. E., Prohovnik, I., & Mayeux, R. (1992). Inverse relationship between education and parietotemporal perfusion deficit in Alzheimer's disease. *Annals of Neurology, 32*(3), 371–375.

Strub, R. L., & Black, F. W. (1985). *The mental status examination in neurology.* Philadelphia: F. A. Davis.

Sumowski, J. F., & Leavitt, V. M. (2013). Cognitive reserve in multiple sclerosis. *Multiple Sclerosis, 19*(9), 1122–1127.

Tucker, M. A., & Stern, Y. (2011). Cognitive reserve in aging. *Current Alzheimer Research, 8*(4), 354–360.

Üstün, T. B., Kostanjsek, N., Chatterji, S., & Rehm, J. (Eds.). (2010). *Measuring health and disability: Manual for WHO disability assessment schedule WHODAS 2.0.* Geneva: World Health Organization.

Venezia, R. G., Gorlyn, M., Burke, A. K., Oquendo, M. A., Mann, J. J., & Keilp, J. G. (2018). The impact of cognitive reserve on neurocognitive performance in major depressive disorder. *Psychiatry Research, 270,* 211–218.

Wechsler, D. (1997). *Wechsler Adult Intelligence Scale—Third Edition (WAIS-III).* San Antonio, TX: Psychological Corporation.

Willis, K. J., & Hakim, A. M. (2013). Stroke prevention and cognitive reserve: Emerging approaches to modifying risk and delaying onset of dementia. *Frontiers in Neurology, 4,* 13.

Yang, L., Krampe, R. T., & Baltes, P. B. (2006). Basic forms of cognitive plasticity extended into the oldest-old: Retest learning, age, and cognitive functioning. *Psychology and Aging, 21*(2), 372–378.

Zakzanis, K. K., Leach, L., & Kaplan, E. (1998). On the nature and pattern of neurocognitive function in major depressive disorder. *Neuropsychiatry, Neuropsychology, and Behavioral Neurology, 11*(3), 111–119.

CHAPTER 7

Learning and Memory Systems

Adam A. Christensen
Margaret O'Connor

Many people with major depressive disorder (MDD) struggle with memory problems that adversely affect educational, occupational, and social functioning. Despite the prevalence of these problems, there is no consensus regarding the extent or pattern of memory loss associated with depression. Moreover, there is no agreement regarding whether the association is causal or correlational. Some people with depression and memory complaints perform normally on objective tests of memory (Dux et al., 2008), underscoring the possible contributions of low self-esteem and/or a lack of self-confidence in their evaluations of their mnestic capabilities (Mohn & Rund, 2016). The association between depression and memory problems is complex and there is no consensus regarding the relative importance of biological or psychological factors. Some people with depression have reduced hippocampal volume and frontal system vulnerabilities that adversely affect memory (Koenigs & Grafman, 2009; McKinnon, Yusel, Nazarov, & MacQueen, 2009). Others may experience reductions in dopamine and serotonin that undermine initial encoding of new information (Kraus, Castrén, Kasper, & Lanzenberger, 2017; Rocchetti et al., 2015). Depression is often associated with increased stress, which may have a deleterious effect on the hypothalamic–pituitary–adrenal axis important for learning and memory. Social introversion and ruminative thinking, common in depression, may undermine a person's ability to attend to and remember new information. Depression may have significant effects on qualitative aspects of memory. People with depression are more likely to learn and retrieve negative information about themselves and the world (Gaddy & Ingram, 2014). In addition to this negative bias, studies have shown that people with depression may have overly generalized memories that lack specific details (Williams et al., 2007).

In this chapter, we review biological and psychological studies focused on the complex interplay between depression and memory. We consider important neurological and emotional factors that give rise to memory loss in people with depression. We discuss the clinical evaluation and pattern of memory problems associated with depression. Finally, we review therapeutically oriented treatment interventions.

NEUROBIOLOGICAL CONTRIBUTIONS TO DEPRESSION-RELATED MEMORY PROBLEMS

Depression-related memory loss may involve dysfunction in neural systems critical for new learning, including medial temporal (e.g., the hippocampus and parahippocampal cortices) and frontal networks. Neuroimaging studies have demonstrated that people with MDD have reduced hippocampal volume (McKinnon et al., 2009). Changes have been noted in specific hippocampal subfields, including CA1-3 and the dentate gyrus, and several studies have demonstrated disproportionate reduction in the posterior hippocampus (Malykhin & Coupland, 2015). The extent of hippocampal volume loss has been associated with lifetime duration of MDD (Bell-McGinty et al., 2002; Travis et al., 2014). However, given the cross-sectional nature of these studies, it remains unclear whether there is a causal relationship between hippocampal volume loss and depression.

Dysfunction in frontal brain regions has been observed in the context of memory problems as well as in depression. Functional imaging studies have shown that depression is associated with ventromedial prefrontal cortex hyperactivity and dorsolateral prefrontal cortex hypoactivity (Koenigs & Grafman, 2009). Of note, these brain regions are critical for encoding and retrieval operations. Abnormal activity in these regions may simultaneously contribute to memory inefficiencies, which may exacerbate depression.

In addition to pathological brain changes, disruptions in neurotransmitter systems may affect both emotional regulation and memory proficiency. Anhedonia is exacerbated by decreased sensitivity in the dopaminergic reward system (Belujon & Grace, 2017). In addition to affecting mood, dopamine plays a key role in modulation of hippocampal synaptic activity (potentiation and depression), which has direct bearing on memory (Rocchetti et al., 2015). There is also a strong connection between dopamine regulation in response to reward for people with MDD and nondepressed individuals (Pizzagalli, Evins, et al., 2008; Pizzagalli, Iosifescu, Hallett, Ratner, & Fava, 2008). The neurotransmitter serotonin, which is associated with mood regulation, mediates brain development and neuroplasticity (Whitaker-Azmitia, 2001). Serotonergic imbalances, per translational preclinical models, may lead to a reduction in hippocampal volume (Kraus et al., 2017). Hence, serotonin has a critical role in mood and memory.

Depression may also be associated with alterations within the stress reactivity system (Wingenfeld & Wolf, 2011). The hypothalamic–pituitary–adrenal (HPA) axis and stress response are regulated by a feedback loop that involves stimulation of corticotropin-releasing factor and adrenocorticotropin, and negative feedback from the release of cortisol to achieve homeostasis. Previous studies have focused on the association between HPA axis functioning and memory. Findings suggest that higher cortisol levels are associated with poor memory performance in individuals with depression and healthy controls (Keller et al., 2017). However, the directionality of this association is not clear: it remains to be determined whether cortisol levels affect cognitive impairment versus whether cognitive impairment impacts cortisol levels (Wingenfeld & Wolf, 2011).

In addition to the above, there is an emerging literature focused on the the link between depression and neurodegenerative brain changes in older individuals. Depression has been cited as a risk factor for cognitive decline (Donovan et al., 2015; Modrego & Ferrández, 2004; Royall & Palmer, 2013). Pathological brain changes associated with different neurodegenerative conditions (e.g., Alzheimer's disease, stroke, and Lewy Body disease), for which memory deficits are often primary in presentation, have been associated with depression. Older adults with increased mood symptoms have a higher burden of amyloid beta, a protein associated with Alzheimer's disease (Donovan et al., 2018). Furthermore, people with increased amyloid are more likely to be diagnosed with depression (Wilson et al., 2016). The direct link between Alzheimer's disease and depression remains elusive. Some studies have shown that even when controlling for AD-related plaque and tangle pathology, depression has an independent and potent effect on memory performance (Royall & Palmer, 2013; Wilson et al., 2003). A postmortem study revealed that depression is associated with increased Lewy bodies and hippocampal volume loss, but not Alzheimer's or cerebrovascular neuropathology (Tsopelas et al., 2011). Other studies that have focused on the effects of cerebrovascular disease have also yielded mixed findings. Depression commonly emerges following cerebrovascular change and stroke, with white matter lesions and disruptions of subcortical circuits potentially affecting neurotransmitter and HPA axis functionality, contributing to mood dysregulation (Robinson & Jorge, 2016). While cerebrovascular change in the form of severe white matter change was associated with a higher liklihood of the presence of depression symptoms (de Groot et al., 2000), investigators have also found that there is no association between extent of subcortical hyperintensities detected by magnetic resonance imaging and depression severity (Salloway et al., 2002).

PSYCHOLOGICAL CONTRIBUTIONS TO DEPRESSION-RELATED MEMORY PROBLEMS

Cognitive and emotional factors have a direct bearing on quantitative and qualitative aspects of memory. People with depression are prone to ruminative thinking, which reduces the ability to allocate cognitive resources to important events in the environment, thereby undermining encoding of new events, as well as the retrieval of previously stored information (Levens, Muhtadie, & Gotlib, 2009). Depression-related problems with motivation and attention negatively impact performance during objective memory testing. Negative affect has been associated with increased subjective memory complaints, but the level of complaints is not always consistent with performance on dementia screening and memory tests. This suggests that some aspect of perceived difficulty is related to the negative thought pattern (Dux et al., 2008).

Studies have shown that depression is often associated with a negative response bias and overly generalized thinking. People with depression tend to retrieve vague rather than specific information in response to a stimulus (Williams & Broadbent, 1986). Their memories of personal events may lack the detailed qualities of those of nondepressed people (Williams et al., 2007). For example, when recounting events, depressed people may recall a broad concept such as playing baseball during a particular decade of life, whereas they are less likely to retrieve unique information about a specfic game. The extent of generalization may predict the course of depression. Research has shown that poor recall of autobiographical events is associated with increased depressive symptoms (Hermans et al., 2008; Liu et al., 2016; Sumner, Griffith, & Mineka, 2010). For individuals with first-episode depression, more overly general memory at baseline predicted persistent depressive symptoms at follow-up, indicating that lack of well-articulated personal memories may have a directional effect on the maintenance of depression (Liu et al., 2016).

Depression-related memory biases operate at an implicit or preconscious level; the individual may not be aware of their negatively skewed thought processes. Studies have shown that people with depression access negative information more readily, whereas nondepressed people demonstrate preferential recall of positive information, even though they are not consciously aware of these tendencies (Gaddy & Ingram, 2014). Emotional biases in depression also impact explicit memory or memory *with* awareness. In these investigations, people with MDD had a distinct bias to learn and retrieve negative words (e.g., cruel, liar) from an array of valenced material more easily, whereas nondepressed controls were more likely to recall positive information (e.g., honest, sincere; Matt, Vazquez, & Campbell, 1992). Viewed systemically, overly generalized memory and negative biases have convergent detrimental effects on memory retrieval. People with depression consistently retrieve negative general memories, which reinforces a negative self-view, exacerbating depression. In turn, they may have less access to neutral and positive experiences, which limits memory specificity (Young, Erickson, & Drevets, 2012). Problems with prospective memory and the generation of potential future events are also negatively reinforced. People with depression tend to imagine negative futures as well as negative self-views. Their access to positive future and self memories are less available and vivid. They tend to judge negative outcomes as more likely. and, in this context, they may feel powerless as agents of change. This "faulty prospection" serves to perpetuate the generation of negative thoughts (Roepke & Seligman, 2016) and adversely impacts learning and memory functions.

CLINICAL APPLICATIONS: THE COGNITIVE PROFILE OF DEPRESSION

In the clinic, it is important to identify the unique contributions of depression on memory performance to ensure accuracy in diagnosis. Memory difficulties in depression can only be understood in the context of the broader neuropsychological profile, as memory inefficiency is potentially exacerbated by weaknesses in other domains. Learning and memory impairments have been observed for individuals with MDD across numerous studies, but there is little agreement regarding the profile of depression-related memory problems (McDermott & Ebmeier, 2009). A number of meta-analytic studies have examined whether there is a cognitive phenotype in depression. Zakzanis, Leach, and Kaplan. (1998) conducted an investigationof 22 studies with 726 patients with MDD and 795 nondepressed controls. Large effect sizes were observed on memory tasks, whereas intermediate effect sizes were observed in other cognitive areas such as processing speed and sustained attention. The Rey Auditory Verbal Learning Test (RAVLT; Rey, 1964) was the most sensitive measure in discriminating between individuals with MDD and controls (mean effect size ranged from Cohen's $d = -1.93$ to -1.24). The RAVLT had greater effects than other memory tests such as the California Verbal Learning Test (CVLT; Delis, Kramer, Kaplan, & Ober, 1987) and the Buschke Selective Reminding Test (BSRT; Buschke & Fuld, 1974), perhaps because the CVLT nad BSRT have semantically integrated word lists that may make learning easier, thereby reducing the sensitivity of these tests. Large effect sizes were also observed on tasks of visual memory, such as the Rey–Osterrieth Complex Figure Test (Osterrieth, 1944; Rey, 1941; English translation, Corwin & Bylsma, 1993) and immediate reproduction (mean effect size Cohen's $d = -1.02$). Other memory measures showed above-average effect sizes, including the Wechsler Memory Scale—Revised Visual Reproduction and Logical Memory subtests (Wechsler, 1987) and the CVLT long delay free recall.

More recently, Ahern and Semkovska (2017) determined the mean effect sizes of cognitive functions for adults with first episode depression across 31 studies and 994 patients. They examined four longitudinal studies that included 92 adults with MDD to assess the mean change effect sizes in cognitive function from the first depressive episode to remission. Twelve cognitive composite domains were examined, six of which were memory domains (autobiographical memory, verbal: learning, delayed memory, recognition, and visual: learning, delayed memory). Patients with MDD had moderate impairment on tasks of autobiographical memory and visual learning, and they had mild impairments in visual and verbal recall. There were no significant differences for verbal learning and recognition. The surprising finding of *insignificant* verbal learning was attributed to sample heterogeneity; notably within that domain, list learning was insignificant, but story learning was moderately impaired. Those adults with MDD in remission showed normalization of visual learning and memory, verbal learning and memory, and autobiographical memory. Another meta-analysis of 15 studies (Lee, Hermens, Porter, & Redoblado-Hodge, 2012) that included 644 adults with first-episode MDD revealed impairments in processing speed, attention, executive functioning, and visual learning and memory. Depression severity accounted for reductions in psychomotor speed and visual learning and memory, which suggested that these deficits were state markers or indicative of acute exacerbation of mood state, whereas attention and executive deficits persisted following remission and were posited to be trait markers, inherent to chronic MDD.

Other studies have highlighted the link between resolution of depression and enhanced memory performance. As per a review of longitudinal studies (30 studies; Douglas & Porter, 2009), improved mood was related to better verbal memory, whereas executive and attentional deficits persisted in younger adults. For older depressed adults (mean age 68–76 across 14 studies), remission has been associated with psychomotor speed improvement. These findings suggest that verbal learning and memory and psychomotor speed are sensitive to clinical state, whereas attention and executive functioning are trait-specific for MDD.

Porter, Bourke, and Gallagher (2007) attributed inconsistencies across studies to heterogeneity in methodology, with different cognitive outcomes and sample characteristics (e.g., clinical subtype, depression severity, age, and medication). Overall, some studies with varied definitions of depression severity have associated increased cognitive dysfunction with frequency of occurrence, duration of episodes, and age at onset, while other studies have shown no learning and memory effects related to the illness course (McClintock, Husain, Greer, & Cullum 2010). One meta-analysis indicated that depression severity was associated with problems in verbal memory, executive functioning, and processing speed, but not visuospatial memory or verbal fluency (McDermott & Ebmeier

2009). In contrast, a large 35-year longitudinal assessment (Franz et al., 2011) of 1237 male twins revealed that depression severity was associated with lower executive functioning, processing speed, and visual memory, but not verbal memory. Low cognitive ability at age 20 was a risk factor for depression susceptibility, partly due to shared genetic influences.

It is important to reconcile differences between these studies. The McDermott and Ebmeier (2009) study indicated that verbal but not nonverbal memory was impaired, whereas Franz and colleagues (2011) found the opposite pattern. These divergent results may simply be due to the fact that they used different tests. The inconsistency in cognitive tests employed in research is a key factor contributing to the lack of consensus across studies examining the effects of depression on memory. The meta-analysis and longitudinal study noted above (Franz et al., 2011; McDermott & Ebmeier, 2009) revealed discrepant results of depression severity on verbal and visual memory but had examined different neuropsychological measures for both of these memory constructs. Consistent with the conclusions of Zakzanis and colleagues (1998), noncontextual verbal memory tests (e.g., RAVLT) with heavy executive and encoding load have been associated with depression severity (McDermott & Ebmeier 2009), while measures with contextual cues (e.g., story memory, CVLT) have been found to be unrelated to depression severity (Franz et al., 2011). Similarly, in a longitudinal study of depression, no impairments in verbal memory were observed at the initial testing timepoint as compared to controls on the CVLT. However, 9 years later, the only significant group difference was observed in short-delay free recall, which declined for depressed individuals but not for controls (Halvorsen, Waterloo, Sundet, Eisemann, & Wang, 2011). Of the several CVLT variables that were examined, short-delay free recall was most similar to recall on the RAVLT in that an examinee had not yet been cued to the presence of categories, and therefore any semantic clustering that occurred to contextualize and aid subsequent retrieval was independent and effortful on the part of the examinee. In the above study, once they were cued to the categories at short- and long-delay recall, individuals with depression and controls showed similar performance.

To address the contribution of test heterogeneity, Rock and colleagues (Rock, Roiser, Riedel, & Blackwell, 2014) assessed 24 studies that used the same cognitive tool, the Cambridge Neuropsychological Test Automated Battery (CANTAB). Persistent executive functioning and attentional impairments, but memory improvements, were observed in patients with remitted depression. Compared to controls, the performance by adults with depression on the CANTAB showed moderate executive, attention, and memory impairment, while adults who remitted continued to show executive and attentional impairment, but nonsignificant small/moderate memory deficits.

The inherent symptomatic heterogeneity of the depressed patient population contributes to reported cognitive differences, but memory impairments appear consistent across depressive subtypes. For instance, melancholic relative to nonmelancholic depressive subtype has been found to have greater attention and executive dysfunction, but both melancholic and nonmelancholic subtypes show similar levels of impaired memory recall (Darcet, Gardier, Gaillard, David, & Guilloux, 2016). Melancholic, atypical, and undifferentiated depressive subtypes all showed visuospatial memory improvement upon remission (Lin et al., 2014).

LEARNING AND MEMORY IN DEPRESSION ACROSS THE ADULT LIFESPAN

Research studies have shown that early-life onset of depression is associated with increased memory impairment. Adolescents and children diagnosed with MDD have more significant deficits in verbal memory as well as attention and executive functions (Wagner, Müller, Helmreich, Huss, & Tadić, 2014). Duration of depressive illness has been shown to have a negative impact on global cognitive functions (Hasselbalch, Knorr, Hasselbalch, Gade, & Kessing, 2013). Specific to memory, a very large study of 8,229 adults (ages 18–97) revealed that those with favorable responses to antidepressant treatment demonstrated an association between reduced duration of illness, fewer episodes, and better performance on memory tests. This finding was driven by the younger age groups (ages 18–47) (Gorwood, Corruble, Falissard, & Goodwin, 2008).

For older adults with depression, verbal learning difficulty is mediated by executive dysfunction, as evidenced in the correlation of word list learning and executive function tests (Elderkin-Thompson, Mintz, Haroon, Lavretsky, & Kumar, 2007). Comparing currently remitted, currently depressed, and never depressed older individuals, all patients with a history of depression showed difficulty in episodic memory and other cognitive domains, whereas executive deficits were similar between depressive groups (Koenig et al., 2015). In a recent study of healthy controls and early-onset depression in elderly adults, recall and recognition memory function were similar between groups. However, results from functional neuroimaging revealed differential neuroactivation. Specifically, the elderly group with depression showed lower activation in the hippocampus, parahippocampal gyrus, insula, and cingulate, and higher activation in the inferior frontal gyrus. The study authors postulated that this region of hyperactivity was essential for memory consolidation (Weisenbach et al., 2014).

See Table 7.1 for a summary of learning and memory in depression across the lifespan.

TREATMENTS, MEMORY, AND COGNITION IN DEPRESSION

A meta-analysis of psychological and pharmacological interventions revealed mild improvement on tasks of verbal memory in concert with improved mood (Bernhardt, Klauke, & Schröder, 2019). Visual and verbal memory improvements have been observed with antidepressant pharmacotherapy (Keefe et al., 2014). Another review found improvement with antidepressant treatment specifically for delayed recall (Rosenblat, Kakar, & McIntyre, 2015). A meta-analysis of 33 studies that investigated antidepressant agents by type (Prado, Watt, & Crowe, 2018) indicated a modest positive effect for immediate and delayed memory recall, as well as other functions, including divided and sustained attention, executive function, and processing speed. Specifically, selective serotonin reuptake inhibitors (SSRIs) demonstrated a significant positive effect on immediate memory, while serotonin modulator and stimulators, serotonin–norepinephrine reuptake inhibitors, and SSRIs had small significant positive effects on delayed memory. Tricyclic antidepressants (TCAs) and atypical antidepressant tianeptine had no significant effects. Antidepressant agents had insignificant effects on memory in nondepressed adults. Randomized control trials have found that certain antidepressants may show cognitive improvement

TABLE 7.1. Summary of Learning and Memory Systems in Depression

Biological contributions to depression-related memory problems	Major depressive disorder (MDD) is associated with hippocampal volume loss, differential activity of the prefrontal cortex, disruption in neurotransmitter systems (dopamine, serotonin), and the stress reactivity system. For older individuals, depression has been linked to some markers for neurodegenerative disease (amyloid beta, Lewy bodies) and variably associated with others (neurofibrillary plaque and tangle pathology, cerebrovascular change).
Psychological contributions to depression-related memory problems	Cognitive and emotional factors, including rumination, anhedonia, negative response bias, and overly general thinking, influence learning and retrieval in implicit and explicit memory processes in MDD.
Clinical applications: the cognitive profile of depression	The nature of learning and memory deficits in the cognitive profile of MDD is varied and debated. Meta-analytic and longitudinal studies are reviewed, which found disparate verbal and visual learning and retrieval memory impairments. Differences in findings are attributable to heterogeneity of methodology and clinical samples. Noncontextual verbal encoding appears to be a consistent area of primary deficit associated with depression across several studies.
Learning and memory in depression across the adult lifespan	Children, adolescents, and younger adults with depression have verbal memory deficiencies in addition to attention and executive dysfunction. For older adults with depression, verbal learning difficulty is mediated by executive dysfunction and functionally related to frontal lobe functioning.
Treatments, memory, and cognition in depression	Pharmacotherapy and psychotherapy can benefit learning and memory for individuals with MDD. Electroconvulsive therapy (ECT) results in transient memory deficits largely circumscribed to the first 3 weeks following treatment. Transcranial magnetic stimulation for MDD is not associated with memory impairment. Cortisol levels after ECT and pharmacotherapy are similar. Small studies of cognitive remediation that include behavioral and computer interventions have shown benefit to verbal memory but require further exploration.

irrespective of mood change for adults with MDD or in those who had depression remission (Bortolato et al., 2016).

Cognitive deficits that follow electroconvulsive therapy (ECT; see Finnegan & McLoughlin, Chapter 20, this volume, for additional information) are time limited. A meta-analysis of 24 cognitive variables across 84 studies and 2,981 adults with MDD-revealed transient verbal memory deficits that resolved within the subsequent 2 weeks post-ECT to pretreatment levels for word list learning and delayed recall, while story memory appeared to be unaffected by ECT (Semkovska & McGloughlin, 2010). Visual learning and memory showed smaller impairments and improved. While ECT can induce memory impairments that tend to be transient (with the exception of persistent retrograde amnesia), no evidence of memory impairment has been observed in adults when MDD was treated with transcranial magnetic stimulation (see Kavanaugh & Croarkin, Chapter 23, this volume, for additional information; O'Connor et al., 2003). Pre- and posttreatment cortisol levels for different antidepressant treatments (e.g., ECT, SSRIs, TCAs) have been found to be similar (meta-analysis of McKay & Zakzanis, 2010). Given that higher cortisol levels are associated with poorer memory (Keller et al., 2017), similar cortisol levels may suggest similar memory functioning before and after treatments.

Cognitive remediation programs, involving aspects of psychoeducation, compensatory behavioral strategies, and computer training, have shown benefit specific to verbal learning and memory for depressed individuals (Bowie et al., 2013; Naismith, Redoblado-Hodge, Lewis, Scott, & Hickie, 2010; Naismith et al., 2011). Given the small sample sizes and varied interventions individualized to each participant's cognitive profile, the degree to which computer drills, behavioral modifications, or other factors contributed to memory test performance improvement remains an area for further exploration.

CONCLUSION

Depression is often associated with learning and memory impairments that have negative functional implications for the person with MDD. Depression-related memory loss is likely a consequence of biological factors that affect the health and efficiency of core neural systems involved in memory. While there is no consensus regarding a specific memory phenotype, there is agreement that depression affects both quantitative and qualitative apects of memory—reducing the amount of information that a person can learn as well as the specificity and emotional valence of their memories. It is essential to acknowledge that memory loss is common in depression and there is a mandate to remediate this problem with individually tailored treatment interventions.

REFERENCES

Ahern, E., & Semkovska, M. (2017). Cognitive functioning in the first episode of major depressive disorder: A systematic review and meta-analysis. *Neuropsychology, 31*(1), 52–72.

Bell-McGinty, S., Butters, M. A., Meltzer, C. C., Greer, P. J., Reynolds III, C. F., & Becker, J. T. (2002). Brain morphometric abnormalities in geriatric depression: Long-term neurobiological effects of illness duration. *American Journal of Psychiatry, 159*, 1424–1427.

Belujon, P., & Grace, A. A. (2017). Dopamine system dysregulation in major depressive disorders. *International Journal of Neuropsychopharmacology, 20*, 1036–1046.

Bernhardt, M., Klauke, S., & Schröder, A. (2019). Longitudinal course of cognitive function across treatment in patients with MDD: A meta-analysis. *Journal of Affective Disorders, 249*, 52–62.

Bortolato, B., Miskowiak, K. W., Köhler, C. A., Maes, M., Fernandes, B. S., Berk, M., et al. (2016). Cognitive remission: A novel objective for the treatment of major depression? *BMC Medicine, 14*(1).

Bowie, C. R., Gupta, M., Holshausen, K., Jokic, R., Best, M., Milev, R. (2013). Cognitive remediation for treatment-resistant depression: Effects on cognition and functioning and the role of online homework, *Journal of Nervous and Mental Disease, 201*(8), 680–685.

Buschke, H., & Fuld, P. A. (1974). Evaluation of storage, retention and retrieval in disordered memory and learning. *Neurology, 11*, 1019–1025.

Corwin, J., & Bylsma, F. W. (1993). Psychological examination of traumatic encephalopathy, *Clinical Neuropsychologist, 7*(1), 3–21.

Darcet, F., Gardier, A. M., Gaillard, R., David, D. J., & Guilloux, J. P. (2016). Cognitive dysfunction in major depressive disorder. A translational review in animal models of the disease. *Pharmaceuticals, 9.*

de Groot, J. C., de Leeuw, F.-E., Oudkerk, M., Hofman, A., Jolles, J., & Breteler. M. M. B. (2000). Cerebral white matter lesions and depressive symptoms in elderly adults. *Archives of General Psychiatry, 57,* 1071–1076.

Delis, D. H., Kramer, J. H., Kaplan, E., & Ober, B. A. (1987). *California Verbal Learning Test.* Cleveland: Psychological Corporation.

Donovan, N. J., Hsu, D. C., Dagley, A. S., Schultz, A. P., Amariglio, R. E., Mormino, E. C., et al. (2015). Depressive symptoms and biomarkers of Alzheimer's disease in cognitively normal older adults. *Journal of Alzheimer's Disease, 46*(1), 63–73.

Donovan, N. J., Locascio, J. J., Marshall, G. A., Gatchel, J., Hanseeuw, B. J., Rentz, D. M., et al. (2018). Longitudinal association of amyloid beta and anxious-depressive symptoms in cognitively normal older adults. *American Journal of Psychiatry, 175*(6), 530–537.

Douglas, K. M., & Porter, R. J. (2009). Longitudinal assessment of neuropsychological function in major depression. *Australian and New Zealand Journal of Psychiatry, 43,* 1105–1117.

Dux, M. C., Woodard, J. L., Calamari, J. E., Messina, M., Arora, S., Chik, H., et al. (2008). The moderating role of negative affect on objective verbal memory performance and subjective memory complaints in healthy older adults. *Journal of the International Neuropsychological Society, 14*(2), 327–336.

Elderkin-Thompson, V., Mintz, J., Haroon, E., Lavretsky, H., & Kumar, A. (2007). Executive dysfunction and memory in older patients with major and minor depression. *Archives of Clinical Neuropsychology, 22,* 261–270.

Franz, C. E., Lyons, M. J., O'Brien, R., Panizzon, M. S., Kim, K., Bhat, R., et al. (2011). A 35-year longitudinal assessment of cognition and midlife depression symptoms: The Vietnam era twin study of aging. *American Journal of Geriatric Psychiatry, 19*(6), 559–570.

Gaddy, M. A., & Ingram, R. E. (2014). A meta-analytic review of mood-congruent implicit memory in depressed mood. *Clinical Psychology Review, 34,* 402–416.

Gorwood, P., Corruble, E., Falissard, B., & Goodwin, G. M. (2008). Toxic effects of depression on brain function: Impairment of delayed recall and the cumulative length of depressive disorder in a large sample of depressed outpatients. *American Journal of Psychiatry, 165,* 731–739.

Halvorsen, M., Waterloo, K., Sundet, K., Eisemann, M., & Wang, C. E. A. (2011). Verbal learning and memory in depression: A 9-year follow-up study. *Psychiatry Research, 188*(3), 350–354.

Hasselbalch, B. J., Knorr, U., Hasselbalch, S. G., Gade, A., & Kessing, L. V. (2013). The cumulative load of depressive illness is associated with cognitive function in the remitted state of unipolar depressive disorder. *European Psychiatry, 28*(6), 349–355.

Hermans, D., Vandromme, H., Debeer, E., Raes, F., Demyttenaere, K., Brunfaut, E., et al. (2008). Overgeneral autobiographical memory predicts diagnostic status in depression. *Behaviour Research and Therapy, 46*(5), 668–677.

Keefe, R. S. E., McClintock, S. M., Roth, R. M., Murali Doraiswamy, P., Tiger, S., & Madhoo, M. (2014). Cognitive effects of pharmacotherapy for major depressive disorder: A systematic review. *Journal of Clinical Psychiatry, 75,* 864–876.

Keller, J., Gomez, R., Williams, G., Lembke, A., Lazzeroni, L., Murphy, G. M., et al. (2017). HPA axis in major depression: Cortisol, clinical symptomatology and genetic variation predict cognition. *Molecular Psychiatry, 22*(4), 527–536.

Koenig, A. M., Delozier, I. J., Zmuda, M. D., Marron, M. M., Begley, A. E., Anderson, S. J., et al. (2015). Neuropsychological functioning in the acute and remitted states of late-life depression. In G. Smith (Ed.) *Handbook of depression in Alzheimer's disease* (pp. 95–106). Amsterdam: IOS Press.

Koenigs, M., & Grafman, J. (2009). The functional neuroanatomy of depression: Distinct roles for ventromedial and dorsolateral prefrontal cortex. *Behavioural Brain Research, 201,* 239–243.

Kraus, C., Castrén, E., Kasper, S., & Lanzenberger, R. (2017). Serotonin and neuroplasticity – Links between molecular, functional and structural pathophysiology in depression. *Neuroscience and Biobehavioral Reviews, 77*, 317–326.

Lee, R. S. C., Hermens, D. F., Porter, M. A., & Redoblado-Hodge, M. A. (2012). A meta-analysis of cognitive deficits in first-episode major depressive disorder. *Journal of Affective Disorders, 140*, 113–124.

Levens, S. M., Muhtadie, L., & Gotlib, I. H. (2009). Rumination and impaired resource allocation in depression. *Journal of Abnormal Psychology, 118*(4), 757–766.

Lin, K., Xu, G., Lu, W., Ouyang, H., Dang, Y., Lorenzo-Seva, U., et al. (2014). Neuropsychological performance in melancholic, atypical and undifferentiated major depression during depressed and remitted states: A prospective longitudinal study. *Journal of Affective Disorders, 168*, 184–191.

Liu, Y., Zhang, F., Wang, Z., Cao, L., Wang, J., Na, A., et al. (2016). Overgeneral autobiographical memory at baseline predicts depressive symptoms at follow-up in patients with first-episode depression. *Psychiatry Research, 243*, 123–127.

Malykhin, N. V., & Coupland, N. J. (2015). Hippocampal neuroplasticity in major depressive disorder. *Neuroscience, 309*, 200–213.

Matt, G. E., Vazquez, C., & Campbell, W. K. (1992). Mood-congruent recall of affectively toned stimuli: A meta-analytic review. *Clinical Psychology Review, 12*, 227–255.

McClintock, S. M., Husain, M. M., Greer, T. L., & Cullum, C. M. (2010). Association between depression severity and neurocognitive function in major depressive disorder: A review and synthesis. *Neuropsychology, 24*(1), 9–34.

McDermott, L. M., & Ebmeier, K. P. (2009). A meta-analysis of depression severity and cognitive function. *Journal of Affective Disorders, 119*, 1–8.

McKay, M. S., & Zakzanis, K. K. (2010). The impact of treatment on HPA axis activity in unipolar major depression. *Journal of Psychiatric Research, 44*, 183–192.

McKinnon, M. C., Yusel, K., Nazarov, A., & MacQueen, G. M. (2009) A meta-analysis examining clinical predictors of hippocampal volume in patients with major depressive disorder. *Journal of Psychiatry and Neuroscience, 31*, 41–54.

Modrego, P. J., & Ferrández, J. (2004). Depression in patients with mild cognitive impairment increases the risk of developing dementia of Alzheimer type: A prospective cohort study. *Archives of Neurology, 61*, 1290–1293.

Mohn, C., & Rund, B. R. (2016). Neurocognitive profile in major depressive disorders: Relationship to symptom level and subjective memory complaints. *BMC Psychiatry, 16*(1), 108.

Naismith, S. L., Diamond, K., Carter, P. E., Norrie, L., Redoblado-Hodge, M. A., Lewis, S. J. G., et al. (2011). Enhancing memory in late-life depression: The effects of a combined psychoeducation and cognitive training program. *American Journal of Geriatric Psychiatry, 19*, 240–248.

Naismith, S. L., Redoblado-Hodge, M. A., Lewis, S. J. G., Scott, E. M., & Hickie, I. B. (2010). Cognitive training in affective disorders improves memory: A preliminary study using the NEAR approach. *Journal of Affective Disorders, 121*, 258–262.

O'Connor, M., Morgan, A., Bloomingdale, K., Thall, M., Vasile, R., & Leone, P. (2003). Relative effects of repetitive transcranial magnetic stimulation and electroconvulsive therapy on mood and memory: A neurocognitive risk-benefit analysis. *Cognitive and Behavioral Neurology, 16*(2), 118–127.

Osterrieth, P. A. (1944). Le test de copie d'une figure complexe. Contribution à l'étude de la perception et de la mémoire. *Archives de Psychologie, 30*, 206–353.

Pizzagalli, D. A., Evins, A. E., Schetter, E. C., Frank, M. J., Pajtas, P. E., Santesso, D. L., et al. (2008). Single dose of a dopamine agonist impairs reinforcement learning in humans: behavioral evidence from a laboratory-based measure of reward responsiveness. *Psychopharmacology, 196*(2), 221–232.

Pizzagalli, D. A., Iosifescu, D., Hallett, L. A., Ratner, K. G., & Fava, M. (2008). Reduced hedonic capacity in major depressive disorder: Evidence from a probabilistic reward task. *Journal of Psychiatric Research, 43*(1), 76–87.

Porter, R. J., Bourke, C., & Gallagher, P. (2007). Neuropsychological impairment in major depression: Its nature, origin and clinical significance. *Australian and New Zealand Journal of Psychiatry, 41*, 115–128.

Prado, C. E., Watt, S., & Crowe, S. F. (2018). A meta-analysis of the effects of antidepressants on cognitive functioning in depressed and non-depressed samples. *Neuropsychology Review, 28*, 32–72.

Rey, A. 1941. L'examen psychologique dans les cas d'encéphalopathie traumatique. *Archives de Psychologie, 28*, 286–340.

Rey, A. (1964). *L' examen clinique en psychologie. [The clinical examination in psychology]*. Paris: Universitaires de France.

Robinson, R. G., & Jorge, R. E. (2016). Post-stroke depression: A review. *American Journal of Psychiatry, 173*(3), 221–231.

Rocchetti, J., Isingrini, E., Dal Bo, G., Sagheby, S., Menegaux, A., Tronche, F., et al. (2015). Presynaptic D2 dopamine receptors control long-term depression expression and memory processes in the temporal hippocampus. *Biological Psychiatry, 77*(6), 513–525.

Rock, P. L., Roiser, J. P., Riedel, W. J., & Blackwell, A. D. (2014). Cognitive impairment in depression: A systematic review and meta-analysis. *Psychological Medicine, 44*, 2029–2040.

Roepke, A. M., & Seligman, M. E. P. (2016). Depression and prospection. *British Journal of Clinical Psychology, 55*(1), 23–48.

Rosenblat, J. D., Kakar, R., & McIntyre, R. S. (2015). The cognitive effects of antidepressants in major depressive disorder: A systematic review and meta-analysis of randomized clinical trials. *International Journal of Neuropsychopharmacology, 19*(2), 1–13.

Royall, D. R., & Palmer, R. F. (2013). Alzheimer's disease pathology does not mediate the association between depressive symptoms and subsequent cognitive decline. *Alzheimer's and Dementia, 9*(3), 318–325.

Salloway, S., Correia, S., Boyle, P., Malloy, P., Schneider, L., Lavretsky, H., et al. (2002). MRI subcortical hyperintensities in old and very old depressed outpatients. *Journal of the Neurological Sciences, 203–204*, 227–233.

Semkovska, M., & McLoughlin, D. M. (2010). Objective cognitive performance associated with electroconvulsive therapy for depression: A systematic review and meta-analysis. *Biological Psychiatry, 68*(6), 568–577.

Sumner, J. A., Griffith, J. W., & Mineka, S. (2010). Overgeneral autobiographical memory as a predictor of the course of depression: A meta-analysis. *Behaviour Research and Therapy, 48*(7), 614–625.

Travis, S., Coupland, N. J., Silversone, P. H., Huang, Y., Fujiwara, E., Carter, R., et al. (2014). Dentate gyrus volume and memory performance in major depressive disorder. *Journal of Affective Disorders, 172*, 159–164.

Tsopelas, C., Stewart, R., Savva, G. M., Brayne, C., Ince, P., Thomas, A., et al. (2011). Neuropathological correlates of late-life depression in older people. *British Journal of Psychiatry, 198*(2), 109–114.

Wagner, S., Müller, C., Helmreich, I., Huss, M., & Tadić, A. (2014). A meta-analysis of cognitive functions in children and adolescents with major depressive disorder. *European Child and Adolescent Psychiatry, 24*, 5–19.

Wechsler, D. (1987). *Wechsler Memory Scale—Revised*. San Antonio, TX: The Psychological Corporation.

Weisenbach, S. L., Kassel, M. T., Rao, J., Weldon, A. L., Avery, E. T., Briceno, E. M., et al. (2014). Differential prefrontal and subcortical circuitry engagement during encoding of semantically related words in patients with late-life depression. *International Journal of Geriatric Psychiatry, 29*(11), 1104–1115.

Whitaker-Azmitia, P. M. (2001). Serotonin and brain development: Role in human developmental diseases. *Brain Research Bulletin, 56*(5), 479–485.

Williams, J. M. G., Barnhofer, T., Crane, C., Hermans, D., Raes, F., Watkins, E., et al. (2007). Autobiographical memory specificity and emotional disorder. *Psychological Bulletin, 133*, 122–148.

Williams, J. M. G., & Broadbent, K. (1986). Autobiographical memory in suicide attempters. *Journal of Abnormal Psychology, 95*, 144–149.

Wilson, R. S., Boyle, P. A., Capuano, A. W., Shah, R. C., Hoganson, G. M., Nag, S., et al. (2016). Late-life depression is not associated with dementia-related pathology. *Neuropsychology, 30*(2), 135–142.

Wilson, R. S., Schneider, J. A., Bienias, J. L., Arnold, S. E., Evans, D. A., & Bennett, D. A. (2003).

Depressive symptoms, clinical AD, and cortical plaques and tangles in older persons. *Neurology,* *61*(8), 1102–1107.

Wingenfeld, K., & Wolf, O. (2011). HPA axis alterations in mental disorders: Impact on memory and its relevance for therapeutic interventions. *CNS Neuroscience and Therapeutics, 17*(6), 714–722.

Young, K. D., Erickson, K., & Drevets, W. C. (2012). Match between cue and memory valence during autobiographical memory recall in depression. *Psychological Reports, 111,* 129–148.

Zakzanis, K., Leach, L., & Kaplan, E. (1998). On the nature and pattern of neurocognitive function in major depressive disorder. *Neuropsychiatry, Neuropsychology, and Behavioral Neurology, 11,* 111–119.

CHAPTER 8

Working Memory in Depression

Ashleigh V. Rutherford
Jutta Joormann

Sustained negative affect and difficulties experiencing positive affect are the hallmark features of depression. Depression, however, is also characterized by deficits and biases in cognition. Indeed, as will be reviewed in this chapter, even though general cognitive deficits have been reported, depressed compared to nondepressed individuals show increased attention and improved memory for mood-congruent material. Concentration difficulties are one of the symptoms listed in the definition of a major depressive episode in the fifth edition of the *Diagnostic and Statistical Manual of Mental Disorders* (American Psychiatric Association, 2013). Depressed patients often report that these difficulties are a particularly disabling feature of depression that often remains after the episode has remitted (Bora, Harrison, Yücel, & Pantelis, 2013). In addition to concentration difficulties, deficits and biases in memory and attention have been reported in depression (for a review, see Trivedi & Greer, 2014). Research on these deficits and biases suggests that they are not only a symptom of a depressive episode but may precede the onset of depression, suggesting that they play a role in vulnerability to this disorder (Goodyer, Herbert, Tamplin, & Altham, 2000). Importantly, cognitive deficits and biases may be linked to the emotional problems that define depression, that is, sustained negative affect and lowered positive affect (Gotlib & Joormann, 2010). In particular, cognitive biases may help explain individual differences in maintenance of negative affect and difficulties with experiencing positive affect, the hallmark features of depression. Mood-congruent biases maintain attention on negative stimuli in the environment, increase accessibility of negative material in memory, and result in negative interpretation of ambiguous material, all of which maintain negative affect and hinder the regulation of negative mood states. Indeed, cognitive processes have been shown to be closely related to individual differences in emotion regulation, and research on working memory in depression has shown important links to emotion regulation ability (see Joormann & Quinn, 2014, for a review).

This finding is important because depression is frequently considered a disorder of emotion dysregulation (e.g., Joormann & Stanton, 2016). Emotion regulation is defined as the ability to manage and modulate one's emotions in response to affective experiences (Gross & Thompson, 2007). It may provide an important bridge to understanding the role cognitive deficits and biases play in the sustained negative affect characteristic of depression. Indeed, emotion regulation deficits have been identified as an important risk factor for and symptom of depression (Durbin & Shafir, 2008), and cognitive processes have been shown to play a critical role in the ability to regulate affective states (see Joormann & Quinn, 2014, for a review). Cognitive reappraisal, for example, has been identified as an important emotion regulation strategy that is closely related to people's ability to exert cognitive control (Oschner & Gross, 2008). Rumination, on the other hand, is a process in which repetitive and perseverative attention is paid to specific thoughts and may reflect a failure of cognitive control in that attention gets stuck on salient but not necessarily goal-relevant aspects of an emotion-eliciting situation (Nolen-Hoeksema, 2000).

As illustrated in these examples, the ability to exert cognitive control and update the contents of working memory may play an important role in understanding individual differences in emotion regulation, which, in turn, may improve our understanding of depression. Cognition and emotion closely interact, and experiencing an affective state will activate mood-congruent thoughts in working memory. The regulation of this affect thus requires updating the content of working memory and exerting control over mood-congruent but goal-irrelevant thoughts so that they can be replaced with goal-relevant information so as to regulate that affective state.

This chapter reviews the current status of work on cognition in depression, with a special focus on working memory and specifically executive control. After providing definitions of the main constructs, reviews are provided focusing on (1) general deficits in working memory and (2) biased processing of emotional information in working memory in depression. The chapter also briefly reviews neurobiological correlates of the identified difficulties and biases and outlines the link of cognitive processing in depression to difficulties in affect, which are the hallmark feature of depression. Ultimately, by identifying depression-specific deficits and biases in working memory and the processing of emotional information, the field may be able to target specific neurocognitive treatments such as cognitive control training (see Koster, Hoorelbeke, Onraedt, Owens, & Derakshan, 2017, for a review) to combat these particularly debilitating symptoms.

WORKING MEMORY

Working memory refers to the cognitive system for temporarily storing, actively maintaining, and manipulating information across a short delay (Cowan, 2008). Working memory is necessary to carry out temporally relevant goal-directed tasks (Miller, 2013). Several different models of the organization of working memory highlight its role in complex cognitive tasks such as learning, reasoning, and comprehension. One widely accepted model of working memory was proposed by Alan Baddeley and Graham Hitch (1974). This three-part model of working memory conceptualizes primary memory (or short-term memory) as existing in a variety of component parts, rather than as one unitary construct. Their model divided working memory into three specific parts: the central executive, which is thought to flexibly redirect new information to aid in necessary processing; the phonological loop, which briefly stores auditory and verbal information; and the visuospatial sketchpad, which is responsible for storing visual information for short-term manipulation.

Most of the work in the realm of psychopathology, specifically depression, focuses on the central executive arm of working memory. Executive functions are defined as "general-purpose control mechanisms that modulate the operation of various cognitive subprocesses and thereby regulate the dynamics of human cognition" (Miyake et al., 2000, p. 50). Many different aspects of executive functions have been proposed, including maintaining information, switching between tasks, inhibiting prepotent behavior, and selecting among different options. Importantly, working memory is capacity-limited, and executive functions play a central role in keeping the limited information that is stored and manipulated in working memory goal-relevant. Updating, shifting, and inhibiting play a critical role in maintaining the goal relevance of the representations stored in working memory, as is outlined in the following ways. Current consensus in the field is that even though there seems to be a general overarching aspect to executive control, different components can be separated. In particular, one frequently cited framework for the structure of executive functions (Friedman et al., 2008; Miyake et al., 2000) is used here to focus on aspects of working memory that go especially awry in major depressive disorder (MDD). This influential model outlines three specific "executive functions" or processes necessary for optimal functioning and successful goal completion: (1) "updating" (adding or removing) of relevant information in working memory, (2) "shifting" between tasks or mental states, and (3) "inhibiting" or suppressing automatic responses to stimuli.

Within their framework, Miyake and colleagues (2000) elaborate on updating the target executive function, to include the "monitoring" of working memory representations (Miyake et al., 2000). This elaboration is particularly important because information within working memory must be continuously monitored and revisited so that newer, more goal-relevant information can replace the older information in working memory that is no longer relevant. Because working memory is capacity limited, it is important that the executive functions continue to update and keep the limited information that can be held in working memory at any given time relevant to current goals. Thus, updating goes beyond passive memory storage by requiring people to actively manipulate information in working memory by both adding and discarding information from working memory on the basis of current task or goal relevance. For example, the n-back task (Kirchner, 1958) is a behavioral paradigm that tests, among other components of working memory, updating ability. In this task, participants are asked to identify whether or not a stimulus (e.g., a number or image) matches that which was shown n (e.g., two) items back, forcing participants to actively decide whether to add or discard information on the basis of its relevance (as instructed by the n).

Distinct from the process of, for example, shifting visual attention, the cognitive shifting outlined by Miyake and colleagues (2000) refers to one's ability to switch, or "shift," attention either between concurrent tasks or information being held in working memory at any given time in order to fulfill a given task at hand. Miyake and associates carefully note that shifting requires more than simply engaging and disengaging with present stimuli or mental sets; shifting also necessitates an ability to overcome the interference of past behavior to perform a new operation. In behavioral paradigms, this skill can be tested in a variety of ways. For example, the Wisconsin Card Sorting Task (WCST; Berg, 1948) is a common measure of shifting that requires new operations (e.g., sorting cards by color instead of by shape) be applied to a set of stimuli several times throughout the task, such that participants are frequently shifting their mental sets on the basis of shifts in rules.

Lastly, within Miyake and collaborators' framework, the process of inhibition refers to the cognitive ability to reject or ignore dominant and automatic responses when necessary to complete a current task or goal. These authors address the idea that the construct of inhibition is used across a variety of contexts and functions, but emphasize that, as it pertains to executive function, it is imperative that inhibition is a deliberate, controlled process (rather than what would otherwise be considered "reactive inhibition"; Miyake et al., 2000). Thus, in common inhibition tasks such as the Stroop Color-Naming Task (Stroop, 1935), individuals are asked to deliberately ignore or suppress dominant and prepotent responses (e.g., naming a color word) in favor of a less automatic response (e.g., stating the color ink the color word was printed in).

The above model of executive functioning provides an essential basis for which to understand many of the various processes involved in working memory. Accordingly, a wealth of research has been done using the aforementioned tasks and various other behavioral paradigms to better understand the cognitive symptoms associated with depression. Frequently reported cognitive symptoms of depression includes difficulty in the ability to concentrate or to think. Indeed, a recent review by Rock, Roiser, Riedel, and Blackwell (2014) examined literature from 24 studies using a working memory psychological test battery (the Cambridge Neuropsychological Test Automated Battery; Robbins et al., 1994) and found that currently depressed individuals performed poorer in tasks that specifically test visuospatial working memory (the Delayed Matching to Sample, Spatial Recognition Memory, and Pattern Recognition Memory tasks).

Findings from Rock and colleagues (2014) corroborate the earlier literature showing a depression-related impairment in the recall of nonaffective, neutral information. For example, Snyder (2013), in a review of the literature on executive functioning deficits in MDD, demonstrates that compared to never-depressed controls, participants with MDD exhibit broad impairments across many areas of executive functioning (e.g., inhibition, shifting, verbal working memory, visuospatial working memory, and verbal fluency). Moreover, when comparing across 112 studies on executive functioning in depression, Snyder found that these executive function deficits in MDD are not better explained by slower processing speed or IQ scores. In an earlier review, Matthews and MacLeod (2005) also found depression-specific biases in selective attention and memory for neutral information.

However, the above findings on executive functioning deficits in depression should be evaluated with caution because, as Burt, Zembar, and Niederehe (1995) noted in her frequently cited meta-analysis, deficits in executive functioning are often seen more frequently for inpatients versus outpatients. Moreover, many of these impairments are also witnessed in comorbid disorders (e.g., schizophrenia, anxiety disorders, substance use). Therefore, these cognitive impairments may be associated with severe psychopathology in general, rather than representing depression-specific impairment (Burt et al., 1995). Indeed, Snyder (2013) also found moderating effects of depression symptom severity, age, and comorbidities in many studies that were reviewed. Likewise, a meta-analysis by McClintock, Husain, Greer, and Cullum (2010) summarized the literature on depression-specific neurocognitive deficits in nonemotional working memory tasks to find widespread heterogeneity in performance on these tasks. These authors also found that working memory deficits were more closely tied to severity of depression as well as a number of hospitalizations than to simply a depression diagnosis.

Taken together, the body of research on nonemotional working memory deficits in depression suggests that they can be observed in large samples of depressed individuals, though they may not be as pervasive as expected, given the frequency with which memory and attentional symptoms are reported. Furthermore, when cognitive deficits are shown in studies, they may reflect other processes (e.g., visuospatial or verbal working memory rather than shifting, inhibition, and updating) that are less closely tied to the cognitive deficits observed in depression. Lastly, certain subgroups (e.g., patients with more severe symptoms and increased hospitalizations) across all psychological disorders are more prone to exhibit general working memory and other cognitive deficits. In this regard, it may be particularly promising to examine the processing of emotional information in depression, as it may be more specific to the disorder itself.

WORKING MEMORY AND EMOTIONAL MATERIAL

In addition to cognitive deficits, depression is characterized by biases in the processing of affective material. Indeed, many studies have reported negative biases in attention, memory, and interpretation, along with a lack of positive biases that is often reported in depressed participants (for a review, see, e.g., Gotlib & Joormann, 2010). Less work has focused on examining working memory for emotional information in depression. Given the link between executive control and emotion regulation, however, this seems a particularly important focus for research on depression, especially in tasks that probe shifting, updating, and inhibition.

To target the first construct within Miyake and colleagues' (2000) framework, studies have used variations of the WCST to assess shifting in the context of emotional material. In an emotional modification of the WCST (the Emotion Card Sort Test), Deveney and Deldin (2006), for example, have probed cognitive shifting in depression by asking participants to sort emotional cards by one dimension (e.g., positive words, neutral words, or negative words) and then to switch sorting by a different dimension upon receiving negative feedback on the current sorting scheme. As compared to a sample of nondepressed participants, Deveney and Deldin found that depressed individuals exhibit less cognitive flexibility when processing negative stimuli. Results of this study suggest that not only are people with MDD attending selectively to negative stimuli, but they are perseverating specifically on negative stimuli far more than participants who are not depressed. Thus, they are less successful at cognitive shifting when presented with negative information.

As outlined by Miyake and colleagues (2000), updating is a second core executive function and represents a process in which working memory representations are monitored and manipulated, to the point that irrelevant information is discarded in favor of newer, goal-relevant stimuli. Research has shown that depressed individuals are more likely to attend to cues in their environment that correspond with negative versus positive or neutral stimuli, even when they are not relevant to their current task or goal (Peckham,

McHugh, & Otto, 2010). As such, it is important to know what happens to the wealth of irrelevant (negative) information that gains access to and occupies working memory space in depression. The Modified Sternberg Task (Joormann & Gotlib, 2008) combines both inhibition and updating with use of emotional information to probe precisely this issue. In this task, participants are asked to memorize a list of both positive and negative words and are then asked to ignore one of the lists. Because participants are then tested on whether a given probe was a member of the relevant list they are supposed to remember, they must both inhibit/expel the list that is no longer relevant and update their current working memory representation to facilitate successful retrieval. Research using this task in MDD and nondepressed samples has shown that individuals with major depression exhibit difficulty removing negative contents of working memory that were once—but are no longer—relevant, and thus show greater intrusion effects for negative words (Joormann & Gotlib, 2008; Li et al., 2018). Thus, not only does negative information make its way into working memory more readily in MDD, but those who are depressed show greater difficulty discarding the irrelevant negative contents of working memory to free capacity for more goal-relevant information.

Similarly, the Emotional n-back (Levens & Gotlib, 2010) is an affective updating task in which participants are presented with a sequence of emotionally valenced stimuli (sad, happy, or neutral faces) and asked to indicate whether the current stimuli match those from n-steps back in the sequence. Indeed, in a study comparing depressed and nondepressed participants, Levens and Gotlib (2010) found that depressed participants integrated (i.e., matched) sad stimuli faster than controls and broke (i.e., unmatched) sets of happy stimuli faster than controls. Thus, these findings suggest that depressed persons are slower to update working memory when removing sad material but disengage with happy stimuli much faster than nondepressed controls. Interestingly, Levens and Gotlib (2015) replicated their previous study in a group of remitted depressed subjects as compared with never-depressed controls. They found that individuals with no current depressive symptoms, but a history of depressive episodes, also disengage from happy material more quickly and from sad material more slowly. These findings suggest that emotional updating deficits in depression may be a trait marker of the disorder rather than tied to a depressed state itself.

The third executive function outlined by Miyake and colleagues (2000), inhibition, is also of interest in depression, as cognitive theories have suggested that ability to ignore as well as shift attention away from negatively valenced stimuli is closely tied to cognitive inhibition (see Gianni, Papadakis, & Pirri, 2012, for a review). One task that probes this core executive function, the Stroop task, requires participants to read the color in which a color word is printed, where the stimulus color is either name congruent or name incongruent. Many studies have shown that participants are susceptible to a "Stroop effect" in which identifying the color of the word takes longer and is more error prone when the name of a color presented is different from the color ink in which it is printed. A variation of this task, the Emotional Stroop Task (Williams, Matthews, & MacLeod, 1996), asks participants to name the color of emotional words, specifically. A wide array of studies have replicated the finding that depressed participants are much slower to respond with the name of a color when shown a depressed word as compared to a nondepressed word (see Epp, Dobson, Dozons, & Frewen, 2012, for a review). This provides evidence for a hypothesis that depressed persons have greater difficulty inhibiting negative information, even when it is not relevant to the task at hand. Kaiser and colleagues (2014) replicated these findings in a functional magnetic resonance imaging (fMRI) study, showing not only that depressive symptoms correlated with poorer performance on the Emotional Stroop Task, but also that brain regions implicated in internally directed attention were activated during exposure to emotional words for persons with greater depressive symptoms. The authors therefore postulated that those experiencing depression may direct thoughts inward when confronted with negative stimuli, subsequently interfering with their ability to complete goal-directed tasks.

Through successful inhibition, less irrelevant information makes its way into working memory to begin with. Furthermore, less irrelevant information is activated within working memory when a given individual is faced with a particular task. The Negative Affective Priming Task (Joormann, 2004) is one such paradigm that assesses an individual's ability to inhibit irrelevant information for the sake of successful task completion. In this task, participants are presented with consecutive pairs of trials (a prime-trial and a test-trial) in which two adjectives are presented (a target and a distractor), along with an instruction to ignore the distractor and respond to the target. In the negative priming condition, distractors in the prime trial and targets in the test trial are words with shared valence, whereas in control conditions, the target words are unrelated. Joormann (2004) found that when comparing MDD and control participants, those who were depressed exhibited reduced inhibition of negative words. Consequently, this points to a depression-specific impairment in inhibiting/ignoring negative emotional material that is irrelevant to the current task.

Another task that engages inhibitory processes, the Flanker Task (Eriksen & Eriksen, 1974), can provide insight into depression-specific difficulties in combating the interference of irrelevant (negative) information. In this task, participants are asked to respond to stimuli that are "flanked," or surrounded by, irrelevant stimuli. Researchers have likewise manipulated this task to study emotional valence, by replacing the standard flanker stimuli with either faces (Fenske & Eastwood, 2006) or words (Zetsche, D'Avanzato, & Joormann, 2012). In both versions of these tasks, participants were tasked with identifying the valence of the stimuli (i.e., negative, positive, or neutral) while ignoring the "flanking" distractors, which were either congruent or incongruent in valence to the target stimulus. Zetsche and colleagues (2012) probed differences between depressed individuals and healthy controls using their emotional Flanker task and found that depression was linked to reduced interference control of irrelevant negative material. Thus, depressed participants were less able to harness the cognitive control necessary to ignore information that was irrelevant to the target stimuli when it was negative in valence. Interestingly, Pe, Vandekerckhove, and Kuppens (2013) conducted follow-up computational analyses to take into account both depression and rumination and showed that rumination accounted for the attentional bias toward negative flankers that was exhibited in depression, suggesting specific links between rumination and inhibition.

Taken together, the body of literature on working memory deficits in depression suggests that working memory deficits in depression are especially pronounced when emotional material is processed. Findings from the above studies represent several depression-related impairments in neurocognitive processes in the face of emotionally valenced material, which, in sum, may help explain how working memory may go awry in this disorder.

LINKING WORKING MEMORY, EXECUTIVE FUNCTIONS, AND DEPRESSION

As previously discussed, the efficient functioning of working memory depends on executive functions to carry out a diverse array of processes, including: limiting the entry of information into working memory (particularly that which is irrelevant and negative), shifting between mental sets as is necessary to complete a given task or goal, and monitoring and updating the contents of working memory by removing information that is no longer relevant to the current task or goal. The work reviewed in the previous section details ways in which these core executive functions are impaired in depression, specifically when emotions (negative vs. positive or neutral) are presented as stimuli. Nevertheless, the question remains as to why biases in emotional processing (as outlined above) are found consistently in MDD samples.

One key link between the described executive function and working memory impairments and depressive symptomatology can be elucidated by examining emotion regulation impairments, which are also hallmark features of MDD. Emotion regulation is defined as the strategic and automatic processes that influence the occurrence, magnitude, and expression of an emotional response (Joormann & Vanderlind, 2014). In individuals with depression as well as in those who have remitted from depression, research has shown an increased tendency to use maladaptive emotion regulation strategies (e.g., rumination), and a decreased tendency to use adaptive emotion regulation strategies (e.g., cognitive reappraisal; Visted, Vøllestad, Nielsen, & Schanche, 2018).

Research by Nolen-Hoeksema (1991) illustrated that an increased tendency to ruminate on negative information, combined with difficulties distracting oneself from such negative material, plays a role in maintaining depressed mood. It is also known that a person's stable tendency to respond to negative life events and negative mood states with ruminative thinking (a ruminative style) is a marker of vulnerability for developing depression. Thus, while inhibitory deficits in the processing of negative information can explain some of the emotional and cognitive symptoms in depression, these same deficits may also represent an important risk factor for developing major depression. Similarly, Yang, Cao, Shields, Teng, and Liu (2017), in a meta-analysis of studies assessing rumination and core executive functions, found negative associations between rumination and both shifting and inhibition abilities. The literature suggests that through rumination, depressed persons not only have too much negative irrelevant information making its way into working memory, but face difficulty switching between mental sets (i.e., away from the negative information) in order to complete necessary goals.

Interestingly, research studies have also shown that even when individuals attempt to use emotion regulation strategies, the efficacy of these strategies in regulating emotional states depends on working memory and executive function capabilities—particularly updating. In their study Pe, Raes, and Kuppens (2013) found that the use of reappraisal was associated with a decrease in arousal toward negative emotions only for individuals with high updating ability, as assessed using the *n*-back task. Likewise, the relationship between negative emotional arousal and rumination was moderated by updating ability within the sample. Thus, especially for depressed individuals who have been shown to engage in decreased cognitive reappraisal and increased rumination, negative affective arousal may be exacerbated by the core executive function impairments in the realm of updating, inhibition, and shifting. On the other hand, this work demonstrates that even for individuals who engage in emotion regulation strategies at normal rates, executive function impairments may preclude them from experiencing the benefits of adaptive emotion regulation (i.e., decreasing negative affect).

Pe and colleagues' (2013) work has important implications for the treatment of depression, as it suggests that cognitive training to bolster executive function and working memory performance can be leveraged in order to target depression-specific impairments in cognition, attention, and emotion regulation.

INSIGHTS FROM NEUROIMAGING

In light of this framework and the aforementioned behavioral task results, there has been increasing interest in understanding what neural mechanisms may underlie the depression-specific cognitive biases shown in emotional working memory tasks.

Matsuo and colleagues (2007) are one of a handful of groups who have studied brain activation in patient populations during working memory tasks. In particular, they focused on an area of the brain called the prefrontal cortex (PFC), which is thought to be integral for successful executive function processes, including working memory, and also for the regulation of mood. Using the *n*-back task in a group of untreated patients with MDD and healthy controls, they found significant hyperactivation in several areas of the PFC (including the dorsolateral cortex and the anterior cingulate cortex) among depressed participants, as compared to never-depressed controls.

These findings replicated earlier work done by Harvey and colleagues (2004) in which MDD participants completing an *n*-back task during fMRI also showed greater activation of the lateral PFC and the anterior cingulate cortex as compared to healthy subjects. In both studies, overall task performance was similar between groups; thus, the authors theorized that MDD might require overrecruitment of PFC to achieve same performance as controls.

Indeed, a recent meta-analysis conducted by Wang and colleagues (2015) examined more broadly the literature on working memory tasks in depression as studied using fMRI. The authors found, across 11 studies, increased activation during working memory tasks in the lateral PFC, as well as a number of surrounding brain regions observed in MDD as compared with controls. For studies where task performance was matched across groups, interestingly, the authors observed hyperactivation only in the PFC. Thus, this study likewise points to abnormal neural engagement in the PFC during working memory tasks, which may reflect compensatory neural processes for patients with MDD to match the behavioral performance of never-depressed individuals.

Another recent fMRI study by Yüksel and colleagues (2018) examined brain activation during an *n*-back working memory task among healthy controls, first-depressed-episode subjects, and recurrent-depressed-episode subjects. The authors found group differences in frontoparietal regions but interestingly showed only differences between the recurrent-depressive-episode subjects and the other two groups. Notably, the first-depressive-episode and healthy control individuals showed similar patterns of brain activity. This suggests that neurobiological differences may also arise over the course of major depression, worsening with subsequent episodes.

Though further work is necessary to gain a better understanding of what other brain regions might contribute to abnormal processing of emotional material (which is the hallmark of depression), these studies have come closer to building a biological framework and to identifying the neural networks involved. In sum, the PFC seems to be highly implicated in emotional processing biases. In addition, executive function deficits and changes in prefrontal cortex activation over the course of the illness may be an important target for future neuroimaging research in depression.

CONCLUSIONS AND FUTURE DIRECTIONS

A better understanding of the roles executive functions and working memory play in depression-specific emotional and cognitive impairments is imperative for building a neurocognitive model of depression that can help to identify targets of treatments as well as risk and vulnerability factors for future development of the disorder. Based on this framework, treatments such as cognitive control therapy (e.g., Koster, Hoorelbeke, Onraedt, Owens, & Derakshan, 2017) have been developed to intervene in cognitive processing at an early stage, with hopes of breaking the cycle of maladaptive emotion regulation strategies that both lead to and perpetuate sustained negative affect.

One notable limitation of this work, however, is the inability to make assumptions about the causal direction of executive function and working memory impairments on depressive symptomatology. Although some studies show working memory impairments that persist throughout remission of a major depressive episodes (e.g., Bartova et al., 2015), others identify working memory impairments as vulnerability markers that proceed upon the onset of a depressive episode (e.g., Huang-Pollock, Shapiro, Falloway-Long, & Weigard, 2016). Thus, it still remains unknown whether depression causes executive function deficits or whether executive function deficits contribute to depression (or both).

Longitudinal work to better uncover the directionality with which executive function deficits co-occur is necessary to gain a better understanding of the temporal and causal nature of these impairments. Similarly, further research to uncover the neural circuitry of "the emotional brain"—that is, how neural circuits that execute working memory interact with/relate to neural circuits involved in emotion regulation—will be useful in creating a more holistic biological model of neurocognition in depression. Lastly, with the promise of cognitive control training, and the important role that shifting, inhibition, and updating each individually play in the larger picture of cognitive deficits in depression, further training targeting these aspects individually may be useful in tailoring treatments specifically and individually to one's neurocognitive needs.

REFERENCES

American Psychiatric Association. (2013). *Diagnostic and statistical manual of mental disorders* (5th ed.). Arlington, VA: Author.

Baddeley, A. D., & Hitch, G. (1974). Working memory. In G. H. Bower (Ed.), *The psychology of learning and motivation: Advances in research and theory* (Vol. 8, pp. 47–89). New York: Academic Press.

Bartova, L., Meyer, B. M., Diers, K., Rabl, U., Scharinger, C., Popovic, A., et al. (2015). Reduced default mode network suppression during a working memory task in remitted major depression. *Journal of Psychiatric Research, 64*(C), 9–18.

Berg, E. A. (1948). A simple objective technique for measuring flexibility in thinking. *Journal of General Psychology, 39*, 15–22.

Bora, E., Harrison, B. J., Yücel, M., & Pantelis, C. (2013). Cognitive impairment in euthymic major depressive disorder: A meta-analysis. *Psychological Medicine, 43*(10), 2017–2026.

Burt, D. B., Zembar, M. J., & Niederehe, G., (1995). Depression and memory impairment: A meta-analysis of the association, its pattern, and specificity. *Psychological Bulletin, 117* (2), 285–305.

Cowan, N. (2008). What are the differences between long-term, short-term and working memory? *Progressive Brain Research, 169*, 323–338.

Deveney, C. M., & Deldin, P. J. (2006). A preliminary investigation of cognitive flexibility for emotional information in major depressive disorder and non-psychiatric controls. *Emotion, 6*(3), 429–437.

Durbin, C. E., & Shafir, D. M. (2008). Emotion regulation and risk for depression. In J. R. Z. Abela & B. L. Hankin (Eds.), *Handbook of depression in children and adolescents* (pp. 149–176). New York: Guilford Press.

Epp, A. M., Dobson, K. S., Dozois, D. J. A., & Frewen, P. A. (2012). A systematic meta-analysis of the Stroop task in depression. *Clinical Psychology Review, 32*(4), 316–328.

Eriksen, B. A., & Eriksen, C. W. (1974). Effects of noise letters upon identification of a target letter in a non-search task. *Perception and Psychophysics, 16*, 143–149.

Fenske, M. J., & Eastwood, J. D. (2006). Affective influences of selective attention. *Current Directions in Psychological Science, 15*(6), 312–316.

Friedman, N. P., Miyake, A., Young, S. E., DeFries, J. C., Corley, R. P., & Hewitt, J. K. (2008). Individual differences in executive functions are almost entirely genetic in origin. *Journal of Experimental Psychology: General, 137*, 201–225.

Gianni, M., Papadakis, P., & Pirri, F. (2012). *Shifting and inhibition in cognitive control.* Paper presented at the IROS 2012 Workshop on Cognitive Neuroscience Robotics, Algarve, Portugal.

Goodyer, I. M., Herbert, J., Tamplin, A., & Altham, P. M. E. (2000). First-episode major depression in adolescents. (2000). *British Journal of Psychiatry, 176*, 142–149.

Gotlib, I. H., & Joormann, J. (2010). Cognition and depression: Current status and future directions. *Annual Review of Clinical Psychology, 6*(1), 285–312.

Gross, J. J., & Thompson, R. A. (2007). Emotion regulation: Conceptual foundations. In J. J. Gross (Ed.), *Handbook of emotion regulation* (pp. 3–24). New York: Guilford Press.

Harvey, P. O., Le Bastard, G., Pochon, J. B., Levy, R., Allilaire, J. F., Dubois, B., et al. (2004). Executive functions and updating of the contents of working memory in unipolar depression. *Journal of Psychiatric Research, 38*, 567–576.

Huang-Pollock, C., Shapiro, Z., Galloway-Long, H., & Weigard, A. (2016). Is poor working memory a transdiagnostic risk factor for psychopathology? *Journal of Abnormal Child Psychology, 45*(8), 1477–1490.

Joormann, J. (2004). Attentional bias in dysphoria: The role of inhibitory processes. *Cognition and Emotion, 18*, 125–147.

Joormann, J., & Gotlib, I. H. (2008). Updating the contents of working memory in depression: Interference from irrelevant negative material. *Journal of Abnormal Psychology, 117*(1), 182.

Joormann, J., & Quinn, M. E. (2014). Cognitive processes and emotion regulation in depression. *Depression and Anxiety, 31*(4), 308–315.

Joormann, J., & Stanton, C. H. (2016). Examining emotion regulation in depression: A review and future directions. *Behaviour Research and Therapy, 86*, 35–49.

Joormann, J., & Vanderlind, W. M. (2014). Emotion regulation in depression. *Clinical Psychological Science, 2*(4), 402–421.

Kaiser, R. H., Andrews-Hanna, J. R., Spielberg, J. M., Warren, S. L., Sutton, B. P., Miller, G. A., et al. (2014). Distracted and down: Neural mechanisms of affective interference in subclinical depression. *Social Cognitive and Affective Neuroscience, 10*(5), 654–663.

Kirchner, W. K. (1958). Age differences in short-term retention of rapidly changing information. *Journal of Experimental Psychology, 55*(4), 352–358.

Koster, E. H. W., Hoorelbeke, K., Onraedt, T., Owens, M., & Derakshan, N. (2017). Cognitive control interventions for depression: A systematic review of findings from training studies. *Clinical Psychology Review, 53*, 79–92.

Levens, S. M., & Gotlib, I. H. (2010). Updating positive and negative stimuli in working memory in depression. *Journal of Experimental Psychology: General, 139*(4), 654–664.

Levens, S. M., & Gotlib, I. H. (2015). Updating emotional content in recovered depressed individuals: Evaluating deficits in emotion processing following a depressive episode. *Journal of Behavior Therapy and Experimental Psychiatry, 48*, 156–163.

Li, M., Feng, L., Xingwang, L., Zhang, M., Fu, B., Wang, G., et al. (2018). Emotional working memory in patients with major depressive disorder. *Journal of International Medical Research, 46*(5), 1734–1746.

Matsuo, K., Glahn, D. C., Peluso, M. A. M., Hatch, J. P., Monkul, E. S., Najt, P., et al. (2007). Prefrontal hyperactivation during working memory task in untreated individuals with major depressive disorder. *Molecular Psychiatry, 12*(2), 158–166.

Matthews, A., & MacLeod, C. M. (2005). Cognitive vulnerability to emotional disorders. *Annual Review of Clinical Psychology, 1*, 167–195.

McClintock, S. A., Husain, M. M., Greer, T. L., & Cullum, C. M. (2010). Association between depression severity and neurocognitive function in major depressive disorder: A review and synthesis. *Neuropsychology, 24*, 9–34.

Miller, E. K. (2013). The "working" of working memory. *Dialogues in Clinical Neuroscience, 15*(4), 411–418.

Miyake, A., Friedman, N. P., Emerson, M. J., Witzki, A. H., Howerter, A., & Wager, T. D. (2000). The unity and diversity of executive functions and their contributions to complex "frontal lobe" tasks: A latent variable analysis. *Cognitive Psychology, 41*(1), 49–100.

Nolen-Hoeksema, S. (1991). Responses to depression and their effects on the duration of depressive episodes. *Journal of Abnormal Psychology, 100*(4), 569–582.

Nolen-Hoeksema, S. (2000). The role of rumination in depressive disorders and mixed anxiety/depressive symptoms. *Journal of Abnormal Psychology, 109*, 504–511.

Ochsner, K. N., & Gross, J. J. (2008). Cognitive emotion regulation: Insights from social cognitive and affective neuroscience. *Current Directions in Psychological Science, 17*(2), 153–158.

Pe, M. L., Raes, F., & Kuppens, P. (2013). The cognitive building blocks of emotion regulation: ability to update working memory moderates the efficacy of rumination and reappraisal on emotion. *PLoS one, 8*(7), 1–12.

Pe, M. L., Vandekerckhove, J., & Kuppens, P. (2013). A diffusion model account of the relationship between the emotional flanker task and rumination and depression. *Emotion, 13*(4), 739–747.

Peckham, A. D., McHugh, R. K., & Otto, W. M. (2010). A meta-analysis of the magnitude of biased attention in depression. *Depression and Anxiety, 27*, 1135–1142.

Robbins, T. W., James, M., Owen, A. M., Sahakian, B. J., McInnes, L., & Rabbitt, P. (1994). Cambridge Neuropsychological Test Automated Battery (CANTAB): A factor analytic study of a large sample of normal elderly volunteers. *Dementia and Geriatric Cognitive Disorders, 5*(5), 266–281.

Rock, P. L., Roiser, J. P., Riedel, W. J., & Blackwell, A. D. (2014). Cognitive impairment in depression: A systematic review and meta-analysis. *Psychological Medicine, 44*(10), 2029–2040.

Snyder, H. R. (2013). Major depressive disorder is associated with broad impairments on neuropsychological measures of executive function: A meta-analysis and review. *Psychological Bulletin, 139*(1), 81–132.

Stroop, J. R. (1935). Studies of interference in serial verbal reactions. *Journal of Experimental Psychology. 18*(6), 643–662.

Trivedi, M. H., & Greer, T. L. (2014). Cognitive dysfunction in unipolar depression: Implications for treatment. *Journal of Affective Disorders, 152–154*(C), 19–27.

Visted, E., Vøllestad, J., Nielsen, M. B., & Schanche, E. (2018). Emotion regulation in current and remitted depression: A systematic review and meta-analysis. *Frontiers in Psychology, 9*(756), 1–20.

Wang, X. L., Du, M. Y., Chen, T. L., Chen, Z. Q., Huang, X. Q., Luo, Y., et al. (2015). Neural correlates during working memory processing in major depressive disorder. *Progress in Neuropsychopharmacology and Biological Psychiatry, 56,* 101–108.

Williams, J. M. G., Mathews, A., & MacLeod, C. (1996). The Emotional Stroop Task and psychopathology. *Psychological Bulletin, 120*(1), 3.

Yang, Y., Cao, S., Shields, G. S., Teng, Z., & Liu, Y. (2017). The relationships between rumination and core executive functions: A meta-analysis. *Depression and Anxiety, 34*(1), 37–50.

Yüksel, D., Dietsche, B., Konrad, C., Dannlowski, U., Kircher, T., & Krug, A. (2018). Neural correlates of working memory in first episode and recurrent depression: An fMRI study. *Progress in Neuro-Psychopharmacology and Biological Psychiatry, 84,* 39–49.

Zetsche, U., D'Avanzato, C., & Joormann, J. (2012). Depression and rumination: Relation to components of inhibition. *Cognition and Emotion, 26*(4), 758–767.

CHAPTER 9

Executive Functions in Depression

Muzaffer Kaser
Barbara J. Sahakian

Patients with major depressive disorder (MDD) and/or significant depressive symptoms often report difficulties in a variety of cognitive domains. Available evidence (Snyder, 2013; Zakzanis, Leach, & Kaplan, 1998) pointed out that higher-order cognitive functions (executive functioning) along with memory are mostly affected. The description of executive functioning is often an umbrella term that would include various cognitive abilities that overlap to a certain extent. In neuropsychological terms, the following domains have been used within the broad definition of executive functions, including cognitive control, planning, cognitive flexibility, response inhibition, problem solving, verbal fluency, and working memory (see Table 9.1). There is no universal consensus about what cognitive domains are regarded as executive functions. The term generally refers to the higher-order cognitive abilities that help the person to deviate from stereotypic behavior locked to the environmental stimuli (Mesulam, 2002). The "higher-order" cognition has a connotation to the hierarchically organized brain systems. Specifically, the prefrontal cortex is invariably associated with executive tasks and is the center of control over other neural structures.

EXECUTIVE FUNCTIONING IN DEPRESSION

At the neuropsychological level, numerous case-control studies with patients with MDD consistently reported poorer performance on executive function tests (e.g., Wisconsin Card Sorting Test, Tower of London Test; Elliott, 1998). There are also a few studies that found no executive deficits in adults with depression (e.g., Grant, Thase, & Sweeney, 2001). In the literature, the assessment methods, definition of executive functions, and the sample size and characteristics varied substantially. Some neuropsychological tests have ceiling effects. Therefore, meta-analytic evidence may provide a more reliable account of depression-related executive function deficits. In a comprehensive review and

TABLE 9.1. Overview of Executive Functions and Relevant Neuropsychological Tests

Executive functions	Neuropsychological tests	References
Planning	Tower of London Test, CANTAB One Touch Stockings test	Owen et al. (1995); Shallice (1982)
Cognitive flexibility	Wisconsin Card Sorting Test, CANTAB ID/ED Set Shifting test	Heaton (1981); Owen et al. (1991)
Decision making	Iowa Gambling Task, CANTAB Cambridge Gambling task	Bechara et al. (1994); Rogers et al. (1999)
Response inhibition	CANTAB Stop Signal Reaction Time task, Stroop Test	Stroop (1935); Turner et al. (2003)
Verbal fluency	Semantic fluency/category fluency	Abwender et al. (2001)
Working memory	Backward Digit Span, *n*-back, CANTAB Spatial Working Memory task	Owen et al. (1990); Wechsler (1981)

meta-analysis (Snyder, 2013), patients with depression had impairments in a number of executive functions, with effect sizes that ranged between small and large (Cohen's d = 0.32–0.97). A striking finding from that meta-analysis was that healthy controls had better performance than patients with depression across all executive function tests. Of all the 113 studies investigated, only a few studies with relatively small samples reported no difference in executive abilities between adult healthy controls and those with depression. Pooled evidence clearly indicated that executive dysfunction in depression was a consistent finding. The results supported the view that patients with depression had impairments in common components of executive function (Miyake et al., 2000). Importantly, slower processing speed, lack of concentration, and differences in IQ and education levels did not account for or impact the results. However, severity of depressive symptoms and use of psychotropic medications were associated with greater executive dysfunction.

Despite the clear presence of executive function cognitive impairments, the degree of such impairments and the extent to which they can be reversed following remission remains to be determined. Depression is by definition a clinically heterogeneous condition (Chen, Eaton, Gallo, & Nestadt, 2000; Fried, 2017). Many different neuropsychological tests were used to assess executive functions in depression. There is a lack of consensus as to which tests tap into which subdomains of executive function and how reliably we can draw comparisons between reports (Jurado & Rosselli, 2007). The variance in the psychometric properties of the tests can also affect sensitivity to change (Porter, Bourke, & Gallagher, 2007). When accounting for interaction between cognition and clinical features, there is an inherent need to control for many confounders. For instance, the results from a young to mid-adult sample with first-episode depression may differ from results from older patients or patients with repeated depressive episodes. Late-life depression is regarded as a possible signal for dementia, and evidence has suggested that while depression does not increase the incidence of dementia, it can speed up the neurodegenerative process (Butters et al., 2008). In a sample of elderly depressed patients, memory was mildly impaired and recovered with antidepressant treatment, while there were residual impairments in tests for planning ability (Beats, Sahakian, & Levy, 1996). A systematic review showed that patients with late-life depression had poorer performance in executive function and processing speed domains relative to their nonelderly counterparts, whereas the patients across those two age groups had similar impairments in episodic memory (Hermann, Goodwin, & Ebmeier, 2007). In a study that investigated elderly (>61 years) and working-age adults (20–60 years) with depression reported more pronounced deficits in executive function in the elderly (Lockwood, Alexopoulos, & van Gorp, 2002). Other studies reported that younger patients outperformed elderly depressed patients only in the processing speed domain, while there was no difference between two groups in memory performance and verbal fluency (Tarbuck & Paykel, 1995). Whether the changes in processing speed were an aging effect or an additive effect of depression and age remains to be elucidated. Residual cognitive impairments into remission may represent a major challenge in managing mood disorders in the elderly (Rubinsztein, Sahakian, & O'Brien, 2019).

EXECUTIVE FUNCTION AND DEPRESSION SEVERITY

In terms of depression severity, while there is mixed evidence (Keilp et al., 2018; McClintock, Husain, Greer, & Cullum, 2010), some studies suggest that patients with more severe depressive symptoms tend to have more marked executive dysfunction (Gohier et al., 2009; McCall & Dunn, 2003), whereas young, unmedicated, mildly depressed patients may show minimal executive function problems (Grant et al., 2001). The evidence was mixed in regards to which cognitive functions (episodic memory or executive functions) were more affected by the severity of the depressive disease (Cataldo, Nobile, Lorusso, Battaglia, & Molteni, 2005; Naismith et al., 2003). Since correlation analysis was the main method used to examine the impact, the role of confounding effects (e.g., hospitalization, age, medication) may not have been addressed properly. A meta-analysis of the studies showed a statistically significant association between executive function, processing speed, and episodic memory and depression severity (McDermott & Ebmeier, 2009). An important aspect is that depression severity cannot be used as a proxy for general cognitive slowing. Indeed, several studies were able to tease apart processing speed and executive dysfunction and concluded that diminished cognitive effort could not explain the extent of executive function deficits in depression (Hammar et al., 2011).

The confounding effects of mood should be taken into consideration when evaluating the cognitive function results, especially in antidepressant treatment studies. The marked heterogeneity in cognitive functions for patients with MDD should also be noted (Hammar & Ardal, 2009). Additionally, the use of insensitive or broad cognitive measures may be unable to detect cognitive impairments. A majority of tests may measure a narrow range of executive functions, but some tests can provide various outcome measures as indices of different executive skills (Jurado & Rosselli, 2007). One example is the Cambridge Neuropsychological Test Automated Battery (CANTAB) One Touch Stockings (OTS) test

(Owen et al., 1995). This cognitive test was based on the widely used Tower of London test (Shallice, 1982) and modified from the Stockings of Cambridge test. The CANTAB OTS is regarded as a test of executive function that measures both spatial planning and working memory. In this task, participants are asked to think about how they can achieve the target pattern with the fewest number of moves. The test provides three primary outcome measures, including the number of corrections (error monitoring), latency (planning), and total number of problems solved within the required number of minimum moves (execution, accuracy; Elliott, 1998). Observations on the performance of patients with depression on the OTS showed that the emotional responses to errors may also be at play (Elliott et al., 1996). A key observation was that depressed patients' performance dipped after they noticed they made a mistake (Beats et al., 1996). Up until the error, the patients were able to respond correctly as the healthy controls, but the response to mistake—also termed the "catastrophic response"—led to a rapid deterioration in performance. The interface between emotional states and cognitive control has been a distinct focus in relation to the neuropsychology of depression. The term *affective cognition* was proposed to conceptualize the dynamic interaction between emotional and cognitive processes (Elliott, Zahn, Deakin, & Anderson, 2011). The link between affective states and executive control is detailed within a relatively recent cognitive neuropsychological model (see Figure 9.1; Roiser, Elliott, & Sahakian, 2012).

FACTORS THAT MAY ACCOUNT FOR EXECUTIVE DYSFUNCTION IN DEPRESSION

The use of standardized neurocognitive testing measures can provide valuable evidence regarding the association between depression and executive function. In a meta-analysis (Rock, Roiser, Riedel, & Blackwell, 2014), the authors included only the studies that used tests from the CANTAB. They reported that patients with current and remitted depression had moderate impairments on executive function tasks. In subgroup analysis, medicated and unmedicated patients had similar levels of executive impairments. The impact of depressive symptoms on neurocognitive function was unassessed in this meta-analysis, but the findings from studies on remitted depression support the view that cognitive impairments are not simply an extension of low mood. Therefore, cognitive function should be a target for treatment in depression (National Academies of Sciences, Engineering, & Medicine, 2015).

The question of whether the executive dysfunction is mood-state-dependent is complex and multilayered. First, a simple dichotomy of state versus trait is not applicable in a common and heterogeneous condition like MDD. One needs to consider vulnerability factors before the depressive onset and the variable outcomes throughout the MDD course. Heritability estimates for depression are around 30–40%, and while genetic mechanisms may play a role in the development of cognitive impairments, other factors also contribute (Naismith et al., 2003). Some authors proposed a more complex endophenotype approach (Hasler, Drevets, Manji, & Charney, 2004) that may be dissected in several emotional and cognitive features that pertain to some executive functions (e.g., inspection time; Tsourtos,

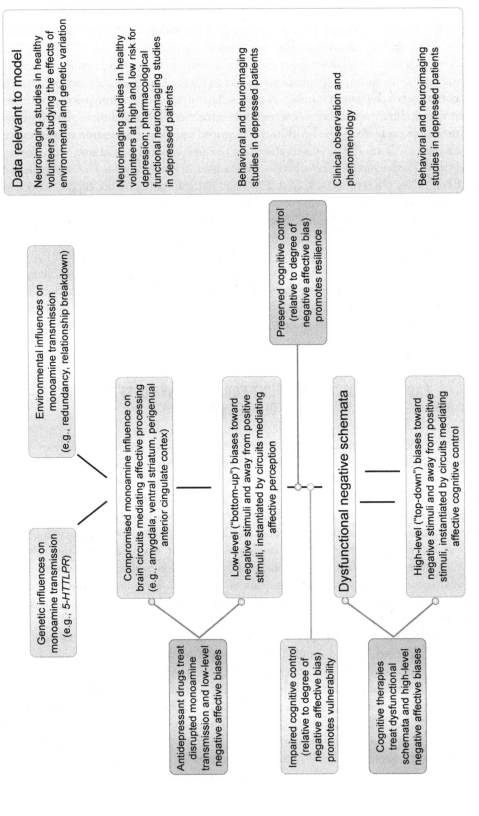

FIGURE 9.1. A cognitive neuropsychological model of depression (Roiser et al., 2012).

Thompson, & Stough, 2002). The evidence on genetic vulnerability in depressed mood should be interpreted with caution, as a recent critique suggested that most genetic studies lack sufficient statistical power (Culverhouse et al., 2018).

From a developmental point of view, it would be invaluable to know if the cognitive impairments were present prior to or at the same time as the onset of depression. There is a paucity of developmental neurocognitive research that has examined the trajectory of the depressive course from childhood to adolescence and then adulthood. Several studies found comparable executive function to controls at the onset of depression (Grant et al., 2001; Kyte, Goodyer, & Sahakian, 2005), whereas some studies reported impairments in patients between the ages of 13 and 25 (Baune, Czira, Smith, Mitchell, & Sinnomon, 2012).

The link between executive dysfunction and repeated depressive episodes is more solidly established. A line of research suggests that depressive episodes have a cumulative negative impact on cognitive abilities, including memory and executive function (Gorwood, Corruble, Falissard, & Goodwin, 2008). Patients with MDD and executive dysfunction at the time of admission to hospital have been found to have poorer psychosocial function at follow-up evaluation (Jaeger, Berns, Uzelac, & Davis-Conway, 2006). Cognitive impairments can persist during remission (Conradi, Ormel, & de Jonge, 2011). In a follow-up study, the impairments in a response inhibition task persisted at 6 months after the patients' depressive symptoms improved (Hammar et al., 2010). The meta-analytic evidence showed that patients in remission had cognitive impairments and that executive function was the most significantly impaired domain (Bora, Harrison, Yücel, & Pantelis, 2013). The effects were independent from major depressive episode duration, number of depressive episodes, presence of residual depressive symptoms, age, or gender. The conclusions on cognitive dysfunction in remitted depression were similar to those reported by another meta-analysis (Rock et al., 2014). Greater effect sizes were evident for executive function than for memory functions in remitted patients. The main clinical implication is that executive dysfunction in remission could be a treatment target (Kaser, Zaman, & Sahakian, 2017).

An important factor relative to the persistence of executive dysfunction is that most antidepressant treatments do not specifically improve cognitive functions (Keefe et al., 2014; Shilyansky et al., 2016). More recently, vortioxetine became the first antidepressant medication with U.S. Food and Drug Administration recognition for improving cognitive performance (see Suarez & Martinez-Kaigi, Chapter 14, this volume, for additional information on the cognitive effects of antidepressant medications). The approval was based on an 8-week study that showed vortioxetine's beneficial effects on processing speed (Mahableshwarkar, Zajecka, Jacobson, Chen, & Keefe, 2015; McIntyre, Lophaven, & Olsen, 2014). The effect sizes for other standard executive function measures (e.g., Trail Making Test Part B, Stroop) were small. The researchers used path analysis to suggest that the improved processing speed effects were independent from positive effects on mood. However, the European Medicines Agency report indicated that the study's reporting bias and lack of an active comparator made it difficult to distinguish the effects of mood on cognition (Koesters, Ostuzzi, Guaiana, Breilmann, & Barbui, 2017). Interestingly, a recent study showed that vortioxetine had no positive effects on cognitive functions in patients with remitted depression (Nierenberg, Loft, & Olsen, 2019).

EXECUTIVE FUNCTION AND WORKING MEMORY

Impairment of working memory, a domain that is thought to be within the executive function framework, is one of the most consistent findings from case-control studies in depression (see Rutherford & Joormann, Chapter 8, this volume, for comprehensive information on working memory). A meta-analysis reported a medium effect (Cohen's $d = 0.54$) on the magnitude of working memory deficits in depression (Rock et al., 2014). Like other higher-order cognitive functions, working memory spans several other abilities. A general definition of working memory is the cognitive skill needed to keep information for a brief period in order to execute a task successfully. A neuropsychological model of working memory is composed of two elements: the central executive and memory maintenance (Baddeley, 1996). Studies of those elements showed that depressed patients had impairments in both, but the effect on the central executive was more pronounced. The role of the prefrontal cortex and its connections is well documented in working memory experiments in humans as well as in nonhuman primates and rodents. (Dalley, Cardinal, & Robbins, 2004; Goldman-Rakic, 1995). Those circuits are also implicated in cognitive deficits in depression. A better understanding of the neural circuits mediating the working memory deficits in depression would help develop targeted treatments.

Working memory is reliably measured by the CANTAB Spatial Working Memory (SWM) task. CANTAB SWM tests the participant's ability to retain spatial information and use remembered items in working memory. The participant is asked to find the correct spatial location of colored squares among several boxes by elimination. The task gets more challenging as the number of boxes is gradually increased. The classical version has up to 8 boxes, while the new version has as many as 12 boxes. Once a token is found under a box, no further tokens are hidden under that particular box (Robbins et al., 1998). Outcome measures include the number of errors while searching for the boxes (up to 8–12 boxes, depending on the version) and a measure of strategy (Sahakian et al., 1988). Strategy measure reflects the search pattern of participants who followed a repetitive sequence to approach the task (Owen, Downes, Sahakian, Polkey, & Robbins, 1990). Participants with a higher number of sequences beginning with different boxes would have a high score, indicating less skillful use of strategy. In one study, during the execution stage of the task, participants showed increased ventrolateral prefrontal activity while spatial searches were associated with mid-dorsolateral prefrontal cortex activation (Owen, Evans, & Petrides, 1996). CANTAB SWM performance is sensitive to pharmacological modulation with dopaminergic agents (Mehta et al., 2000) via activation of the dorsolateral prefrontal cortex.

HOT AND COLD EXECUTIVE FUNCTIONS

Cognitive processes in depression can be conceptualised as "hot" (linked to emotional processes) or "cold" (information processing in the absence of emotional influence; Roiser & Sahakian, 2013). Conventional neuropsychological testing tools that showed deficits in patients with depression are usually regarded as measures of cold cognitive processes where the stimuli required are neutral (e.g., Trail Making Test, Wisconsin Card Sorting

Test). Brain circuits that mediate cold executive functions are complex and involve critical structures such as the dorsolateral prefrontal cortex, anterior cingulate cortex, and hippocampus. As described in the context of affective cognition, some executive processes are linked to emotions and are described as "hot executive functions." Altered emotions in the context of depressed mood affect top-down and bottom-up information processes that eventually lead to deficits in executive functions. One example is the CANTAB Affective Go/No-Go test, where the participants are required to respond to words with one type of emotional valence (negative or positive) while controlling their urge to respond to other type of valence. Patients with depression respond more quickly to the negative words in this test that demonstrates the impact of negative emotional bias on decisions (Murphy, Michael, Robbins, & Sahakian, 2003).

Cognitive control over emotion-laden cognitive processes (i.e., hot cognition) is mediated by top-down executive functions (Roiser et al., 2012). Patients with depression tend to show negative biases to emotional stimuli. That is, they tend to respond at a much quicker rate to negative words or faces relative to positive or neutral ones (Harmer et al., 2011; Robinson & Sahakian, 2013). When cognitive control is suboptimal, the negative biases can lead to maintenance of the depressive state. Alternatively, bottom-up processes may interfere with optimal performance on executive function tasks. For example, patients with depression had impairments on a planning task that was linked to a catastrophic response to negative feedback (Elliott, Sahakian, Herrod, Robbins, & Paykel, 1997). In the conditions where the participant was asked to make selections based on winning or losing, individuals with depression demonstrated sensitivity to losses and any negative feedback (Murphy et al., 2003). Similar patterns of cognitive control impairments on negative biases were reported in an adolescent sample with first episode depression (Kyte et al., 2005).

Reciprocal links between factors involved in depressive state were formulated in a cognitive neuropsychological model of depression (see Figure 9.1). According to this model, dysfunctional executive control contributes to negative attentional biases, which in turn reinforce the depressive symptoms. The model accounts for complexities such as genetic influences and adverse life events, as well as positive factors (e.g., resilience). Psychological treatments (e.g., cognitive-behavioral therapy) or the role of pharmacological interventions in the model help to mitigate negative biases through reinforcement of the cognitive control that eventually leads to remission of the depressive state. At the neural level, interference by emotional stimuli on cognitive control was demonstrated in functional magnetic resonance imaging studies. Patients with depression showed increased prefrontal activation when they did not need to attend to emotional cues (Dichter, Felder, & Smoski, 2009). Active efforts to dismiss emotional stimuli led to decreased prefrontal responses, which suggested that there was a role for executive function impairments (Fales et al., 2008). The anterior cingulate cortex (ACC) is also implicated in error monitoring and is regarded as a critical juncture between emotional processing and higher-order control. Patients with depression have been found to have altered activation in the ACC (Elliott, Rubinsztein, Sahakian, & Dolan, 2002). Executive function impairments have been associated with dysfunctional neural circuits, mainly in the prefrontal areas. A proposed model emphasizes the roles of different prefrontal systems (ventral and dorsal) in the pathophysiology of MDD (Mayberg et al., 1997; Phillips, Drevets, Rauch, & Lane, 2003). According to this model, the ventral prefrontal cortex and its connections with the brainstem, paralimbic, and subcortical regions comprise the ventral system that is linked to the vegetative symptoms of depression. The dorsal system involves the dorsolateral prefrontal cortex (DLPFC) and midline brain structures (e.g., anterior cingulate) that mediate the cognitive features of depression. Further evidence from neuroimaging studies shows that DLPFC is recruited in response to reappraisal of negative affect (Phan et al., 2005), suggesting that DLPFC dysfunction in depression may be related to a broader effect in addition to a lack of cognitive control (Koenigs & Grafman, 2009).

NEUROTRANSMITTERS AND EXECUTIVE FUNCTION

Neurochemical modulation of executive functions can be traced to prefrontal and striatal neurocircuits. Dopamine is the key neurotransmitter regarding working memory and executive functions (Robbins, 2000). As such, dopamine agonists or antagonists could improve or impair spatial working memory functions (Mehta, Sahakian, McKenna, & Robbins, 1999; Müller, von Cramon, & Pollmann, 1998), respectively. However, the direction of the association is nonlinear. For instance, methylphenidate that acts on dopamine transporter protein facilitates performance on easier versions but worsens performance on challenging versions of a planning task (Elliott, Sahakian, Matthews, et al., 1997). The modulation of striatal dopamine and cortical dopamine by methylphenidate may explain the discrepancy in executive function performance. Specifically, the effects on striatal dopamine will produce quicker reaction times at the cost of poorer accuracy that is mediated by cortical dopamine.

Catecholamine levels and receptors are dynamic in the crucial brain areas for cognition, and correspondingly executive processes are particularly sensitive to multiple factors, including stress, arousal, and motivation (Robbins & Arnsten, 2009). Increased stress levels may impair prefrontal functions through activation of low-affinity noradrenergic receptors (Arnsten, 2000). Executive function impairments induced by acute stress can be reversed by glucocorticoid receptor blocking agents (Butts, Weinberg, Young, & Phillips, 2011). Arousal can lead to increased levels of noradrenaline, and prefrontal functions are optimal at moderate levels of noradrenaline through activation of postsynaptic high-affinity alpha 2 receptors. Understanding the U-shaped effect of dopaminergic function in prefrontal–striatal areas would be important to investigate executive functions as treatment targets.

Another neurotransmitter that has been implicated in executive functions is serotonin (Skandali et al., 2018). In experimental models, decreased serotonin (via tryptophan depletion) led to cognitive inflexibility (Clarke, Dalley, Crofts, Robbins, & Roberts, 2004) and impairments in response inhibition (Hayward, Goodwin, Cowen, & Harmer, 2005). However, some effects may be indirect and possibly via glutamatergic and GABA-ergic stimulation (Pehrson et al., 2015). Serotonergic medication was shown to have a positive impact on executive processes such as impulse control (Skandali et al., 2018). The proposed mechanism is that serotonergic modulation can alter stress-induced sensitization, possibly at the level of postsynaptic serotonin receptors (e.g., 5-HT1A) (McAllister-Williams, Ferrier, & Young, 1998; Watanabe, Sakai, McEwen, & Mendelson, 1993). Stress effects can also impair 5-HT1A activity, which can eventually lead to hypothalamus–pituatry–adrenal system dysregulation and neuropsychological impairment.

A more general sensitivity to external stimuli might influence diverse outcomes in emotional and cognitive context. The role of serotonin transporter protein polymorphism on emotional circuits was also proposed in the context of stress vulnerability (Borg et al., 2009). However, the literature on serotonin transporter protein and depression should be read with caution based on a recent meta-analysis that suggested no interaction between the short allele of the serotonin transporter gene and development of depression (Culverhouse et al., 2018). The variable effects of serotonin on emotional circuits and higher-order cognitive systems may be an underlying factor showing that serotonergic antidepressants lack procognitive effects despite their consistent positive effects on reducing negative biases in patients with depression. Evidence from preclinical (Dale et al., 2016) and clinical (Harmer, Shelley, Cowen, & Goodwin, 2004) studies support the view that emotion-laden cognitive functions (hot cognition) may be more sensitive to serotonin modulation. Specifically, participants receiving selective serotonin reuptake inhibitors (e.g., citalopram) showed altered bias to emotional faces (Harmer et al., 2003). Experimental modulation of serotonin levels with tryptophan depletion leads to more negative bias in affective information processing (Feder et al., 2011).

PHARMACOLOGICAL MODULATION OF EXECUTIVE FUNCTION

Pharmacological modulation of executive functions in patients with depression has received limited investigation, as treatment studies rarely focus on agents that act specifically on cognitive functions. Several candidate drugs could help improve cognitive abilities in depression (Miskowiak, Ott, Petersen, & Kessing, 2016). For example, modafinil is a wakefulness-promoting agent that has shown promising effects on cognition. Although originally licenced for narcolepsy and shift-work sleep disorder, modafinil has been a research focus due to its procognitive efficacy. Previous work from our laboratory showed that modafinil can improve inhibitory control (Turner et al., 2003) and planning performance (Müller et al., 2013; Winder-Rhodes et al., 2010) in healthy adults. Modafinil led to better performance in psychomotor speed and executive functions in sleep-deprived individuals (Bonnet et al., 2005; Wesensten, 2006), including doctors after a night's sleep deprivation (Sugden, Housden, Aggarwal, Sahakian, & Darzi, 2012). A systematic review of studies on the use of modafinil in healthy adults indicated that the beneficial effects of this drug on executive functions have been consistently replicated across several samples (Battleday & Brem, 2015). Although the exact mechanism by which modafinil exerts its effects remains unclear, the effects on working memory may be associated with action on catecholaminergic transmission in the prefrontal cortex (de Saint Hilaire, Orosco, Rouch, Blanc, & Nicolaidis, 2001; Minzenberg & Carter, 2008).

In clinical samples, modafinil has been found to have favorable effects on a range of executive functions. Patients with schizophrenia treated with modafinil had better performance on cognitive measures of working memory (Rosenthal & Bryant, 2004), inhibitory control, and set-shifting (Minzenberg, Watrous, Yoon, Ursu, & Carter, 2008; Turner, Clark, Dowson, Robbins, & Sahakian, 2004). Modafinil has been found to improve spatial working memory in patients with first-episode psychosis (Scoriels, Barnett, Soma, Sahakian, & Jones, 2012), and it had beneficial effects on planning and response inhibition in adults with attention-deficit/hyperactivity disorder (Turner, Clark, Pomarol-Clotet, et al., 2004). Previously, an open-label study showed that patients with depression who were treated with add-on modafinil, in addition to resolution of depressive symptoms, had improved performance on the Stroop test (DeBattista, Lembke, Solvason, Ghebremichael, & Poirier, 2004).

The results from treatment studies in MDD that measure cognitive function need to be appraised regarding pseudospecificity, that is, to determine if the improvements in cognition are independent from change in depressive symptoms. In a systematic review and meta-analysis of randomised controlled trials, Goss, Kaser, Costafreda, Sahakian, and Fu (2013) showed that augmentation with modafinil was superior to placebo for depressive symptom improvement. The studies included in this meta-analysis did not have any specific outcomes on cognition. However, the additional positive impact of modafinil on fatigue symptoms was noteworthy. One should consider its beneficial effects on depressive symptoms in terms of future feasibility. From a more mechanistic point of view, a useful approach to test the independent effects of a potential precognitive agent is to include patients with remitted depression. We adopted this approach and conducted a placebo-controlled, randomized controlled study that showed the beneficial effects of modafinil on working memory and episodic memory in patients with depression who remitted (Kaser, Deakin, et al., 2017). Patients who received placebo produced more errors on the CANTAB Spatial Working Memory task with a medium effect size. We have evidence that modafinil showed benefits for patients with remitted depression (Kaser, Deakin, et al., 2017) and in healthy adults free of depression (Müller et al., 2013). Therefore, the improvements in cognitive function cannot be attributed to improvements in mood alone. In other words, the cognitive improvements attained with modafinil cannot be attributed to pseudospecificity. A longer-term study is underway to test the efficacy of modafinil on residual cognitive dysfunction in patients with remitted depression (*clinicaltrials.gov* identifier NCT03620253). Another study with modafinil has identified cognitive function as a primary outcome in a sample of patients with remitted bipolar disorder (*clinicaltrials.gov* identifier NCT01965925). Further research will help clarify the feasibility of modafinil for cognitive dysfunction in depression.

FUTURE RESEARCH DIRECTIONS WITH COMPUATIONAL MODELING

The emerging research evidence from computational modeling can offer additional understanding of the complex relationship between executive function and depression (Chen, Takahashi, Nakagawa, Inoue, & Kusumi, 2015). The main body of literature is in relation to the reinforcement learning paradigms that are mathematically formulated to understand the latent variables in learning and decision making. Those cognitive abilities are closely linked to executive control and are in constant interaction. According to the reinforcement learning models, the brain constantly produces a model of the world outside, and decisions are shaped based on the gains and losses. In test conditions, the computational modeling algorithm learns the subjective value of an action (or stimulus) through trial and error. Specifically, the reinforcement model iteratively learns the reward value associated with an action. Through external stimuli, the updates can identify the mismatch between the experienced and expected outcome of the current action (prediction error). One problem with the decision-making difficulties that adult patients with MDD report could be related to the relative blunting of rewards and sensitivity to losses. This can translate into daily living as increased avoidance and also reinforcement of negative views toward the world. Patients with depression may be more predisposed to diminished model-based (goal-directed) reinforcement learning. A vicious cycle is then completed with the increased stress levels. Higher cortisol levels lead to poorer executive functions and working memory that further reduce the use of goal-directed choices (model-based reinforcement learning; Otto, Gershman, Markman, & Daw, 2013; Radenbach et al., 2015). Computational modeling can provide the latent variables underlying those cognitive impairments in decision making. This line of research can help develop more refined measures of behavioral change. Thus, the use of computational modeling can advance understanding of how depression affects cognition and motivation, as well as their interaction to promote the development of new, more effective treatments.

CONCLUSION

In this chapter, we reviewed key aspects of executive functions in depression. Evidence consistently suggests that a broad range of executive functions are affected in patients with depression. Clinical factors, methodological differences, and sensitivity of neuropsychological measures impact the findings. Executive functions are in constant interaction with emotional processes that are key to understanding the behavioral brain mechanism implicated in depression. The interaction was formulated in a cognitive neuropsychological model. According to the model, impaired top-down cognitive control and altered emotional biases can affect depressed mood. Pharmacological modulation of emotional biases can lead to positive changes in the integration of emotion and cognition, and psychological treatments, such as cognitive-behavioral therapy, can improve cognitive control of emotion regulation. Our own research shows that modafinil is feasible as a treatment. Finally, future directions are set out on executive functions in depression, particularly in relation to computational modeling of behavior.

ACKNOWLEDGMENTS

We acknowledge funding from the NIHR Cambridge Biomedical Research Centre Mental Health theme. Dr. Kaser was supported by an NIHR Clinical Lectureship.

REFERENCES

Abwender, D. A., Swan, J. G., Bowerman, J. T., & Connolly, S. W. (2001). Qualitative analysis of verbal fluency output: Review and comparison of several scoring methods. *Assessment, 8*(3), 323–338.

Arnsten, A. F. (2000). Stress impairs prefrontal cortical function in rats and monkeys: Role of dopamine D1 and norepinephrine α-1 receptor mechanisms. *Progress in Brain Research, 126,* 183–192.

Baddeley, A. (1996). Exploring the central executive. *Quarterly Journal of Experimental Psychology Section A, 49*(1), 5–28.

Battleday, R. M., & Brem, A. K. (2015). Modafinil for cognitive neuroenhancement in healthy non-sleep-deprived subjects: A systematic review. *European Neuropsychopharmacology, 25*(11), 1865–1881.

Baune, B. T., Czira, M. E., Smith, A. L., Mitchell, D., & Sinnamon, G (2012). Neuropsychological performance in a sample of 13–25 year olds with a history of non-psychotic major depressive disorder. *Journal of Affective Disorders, 141*(2–3), 441–448.

Beats, B. C., Sahakian, B. J., & Levy, R. (1996). Cognitive performance in tests sensitive to frontal lobe dysfunction in the elderly depressed. *Psychological Medicine, 26*(3), 591–603.

Bechara, A., Damasio, A. R., Damasio, H., & Anderson, S. W. (1994). Insensitivity to future consequences following damage to human prefrontal cortex. *Cognition, 50,* 1–3.

Bonnet, M. H., Balkin, T. J., Dinges, D. F., Roehrs, T., Rogers, N. L., & Wesensten, N. J. (2005). The use of stimulants to modify performance during sleep loss: A review by the Sleep Deprivation and Stimulant Task Force of the American Academy of Sleep Medicine. *Sleep, 28*(9), 1163–1187.

Bora, E., Harrison, B. J., Yücel, M., & Pantelis, C. (2013). Cognitive impairment in euthymic major depressive disorder: A meta-analysis. *Psychological Medicine, 43*(10), 2017–2026.

Borg, J., Henningsson, S., Saijo, T., Inoue, M., Bah, J., Westberg, L., et al. (2009). Serotonin transporter genotype is associated with cognitive performance but not regional 5-HT1A receptor binding in humans. *International Journal of Neuropsychopharmacology, 12*(6), 783–792.

Butters, M. A., Young, J. B., Lopez, O., Aizenstein, H. J., Mulsant, B. H., Reynolds III, C. F., et al. (2008). Pathways linking late-life depression to persistent cognitive impairment and dementia. *Dialogues in Clinical Neuroscience, 10*(3), 345.

Butts, K. A., Weinberg, J., Young, A. H., & Phillips, A. G. (2011). Glucocorticoid receptors in the prefrontal cortex regulate stress-evoked dopamine efflux and aspects of executive function. *Proceedings of the National Academy of Sciences, 108*(45), 18459–18464.

Cataldo, M. G., Nobile, M., Lorusso, M. L., Battaglia, M., & Molteni, M. (2005). Impulsivity in depressed children and adolescents: A comparison between behavioral and neuropsychological data. *Psychiatry Research, 136*(2–3), 123–133.

Chen, C., Takahashi, T., Nakagawa, S., Inoue, T., & Kusumi, I. (2015). Reinforcement learning in depression: A review of computational research. *Neuroscience and Biobehavioral Reviews, 55,* 247–267.

Chen, L. S., Eaton, W. W., Gallo, J. J., & Nestadt, G. (2000). Understanding the heterogeneity of depression through the triad of symptoms, course and risk factors: A longitudinal, population-based study. *Journal of Affective Disorders, 59*(1), 1–11.

Clarke, H. F., Dalley, J. W., Crofts, H. S., Robbins, T. W., & Roberts, A. C. (2004). Cognitive inflexibility after prefrontal serotonin depletion. *Science, 304*(5672), 878–880.

Conradi, H. J., Ormel, J., & de Jonge, P. (2011). Presence of individual (residual) symptoms during depressive episodes and periods of remission: A 3-year prospective study. *Psychological Medicine, 41*(6), 1165–1174.

Culverhouse, R. C., Saccone, N. L., Horton, A. C., Ma, Y., Anstey, K. J., Banaschewski, T., et al. (2018). Collaborative meta-analysis finds no evidence of a strong interaction between stress and 5-HTTLPR genotype contributing to the development of depression. *Molecular Psychiatry, 23*(1), 133.

Dale, E., Pehrson, A. L., Jeyarajah, T., Li, Y., Leiser, S. C., Smagin, G., et al. (2016). Effects of serotonin in the hippocampus: How SSRIs and multimodal antidepressants might regulate pyramidal cell function. *CNS Spectrums, 21*(2), 143–161.

Dalley, J. W., Cardinal, R. N., & Robbins, T. W. (2004). Prefrontal executive and cognitive functions in rodents: Neural and neurochemical substrates. *Neuroscience and Biobehavioral Reviews, 28*(7), 771–784.

de Saint Hilaire, Z., Orosco, M., Rouch, C., Blanc, G., & Nicolaidis, S. (2001). Variations in extracellular monoamines in the prefrontal cortex and medial hypothalamus after modafinil administration: A microdialysis study in rats. *Neuroreport, 12*(16), 3533–3537.

DeBattista, C., Lembke, A., Solvason, H. B., Ghebremichael, R., & Poirier, J. (2004). A prospective trial of modafinil as an adjunctive treatment of major depression. *Journal of Clinical Psychopharmacology, 24*(1), 87–90.

Dichter, G. S., Felder, J. N., & Smoski, M. J. (2009). Affective context interferes with cognitive control in unipolar depression: An fMRI investigation. *Journal of Affective Disorders, 114*(1–3), 131–142.

Elliott, R. (1998). The neuropsychological profile in unipolar depression. *Trends in Cognitive Sciences, 2*(11), 447–454.

Elliott, R., Rubinsztein, J. S., Sahakian, B. J., & Dolan, R. J. (2002). The neural basis of mood-congruent processing biases in depression. *Archives of General Psychiatry, 59*(7), 597–604.

Elliott, R., Sahakian, B. J., Herrod, J. J., Robbins, T. W., & Paykel, E. S. (1997). Abnormal response to negative feedback in unipolar depression: Evidence for a diagnosis specific impairment. *Journal of Neurology, Neurosurgery and Psychiatry, 63*(1), 74–82.

Elliott, R., Sahakian, B. J., Matthews, K., Bannerjea, A., Rimmer, J. & Robbins, T. W. (1997). Effects of methylphenidate on spatial working memory and planning in healthy young adults. *Psychopharmacology, 131*(2), 196–206.

Elliott, R., Sahakian, B. J., McKay, A. P., Herrod, J. J., Robbins, T. W., & Paykel, E. S. (1996). Neuropsychological impairments in unipolar depression: The influence of perceived failure on subsequent performance. *Psychological Medicine, 26*(5), 975–989.

Elliott, R., Zahn, R., Deakin, J. W., & Anderson, I. M. (2011). Affective cognition and its disruption in mood disorders. *Neuropsychopharmacology, 36*(1), 153–182.

Fales, C. L., Barch, D. M., Rundle, M. M., Mintun, M. A., Snyder, A. Z., Cohen, J. D., et al. (2008). Altered emotional interference processing in affective and cognitive-control brain circuitry in major depression. *Biological Psychiatry, 63*(4), 377–384.

Feder, A., Skipper, J., Blair, J. R., Buchholz, K., Mathew, S. J., Schwarz, M., et al. (2011). Tryptophan depletion and emotional processing in healthy volunteers at high risk for depression. *Biological Psychiatry, 69*(8), 804–807.

Fried, E. I. (2017). The 52 symptoms of major depression: Lack of content overlap among seven common depression scales. *Journal of Affective Disorders, 208*, 191–197.

Gohier, B., Ferracci, L., Surguladze, S. A., Lawrence, E., El Hage, W., Kefi, M. Z., et al. (2009). Cognitive inhibition and working memory in unipolar depression. *Journal of Affective Disorders, 116*(1), 100–105.

Goldman-Rakic, P. S. (1995). Cellular basis of working memory. *Neuron, 14*(3), 477–485.

Gorwood, P., Corruble, E., Falissard, B., & Goodwin, G. M. (2008). Toxic effects of depression on brain function: Impairment of delayed recall and the cumulative length of depressive disorder in a large sample of depressed outpatients. *American Journal of Psychiatry, 165*(6), 731–739.

Goss, A. J., Kaser, M., Costafreda, S. G., Sahakian, B. J., & Fu, C. H. (2013). Modafinil augmentation therapy in unipolar and bipolar depression: A systematic review and meta-analysis of randomized controlled trials. *Journal of Clinical Psychiatry, 74*(11), 1101–1107.

Grant, M. M., Thase, M. E., & Sweeney, J. A. (2001). Cognitive disturbance in outpatient depressed younger adults: Evidence of modest impairment. *Biological Psychiatry, 50*(1), 35–43.

Hammar, Å., & Årdal, G. (2009). Cognitive functioning in major depression–a summary. *Frontiers in Human Neuroscience, 3*, 26.

Hammar, Å., Sorensen, L. I. N., Årdal, G., Oedegaard, K. J., Kroken, R., Roness, A., et al. (2010). Enduring cognitive dysfunction in unipolar major depression: A test–retest study using the Stroop paradigm. *Scandinavian Journal of Psychology, 51*(4), 304–308.

Hammar, Å., Strand, M., Årdal, G., Schmid, M., Lund, A. & Elliott, R. (2011). Testing the cognitive effort hypothesis of cognitive impairment in major depression. *Nordic Journal of Psychiatry, 65*(1), 74–80.

Harmer, C. J., Bhagwagar, Z., Perrett, D. I., Völlm, B. A., Cowen, P. J., & Goodwin, G. M. (2003). Acute SSRI administration affects the processing of social cues in healthy volunteers. *Neuropsychopharmacology, 28*(1), 148–152.

Harmer, C. J., O'Sullivan, U., Favaron, E., Massey-Chase, R., Ayres, R., Reinecke, A., et al. (2009). Effect of acute antidepressant administration on negative affective bias in depressed patients. *American Journal of Psychiatry, 166*(10), 1178–1184.

Harmer, C. J., Shelley, N. C., Cowen, P. J., & Goodwin, G. M. (2004). Increased positive versus negative affective perception and memory in healthy volunteers following selective serotonin and norepinephrine reuptake inhibition. *American Journal of Psychiatry, 161*(7), 1256–1263.

Hasler, G., Drevets, W. C., Manji, H. K., & Charney, D. S. (2004). Discovering endophenotypes for major depression. *Neuropsychopharmacology, 29*(10), 1765–1781.

Hayward, G., Goodwin, G. M., Cowen, P. J., & Harmer, C. J. (2005). Low-dose tryptophan depletion in recovered depressed patients induces changes in cognitive processing without depressive symptoms. *Biological psychiatry, 57*(5), 517–524.

Heaton, R. K. (1981). *Wisconsin Card Sorting Test manual.* Odessa, FL: Psychological Aassessment Resources.

Herrmann, L. L., Goodwin, G. M., & Ebmeier, K. P. (2007). The cognitive neuropsychology of depression in the elderly. *Psychological Medicine, 37*(12), 1693–1702.

Jaeger, J., Berns, S., Uzelac, S., & Davis-Conway, S. (2006). Neurocognitive deficits and disability in major depressive disorder. *Psychiatry Research, 145*(1), 39–48.

Jurado, M. B., & Rosselli, M. (2007). The elusive nature of executive functions: A review of our current understanding. *Neuropsychology Review, 17*(3), 213–233.

Kaser, M., Deakin, J. B., Michael, A., Zapata, C., Bansal, R., Ryan, D., et al. (2017). Modafinil improves episodic memory and working memory cognition in patients with remitted depression: A double-blind, randomized, placebo-controlled study. *Biological Psychiatry: Cognitive Neuroscience and Neuroimaging, 2*(2), 115–122.

Kaser, M., Zaman, R., & Sahakian, B. J. (2017). Cognition as a treatment target in depression. *Psychological Medicine, 47*(6), 987–989.

Keefe, R. S., McClintock, S. M., Roth, R. M., Doraiswamy, P. M., Tiger, S., & Madhoo, M. (2014). Cognitive effects of pharmacotherapy for major depressive disorder: A systematic review. *Journal of Clinical Psychiatry, 75*(8), 1–478.

Keilp, J. G., Madden, S. P., Gorlyn, M., Burke, A. K., Oquendo, M. A., & Mann, J. J. (2018). The lack of meaningful association between depression severity measures and neurocognitive performance. *Journal of Affective Disorders, 241*, 164–172.

Koenigs, M., & Grafman, J. (2009). The functional neuroanatomy of depression: Distinct roles for ventromedial and dorsolateral prefrontal cortex. *Behavioural Brain Research, 201*(2), 239–243.

Koesters, M., Ostuzzi, G., Guaiana, G., Breilmann, J., & Barbui, C. (2017). Vortioxetine for depression in adults. *Cochrane Database of Systematic Reviews*, Issue 7, CD011520.

Kyte, Z. A., Goodyer, I. M., & Sahakian, B. J. (2005). Selected executive skills in adolescents with recent first episode major depression. *Journal of Child Psychology and Psychiatry, 46*(9), 995–1005.

Lockwood, K. A., Alexopoulos, G. S., & van Gorp, W. G. (2002). Executive dysfunction in geriatric depression. *American Journal of Psychiatry, 159*(7), 1119–1126.

Mahableshwarkar, A. R., Zajecka, J., Jacobson, W., Chen, Y., & Keefe, R. S. (2015). A randomized, placebo-controlled, active-reference, double-blind, flexible-dose study of the efficacy of vortioxetine on cognitive function in major depressive disorder. *Neuropsychopharmacology, 40*(8), 2025–2037.

Mayberg, H. S., Brannan, S. K., Mahurin, R. K., Jerabek, P. A., Brickman, J. S., Tekell, J. L., et al. (1997). Cingulate function in depression: A potential predictor of treatment response. *Neuroreport, 8*(4), 1057–1061.

McAllister-Williams, R. H., Ferrier, I. N., & Young, A. H. (1998). Mood and neuropsychological function in depression: The role of corticosteroids and serotonin. *Psychological Medicine, 28*(3), 573–584.

McCall, W. V., & Dunn, A. G. (2003). Cognitive deficits are associated with functional impairment in severely depressed patients. *Psychiatry Research, 121*(2), 179–184.

McClintock, S. M., Husain, M. M., Greer, T. L., & Cullum, C. M. (2010). Association between depression severity and neurocognitive function in major depressive disorder: A review and synthesis. *Neuropsychology, 24*(1), 9–34.

McDermott, L. M., & Ebmeier, K. P. (2009). A meta-analysis of depression severity and cognitive function. *Journal of Affective Disorders, 119*(1), 1–8.

McIntyre, R. S., Lophaven, S., & Olsen, C. K. (2014). A randomized, double-blind, placebo-controlled study of vortioxetine on cognitive function in depressed adults. *International Journal of Neuropsychopharmacology, 17*(10), 1557–1567.

Mehta, M. A., Owen, A. M., Sahakian, B. J., Mavaddat, N., Pickard, J. D., & Robbins, T. W. (2000). Methylphenidate enhances working memory by modulating discrete frontal and parietal lobe regions in the human brain. *Journal of Neuroscience, 20*(6), RC65.

Mehta, M. A., Sahakian, B. J., McKenna, P. J., & Robbins, T. W. (1999). Systemic sulpiride in young adult volunteers simulates the profile of cognitive deficits in Parkinson's disease. *Psychopharmacology, 146*(2), 162–174.

Mesulam, M. M. (2002). The human frontal lobes: Transcending the default mode through contingent encoding. In D. T. Stuss & R. T. Knight (Eds.), *Principles of frontal lobe function* (pp. 8–30). Oxford, UK: Oxford University Press.

Minzenberg, M. J., & Carter, C. S. (2008). Modafinil: A review of neurochemical actions and effects on cognition. *Neuropsychopharmacology, 33*(7), 1477–1502.

Minzenberg, M. J., Watrous, A. J., Yoon, J. H., Ursu, S., & Carter, C. S. (2008). Modafinil shifts human locus coeruleus to low-tonic, high-phasic activity during functional MRI. *Science, 322,* 1700–1702.

Miskowiak, K. W., Ott, C. V., Petersen, J. Z., & Kessing, L. V. (2016). Systematic review of randomized controlled trials of candidate treatments for cognitive impairment in depression and methodological challenges in the field. *European Neuropsychopharmacology, 26*(12), 1845–1867.

Miyake, A., Friedman, N. P., Emerson, M. J., Witzki, A. H., Howerter, A., & Wager, T. D. (2000). The unity and diversity of executive functions and their contributions to complex "frontal lobe" tasks: A latent variable analysis. *Cognitive Psychology, 41*(1), 49–100.

Müller, U., Rowe, J. B., Rittman, T., Lewis, C., Robbins, T. W., & Sahakian, B. J. (2013). Effects of modafinil on non-verbal cognition, task enjoyment and creative thinking in healthy volunteers. *Neuropharmacology, 64,* 490–495.

Müller, U., von Cramon, D. Y., & Pollmann, S. (1998). D1- versus D2-receptor modulation of visuospatial working memory in humans. *Journal of Neuroscience, 18*(7), 2720–2728.

Murphy, F. C., Michael, A., Robbins, T. W., & Sahakian, B. J. (2003). Neuropsychological impairment in patients with major depressive disorder: The effects of feedback on task performance. *Psychological Medicine, 33*(3), 455–467.

Naismith, S. L., Hickie, I. B., Turner, K., Little, C. L., Winter, V., Ward, P. B., et al. (2003). Neuropsychological performance in patients with depression is associated with clinical, etiological and genetic risk factors. *Journal of Clinical and Experimental Neuropsychology, 25*(6), 866–877.

National Academies of Sciences, Engineering, and Medicine. (2015). *Enabling discovery, development, and translation of treatments for cognitive dysfunction in depression: Workshop summary.* Washington, DC: National Academies Press.

Nierenberg, A. A., Loft, H., & Olsen, C. K. (2019). Treatment effects on residual cognitive symptoms among partially or fully remitted patients with major depressive disorder: A randomized, double-blinded, exploratory study with vortioxetine. *Journal of Affective Disorders, 250,* 35–42.

Otto, A. R., Gershman, S. J., Markman, A. B., & Daw, N. D. (2013). The curse of planning: dissecting multiple reinforcement-learning systems by taxing the central executive. *Psychological Science, 24*(5), 751–761.

Owen, A. M., Downes, J. J., Sahakian, B. J., Polkey, C. E., & Robbins, T. W. (1990). Planning and spatial working memory following frontal lobe lesions in man. *Neuropsychologia, 28*(10), 1021–1034.

Owen, A. M., Evans, A. C., Petrides, M. (1996). Evidence for a two-stage model of spatial working memory processing within the lateral frontal cortex: A positron emission tomography study. *Cerebral Cortex, 6*(1), 31–38.

Owen, A. M., Roberts, A. C., Polkey, C. E., Sahakian, B. J., & Robbins, T. W. (1991). Extra-dimensional versus intra-dimensional set shifting performance following frontal lobe excisions, temporal lobe excisions or amygdalo-hippocampectomy in man. *Neuropsychologia, 29*(10), 993–1006.

Owen, A. M., Sahakian, B. J., Hodges, J. R., Summers, B. A., Polkey, C. E., & Robbins, T. W. (1995). Dopamine-dependent frontostriatal planning deficits in early Parkinson's disease. *Neuropsychology, 9*(1), 126.

Pehrson, A. L., Leiser, S. C., Gulinello, M., Dale, E., Li, Y., Waller, J. A., et al. (2015). Treatment of cognitive dysfunction in major depressive disorder—a review of the preclinical evidence for efficacy of selective serotonin reuptake inhibitors, serotonin–norepinephrine reuptake inhibitors and the multimodal-acting antidepressant vortioxetine. *European Journal of Pharmacology, 753,* 19–31.

Phan, K. L., Fitzgerald, D. A., Nathan, P. J., Moore, G. J., Uhde, T. W., & Tancer, M. E. (2005). Neural substrates for voluntary suppression of negative affect: A functional magnetic resonance imaging study. *Biological Psychiatry, 57*(3), 210–219.

Phillips, M. L., Drevets, W., Rauch, S. L., & Lane, R. (2003). Neurobiology of emotion perception I: The neural basis of normal emotion perception. *Biological Psychiatry, 54*(5), 504–514.

Porter, R. J., Bourke, C., & Gallagher, P. (2007). Neuropsychological impairment in major depression: Its nature, origin and clinical significance. *Australian & New Zealand Journal of Psychiatry, 41*(2), 115–128.

Radenbach, C., Reiter, A. M., Engert, V., Sjoerds, Z., Villringer, A., Heinze, H. J., et al. (2015). The interaction of acute and chronic stress impairs model-based behavioral control. *Psychoneuroendocrinology, 53,* 268–280.

Robbins, T. W. (2000). From arousal to cognition: the integrative position of the prefrontal cortex. *Progress in Brain Research, 126,* 469–483.

Robbins, T. W., & Arnsten, A. F. (2009). The neuropsychopharmacology of fronto-executive function: monoaminergic modulation. *Annual Review of Neuroscience, 32,* 267–287.

Robbins, T. W., James, M., Owen, A. M., Sahakian, B. J., Lawrence, A. D., McInnes, L., et al. (1998). A study of performance on tests from the CANTAB battery sensitive to frontal lobe dysfunction in a large sample of normal volunteers: Implications for theories of executive functioning and cognitive aging. *Journal of the International Neuropsychological Society, 4*(5), 474–490.

Robinson, O. J., & Sahakian, B. J. (2013). Cognitive biomarkers in depression. In H. Lavretsky, M. Sajatovic, & C. F. Reynolds III (Eds.), *Late-life mood disorders* (pp. 606–626). New York: Oxford University Press.

Rock, P. L., Roiser, J. P., Riedel, W. J., & Blackwell, A. D. (2014). Cognitive impairment in depression: A systematic review and meta-analysis. *Psychological Medicine, 44*(10), 2029–2040.

Rogers, R. D., Everitt, B. J., Baldacchino, A., Blackshaw, A. J., Swainson, R., Wynne, K., et al. (1999). Dissociable deficits in the decision-making cognition of chronic amphetamine abusers, opiate abusers, patients with focal damage to prefrontal cortex, and tryptophan-depleted normal volunteers: Evidence for monoaminergic mechanisms. *Neuropsychopharmacology, 20*(4), 322–339.

Roiser, J. P., Elliott, R., & Sahakian, B. J. (2012). Cognitive mechanisms of treatment in depression. *Neuropsychopharmacology, 37*(1), 117–136.

Roiser, J. P., & Sahakian, B. J. (2013). Hot and cold cognition in depression. *CNS spectrums, 18*(3), 139–149.

Rosenthal, M. H., & Bryant, S. L. (2004). Benefits of adjunct modafinil in an open-label, pilot study in patients with schizophrenia. *Clinical Neuropharmacology, 27*(1), 38–43.

Rubinsztein, J. S., Sahakian, B. J. & O'Brien, J. T. (2019). Understanding and managing cognitive impairment in bipolar disorder in older people. *BJPsych Advances 25*(3), 150–156.

Sahakian, B. J., Morris, R. G., Evenden, J. L., Heald, A., Levy, R., Philpot, M., & Robbins, T. W. (1988). A comparative study of visuospatial memory and learning in Alzheimer-type dementia and Parkinson's disease. *Brain, 111*(3), 695–718.

Scoriels, L., Barnett, J. H., Soma, P. K., Sahakian, B. J., & Jones, P. B. (2012). Effects of modafinil on cognitive functions in first episode psychosis. *Psychopharmacology, 220*(2), 249–258.

Shallice, T. (1982). Specific impairments of planning. *Philosophical Transactions of the Royal Society of London B: Biological Sciences, 298,* 199–209.

Shilyansky, C., Williams, L. M., Gyurak, A., Harris, A., Usherwood, T., & Etkin, A. (2016). Effect of antidepressant treatment on cognitive impairments associated with depression: A randomised longitudinal study. *Lancet Psychiatry, 3*(5), 425–435.

Skandali, N., Rowe, J. B., Voon, V., Deakin, J. B., Cardinal, R. N., Cormack, F., et al. (2018). Dissociable effects of acute SSRI (escitalopram) on executive, learning and emotional functions in healthy humans. *Neuropsychopharmacology 43,* 2645–2651.

Snyder, H. R. (2013). Major depressive disorder is associated with broad impairments on neuropsychological measures of executive function: A meta-analysis and review. *Psychological Bulletin, 139*(1), 81.

Stroop, J. R. (1935). Studies of interference in serial verbal reactions. *Journal of Experimental Psychology, 18*(6), 643.

Sugden, C., Housden, C. R., Aggarwal, R., Sahakian, B. J., & Darzi, A. (2012). Effect of pharmacological enhancement on the cognitive and clinical psychomotor performance of sleep-deprived doctors: a randomized controlled trial. *Annals of Surgery, 255*(2), 222–227.

Tarbuck, A. F., & Paykel, E. S. (1995). Effects of major depression on the cognitive function of younger and older subjects. *Psychological Medicine, 25*(2), 285–295.

Tsourtos, G., Thompson, J. C., & Stough, C. (2002). Evidence of an early information processing speed deficit in unipolar major depression. *Psychological Medicine, 32*(2), 259–265.

Turner, D. C., Clark, L., Dowson, J., Robbins, T. W., & Sahakian, B. J. (2004). Modafinil improves cognition and response inhibition in adult attention-deficit/hyperactivity disorder. *Biological Psychiatry, 55*(10), 1031–1040.

Turner, D. C., Clark, L., Pomarol-Clotet, E., McKenna, P., Robbins, T. W., & Sahakian, B. J. (2004). Modafinil improves cognition and attentional set shifting in patients with chronic schizophrenia. *Neuropsychopharmacology, 29*(7), 1363–1373.

Turner, D. C., Robbins, T. W., Clark, L., Aron, A. R., Dowson, J., & Sahakian, B. J. (2003). Cognitive enhancing effects of modafinil in healthy volunteers. *Psychopharmacology, 165*(3), 260–269.

Watanabe, Y., Sakai, R. R., McEwen, B. S., & Mendelson, S. (1993). Stress and antidepressant effects on hippocampal and cortical 5-HT 1A and 5-HT 2 receptors and transport sites for serotonin. *Brain Research, 615*(1), 87–94.

Wechsler, D. (1981). *Wechsler Adult Intelligence Scale—Revised (WAIS-R)*. New York: Psychological Corporation.

Wesensten, N. J. (2006). Effects of modafinil on cognitive performance and alertness during sleep deprivation. *Current Pharmaceutical Design, 12*(20), 2457–2471.

Winder-Rhodes, S. E., Chamberlain, S. R., Idris, M. I., Robbins, T. W., Sahakian, B. J., & Müller, U. (2010). Effects of modafinil and prazosin on cognitive and physiological functions in healthy volunteers. *Journal of Psychopharmacology, 24*(11), 1649–1657.

Zakzanis, K. K., Leach, L., & Kaplan, K. (1998). On the nature and pattern of neurocognitive function in major depressive disorder. *Neuropsychiatry, Neuropsychology, and Behavioral Neurology, 11*(3), 111–119.

PART III

CLINICAL AND NEUROPSYCHOLOGICAL ASSESSMENT

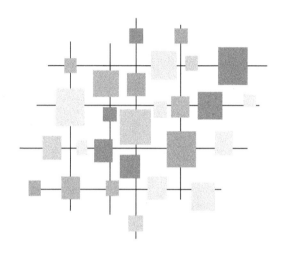

CHAPTER 10

Major Depressive Disorder Diagnostic and Depressive Symptom Metrics

Benjamin D. Pace
Mustafa M. Husain

Major depressive disorder (MDD) is a heterogeneous condition that shares symptoms that are concurrently present in other health disorders. For instance, flat affect and cognitive problems are common concerns for those suffering from MDD; however, without proper assessment and diagnosis, an elderly individual could be misdiagnosed with dementia. For this reason, diagnostic measures such as the Mini-International Neuropsychiatric Interview (MINI; Sheehan et al., 1998) and the Structured Clinical Interview for DSM-5 (SCID; First, 2015) are necessary to properly diagnose health conditions in vulnerable populations (see Tureson, Gold, & Thames, Chapter 13, this volume, for additional information). From diagnosis, the severity of depressive symptoms helps determine the treatment options and course.

Over the past several decades, approximately 280 different assessment tools have been developed to assess depression symptom severity (Santor, Gregus, & Welch, 2006). Consequently, a main problem in the neuropsychiatric field is not the paucity of a depression severity assessment instrument, but rather which psychometrically sound instruments are to be used in clinical and research practices. This chapter reviews seven depression symptom severity assessment scales that are most frequently used in comparative studies of depression rating scales for MDD as well as the measures that are most often cited in the published literature (Fried, 2017).

These seven depression severity rating scales are the Hamilton Rating Scale for Depression (Hamilton, 1960); Montgomery–Åsberg Depression Rating Scale (Montgomery & Åsberg, 1979); Beck Depression Inventory–II (BDI-II; Strunk & Lane, 2016); Inventory of Depressive Symptomatology (IDS; Trivedi et al., 2004); Quick Inventory of Depressive Symptomatology (Rush et al., 2003); Zung Self-Rating Depression Scale (Zung SDS; Zung, 1965); and Center for Epidemiologic Studies Depression Scale (Radloff, 1977). Information on inclusion and diversity for some of these depression rating scales can be found in Tureson, Gold, and Thames (Chapter 13, this volume).

This chapter focuses on diagnostic and depression symptom severity rating scales for general adults with MDD and depression. Accordingly, other diagnostic or depression severity scales for other populations are beyond the scope of this review. However, it should be noted that there are many assessment scales designed to assess depression severity in other populations. For instance, for elderly adults, rating scales include the Geriatric Depression Scale (Yesavage, 1988; Yesavage et al., 1982); Brief Assessment Schedule Depression Cards (Adshead, Day Cody, & Pitt, 1992); Cornell Scale for Depression in Dementia (Alexopoulos, Abrams, Young, & Shamoian, 1988); and Geriatric Mental State Schedule (Burns, Lawlor, & Craig, 2002). For child and adolescent populations, depression severity scales include the Children's Depression Rating Scale (CDRS and CDRS-R; Poznanski, Cook, & Carroll, 1980; Poznanski, Mokros, Grossman, & Freeman, 1985); Kutcher Adolescent Depression Scale (Brooks, 2004); Children's Depression Inventory (Kovacs, 1985); Child Depression Scale (Reynolds & Graves, 1989); and Beck Youth Inventories of Emotional and Social Impairment (Steer, Kumar, Beck, & Beck, 2001). For patients with medical illnesses, depression rating scales include the Hospital Anxiety and Depression Scale (Zigmond & Snaith, 1983) and Beck Depression Inventory for Primary Care (Steer, Cavalieri, Leonard, & Beck, 1999). Lastly, for women with postpartum depression, the Edinburgh Postnatal Depression Scale (EPDS; Cox, Holden, & Sagovsky, 1987) is the primary depression severity measure.

DEPRESSION DIAGNOSTIC INSTRUMENTS

As mentioned above, the two main diagnostics tools are the MINI (Sheehan et al., 1998) and the SCID (First, 2015). These instruments offer semi-structured interview formats to derive a neuropsychiatric diagnosis. In terms of diagnosis of depressive disorders, the SCID had an average sensitivity/specificity of 85%/92%, while the MINI had an average sensitivity/specificity of 95%/84% (Pettersson, Boström, Gustavsson, & Ekselius, 2015).

DEPRESSION SYMPTOM SEVERITY RATING SCALES

In this section, we describe depression symptom severity rating scales in terms of their symptom content, method of administration (e.g., self-report, clinician-rated), scoring, psychometric properties, and strengths and limitations. For the description of the content of the scales, we follow the framework provided by Fried's (2017) study. Specifically, Fried analyzed the content of the seven rating scales (125 total items) and concluded that collectively these scales contained 52 specific depression symptoms (see Table 10.1).

Hamilton Rating Scale for Depression

Max Hamilton published the first version of this scale in 1960 (Hamilton, 1960). The Hamilton Rating Scale for Depression (HRSD) is a clinician-rated scale. Hamilton noted that this scale was developed for use only in adult patients who were already diagnosed

TABLE 10.1. Symptoms Evaluated by the Seven Selected Depression Rating Scales

Early insomnia	Appetite decrease	Psychomotor agitation
Middle insomnia	Appetite increase	Psychomotor retardation
Late insomnia	Weight decrease	Somatic complaints
Hypersomnia	Weight increase	Sympathetic arousal
Sad mood	Concentration difficulty	Gastrointestinal dysfunction
Anxiousness	Indecisiveness	Interpersonal sensitivity
Panic	Guilt	Leaden paralysis
Irritability	Worthlessness	Past failure
Mood reactivity	Pessimism	Self-punishment
Diurnal variation	Suicidal ideation	Self-dislike
Grief	Interest loss	Self-criticalness
Fatigue	Pleasure loss	Crying
Energy loss	Decreased libido	Feeling of being lonely
Effort	Talked less	People are unfriendly
People dislike me	Feeling bothered	Feeling good
Feeling happy	Feeling needed	Life is full
Inner tension	Inability to feel	Hypochondriasis
Loss of insight		

with depression. Accordingly, the scale is best suited for assessing depression symptom severity, antidepressant treatment effects, and recovery from depression (Hedlund & Vieweg, 1979).

The HRSD captures 22 of the 52 main depression symptoms (Fried, 2017). Of those 22, 12 symptoms are assessed directly (early insomnia, middle insomnia, late insomnia, sad mood, appetite decrease, weight decrease, suicidal ideation, decreased libido, retardation, agitation, hypochondriasis, and loss of insight) and 10 symptoms are assessed indirectly (anxiousness, panic, irritability, guilt, interest loss, pleasure loss, fatigue, energy loss, sympathetic arousal, and gastrointestinal dysfunction).

The HRSD was revised by Hamilton several times, including in 1966, 1967, 1969, and 1980. While the original HRSD scored 17 items, later versions include up to 30 items.

Administration Method

To assess depression severity, clinicians conduct a semi-structured interview with patients. Williams (1988) developed a structured interview guide for the HRSD that takes approximately 15–20 minutes to complete. This widely used guide helps to improve inter-rater reliability.

Scoring and Interpretation

Eight items of the HRSD have a 5-point rating scale that ranges from 0 to 4, and nine items have a 3-point rating scale that ranges from 0 to 2. The final (total) score is equal to the sum of scores for individual items, ranging from 0 to 54. The total score between

0 and 7 indicates the absence of depression; between 8 and 16, mild depression severity; between 17 and 23, moderate depression severity; and scores equal to or greater than 24, severe depression severity (Zimmerman, Martinez, Young, Chelminski, & Dalrymple, 2013).

Psychometric Properties

The correlations of the HRSD with other clinician-rated measures of depression (convergent validity) range from .65 to .90 (Cusin, Yang, & Yeung, 2009). Although the values of Cronbach's α (internal consistency) range from 0.46 to 0.92 in most studies, the coefficients have mainly been reported to be above 0.70 (Bagby, Ryder, Schuller, & Marshall, 2004). The test–retest reliability ranges from 0.81 to 0.98 (Bagby et al., 2004).

Limitations

The HRSD has been found to have multiple limitations, including uneven weights attributed to different symptom domains. One group of symptoms is rated on a 5-point scale, while other symptoms are rated on a 3-point scale (Cusin et al., 2009). Additionally, the scale overestimates insomnia and underestimates suicidality as indicators of depression severity. (Morgan, 2016). Finally, the 17-, 21-, and 24-item versions of the HRSD do not measure the atypical depressive items (e.g., mood reactivity, hypersomnia) and thus fail to document the presence or absence of atypical depressive symptoms.

Strengths

The HRSD is considered the gold standard of depression severity scales. As such, it has been extensively studied and is frequently used in clinical trials and clinical practice to assess depression severity.

Montgomery–Åsberg Depression Rating Scale

The Montgomery–Åsberg Depression Rating Scale (MADRS) is a 10-item depression severity scale developed by Swedish and British researchers in 1979 (Montgomery & Åsberg, 1979). The scale is administered by a clinician and was designed to provide equivalent weighting of depressive items, measurement of a unitary construct of depression, and sensitivity to change with antidepressant treatment.

The MADRS primarily focuses on psychological (e.g., sadness. guilt) rather than somatic (e.g., physical consequences of anxiety, eating changes) aspects of depression (Montgomery & Åsberg, 1979). The MADRS captures 12 of the 52 main symptoms of depression (Fried, 2017). Seven of the 12 symptoms are directly assessed (pessimism, agitation, concentration difficulties, sad mood, appetite decrease, inner tension, and inability to feel) and 5 are indirectly assessed (energy loss, early insomnia, middle insomnia, late insomnia, and fatigue).

Administration Method

To assess the severity of the depression symptoms, clinicians conduct a semi-structured interview with adult patients. There are several published and available semi-structured interview guides for the MADRS (Fleck, Guelfi, Poirier-Littré, & Lôo, 1994; Takahashi, Tomita, Higuchi, & Inada, 2004; Williams & Kobak, 2008). The sem-istructured interview takes approximately 15–20 minutes to complete.

Scoring and Interpretation

All items of the MADRS have a 7-point rating scale that ranges from 0 to 6 (0 = no abnormality to 6 = severe). The total score is equal to the sum of the scores for individual items, with a total score that can range from 0 to 60. Scores from 0 to 8 indicate the absence of depression; scores from 9 to 17, mild depression severity; scores from 18 to 35, moderate depression severity; and scores equal to or greater than 36, severe depression (Müller et al., 2000).

Psychometric Properties

The MADRS has strong convergent validity based on correlations with the HRSD that range from .80 to .90 (Müller, Himmerich, Kienzle, & Szegedi, 2003) and the clinician version of the IDS (IDS-C) at .81 (Cusin et al., 2009). The internal consistency of the MADRS was reported to be .95 (Galinowski & Lehert, 1995); test–retest reliability was .93 (Williams & Kobak, 2008); and the interrater reliability ranged from .89 to .97 (Montgomery & Åsberg, 1979).

Limitations

The MADRS is limited by the small number of depressive symptoms it captures as well as its inability to measure atypical depressive symptoms and to assess all MDD symptom domains (e.g., decreased concentration) in the fifth edition of the *Diagnostic and Statistical Manual of Mental Disorders* (American Psychiatric Association, 2013).

Strengths

The MADRS is a brief, widely used scale that measures the core symptoms of depression.

Beck Depression Inventory

The Beck Depression Inventory (BDI) is a self-rating depression symptom severity scale. It was developed by Aaron T. Beck to assess the efficacy of psychotherapy in adults with MDD. There are three primary versions of the BDI for physically healthy adult individuals, including the first edition (BDI-I; Beck, Ward, Mendelson, Mock, & Erbaugh, 1961; BDI-IA: Beck, Rush, Shaw, & Emery, 1979) and the second edition (BDI-II; Beck, Steer, & Brown, 1996).

In the first revision of the initial BDI, Beck improved the wording of items. For instance, he clarified the endorsement of symptoms for the previous 2 weeks (Beck, Steer, Ball, & Ranieri, 1996). In the second edition, the author ensured that the BDI correlated with the fourth edition of the *Diagnostic and Statistical Manual of Mental Disorders* (DSM-IV) (Beck, Steer, Ball, & Ranieri, 1996). As such, items related to agitation, worthlessness, concentration difficulty, and loss of energy were included, and items related to body image, hypochondria, and working difficulties were removed.

The BDI-II captures the following 25 symptoms of depression (Fried, 2017). It directly assesses 19 symptoms (sad mood, fatigue, punishment, self-dislike, self-criticalness, past failure, worthlessness, crying, irritability, indecisiveness, guilt, interest loss, decreased libido, pessimism, agitation, concentration difficulty, suicidal ideation, loss of pleasure, loss of energy) and indirectly assesses 6 symptoms (early insomnia, middle insomnia, late insomnia, appetite decrease, appetite increase, hypersomnia).

Administration Method

The BDI-II takes approximately 5–10 minutes to complete. The measure is copyrighted, licensed, and is available for purchase by Pearson (San Antonio, Texas).

Scoring and Interpretation

Each item of the BDI-II has four response options that range from 0 to 3. The sum of all items, ranging from 0 to 63, is used to indicate the level of depression severity. Specifically, scores from 0 to 13 indicate the absence of depression severity; scores from 14 to 19, mild depression severity; scores from 20 to 28, moderate depression severity; and scores equal to or greater than 29, severe depression (Smarr & Keefer, 2011).

Psychometric Properties

In adult patients with psychiatric illnesses, the mean correlation of the BDI-II with clinical ratings (*criterion validity*) is 0.72 (Beck, Steer, & Carbin, 1988). As for *convergent validity*, the BDI-II is positively correlated with the 17-item HRSD (.71; Smarr & Keefer, 2011) and the Zung SDS (0.57–0.83; Cusin et al., 2009). The BDI-II has been found to have high *internal consistency* with a reported Cronbach's α of 0.92 for adult outpatients and 0.93 for college students (Smarr & Keefer, 2011). The *test–retest reliability* has been reported to range from 0.60 to 0.90 for adult patients without psychiatric illnesses and from 0.64 to 0.90 for college students (Beck et al., 1988).

Limitations

The BDI-II has two main limitations: (1) The item content has an overlap between somatic symptoms and depressive symptoms (Smarr & Keefer, 2011) and (2) as is true of most self-rating instruments, it is subjective, and the person completing the questionnaire can maximize or minimize the rating of each item.

Strengths

The BDI has strong psychometric properties and, thus, can be used alongside clinician-rated scales to bolster scoring validity.

Inventory for Depressive Symptomatology

The Inventory for Depressive Symptomatology (IDS) was developed by A. John Rush and colleagues (Rush et al., 1986; Rush, Gullion, et al., 1996) to overcome the limitations of the HRSD and the MADRS, namely, to include all DSM-IV diagnostic criterion items required to diagnose MDD (including the melancholic and atypical subtype classifiers) and to provide equivalent weighting for each symptom item. The IDS is a 30-item scale that is available in both a clinician-rated and self-report format.

The IDS captures 33 depressive symptoms. Of those, 23 symptoms are directly assessed (early insomnia, middle insomnia, late insomnia, hypersomnia, sad mood, anxiousness, panic, irritability, mood reactivity, diurnal variation, grief, pessimism, suicidal ideation, interest loss, pleasure loss, decreased libido, retardation, agitation, somatic complaints, sympathetic arousal, gastrointestinal dysfunction, interpersonal sensitivity, and leaden paralysis), and 10 are indirectly assessed (appetite decrease, appetite increase, weight decrease, weight increase, concentration difficulty, indecisiveness, guilt, worthlessness, fatigue, and energy loss; Fried, 2017).

Administration Method

The IDS takes approximately 15–20 minutes to complete when it is administered by a clinician and 10–15 minutes when it is completed by patient self-report. The clinician conducts a semi-structured interview with patients in which the patient is asked to endorse a score on each item. All items are scaled from 0 to 3.

Scoring and Interpretation

The IDS is scored by summing responses to 28 of the 30 items to obtain a total score. Two symptoms (appetite and weight change) have an option to choose between either an increase or decrease of those specific items. Either appetite increase or decrease is used to calculate the total score. Likewise, weight increase or decrease is used to calculate the total score (Rush, Gullion, et al., 1996). The total score ranges from 0 to 84. The scores from 0 to 11 indicate the absence of depression severity; scores from 12 to 23, mild depression severity; scores from 24 to 36, moderate depression severity; scores from 37 to 46, severe depression severity; and scores equal to or greater than 47, very severe depression.

Psychometric Properties

The correlations (convergent validity) of the IDS-C with the HRSD and BDI have been reported to be .94 and .83, respectively (Rush, Gullion, et al., 1996). The internal consistency of the IDS-C (Cronbach's α) was 0.94 for a sample of 456 adults (338 adult outpatients with MDD and 118 healthy controls; Rush, Gullion, et al., 1996) and 0.90 for a sample of 544 adult patients with MDD (Trivedi et al., 2004).

The convergent validity of the self-rated version of the IDS (IDS-SR) with the HRSD and BDI has been reported to be 0.85 and 0.92, respectively (Rush, Gullion, et al., 1996). The internal consistency of the IDS-SR (Cronbach's α) was 0.94 for a sample of 456 adults (338 adult outpatients with MDD and 118 healthy controls; Rush, Gullion, et al., 1996) and 0.92 for a sample of 544 adult patients with MDD (Trivedi et al., 2004).

Limitations

The IDS-SR is limited by its subjective assessment of symptoms. A 28-item scale may prove taxing to the patient working on a self-report measure.

Strengths

The IDS queries core and atypical depressive symptoms with weighting (0–3 scoring system) and has matched clinician and self-rated questionnaires, offering strong psychometric value as a measure. The IDS-C is reported to be highly sensitive to change and could be beneficial to use in cases of antidepressant medication management (Corruble, Legrand, Duret, Charles, & Guelfi, 1999).

Quick Inventory of Depressive Symptomatology

The Quick Inventory of Depressive Symptomatology (QIDS) is available in both a clinician-rated and self-report format. The QIDS is composed of 16 items from the 30-item IDS (Rush et al., 2003). The rationale for developing the QIDS was predicated on the need to provide a shorter, time-efficient, unifactorial measure of depression severity (as the IDS is a two-factor measure that assesses both depressive and anxiety content (McClintock et al., 2011). The QIDS captures 20 of 52 specific depressive symptoms (Fried, 2017). Two of the symptoms are directly assessed (sad mood and concentration difficulty), and 18 are indirectly assessed (early insomnia, middle insomnia, late insomnia, hypersomnia, anxiousness, appetite decrease, appetite increase, weight decrease, weight increase, indecisiveness, guilt, worthlessness, pessimism, interest loss, pleasure loss, fatigue, energy loss, agitation).

Administration Method

The QIDS takes approximately 5–7 minutes to complete by clinician and 5–10 minutes by patient self-report. The clinician conducts a semi-structured interview with the patient and asks the patient to report on each item. Like the IDS, all items are scaled from 0 to 3.

Scoring and Interpretation

The total score ranges from 0 to 27. The calculation of the total score is obtained by summing the scores on each of the nine symptom domains: depressed mood, loss of interest or pleasure, concentration/decision making, self-outlook, suicidal ideation, energy/fatigability, sleep, weight/appetite change, and psychomotor changes (Rush et al. 2003).

With regard to interpretation, total scores from 0 to 5 indicate the absence of depression, scores from 6 to 10, mild depression severity, scores from 11 to 15, moderate depression severity, scores from 16 to 20, severe depression, and scores equal to or greater than 21, very severe depression.

Psychometric Properties

Research has found that the correlations between the QIDS-SR and IDS-SR, 17-item HRSD, 21-item HRSD, and 24-item HRSD were 0.96, 0.81, 0.82, and 0.84, respectively (Rush et al., 2003), which suggests strong convergent validity. A recent literature review demonstrated moderate to high *internal consistency* for the QIDS-C, as Cronbach's α ranged from 0.65 to 0.87, while Cronbach's α for the QIDS-SR ranged from 0.69 to 0.89 (Reilly, MacGillivray, Reid, & Cameron, 2015). Furthermore, Trivedi and colleagues (2004) showed that the Cronbach's α for the QIDS-SR was 0.86 and 0.85 for the QIDS-C in patients with MDD.

Limitations

The QIDS's main limitation is its inability to document the presence or absence of MDD subtype symptoms, including atypical, melancholic, or psychotic features.

Strengths

By curtailing the IDS, the QIDS retains strong psychometric measurement of core depressive symptoms while minimizing time demands on the patient. Like the full IDS, the QIDS has matched self-report and clinician-rated scales.

Zung Self-Rating Depression Scale

The Zung Self-Rating Depression Scale (Zung SDS) is a 20-item scale for depression that is completed by the patient (Zung, 1965). Zung developed this inventory as a relatively quick and easy measure to screen for the presence or absence of depressive symptoms. The scale can also be used for monitoring changes in depression severity over time.

The Zung SDS captures 23 specific symptoms of depression. Of those symptoms, 18 are directly assessed (sad mood, irritability, diurnal variation, weight decrease, concentration difficulty, indecisiveness, pessimism, suicidal ideation, pleasure loss, fatigue, decreased libido, agitation, sympathetic arousal, gastrointestinal dysfunction, crying, effort, feeling needed, fullness of life) and 5 are indirectly assessed (early insomnia, middle insomnia, late insomnia, appetite decrease, appetite increase; Fried, 2017).

Administration Method

The questionnaire takes approximately 5–7 minutes to complete. Each item is rated according to how each applied to patients within the past week, using a 4-point scale ranging from 1 (none, or a little of the time) to 4 (most, or all of the time).

Scoring and Interpretation

The sum of the items score indicates the severity of the depressive symptoms. The total score ranges from 20 to 80. Total scores between 20 and 49 indicate the absence of depression, scores from 50 to 59, mild depression severity, scores from 60 to 69, moderate depression severity, and scores equal to or greater than 70, severe depression severity.

Psychometric Properties

Research has suggested that the Zung SDS has satisfactory validity. Zung (1967) found statistically significant correlations between the Zung SDS and the Minnesota Multiphasic Personality Inventory—Depression Scale (.65). The Zung SDS and the HRSD have correlations ranging between 0.68 and 0.79 (Biggs, Wylie, & Ziegler, 1978). The internal consistency of the Zung SDS was found to be high, with a Cronbach's α of 0.79 (Knight, Waal-Manning, & Spears, 1983) and 0.81 (Kaneda, 1999). The test–retest *reliability* coefficient for the Zung SDS was reported to be 0.87 (Kaneda, 1999).

Limitations

As with many self-report questionnaires, it is subjective and individual perception plays a role in over- or underreporting symptoms of depression. A structured interview would be suggested to confirm the accuracy of the ratings.

Strengths

The Zung SDS is easy to administer and simple to interpret.

Center for Epidemiologic Studies Depression Scale

The Center for Epidemiologic Studies Depression Scale (CES-D) is a 20-item scale for depression developed by Lenore Radloff (1977) and is completed by patient self-report. The CES-D captures 21 specific symptoms of depression (Fried, 2017). Of those symptoms, 16 are assessed directly (sad mood, anxiousness, appetite decrease, concentration difficulty, pessimism, pleasure loss, past failure, crying, feeling of being lonely, effort, talked less, people are unfriendly, people dislike me, feeling bothered, feeling good, and feeling happy), and five are assessed indirectly (early insomnia, middle insomnia, late insomnia, fatigue, and energy loss).

Administration Method

The CES-D takes approximately 5–10 minutes to complete. Each item has a 4-point scale: 0 = rarely or none of the time, 1 = some or a little of the time, 2 = occasionally or a moderate amount of time, and 3 = most or all of the time.

Scoring and Interpretation

The item scores are summed to obtain a total score that ranges from 0 to 60. While a total score of 16 and higher has been used to classify the presence or absence of depression, this cutoff can result in a high rate of false positives (Smarr & Keefer, 2011). As such, the optimal cutoff total score classifying the presence or absence of depression is 19 (Smarr & Keefer, 2011).

Psychometric Properties

The correlations of the CES-D with other measures of depression severity and clinical interviews have been found to range from 0.49 to 0.61; the Cronbach's α has been reported to range from 0.85 to 0.90; and the test–retest reliability of the CES-D ranges from 0.45 to 0.70 (Smarr & Keefer, 2011).

Limitations

The CES-D has a high rate of false positives for depressive symptoms. Like other self-report scales, subjectivity can artificially inflate or limit endorsement of symptoms.

Strengths

The CES-D is free for public use and aligns well with other commonly used scales.

For a comparison of the selected seven depression rating scales, see Table 10.2.

CONCLUSION

We described the most frequently used rating scales for depression and provided information concerning their coverage of the main symptoms of depression, administration method, scoring and interpretation procedure, psychometric properties, and limitations. Multiple factors may determine which scales are selected. A small, busy clinic may opt for a self-report measure that has a strong correlation with a clinician-rated scale to save time and personnel, while retaining psychometric utility. In a research setting, it may be wise

TABLE 10.2. Comparing the Selected Seven Depression Rating Scales

Scale	Clinician-rated or self-rating?	Depressive symptoms rated	Time to administer	Psychometric properties	Total score range	Score interpretation
HRSD-30	Clinician	22	15–20 min	Moderate to excellent	0–54	0–7 = absence of depression 8–16 = mild depression 17–23 = moderate depression 24+ = severe depression
MADRS	Clinician	12	15–20 min	Good to excellent	0–60	0–8 = absence of depression 9–17 = mild depression 18–35 = moderate depression 36+ = severe depression
BDI-II	Self	25	5–10 min	Moderate to excellent	0–63	0–13 = absence of depression 14–19 = mild depression 20–28 = moderate depression 29+ severe depression
IDS-C IDS-SR	Clinician Self	33 33	15–20 min 10–15 min	Good to excellent Good to excellent	0–84	0–11 = absence of depression 12–23 = mild depression 24–36 = moderate depression 37–46 = severe depression 47+ = very severe depression
QIDS-C QIDS-SR	Clinician Self	20 20	5–7 min 5–10 min	Moderate to excellent Moderate to excellent	0–27	0–5 = absence of depression 6–10 = mild depression 11–15 = moderate depression 16–20 = severe depression 21+ = very severe depression
Zung SDS	Self	23	5–7 min	Moderate to good	20–80	20–49 = absence of depression 50–59 = mild depression 60–69 = moderate depression 70+ = severe depression
CES-D	Self	21	5–10 min	Poor to excellent	0–60	19+ = presence of depression

to employ multiple measures (e.g., both self-rated and clinician-rated) to have perspective and, most importantly, validity in ratings.

REFERENCES

Adshead, F., Day Cody, D., & Pitt, B. (1992). BASDEC: A novel screening instrument for depression in elderly medical inpatients. *British Medical Journal, 305*, 397.

Alexopoulos, G. S., Abrams, R. C., Young, R. C., & Shamoian, C. A. (1988). Cornell Scale for Depression in Dementia. *Biological Psychiatry, 23*(3), 271–284.

American Psychiatric Association. (2013). *Diagnostic and statistical manual of mental disorders* (5th ed.). Arlington, VA: Author.

Bagby, R. M., Ryder, A. G., Schuller, D. R., & Marshall, M. B. (2004). The Hamilton Depression Rating Scale: Has the gold standard become a lead weight? *American Journal of Psychiatry, 161*(12), 2163–2177.

Beck, A. T., Rush, A. J., Shaw, B. F., & Emery, G. (1979). *Cognitive Theory of Depression.* New York: Guilford Press.

Beck, A. T., Steer, R. A., Ball, R., & Ranieri, W. F. (1996). Comparison of Beck Depression Inventories -IA and -II in psychiatric outpatients. *Journal of Personality Assessment, 67*(3), 588–597.

Beck, A. T., Steer, R. A., & Brown, G. K. (1996). *Manual for the Beck Depression Inventory-II.* San Antonio, TX: Psychological Corporation.

Beck, A. T., Steer, R. A., & Carbin, M. G. (1988). Psychometric properties of the Beck Depression Inventory: Twenty-five years of evaluation. *Clinical Psychology Review, 8*(1), 77–100.

Beck, A. T., Ward, C. H., Mendelson, M., Mock, J., & Erbaugh, J. (1961). An Inventory for Measuring Depression. *Archives of General Psychiatry, 4*(6), 561–571.

Biggs, J. T., Wylie, L. T., & Ziegler, V. E. (1978). Validity of the Zung Self Rating Depression Scale. *British Journal of Psychiatry, 132*(4), 381–385.

Brooks, S. (2004). The Kutcher Adolescent Depression Scale (KADS). *Child and Adolescent Psychopharmacology News, 9*(5), 4–6.

Burns, A., Lawlor, B., & Craig, S. (2002). Rating scales in old age psychiatry. *British Journal of Psychiatry, 180*, 161–167.

Corruble, E., Legrand, J. M., Duret, C., Charles, G., & Guelfi, J. D. (1999). IDS-C and IDS-SR: Psychometric properties in depressed in-patients. *Journal of Affective Disorders, 56*(2–3), 95–101.

Cox, J. L., Holden, J. M., & Sagovsky, R. (1987). Detection of Postnatal Depression: Development of the 10-item Edinburgh Postnatal Depression Scale. *British Journal of Psychiatry, 150*, 782–786.

Cusin, C., Yang, H., Yeung, A., & Fava, M. (2009). Rating Scales for Depression. In L. Baer & M. A. Blais (Eds.), *Handbook of Clinical Rating Scales and Assessment in Psychiatry and Mental Health* (pp. 7–35). Boston: Humana Press.

First, M. B. (2015). Structured Clinical Interview for the DSM (SCID). In R. L. Cautin & S. O. Lilienfeld (Eds.), *The encyclopedia of clinical psychology.* Hoboken, NJ: Wiley.

Fleck, M. P., Guelfi, J. D., Poirier-Littré, M. F., & Lôo, H. (1994). Application d'un guide pour l'entretien structuré adapté à quatre échelles de dépression [Application of a structured interview guide adapted to 4 depression scales]. *Encephale, 20*(5), 479–486.

Fried, E. I. (2017). The 52 symptoms of major depression: Lack of content overlap among seven common depression scales. *Journal of Affective Disorders, 208*, 191–197.

Galinowski, A., & Lehert, P. (1995). Structural validity of MADRS during antidepressant treatment. *International Clinical Psychopharmacology, 10*(3), 157–161.

Hamilton, M. (1960). A rating scale for depression. *Journal of Neurology, Neurosurgery, and Psychiatry, 23*(1), 56–62.

Hamilton, M. (1966). Assessment of change in psychiatric state by means of rating scales. *Proceedings of the Royal Society of Medicine, 59*(Suppl. 1), 10–13.

Hamilton, M. (1967). Development of a rating scale for primary depressive illness. *British Journal of Social and Clinical Psychology, 6*(4), 278–296.

Hamilton M. (1969). Standardised assessment and recording of depressive symptoms. *Psychiatria, Neurologia, Neurochirurgia, 72*(2), 201–205.

Hamilton, M. (1980). Rating depressive patients. *Journal of Clinical Psychiatry, 41*(12, Part 2), 21–24.

Hedlund, J. L., & Vieweg, B. W. (1979). The Hamilton Rating Scale for Depression: A comprehensive review. *Journal of Operational Psychiatry, 10,* 149–165.

Kaneda, Y. (1999). Usefulness of the Zung Self-Rating Depression Scale for schizophrenics. *Journal of Medical Investigation, 46*(1–2), 75–78.

Knight, R. G., Waal-Manning, H. J., & Spears, G. F. (1983). Some norms and reliability data for the State-Trait Anxiety Inventory and the Zung Self-Rating Depression scale. *British Journal of Clinical Psychology, 22*(4), 245–249.

Kovacs, M. (1985). The Children's Depression Inventory (CDI). *Psychopharmacology Bulletin, 21,* 995–998.

McClintock, S. M., Husain, M. M., Bernstein, I. H., Wisniewski, S. R., Trivedi, M. H., Morris, D., et al. (2011). Assessing anxious features in depressed outpatients. *International Journal of Methods in Psychiatric Research, 20*(4), e69–e82.

Montgomery, S. A., & Åsberg, M. (1979). A new depression scale designed to be sensitive to change. *British Journal of Psychiatry, 134*(4), 382–389.

Morgan, J. H. (2016). Depression Measurement Instruments: An Overview of the Top Depression Rating Scales. *Preprints, December,* 1–12.

Müller, M. J., Himmerich, H., Kienzle, B., & Szegedi, A. (2003). Differentiating moderate and severe depression using the Montgomery–Åsberg Depression Rating Scale (MADRS). *Journal of Affective Disorders, 77*(3), 255–260.

Müller, M. J., Szegedi, A., Wetzel, H., & Benkert, O. (2000). Moderate and severe depression—Gradations for the Montgomery–Asberg Depression Rating Scale. *Journal of Affective Disorders, 60*(2), 137–140.

Pettersson, A., Boström, K. B., Gustavsson, P., & Ekselius, L. (2015). Which instruments to support diagnosis of depression have sufficient accuracy?: A systematic review. *Nordic Journal of Psychiatry, 69*(7), 497–508.

Poznanski, E. O., Cook, S. C., & Carroll, B. J. (1980). A depression rating scale for children. *Journal of the American Academy of Child Psychiatry, 19*(3), 540.

Poznanski, E. O., Mokros, H. B., Grossman, J., & Freeman, L. N. (1985). Diagnostic criteria in childhood depression. *American Journal of Psychiatry, 142*(10), 1168–1173.

Radloff, L. S. (1977). The CES-D Scale: A Self-Report Depression Scale for research in the general population. *Applied Psychological Measurement, 1*(3), 385–401.

Reilly, T. J., MacGillivray, S. A., Reid, I. C., & Cameron, I. M. (2015). Psychometric properties of the 16-item Quick Inventory of Depressive Symptomatology: A systematic review and meta-analysis. *Journal of Psychiatric Research, 60,* 132–140.

Reynolds, W. M., & Graves, A. (1989). Reliability of children's reports of depressive symptomatology. *Journal of Abnormal Child Psychology, 17*(6), 647–655.

Rush, A. J., Giles, D. E., Schlesser, M. A., Fulton, C. L., Weissenburger, J., & Burns, C. (1986). The inventory for depressive symptomatology (IDS): Preliminary findings. *Psychiatry Research, 18*(1), 65–87.

Rush, A. J., Gullion, C. M., Basco, M. R., Jarrett, R. B., & Trivedi, M. H. (1996). The Inventory of Depressive Symptomatology (IDS): Psychometric properties. *Psychological Medicine, 26*(3), 477–486.

Rush, A. J., Trivedi, M. H., Ibrahim, H. M., Carmody, T. J., Arnow, B., Klein, D. N., et al. (2003). The 16-item Quick Inventory of Depressive Symptomatology (QIDS), clinician rating (QIDS-C), and self-report (QIDS-SR): A psychometric evaluation in patients with chronic major depression. *Biological Psychiatry, 54*(5), 573–583.

Santor, D. A., Gregus, M., & Welch, A. (2006). Eight decades of measurement in depression. *Measurement: Interdisciplinary Research and Perspective, 4*(3), 135–155.

Sheehan, D. V., Lecrubier, Y., Sheehan, K. H., Amorim, P., Janavs, J., Weiller, E., et al. (1998). The Mini-International Neuropsychiatric Interview (M.I.N.I.): The development and validation of a structured diagnostic psychiatric interview for DSM-IV and ICD-10. *Journal of Clinical Psychiatry, 59*(Suppl. 20), 22–33;quiz 34–57.

Smarr, K. L., & Keefer, A. L. (2011). Measures of depression and depressive symptoms: Beck Depression Inventory–II (BDI-II), Center for Epidemiologic Studies Depression Scale (CES-D), Geriatric Depression Scale (GDS), Hospital Anxiety and Depression Scale (HADS), and Patient Health Questionna. *Arthritis Care and Research, 63*(Suppl. 11), S454–S466.

Steer, R. A., Cavalieri, T. A., Leonard, D. M., & Beck, A. T. (1999). Use of the Beck Depression Inventory for primary care to screen for major depression disorders. *General Hospital Psychiatry, 21*(2), 106–111.

Steer, R. A., Kumar, G., Beck, J. S., & Beck, A. T. (2001). Evidence for the construct validities of the Beck Youth Inventories with child psychiatric outpatients. *Psychological Reports, 89*(3), 559–565.

Strunk, K. K., & Lane, F. C. (2016). The Beck Depression Inventory, Second Edition (BDI-II). *Measurement and Evaluation in Counseling and Development, 50*(1–2), 693–712.

Takahashi, N., Tomita, K., Higuchi, T., & Inada, T. (2004). The inter-rater reliability of the Japanese version of the Montgomery–Asberg Depression Rating Scale (MADRS) using a structured interview guide for MADRS (SIGMA). *Human Psychopharmacology: Clinical and Experimental, 19*(3), 187–192.

Trivedi, M. H., Rush, A. J., Ibrahim, H. M., Carmody, T. J., Biggs, M. M., Suppes, T., et al. (2004). The Inventory of Depressive Symptomatology, Clinician Rating (IDS-C) and Self-Report (IDS-SR), and the Quick Inventory of Depressive Symptomatology, Clinician Rating (QIDS-C) and Self-Report (QIDS-SR) in public sector patients with mood disorders: a psych. *Psychological Medicine, 34*(1), 73–82.

Williams, J. B. W. (1988). A structured interview guide for the Hamilton Depression Rating Scale. *Archives of General Psychiatry, 45*(8), 742.

Williams, J. B. W., & Kobak, K. A. (2008). Development and reliability of a structured interview guide for the Montgomery–Åsberg Depression Rating Scale (SIGMA). *British Journal of Psychiatry, 192*(1), 52–58.

Yesavage, J. A. (1988). Geriatric Depression Scale (Short Version). *Psychopharmacology Bulletin.* 24(4), 709–710.

Yesavage, J. A., Brink, T. L., Rose, T. L., Lum, O., Huang, V., Adey, M., et al. (1982). Development and validation of a geriatric depression screening scale: A preliminary report. *Journal of Psychiatric Research, 17*(1), 37–49.

Zigmond, A. S., & Snaith, R. P. (1983). The Hospital Anxiety and Depression Scale. *Acta Psychiatrica Scandinavica, 67*(6), 361–370.

Zimmerman, M., Martinez, J. H., Young, D., Chelminski, I., & Dalrymple, K. (2013). Severity classification on the Hamilton Depression Rating Scale. *Journal of Affective Disorders, 150*(2), 384–388.

Zung, W. W. K. (1965). A Self-Rating Depression Scale. *Archives of General Psychiatry, 12*(1), 63.

Zung, W. W. K. (1967). Depression in the normal aged. *Psychosomatics, 8*(5), 287–292.

CHAPTER 11

Clinical Neuropsychological Assessment of the Patient with Depression

C. Munro Cullum
David A. Denney
K. Chase Bailey

INTRODUCTION

Much has been written about the neuropsychology of depression (e.g., see Chapters 7–10 and 12, this volume), and it is clear that this is a complicated area of investigation due to the multitude of factors involved. While depression has a deleterious effect on patients' lives in many ways, the effects on neuropsychological functioning in the everyday world versus neuropsychological test performance often vary. As with other conditions, knowing that a patient is suffering from "depression" only conveys so much information about an individual, as the symptoms vary across individuals and over time, and related factors such as severity of depression must be considered. Because current neuropsychological techniques rely on patient test responses and engagement during examination, non-neurological factors and conditions such as depression may adversely influence test results at times. It is thus incumbent on the clinician to be aware of the factors that must be considered in evaluating patients with depression, engendering adequate effort during testing, and appropriately interpreting test results. Despite the extensive literature on the neuropsychology of depression, much less attention has been paid to neuropsychological assessment procedures as applied to patients with depression, despite the fact that special considerations may be in order when it comes to clinical examination, neuropsychological assessment, and test interpretation. This chapter summarizes a number of key points for consideration in the clinical evaluation of the patient with depression, including aspects of interviewing, neuropsychological assessment, special situations, and test interpretation. Many of the assessment concepts covered are not unique to depression per se and are applicable in other clinical populations and conditions.

CLINICAL PRESENTATION OF DEPRESSION

It has long been recognized that various neuropsychiatric conditions, including depression, can adversely impact cognitive and neurobehavioral functioning and, in some cases, can be associated with symptoms that, at least at some level, may mimic a neurodegenerative dementia. Whereas the term *pseudodementia* has become less common and has largely fallen out of favor in recent years, it is often attributed to Leslie Kiloh (1961), who used it in reference to cases (many with depression) where dementia was "very closely mimicked" by depression-related behaviors. The primary rationale for this terminology was to instill hope in both patients and providers and to suggest the condition was amenable to treatment. It is obviously essential to identify potentially treatable causes of dementia; in fact, such conditions should be carefully explored and ruled out before a neurodegenerative diagnosis is rendered. Dementia often goes underrecognized in primary care and other settings (Romano, Carter, Anderson, & Monroe, 2019), and even well-trained health care providers make false-positive or false-negative diagnostic errors or delay diagnosis for various reasons. A recent systematic review of outcomes of patients with pseudodementia using various neuropsychiatric search terms revealed 18 studies reporting follow-up data, with a majority of cases (84%) having a diagnosis of depression (Connors, Quinto, & Brodaty, 2019). This finding was consistent with the notion that many cases of so-called pseudodementia in fact reflect the influence of depression. It is also worth noting that a sizeable proportion of all cases identified (33%) developed evidence of an irreversible dementia upon follow-up, however, thereby underscoring the notion that neuropsychiatric symptom presentation (particularly depression) may in some cases presage the development of dementia (Connors et al., 2019).

Clinical practice must be informed by research to provide the highest quality patient care. As described in Kasham and Ajilore (Chapter 4) and in Howe-Martin, Knox-Rice, Denman, and Brown (Chapter 5, this volume), depressive symptoms are often but one data point in a context of additional psychiatric and/or medical conditions. Clinicians are often challenged with sorting through a host of symptoms, risk factors, and neurodiagnostic findings (or lack thereof) and may be left with a rank-order list of differential diagnoses to deliver to a patient and their loved ones. To utilize a research analogy, this complexity could lead to either type I or type II errors. In this context, avoidance of a type I error (i.e., concluding a condition is present, when in fact it is not) is paramount. Clinicians are faced with an unknown diagnostic "significance level" and therefore are left with difficult questions and decisions:

- "Am I confident enough that this is NOT a neurodegenerative process?"
- "Maybe the depression is a symptom of a dementia . . . ?"
- "Do I let this person know that I think they have a fatal neurodegenerative process now, or do I wait for more time and data to confirm my impression?"

Diagnosing dementia when in fact a modifiable condition such as depression is the primary contributor to the patient's clinical status would be a potentially devastating type I error. Here is a brief hypothetical example to summarize.

A woman in her mid-60s presents with cognitive complaints, notably regarding memory, reduced engagement in instrumental activities of daily living (IADLs), and loss of interest in activities. You also learn that she is coping with the recent death of her father. She was serving as his primary caregiver in the final years of his life before he died due to complications secondary to Alzheimer's disease. There is arguably evidence for the presence of a depressive episode, but there is also potential evidence for a dementia if the clinician is concerned based on her complaint and family history.

If the reader were to put themselves in the shoes of this patient, what would the ramifications be of receiving an erroneous diagnosis of dementia? How might you anticipate behaving in the following months after this diagnosis was delivered? These questions are posed to highlight the importance of clinical decision making informed by concern for very real iatrogenic effects if a type I error is made. The following points serve as a general reference to assist clinicians in differentiating these conditions.

Key points that may aid in distinguishing depression from dementia:

- Onset/course of cognitive complaints correlated with mood/life events
- Accurate historian, with emphasis on failures/cognitive difficulties
- Complaints often far worse than suggested by objective neuropsychological test results
- Level of neuropsychological impairment on testing inconsistent with everyday functioning
- Reduced interest/pleasure in activities (distinguished from apathy or inability)
- Inconsistent functioning/cognitive symptoms
- Cuing assists with recall of information

INTERVIEWING AND DEPRESSION IN NEUROPSYCHOLOGICAL EVALUATION

The relationship between a person's emotional state and their subjective experience of cognitive functioning is complicated (Weber & Maki, 2016). Although an association between depression and neuropsychological dysfunction is well established, particularly among older adults (e.g., Boone et al., 1995; Koenig et al., 2015; Luciano et al., 2015; O'Shea et al., 2015), the phenomenon of "symptom overreporting" has repeatedly been associated with depression and anxiety among patients with neurological and psychiatric disorders (Fargo et al., 2004; Prigatano & Hill, 2018; Prigatano & Kirlin, 2009), in addition to healthy older adults (Steinberg et al., 2013). Findings from a cross-sectional study exploring the associations between self-rated memory reports, depressive symptoms, and objective memory performance indicates that individual differences in self-efficacy may attenuate the strength and influence of depressive symptoms on objective neuropsychological functioning, even in the presence of subjectively reported "poor memory" (O'Shea et al., 2016). Patients are often referred for neuropsychological evaluation based solely on the presence of subjective memory complaints; thus, understanding how to interpret a patient's subjective report of memory loss is an important task for the clinical neuropsychologist (Denney & Prigatano, 2019). This is best accomplished in its initial stages during the clinical interview.

The clinical interview provides the clinician with an opportunity to directly gather information from the patient about the nature of their concerns. For the purposes of a neuropsychological evaluation, a significant portion of the interview may be spent taking an account of patients' perceived cognitive difficulties; such issues are often precipitants for referrals made regardless of the presence or absence of potential factors that may contribute to neuropsychological dysfunction (e.g., traumatic brain injury, neurodegenerative diseases, psychiatric disturbance). Because subjective memory complaints are notoriously poor predictors of actual memory performance on objective neuropsychological tests (Denney & Prigatano, 2019; Jungwirth et al., 2004; Smith, Petersen, Ivnik, Malec, & Tangalos, 1996; Sunderland, Watts, Baddeley, & Harris, 1986), and because of the growing body of literature reporting the tendency of patient groups with elevated depression to overestimate their cognitive dysfunction (Galioto, Blum, & Tremont, 2015; O'Shea et al., 2016; Prigatano & Hill, 2018; Santangelo et al., 2014; Singh-Manoux et al., 2014; Zlatar, Moore, Palmer, Thompson, & Jeste, 2014), the clinician should evaluate with each patient the extent to which emotional disturbances are also present, particularly if the patient endorses diffuse cognitive difficulties. This may help elucidate for the patient/family member and clinician the domains of dysfunction that are perceived as most prominent and perhaps of chief concern to the patient and/or family member, all of which can aid in treatment planning and patient management. Although acquisition of this information may be readily achieved in many cases, some patients have difficulty recognizing, appreciating, and/or reporting the presence of depression and other emotional distress for various reasons (e.g., reluctance to share information about emotional experiences, emotional desensitization as a result of chronic distress, poor insight into emotional functioning).

If the presence of a disruptive depressive experience is suspected, the clinician may need to approach gathering information about emotional disturbances using a multifaceted method. Commonly employed strategies include asking the patient:

- If they currently feel (or believe they are) "depressed," "sad a lot," or "feeling down" or that "life isn't worth living"
- About recent/current problems associated with the "cardinal symptoms" of a major depressive episode [e.g., sad/depressed mood and/or loss of interest or pleasure (American Psychiatric Association, 2013)]
- To rate their current level of depression on a scale from 0 to 10 (with 0 meaning no complaint and 10 meaning the worse they have ever felt), in addition to, and in comparison with, standard depression questionnaire responses
- To describe their recent (i.e., over the previous two weeks) mood state
- Whether they have noticed that their cognitive problems (assuming these have been reported) seem to be correlated with their mood ups and downs
  - If they report cognitive problems, are these problems consistently experienced, or are there days when their thinking seems to be back to normal?

Asking a reliable patient informant these same questions about the patient as another source of information can be informative, with careful attention to discrepancies. Inquiring about possible suicidal ideation (past and present) can also be illuminating and can be asked about directly. Although employing these strategies is likely overkill for any one patient encounter, the importance of gathering information about depressive/emotional disturbance and the impact on daily functionging in multiple ways is emphasized. Making use of subjective ratings (i.e., 0 to 10) as a screening technique (for both cognitive and depressive symptoms) has proven particularly useful in older populations. Indeed, a recent study demonstrated that patients with subjective memory complaints but normal neuropsychological performance reported significantly higher levels of emotional disturbance than patients with amnestic mild cognitive impairment (Denney & Prigatano, 2019). The authors note that patients with subjective memory complaints generally rated emotional/behavioral difficulties (e.g., "anxiety" and "fatigue") as more problematic than cognitive difficulties (e.g., memory, concentration, word finding, directionality), despite their presenting concern being a "memory problem." Furthermore, these ratings provided information about what aspects of functioning most concerns patients, which is valuable for delivering feedback and patient management regardless of neuropsychological test findings. Also, subjective memory complaints are the topic of much ongoing research, as some studies have suggested that at least for some individuals, such complaints, when carefully and reliably assessed, may be a harbinger of future cognitive decline (Buckley et al., 2016; van Harten et al., 2018). Thus, over time, serial neuropsychological evaluations may be useful in documenting level of functioning and may help assess the potential impact of depression on cognition as well as determining whether a neurodegenerative condition may be present.

COGNITIVE SCREENING

Managed care requirements and increasing demands on hospital-based clinicians add to the burden of clinical practice and associated documentation. In reality, this can limit the amount of time a provider has with a patient to focus on quantifying and clarifying subjective cognitive complaints. Providers then have to decide whether to personally administer a cognitive screening test to patients with cognitive complaints prior to referring them for a more comprehensive neuropsychological evaluation. Two of the more commonly used cognitive screening tests are the Montreal Cognitive Assessment (MoCA; Nasreddine et al., 2005) and the Mini-Mental State Examination (MMSE; Folstein, Folstein, & McHugh, 1975). Given that the MoCA is currently offered as open access (*www.mocatest. org*), is available in multiple languages, and has demographically adjusted normative cutoffs (e.g., see Rossetti, Lacritz, Cullum, & Weiner, 2011), it may be more easily accessible for referring providers, though many other brief cognitive screening tasks are available. One benefit of the referring provider administering a cognitive screening measure and documenting the findings (assuming that test administration and scoring are correct!) is that it allows the neuropsychologist a snapshot of gross cognitive functioning at a discrete timepoint. For example, if a patient is referred for evaluation with a MoCA score of 26 versus 10, a different approach and plan for evaluation can be readily adopted. As discussed later in this chapter, insight into potential variability within and across cognitive tests is very important and allows for more confident clinical decision making regarding contributing etiology/etiologies. The total score on the MoCA and MMSE is not likely to discriminate between patients with depression versus healthy controls if effort during testing is good (Blair et al., 2016; Moirand et al., 2018). However, if referring providers are able to delineate areas of apparent impairment (e.g., attention, verbal fluency, visuospatial, memory), the literature does suggest that patients with depression are more likely to perform worse in these domains, a situation that may help guide the neuropsychologist in their test selection. It should be underscored that brief cognitive screening tests tend to be insensitive to subtle cognitive impairment, though poor performance or "failure" on individual item(s) may not be reflective of neurological impairment, as there is significant variability on simple cognitive tasks such as three-word recall even among cognitively intact older individuals (Cullum, Thompson, & Smernoff, 1993). For example, if a patient is not fully attending when words are presented for learning, failure to recall the words later may not reflect an impairment in episodic memory. Nevertheless, cognitive complaints and poor performance on cognitive screening examinations may be helpful indicators for further evaluation. Fortunately, formal neuropsychological assessment provides a much more detailed and reliable index of actual cognitive functional capacity and often includes indices of effort.

As a rule, clinicians must consider demographic variables (e.g., age, education, sociodemographic background) when interpreting neuropsychological test results. This *includes cognitive screening measures*, as these factors are known to influence test performance. To illustrate, a study by Rossetti and colleagues (2011) provides normative data for the MoCA based on some of these dimensions. This information allows clinicians to calculate a normatively adjusted Z score by taking the patient's total raw score, subtracting by the appropriate mean, and dividing by the standard deviation. For example, if a 55-year-old patient with 8 years of education were to attain a 21 on the MoCA, the formula would read (21-19.94) / 4.34, producing a Z-score of 0.24. Thus, although this score is below the originally recommended cutoff of 26, this patient is performing in the average range relative to a normative reference group. Additionally, to aid clinicians in comparing across instruments, MMSE-MoCA conversion tables are available (e.g., Bergeron et al., 2017), though it must be noted that these and similar tables provide only general comparisons. Importantly, individuals who differ sociodemographically from the normative samples may require different cutoff scores to provide the most appropriate interpretive guidelines (Rossetti et al., 2017).

NEUROPSYCHOLOGICAL TEST SELECTION

As is the case for neuropsychological evaluation in the context of any clinical condition or setting, test selection for patients with depression should be guided by the referral question and the pertinent information related to each patient's individual clinical status. The nature of depression and its symptoms can sometimes create obstacles to gathering valid information about neuropsychological functioning on objective testing, and their impact should also be considered when determining test batteries and procedures. For patients with prominent neurovegetative depressive symptoms (e.g., low energy/fatigue, insomnia, poor concentration), multiple hours of neuropsychological testing may be unnecessary and unduly burdensome, potentially resulting in suboptimal or fluctuating test engagement. In these situations, a shift in priorities away from assessing nuanced cognitive dysfunction may be more appropriate. Briefer, targeted evaluations may be called for in order to obtain information about the patient's global cognitive status in lieu of spending an extended amount of time essentially oversampling cognitive domains. In fact, data gathered from lengthier test batteries may be more prone to artificially low scores as a result of low energy/fatigue, and poor or variable sustained attention in patients with depression.

Clinical experience shows that some depressed patients are more prone to give "I don't know" responses during neuropsychological evaluation. This presents another challenge, particularly for examiners whose objective is to elicit patients' optimal performance. Examiners must utilize their clinical skill to identify when "I don't know" responses are valid or reflect the patient's apathy or attempts to avoid or curtail the examination. Thus, such responses should be queried and prompted in order to enhance the validity of the test results. Too many "I don't know" responses should cue the examiner that motivation may be an issue. Patients may respond favorably to an examiner who waits patiently while providing gentle encouragement (e.g., "Take your time," "What's your best guess?"). Another example includes the examiner who adopts the "cheerleader" style, who is active in making comments such as "keep going" or "give me more" *while* the patient is responding. Any particular style in which a patient is being prompted to do more than what comes naturally may also be perceived as patronizing and consequently have a detrimental effect on rapport if done excessively. While not ideal due to the nature of standardized testing, adjusting test administration procedures may help to bolster a patient's engagement. Beginning the evaluation with more straightforward, simple tasks, or activities on which patients may perceive they are doing well, can provide a subtle boost to patients' confidence and result in subtle changes in attitude toward testing and their engagement in it. Another example would be for the examiner to acknowledge "that was a tough one" in reference to a test on which the patient clearly struggled, and then provide a smooth transition to the next by smiling and saying, "let's move to the next one."

Ultimately, determining what/if modifications to a test battery or procedure should be made rests on clinical judgment. When the results do not make sense (e.g., findings are too impaired to reflect actual cognitive function), consider what can be accomplished with further testing. It may be helpful for examiners to put themselves in the patient's mindset by, for example, considering one of the saddest times of their life and how it may seem to a depressed patient to be asked to recite numbers backwards or remember details of a seemingly irrelevant story at that particular point in time. In the throes of mental anguish, how relevant do some of these tasks appear to the patient? What is their frame of mind? What is their understanding of the purpose of the evaluation? The clinical neuropsychologist should always be respectful of the patient's situation and be willing to limit, modify, or discontinue testing as appropriate.

KEY POINTS

- In some cases, particularly when patients are minimally testable, the neuropsychological evaluation becomes necessarily brief and may not rely much on "standard" tests and procedures.

- Deviating from standard administration protocol/test interpretation could be warranted if clinical judgment indicates that a patient needs encouragement to demonstrate best/true performance.

- Integration of inconsistent but pertinent data is crucial to minimize the risk of inaccurate diagnosis (e.g., when cognitive testing data are incongruent with a neurodegenerative process).

- Test engagement (i.e., performance validity) could be reduced/variable and contribute to higher than normal rates of low scores.

- Normal performance on symptom validity/effort tests does not guarantee the validity of all results from a test session.

- Some "low" or "impaired" test scores may not represent cerebral dysfunction.

- Be attentive to qualitative features of responses.
  - In drawings, for example, note whether the patient is taking a careful versus hasty or haphazard approach. In some cases, asking them to redraw may be in order.
  - Some patients may make "sketchy" representations of single straight lines or adopt an atypical approach to copying figures, which should be noted, as such factors may impact the accuracy of delayed recall production.

- Be aware of the potential lingering effects of recent electroconvulsive therapy, as attention and memory may be impacted by recent treatments. See Finnegan and McLoughlin (Chapter 20, this volume) for specifics.

INTERPRETING NEUROPSYCHOLOGICAL RESULTS IN THE DEPRESSED PATIENT

Overall, research has demonstrated an inconsistent relationship between neuropsychological test findings and depression. Some studies have shown reduced test scores in depressed groups, and others have shown no relationship. The review of depression and neurocognitive function by McClintock, Husain, Greer, and Cullum (2010) revealed significant heterogeneity across study samples and measures in the literature and drew attention to the complexities involved in studying this relationship. When low scores are found in depressed populations, the cognitive domains found to be most commonly impaired include executive functioning, information-processing speed, and verbal learning and memory (Koenig, Bhalla, & Butters, 2014; Lockwood, Alexopoulos, Kakuma, & Van Gorp, 2000; McDermott & Ebmeier, 2009). See Table 11.1 for characteristic neuropsychological performance tendencies among depressed patients and those with a clinical diagnosis of Alzheimer's disease. Awareness of these trends is critical for proper interpretation of neuropsychological test results in the context of depression. Indeed, among the more challenging concepts required for competent interpretation of neuropsychological test results is not to know when a score or scores are "low," but to know what "low" scores to *ignore*.

TABLE 11.1. Neuropsychological Performance Characteristics That May Help Distinguish between Depression and Alzheimer's Disease

Neuropsychological domain	Depression	Alzheimer's disease
Performance validity	+/–	**Usually WNL**
Processing speed	↓	↓
Attention	↓	↓
Language	**WNL**	↓↓
Memory		
Encoding	+/–	↓
Storage	WNL	↓↓↓
Retrieval	**WNL or +/–**	↓↓↓
Errors	**Few**	**Intrusions common**
Executive functioning	+/–	↓↓

Note. Discrepant findings **bolded**; ↓, mild impairment; ↓↓, moderate impairment; ↓↓↓, major impairment; +/–, variable; WNL, within normal limits.

A recent study of late-life depression found that half of the sample ($N = 121$) demonstrated average or slightly above-average performance across neuropsychological tests, while the other half largely performed less than one standard deviation below the general population (Morin et al., 2019). It is important to note, however, that even though these groups significantly differed in their performance across all neuropsychological measures studied, most of the scores in the lower-functioning group were still *within normal limits.* Morin and colleagues (2019) hypothesized that the lower-scoring group may be experiencing a relative decline from a higher-functioning baseline and may be more likely to decline than the higher-functioning group. This hypothesis was supported by their finding that the presence of an *APOE* e4 allele predicted membership in the lower-cognitive-function group. This study underscores clinical impressions from working with depressed patients insofar as there are clearly neuropsychological subgroups and some cases may require serial testing and/or other clinical studies to improve etiologic attribution of (even relative) cognitive dysfunction.

It is essential for clinicians to keep in mind that while depression and other neuropsychiatric conditions *may* influence neuropsychological test results in *some* individual cases, in the absence of reduced effort or potentially confounding comorbid conditions, patients with depression often score normally on formal testing even in the face of cognitive complaints (Rohling, Green, Allen, & Iverson, 2002). Within the context of a neuropsychological evaluation, many patients are able to focus on the tasks at hand and may do surprisingly well, in fact. The neuropsychological evaluation may represent a break in the context of their ruminative thinking and, with a supportive and skilled examiner, may be able to muster their effort and do well on performance validity/cognitive testing. Even in patients with severe depression, neuropsychological results may be normal or reflect only some mildly reduced test scores (e.g., see McClintock et al., 2010).

When depression does influence test results, it may be reflected by inter- and/or intratest variability. Along these lines, neuropsychologists must be aware of the relationships between test scores in a battery of tests as well as the typical test–retest reliabilities of their measures and when variations in scores may suggest the influence of non-neurologic factors. To illustrate, if a patient demonstrates an inability to repeat three digits forward, yet they can repeat six in reverse and show normal verbal learning, the digits-forward performance reflects an anomaly that cannot be explained based on known brain–behavior relationships. If a clinician were to infer a deficit in attention within this context, that would be an error in clinical judgement, as a neurologically-based impairment in attention would have an impact on other tests as well. Similarly, if test results vary significantly over time (e.g., going from impaired to normal, to impaired), this should also be grounds for a careful review of the factors that may be influencing test performance (e.g. motivation, test engagement, level of depression/distress). Test–retest variability that reflects increases as well as decreases in performance over time may be another important indicator of the extent to which non-neurologic factors may be affecting test results (e.g., see Cullum, Heaton, & Grant, 1991).

CONCLUSION

Clinical experience and research support the notion that individuals experiencing depression, particularly major depressive disorder, often show a variety of functional limitations that can adversely impact cognitive efficiency. The term *pseudodementia* was introduced to reflect the idea that some individuals with non-neurologic conditions may present with symptoms that may mimic aspects of dementia. In such cases, it is essential to identify and rule out potentially treatable causes of cognitive impairment through comprehensive neurodiagnostic evaluation that includes neuropsychological assessment. The relationship between depression and neuropsychological functioning is complex and requires consideration of an array of factors and careful clinical examination and interpretation. While neuropsychological findings vary widely across individuals, the literature in this area reveals small- to medium-effect sizes in the domains of attention, memory, and executive functioning in group studies of patients with depression. Nevertheless, many patients with depression show normal neuropsychological performance on formal examination, regardless of cognitive complaints. Along these lines, clinical evaluation of patients with depression poses a variety of challenges, as low mood, distractibility, reduced attention, psychomotor retardation, and variable engagement in the neuropsychological evaluation process can contribute to unreliable test results. Further complicating the clinical picture is the fact that depression often occurs within the context of neurological disorders and may in some cases reflect awareness of emerging deficits or be a harbinger of cognitive decline. Awareness of when and how depression may adversely impact neuropsychological findings is essential in interpretation of test results, as well as familiarity with common neuropsychological profiles that characterize various cognitive disorders.

Clinicians must attempt to tease out which test results validly reflect underlying brain–behavior dysfunction versus situational or test-engagement-related issues that may contribute to low test scores in some individuals. Examiners must be acutely aware of encouraging good effort throughout the assessment process as well as noting when behavioral/engagement issues arise that may compromise test validity. Cognitive screening may be useful in cases of known or suspected depression when there is a cognitive complaint or evidence of impairment, although in order to ensure valid results, such screening tasks are inherently limited and also rely on patient engagement and proper administration. Careful attention to test results in light of the patient's clinical presentation and extent of depression is also necessary, as not all test scores that fall below the expected level necessarily reflect cognitive impairment per se. Along these lines, familiarity with the base rates of low scores and test–retest reliability and interrelationships among tests is critical. Evaluation of consistency of test results within and across evaluations can provide important information regarding the presence/absence of cognitive impairment and help determine the extent to which mood-related factors may be contributing to reduced test scores. Last, even though many individuals with depression obtain normal neuropsychological test results, depression often accompanies cognitive disorders and can accentuate deficits when present. Thus, clinical experience and familiarity with the potential influence of such factors on cognitive outcome measures are paramount in examining the depressed patient.

REFERENCES

American Psychiatric Association. (2013). *Diagnostic and statistical manual of mental disorders* (5th ed.). Arlington, VA: Author.

Bergeron, D., Flynn, K., Verret, L., Poulin, S., Bouchard, R. W., Bocti, C., et al. (2017). Multicenter validation of an MMSE-MoCA conversion table. *Journal of the American Geriatrics Society, 65*(5), 1067–1072.

Blair, M., Coleman, K., Jesso, S., Desbeaumes Jodoin, V., Smolewska, K., Warriner, E., et al. (2016). Depressive symptoms negatively impact montreal cognitive assessment performance: A memory clinic experience. *Canadian Journal of Neurological Sciences. Le Journal Canadien Des Sciences Neurologiques, 43*(4), 513–517.

Boone, K. B., Lesser, I. M., Miller, L. B., Wohl, M., Berman, N., Lee, A., et al. (1995). Cognitive functioning in older depressed outpatients: Relationship of presence and severity of depression to neuropsychological test scores. *Neuropsychology, 9*, 390–398.

Buckley, R. F., Maruff, P., Ames, D., et al. (2016). Subjective memory decline predicts greater rates of progression in preclinical Alzheimer's disease. *Alzheimer's Dementia, 12*(7), 795–804.

Connors, M, H., Quinto, L., & Brodaty, H. (2019). Longitudinal outcomes of patients with pseudodementia: A systematic review. *Psychological Medicine, 49*, 727–737.

Cullum, C. M., Heaton, R. K., & Grant, I. (1991). Psychogenic factors influencing neuropsychological performance: Somatoform disorders, factitious disorders, and malingering. In H. O. Doerr & A. Carlin (Eds.), *Forensic neuropsychology* (pp. 141–171). New York: Guilford Press.

Cullum, C. M., Thompson, L. L., & Smernoff, E. N. (1993). Three word recall as a measure of memory. *Journal of Clinical and Experimental Neuropsychology, 15*, 321–329.

Denney, D. A., & Prigatano, G. P. (2019). Subjective ratings of cognitive and emotional functioning in patients with mild cognitive impairment and patients with subjective memory complaints but normal cognitive functioning. *Journal of Clinical and Experimental Neuropsychology, 41*, 565–575.

Fargo, J. D., Schefft, B. K., Szaflarski, J. P., Dulay, M. F., Testa, S. M., Privitera, M. D., & Yeh, H. S. (2004). Accuracy of self-reported neuropsychological functioning in individuals with epileptic or psychogenic nonepileptic seizures. *Epilepsy and Behavior, 5*, 143–150.

Folstein, M. F., Folstein, S. E., & McHugh, P. R. (1975). "Mini-mental state": A practical method for grading the cognitive state of patients for the clinician. *Journal of Psychiatric Research, 12*(3), 189–198.

Galioto, R., Blum, A. S., & Tremont, G. (2015). Subjective cognitive complaints versus objective neuropsychological performance in older adults with epilepsy. *Epilepsy and Behavior,51,* 48–52.

Jungwirth, S., Fischer, P., Weissgram, S., Kirchmeyr, W., Bauer, P., & Tragl, K. H. (2004). Subjective memory complaints and objective memory impairment in the Vienna-Transdanube aging community. *Journal of the American Geriatrics Society, 52*(2), 263–268.

Kiloh, L. G. (1961). Pseudo-dementia. *Acta Psychiatrica Scandinavica, 37*(4), 336–351.

Koenig, A. M., Bhalla, R. K., & Butters, M. A. (2014). Cognitive functioning and late-life depression. *Journal of International Neuropsychological Society, 20,* 461–467.

Koenig, A. M., DeLozier, I. J., Zmuda, M. D., Marron, M. M., Begley, A. E., Anderson, S. J., et al. (2015). Neuropsychological functioning in the acute and remitted states of late-life depression. *Journal of Alzheimer's Disease, 45,* 175–185.

Lockwood, K. A., Alexopoulos, G. S., Kakuma, T., & Van Gorp, W. G. (2000). Subtypes of cognitive impairment in depressed older adults. *American Journal of Geriatric Psychiatry, 8,* 201–208.

Luciano, M., Pujals, A. M., Marioni, R. E., Campbell, A., Hayward, C., MacIntyre, D. J., et al. Generation Scotland Investigators. (2015). Current versus lifetime depression, APOE variation, and their interaction on cognitive performance in younger and older adults. *Psychosomatic Medicine, 77,* 480–492.

McClintock, S. M., Husain, M. M., Greer, T. L., & Cullum, C. M. (2010). Association between depression severity and neurocognitive function in major depressive disorder: A review and synthesis. *Neuropsychology, 24,* 9–34.

McDermott, L. M., & Ebmeier, K. P. (2009). A meta-analysis of depression severity and cognitive function. *Journal of Affective Disorders, 119,* 1–3.

Moirand, R., Galvao, F., Lecompte, M., Poulet, E., Haesebaert, F., & Brunelin, J. (2018). Usefulness of the Montreal Cognitive Assessment (MoCA) to monitor cognitive impairments in depressed patients receiving electroconvulsive therapy. *Psychiatry Research, 259,* 476–481.

Morin, R. T., Insel, P., Nelson, C., Butters, M., Bickford, D., Landau, S., et al. Depression Project. (2019). Latent classes of cognitive functioning among depressed older adults without dementia. *Journal of International Neuropsychological Society, 25,* 811–820.

Nasreddine, Z. S., Phillips, N. A., Bedirian, V., Charbonneau, S., Whitehead, V., Collin, I., et al. (2005). The Montreal Cognitive Assessment, MoCA: A brief screening tool for mild cognitive impairment. *Journal of the American Geriatrics Society, 53*(4), 695–699.

O'Shea, D. M., Fieo, R. A., Hamilton, J. L., Zahodne, L. B., Manly, J. J. & Stern, Y. (2015). Examining the association between late-life depressive symptoms, cognitive function, and brain volumes in the context of cognitive reserve. *International Journal of Geriatric Psychiatry, 6,* 614–622.

O'Shea, D. M., Dotson, V. M., Fieo, R. A., Tsapanou, A., Zahodne, L. & Stern, Y. (2016). Older adults with poor self-rated memory have less depressive symptoms and better memory performance when perceived self-efficacy is high. *International Journal of Geriatric Psychiatry, 7,* 783–790.

Prigatano, G. P., & Hill, S. (2018). Cognitive complaints, affect disturbances, and neuropsychological functioning in adults with psychogenic nonepileptic seizures. In S. C. Schacter & W. C. LaFrance Jr. (Eds.), *Gates and Rowan's nonepileptic seizures* (pp. 158–164). New York: Cambridge University Press.

Prigatano, G. P., & Kirlin, K. A. (2009). Self-appraisal and objective assessment of cognitive and affective assessment of cognitive and affective functioning in persons with epileptic and nonepileptic seizures. *Epilepsy and Behavior, 14,* 387–392.

Rohling, M. L., Green, P., Allen, L. M., & Iverson, G. L. (2002). Depressive symptoms and neurocognitive test scores in patients passing symptom validity tests. *Archives of Clinical Neuropsychology, 17,* 205–222.

Romano, R. R., Carter, M. A., Anderson, A. R., & Monroe, T. B. (2019). An integrative review of system-level factors influencing dementia detection in primary care. *Journal of the American Association of Nurse Practitioners, 32,* 299–305.

Rossetti, H. C., Lacritz, L. H., Cullum, C. M., & Weiner, M. F. (2011). Normative data for the Montreal Cognitive Assessment (MoCA) in a population-based sample. *Neurology, 77*(13), 1272–1275.

Rossetti, H. C., Lacritz, L. H., Hynan, L. S., Cullum, C. M., Van Wright, A., & Weiner, M. F. (2017). Montreal Cognitive Assessment performance among community-dwelling African Americans. *Archives of Clinical Neuropsychology, 32*(2), 238–244.

Santangelo, G., Vitale, C., Trojano, L., Angrisano, M. G., Picillo, M., Errico, D., Agosti, V. . . . & Barone, P. (2014). Subthreshold depression and subjective cognitive complaints in Parkinson's disease. *European Journal of Neurology, 21*, 541–544.

Singh-Manoux, A., Dugravot, A., Ankri, J., Nabi, H., Berr, C., Goldberg, M., Zins, M., et al. (2014). Subjective cognitive complaints and mortality: Does the type of complaint matter. *Journal of Psychiatric Research, 48*, 73–78.

Smith, G. E., Petersen, R. C., Ivnik, R. J., Malec, J. F., & Tangalos, E. G. (1996). Subjective memory complaints, psychological distress, and longitudinal change in objective memory performance. *Psychology and Aging, 11*(2), 272.

Steinberg, S. I., Negash, S., Sammel, M. D., Bogner, H., Harel, B. T., Livney, M. G., et al. (2013). Subjective memory complaints, cognitive performance, and psychological factors in healthy older adults. *American Journal of Alzheimer's Disease and Other Dementias, 28*, 778–783.

Sunderland, A., Watts, K., Baddeley, A. D., & Harris, J. E. (1986). Subjective memory assessment and test performance in elderly adults. *Journal of Gerontology, 41*, 376–384.

Van Harten, A. C., Mielke, M. M., Swenson-Dravis, D. M. Hagen, C. E., Edwards, K. K., Roberts, R. O., et al. (2018). Subjective cognitive decline and risk fo MCI: The Mayo Clinic Study of Aging. *Neurology, 91*, e300–e312.

Weber, M. T., & Maki, P. M. (2016). Subjective memory complaints and objective memory performance. In L. L. Sievert & D. E. Brown (Eds.), *Biological measures of human experience across the lifespan* (pp. 275–299). Cham, Switzerland: Springer.

Zlatar, Z. Z., Moore, R. C., Palmer, B. W., Thompson, W. K., & Jeste, D. V. (2014). Cognitive complaints correlate with depression rather than concurrent objective cognitive impairment in the successful aging evaluation baseline sample. *Journal of Geriatric Psychiatry and Neurology, 27*, 181–187.

CHAPTER 12

Assessment of Actual versus Feigned Depression with Symptom and Performance Validity Tests

Kyle Brauer Boone

THE IMPORTANCE OF PSYCHOLOGICAL TESTING IN THE DIAGNOSIS OF DEPRESSION

Psychologists and clinical neuropsychologists are included the category of mental health practitioners, which also encompasses psychiatrists, clinical social workers, and marriage and family therapists. What psychologists "bring to the table" is relatively unique to the mental health field: formal psychological assessment using objective and well-validated psychometric measures. Other practitioners may use personality and psychiatric inventories, but psychologists are taught test construction and psychometric properties of tests in addition to test administration and interpretation, and that interpretation of the psychological measures must be grounded in authoritative scientific literature.

Many mental health professionals commonly diagnose depressive disorders, but nonpsychologists generally base diagnoses on data gathered in an interview of patients, whereas psychologists are more likely to include in their diagnostic formulations the results of formal personality testing, including validity checks regarding the accuracy of patient report. If patient self-reported symptoms are inaccurate, then resulting diagnoses based on those reports will accordingly be inaccurate. Validated personality inventories provide information as to the nature and extent of psychiatric symptoms, as well as the likelihood that patients are reporting symptoms in a plausible manner. As shown in the case examples at the conclusion of this chapter, performance validity tests also have a role in identification of noncredible neurocognitive symptoms in patients with claimed depressive symptoms.

Research has shown that feigning of depression is common in compensation-seeking contexts. For example, in a survey published in 2002, board-certified clinical neuropsychologists estimated that the rate of malingering in compensation-seeking contexts in individuals claiming depression was approximately 15% (Mittenberg, Patton, Canyock,

& Condit, 2002). More recently, in an investigation of 127 compensation-seekers in Germany diagnosed with major depressive disorder (MDD) by treaters (Stevens, Schmidt, & Hautzinger, 2018), 52% were subsequently judged to meet Slick, Sherman, and Iverson (1999) criteria for possible malingering and 33% met criteria for probable malingering; 33% failed the Word Memory Test and 13% failed the Dot Counting Test, while 40% failed a symptom validity inventory (Self-Report Symptom Inventory), and 22% showed nonplausible findings on a physical exam.

Depressive symptoms are relatively easy to feign because nearly everyone has likely experienced some depressive thoughts and feelings from time to time, and thus have personal awareness as to what are actual depressive characteristics. As a result, plausible symptoms can be easily reported even if such symptoms are currently absent. What methods are available then to identify whether a patient actually has significant depression or, alternatively, is feigning depression?

SYMPTOM VALIDITY VERSUS PERFORMANCE VALIDITY

Symptom Validity Tests

Symptom validity tests (SVTs) are psychological tests that incorporate validity scales designed specifically to identify noncredible overreport of symptoms. Tests such as the Minnesota Multiphasic Personality Inventory–2—Restructured Form (MMPI-2-RF), and more recently, the Minnesota Multiphasic Personality Inventory – 3 (MMPI-3), Personality Assessment Inventory (PAI), and Millon Clinical Multiaxial Inventory–3rd Edition (MCMI-III) contain a large array of scales to measure symptoms of such conditions as depression, anxiety, posttraumatic stress disorder (PTSD), psychosis, bipolar illness, substance abuse, somatoform disorder, and personality disorder. These inventories also include validity under- and overreport scales to provide information as to the accuracy and reliability of symptom report. In contrast, tests such as the Structured Interview of Reported Symptoms–2 (SIRS-2), Miller Forensic Assessment of Symptoms Test (M-FAST), and Structured Inventory of Malingered Symptomatology (SIMS) are designed solely to assess for credibility of symptom report. As the SIRS-2 and M-FAST primarily measure feigned severe psychopathology in a correctional setting, they will not be discussed here.

In the following sections, studies are reviewed that examined the effectiveness of various psychological instruments in identifying feigned depression. Simulation studies (involving instruction of subjects to feign depression) are not reviewed due to problematic generalizability of results to clinical contexts. Indeed, study participants instructed to feign tend to fabricate in more blatant ways than "real-world" noncredible patients (for additional information, see discussion in Boone, 2013). Given that the MMPI-2-RF has now been available for more than 10 years and has been shown to be superior to the MMPI-2, only the MMPI-2-RF studies and initial MMPI-3 studies are discussed.

MMPI-2-RF

The 338-item MMPI-2-RF was published in 2008 (Ben-Porath & Tellegen, 2008) and represents an advance over the MMPI-2 in terms of psychometric properties (e.g., removal of the contaminating effect of demoralization on clinical scales; no overlapping items across clinical scales, which ensures that more pure psychological symptoms are measured by the scales), and more overreport validity scales. Specifically, the MMPI-2-RF contains not only general/psychiatric overreport scales (F-r, Fp-r) and a revision of FBS (FBS-r; a somatic and/or cognitive symptoms overreport scale), but also an additional somatic over-report scale (Fs) and a memory overreport scale (RBS). The MMPI-2-RF has a total of nine validity scales (two noncontent-based validity scales, five overreport scales, and two underreport scales) and 42 substantive scales.

A few studies have specifically investigated the effectiveness of the MMPI-2-RF overreport validity scales in differentiating actual versus feigned nonpsychotic psychiatric symptoms. Wygant and colleagues (2009) examined four MMPI-2-RF overreport validity scales in a large sample of compensation-seekers ($n = 151$), 42% of whom claimed work-related "stress" (the remainder were mild traumatic brain injury [33%], orthopedic injury [16%], and neurological injury [7%]). The patients were divided according to performance validity test (PVT) failure (no failures vs. two or more failures), and when cutoffs were selected to maintain at least 90% specificity (F-r ≥ 90T, Fp-r ≥ 60T, FBS-r ≥ 90T, Fs ≥ 80T), sensitivity ranged from 38.5% (F-r, Fp-r, and FBS-r) to 61.5% (Fs).

Rogers, Gillard, Berry, and Granacher (2011) reported the following mean MMPI-2-RF overreport validity scale data for 120 disability-seeking patients with MDD who passed the SIRS/SIRS-2: F-r = 83.23, Fp-r = 53.64, Fs = 68.83, FBS-r = 80.17, and RBS = 81.22. However, cutoffs that maintained specificity of at least 90% in credible depression were not provided.

Tarescavage, Wygant, Gervais, and Ben-Porath (2013) examined the MMPI-2-RF overreport validity scales in 916 non-head-injured disability claimants, 71% of whom either had a depression (41%) or anxiety (30%) diagnosis (with most of the remainder diagnosed with chronic pain [24%]). Using Slick and colleagues (1999) criteria for malingered neuro-cognitive dysfunction (MND), 436 patients passed PVTs and were judged to be "incentive only," while 240 patients fell within the "suspect malingering" category, 171 patients met criteria for "probable malingering," and 16 were assigned to the "definite malingering" category. The two latter groups were combined, and the "suspect malingering" group was excluded, in computation of classification statistics. Using cutoffs selected for ≥90% specificity, sensitivity for F-r (≥110T) was 34%, for Fp-r (≥80T) was 17%, for Fs (≥100T) was 20%, for FBS-r (≥100T) was 10%, and for RBS (≥100T) was 34%.

Nguyen, Green, and Barr (2015) used the MMPI-2-RF in a large sample of patients with medical, neurological, or psychiatric conditions evaluated in the context of compensation-seeking. Within the psychiatric sample ($n = 66$), 17% met criteria for noncredible performance ($n = 11$; i.e., failure on at least 2 PVTs). When MMPI-2-RF overreport validity scale cutoffs were selected to approximate 90% specificity, sensitivity for F-r (≥120T) was 27.3%, for Fs (≥115T) was 36.4%, for FBS-r (≥ 105) was 18.2%, and for RBS (≥114) was 18.2%.

Schroeder, Baade, and colleagues (2012) investigated the MMPI-2-RF overreport validity scales in various groups, including nonlitigating psychiatric patients passing PVTs ($n = 21$), two-thirds (67%) of whom were diagnosed with depression (versus 19% with anxiety and 14% with psychosis). The overreport validity scale cutoffs associated with at least 90% specificity in the psychiatric group were as follows: F-r = 107T, Fp-r = 78T, Fs = 92T, FBS-r = 84T, and RBS = 106T.

The MMPI-3 was introduced in 2020 (Ben-Porath & Tellegen, 2020) and remains comparable to the MMPI-2-RF in terms of overreport validity scales. Tylicki, Rai, Arends, Gervais, and Ben-Porath (2021) reported data on 550 compensation-seeking (primarily worker's compensation) psychiatric patients; nearly 20% were diagnosed with depression, with an additional 44% diagnosed with an adjustment disorder, 7% with PTSD, 3% with an anxiety disorder, and remaining diagnostic categories each representing less than 3% of the sample. One hundred and sixty patients met possible MND criteria, and 133 met criteria for probable/definite MND. The overreport scale cutoffs associated with at least 90% specificity in the incentive-only ($n = 257$) group were F ≥ 85 (36% sensitivity in possible MND; 47% sensitivity in probable/definite MND), Fp ≥ 67 (29% sensitivity in possible MND; 34% sensitivity in probable/definite MND), Fs ≥ 86 (34% sensitivity in possible MND; 47% sensitivity in probable/definite MND), FBS ≥ 86 (14% in possible MND; 32% sensitivity in probable/definite MND), and RBS ≥ 87 (25% sensitivity in possible MND; 45% sensitivity in probable/definite/MND).

As can be seen, cutoffs associated with at least 90% specificity varied widely across MMPI-2-RF studies (90T to 120T for F-r, 60T to 80T for Fp-r, 80T to 115T for Fs, 84T to 105T for FBS-r, and 100T to 114T for RBS), while in the one preliminary study on the MMPI-3, overreport cutoffs that achieved at least 90% specificity were all <90T, and the cutoff for Fp was <70T.

A concern for some of the above MMPI-2-RF studies (e.g., Nguyen et al., 2015; Tarescavage et al., 2013; Wygant et al., 2009) was that all participants had motive to feign, and some of the grouping PVTs used in these studies had low sensitivity (≤50%; Test of Memory Malingering [TOMM]—Greve, Ord, Curtis, Bianchini, & Brennan, 2008; California Verbal Learning Test—Second Edition [CVLT-II]—Root, Robbins, Chang, & van Gorp, 2006; Digit Span—Babikian, Boone, Lu, & Arnold, 2006, and Schroeder, Twumasi-Ankrah, Baade, & Marshall, 2012; Wisconsin Card Sorting Test [WCST] failure to maintain set and Bernard formula—Greve, Heinly, Bianchini, & Love, 2009; Dot Counting Test E-score [>18]—McCaul et al., 2018) or sensitivity only established in experimental simulators (i.e., Computerized Assessment of Response Bias—Dunn, Shear, Howe, & Ris, 2003). Furthermore, in the Rogers and colleagues (2011) study of compensation-seekers, the SIRS-2 was used to exclude noncredible patients from the credible group, but the SIRS/SIRS-2 are primarily used to identify feigned severe psychopathology in a criminal setting and their utility in identifying feigned depression is unclear. Due to these methodological issues, noncredible patients were likely assigned to credible groups, resulting in compromise to accuracy of both specificity and sensitivity data. Additionally, in several studies, patients with indeterminant PVT and SVT data were excluded from analyses (e.g., Rogers et al., 2011; Tarescavage et al., 2013; Wygant et al., 2009), which raises questions regarding generalizability of the findings (i.e., classification statistics may be inaccurate in that cutoffs did not have to assign indeterminant cases).

Also, sample sizes in credible (e.g., Schroeder et al., 2012) and noncredible (e.g., Nguyen et al., 2015) groups were often small, which may have introduced unreliability into the classification statistics. Additionally, some of the credible groups included patients with neurologic (e.g., Wygant et al., 2009) or pain (e.g., Tarescavage et al., 2013; Wygant et al., 2009) conditions, in addition to those with psychiatric conditions, which may limit generalizability of cutoffs to groups solely with depression.

Furthermore, for the studies that provided sensitivity data, patients were assigned to noncredible groups based on failed PVTs. This means that the derived MMPI-2-RF cutoffs were those that identified noncredible patients who claimed psychiatric symptoms and also feigned cognitive complaints. How well the cutoffs would have detected patients who did not feign cognitive dysfunction as a part of a noncredible psychiatric presentation is not known. Research has shown that SVTs and PVTs load on differing factors (van Dyke, Millis, Axelrod, & Hanks, 2013). This suggests that a substantial portion of individuals found to be credible on PVTs will respond in a noncredible manner in symptom reports.

In conclusion, the more that the MMPI-2-RF and MMPI-3 overreport validity *T*-scores exceed 60 for Fp/Fp-r, 80 for Fs, and 90 for F-r, FBS-r, and RBS on the MMPI-2-RF and 85 for F, FBS, and RBS on the MMPI-3, the more confidence can be placed in conclusions regarding overreport of depressive symptoms. Research has shown that when the MMPI-2-RF overreport scales are elevated, scores on the MMPI-2-RF substantive scales and other psychological measures are also elevated, which cautions that information from such inventories as the Beck Depression Inventory–II will be similarly exaggerated and unreliable (Forbey, Lee, Ben-Porath, Arbisi, & Gartland, 2013; Wiggins, Wygant, Hoelzle, & Gervais, 2012).

More research has been conducted on overreport validity scales in depression for the MMPI-2-RF than for the other psychological tests discussed below. With the introduction of the MMPI-3, additional studies are needed, particularly for large samples of noncompensation-seeking patients with depression, in order to establish reliable MMPI-3 cutoff scores that maintain adequate specificity. These cutoffs can then be used to determine sensitivity rates for noncredible depression, although how noncredible depression samples are to be identified for sensitivity studies remains unclear. To date, noncredible depression/psychiatric samples have been constituted either through failure on PVTs or abnormal performance on the SIRS/SIRS-2. These methods are not ideal, however, because PVT failure only captures noncredible depressed patients who are feigning cognitive symptoms as part of their presentation, and the SIRS/SIRS-2 identifies patients who are feigning severe psychopathology/psychosis rather than depression.

Personality Assessment Inventory

The PAI (Morey, 1991) is composed of 344 items that are rated on a 4-point Likert scale and organized into 22 nonoverlapping scales, including four validity scales (Inconsistency, Infrequency, Negative Impression, Positive Impression), 11 clinical scales, five treatment consideration scales, and two interpersonal scales. Three additional overreport scales have subsequently been published: the Malingering Index (Morey, 1996), Rogers Discriminant Function (RDF; Rogers, Sewell, Morey, & Ulstad, 1996), and Negative Distortion Scale (Mogge, Lepage, Bell, & Ragatz, 2010). All of the overreport scales are primarily intended to identify feigned severe psychopathology in criminal defendants and/or psychiatric inpatients, although one study suggested that the RDF scale may have particular utility in detecting feigned depression.

Sumanti, Boone, Savodnik, and Gorsuch (2006) examined the PAI protocols of a large workers compensation sample claiming work-related "stress"; 9% exceeded the Negative Impression Management (NIM) cutoff (≥84T), 16% fell beyond the Malingering Index (MAL) cutoff (≥3), and 29% failed RDF (≥60T). NIM and MAL were moderately correlated with each other (35% shared variance), but neither was related to RDF (<1% shared variance). Higher NIM and MAL scores were associated with elevations on the majority of PAI clinical scales, which is consistent with indiscriminate endorsement of psychiatric symptoms. In contrast, patients who scored high on RDF showed no global psychopathology, but rather obtained only elevated Depression and Paranoia scales. Thus, RDF appears to measure unique parameters of response distortion, distinct from those tapped by NIM and MAL, and is likely to be more appropriate for identification of specific work stress symptoms (e.g., depression and persecutory ideations).

Tylicki and colleagues (2020) compared MMPI-3 overreport validity scales and a recently developed PAI overreport scale designed to detect noncredible memory symptom report (Cognitive Bias Scale [CBS]; Gaasedelen, Whiteside, Altmaier, Welch, & Basso, 2019) in 588 disability and worker's compensation claimants (using a sample that overlapped with Tarescavage et al., 2013, above); 32% had diagnoses of depression, while 41% were diagnosed with an anxiety-related disorder and 21% had chronic pain. When utilizing incentive-only and probable/definite MND groups (total $n = 434$), and setting cutoffs to maintain at least 90% specificity, RBS was more effective than the remaining MMPI-3 overreport scales. An RBS cutoff of 97 detected 33% of noncredible patients, while a CBS cutoff of 20 was associated with 32% sensitivity, indicating that the two measures were comparable in detecting nonplausible memory symptom report in a primarily psychiatric compensation-seeking sample.

In conclusion, minimal research is available regarding the PAI's ability to detect feigned depression; RDF shows promise, as does the CBS when noncredible depression presentations include nonplausible memory symptom report.

Millon Clinical Multiaxial Inventory—3rd Edition

The MCMI–III (Millon, 1996) consists of 175 true–false items divided into 11 clinical personality pattern scales, three severe personality pathology scales, seven clinical syndrome scales, three severe syndromes scales, and four "modifying indices": V (a "validity" scale consisting of three improbable, low-endorsement items used to detect random responding or content-nonresponsive dissimulation); X (a Disclosure Index reflecting self-revealing inclinations toward symptoms); Y (a Desirability Index measuring fake good responding); Z (a Debasement Index to identify fake bad responding); and W (an Inconsistency scale). The test items are mostly "face-valid"; 84% of diagnostic criteria in the fourth edition of the *Diagnostic and Statistical Manual of Mental Disorders* (DSM-IV; American Psychiatric Association, 1994) (105 of 125) have a directly corresponding item on the MCMI-III, and the inventory was deliberately developed to include "obvious" items and to exclude "subtle" criteria.

Search of the published literature revealed a single study of MCMI-III validity scales in "real-world" psychiatric patients with depression; Morgan, Schoenberg, Dorr, and Burke (2002) compared the MCMI-III X scale to MMPI-2 F and Fp scales in a large sample of psychiatric inpatients, two-thirds of whom were diagnosed with a mood disorder (versus 15.5% with anxiety disorder). The X scale remained valid until the MMPI-2 F scale approached 120T and Fp exceeded 105T, and the MMPI-2 was invalid due to overreport at a rate 29 times greater than the MCMI-III. The study authors concluded that the MCMI-III has a "very high tolerance for overreport" (p. 288). Sellbom and Bagby (2008) argued that due to the paucity of research on the effectiveness of the MCMI-III modifying indices, "this shortage precludes the use of these scales for the classification of defensiveness and malingering . . . we do not recommend routine use of these scales in ruling in or ruling out malingering" (p. 188). They ultimately caution: "Under no circumstances should practitioners use this measure in forensic evaluations to determine response styles" (p. 205).

In conclusion, when using the MMPI-2 F and Fp scales as the criterion, available data have indicated that the MCMI-III has minimal effectiveness in identifying noncredible report of depressive symptoms. A new version (MCMI-IV; Millon, Grossman, & Millon, 2015) was published in 2015, but no peer-reviewed literature could be identified in which utility of MCMI-IV overreport scales to detect feigned depression was reported.

Structured Inventory of Malingered Symptomatology

The SIMS (Widows & Smith, 2005) consists of 75 true–false items assigned to five non-overlapping subscales: low intelligence, neurological impairment, psychosis, amnestic disorders, and affective disorders. Individual scores are calculated for each subscale, as well as a total score; a cutoff score of ≥14 has been recommended for the total score to identify noncredible symptom report. However, data from real-world samples indicated that this cutoff is associated with unacceptable specificity (e.g., ≤65%; see Boone, 2013, for a review). Dandachi-Fitzgerald, Ponds, Peters, and Merckelbach (2011) reported that among patients with mood and anxiety disorders who were not seeking compensation (n = 34), 21% (n = 7) exceeded a SIMS cutoff of 16 (and even lower specificity would be expected with the cutoff of ≥14). Individual SIMS subscales were not validated in terms of detecting the specific symptoms/conditions measured by the scales, although clinicians likely assume that if a patient falls beyond cutoffs for a particular scale, they are feigning symptoms specific to that scale. In the only study that examined the SIMS total score and affective disorders scale sensitivity and specificity in psychiatric patients (n = 56; the majority with mood disorder diagnosis) undergoing disability evaluations (Clegg, Fremouw, & Mogge, 2009), even a cutoff of >20 failed to achieve adequate specificity (71%; sensitivity of 85%). An affective disorders scale cutoff of >5 reached 100% sensitivity, but specificity was markedly inadequate (29%). The study was problematic in that patients were judged noncredible (n = 20) based on the SIRS, but the SIRS was developed to identify feigned severe psychopathology/psychosis, not depression. Thus, it is likely that group assignment was inaccurate, which led to unreliable specificity and sensitivity data.

In conclusion, the minimal data on the effectiveness of the SIMS total score and the affective disorders subscale in identifying feigned depression indicate that false-positive rates are likely unacceptably high.

Assessment of Depression Inventory

Mogge and LePage (2004) developed a 39-item instrument in which test takers rate how often they experienced symptoms within the previous 2 weeks. The nine criteria for depression contained in the DSM-IV were used in constructing the Assessment of Depression Inventory (ADI). The ADI also includes three validity scales: a Feigning Scale (Fg) that contains eight items reflecting extreme, bizarre, or atypical content not found in "real" depression; a Random scale (Rd) that consists of four statements with obvious answers that can only be accurately answered in one direction; and a Reliability scale (Rel) that includes six highly correlated pairs of items. Validation of the Fg scale involved use of simulators instructed to feign depression, which renders the scale problematic for use in actual clinical settings. In a subsequent study (Mogge, 2006), the Fg scale was found to have high concordance with the PAI NIM and MAL scores, and in a later publication (Mogge, Steinberg, Fremouw, & Messer, 2008), correlations of .598 and .331, respectively, were found between the Fg and NIM and MAL scores. However, as discussed above, NIM and MAL identify feigned psychopathology involving multiple symptom complaints, not just depression.

In conclusion, while the ADI may have promise in identifying nonplausible symptoms of depression, validation studies involving "real-world" noncredible populations claiming depression are required before the measure can be used in clinical contexts.

Self-Report Symptom Inventory

The Self-Report Symptom Inventory (SRSI; Merten, Merckelbach, Giger, & Stevens, 2016) is a 107-item scale that consists of five self-report scales measuring genuine symptoms (cognitive, depressive, pain, PTSD/anxiety, and nonspecific somatic), and five pseudo-symptom scales reflecting nonplausible symptom report of anxiety/depression (including PTSD), cognitive/memory complaints, pain, motor neurological complaints, and sensory neurological complaints. In the initial validation study, pseudosymptom scores were highly correlated with SIMS scores ($r = .82$) and negatively correlated with the Word Memory Test ($r = -.45$). Using a SIMS total score >16 as the criterion for noncredible report, a total pseudosymptom score of >6 was associated with 91% specificity and 83% sensitivity. However, as discussed above, the SIMS, even at a cutoff of >16, has an unacceptable false-positive rate. Thus, SRSI scores may closely approximate SIMS scores, but this does not mean that the SRSI accurately differentiates valid versus invalid symptom report.

Other Techniques

New experimental methods for identification of feigned depression have been described, including machine learning models applied to time to perform computer-mouse-based tasks in combination with overreport of depression and nondepression psychiatric symptoms (Monaro et al., 2018) and speech content analysis (Cannizzaro, Reilly, & Snyder, 2004). These new techniques are not recommended at this time, as they require validation and confirmation in real-world clinical and noncredible populations.

Performance Validity Tests

PVTs are measures that assess whether a patient is performing to true ability level on cognitive and motor/sensory tasks. PVTs that have a single purpose in documenting veracity of performance on neurocognitive tests are referred to as *free-standing, standalone*, or *dedicated*, whereas performance validity measures derived from standard neuropsychological tests are termed *embedded*. The question arises as to why use of PVTs would be relevant in the evaluation of depression. The text revision of DSM-IV, the fifth edition of

DSM (DSM-5), and *International Classification of Diseases* (ICD-10) criteria for depressive disorders include cognitive symptoms and slowed psychomotor function. For example, DSM-IV-TR criteria for MDD refer to problems in concentration, such as "diminished ability to think or concentrate, or more indecisiveness," as well as psychomotor retardation, which could include reduced processing speed. In DSM-5 (see Salem, Soares, & Selvaraj, Chapter 1, this volume, for additional information), the criteria for MDD cite "diminished ability to think or concentrate, or indecisiveness, nearly every day" and psychomotor retardation (slowed speech, thinking, and/or body movements, speech that is decreased in volume or amount, observable by others) or agitation. Criteria for MDD in ICD-10 also refer to "diminished ability to concentrate or think, accompanied by indecisiveness or vacillation," and "change in psychomotor activity, with agitation or inhibition."

Before identification of feigned cognitive function in depression can be addressed, the actual impact of depression on cognitive and motor/sensory function must be considered. In a comparison of 73 older, medication-free patients with MDD and 110 controls (Boone et al., 1995), with both groups screened for significant neurologic/imaging abnormalities, patients with MDD scored significantly worse than controls in four of nine cognitive domains: processing speed, executive skills, visuospatial intelligence, and visual memory (verbal memory, attention, verbal intelligence, constructional ability, and language skills were comparable). The declines were mild, and the losses in visuospatial intelligence/visual memory appeared to be trait findings (unrelated to depression severity), while losses in processing speed and executive skills appeared to be state findings (moderated by current depression severity). While no declines in verbal memory were detected in this study, other investigations have reported lowered learning/recall of rote verbal information in MDD (Basso & Bornstein, 1999; Otto et al., 1994).

The question arises as to whether the mild cognitive losses associated with depression are pronounced enough to cause failure on PVTs. The research has been nearly uniform and unequivocal in demonstrating that depression has no impact on performance validity indicators. For example, in a study that included most of the patients in the Boone and colleagues (1995) publication described above, false-positive rates were low on the Dot Counting Test and Rey 15-Item Test scores, and depression severity was unrelated to test scores (Lee et al., 2000). In reviews of the impact of depression on dedicated and embedded PVTs (Goldberg, Back-Madruga, & Boone, 2007; Goldberg & Birath, 2021), no effects of depression were found for Digit Span variables, Warrington Recognition Memory Test, Dot Counting Test, Digit Memory Test/Hiscock Forced-Choice Memory Test, TOMM, Rey 15-Item Test, Finger Tapping Test, b Test, Letter Memory Test, 21-Item Test, Victoria Symptom Validity Test, WCST Failure to Maintain Set, California Verbal Learning Test–II, Rey Complex Figure, and Sentence Repetition. Additionally, several studies from our lab have failed to detect a relationship between diagnoses of depression and risk of failure on such PVTs as the Wechsler Adult Intelligence Scale–3rd edition (WAIS-III) Picture Completion Most Discrepant Index (Solomon et al., 2010), WAIS-III Digit Symbol recognition equation (Kim et al., 2010), Rey–Osterrieth Complex Figure Test effort equation (Reedy et al., 2013), Rey Auditory Verbal Learning Test (Boone et al., 2021), and Rey Word Recognition Test (Bell-Sprinkel et al., 2013), although adjustment to PVT cutoffs may be needed for Stroop rapid word reading and color naming in patients with MDD (Arentsen et al., 2013).

Some research has suggested that PVTs may differ in sensitivity to various diagnoses. Specifically, verbal memory PVTs may be particularly sensitive to feigned cognitive presentations associated with claimed long-term residuals from traumatic brain injury (Rey Word Recognition Test; Nitch, Boone, Wen, Arnold, & Alfano, 2006), while processing speed and visual attention/memory PVTs appear to be more sensitive to feigned cognitive dysfunction in the context of claimed psychiatric conditions. For example, a 76–80% sensitivity rate was found for the b Test, Dot Counting Test, and Rey 15-Item plus recognition score in compensation-seeking patients claiming depression and who were documented to have performed below true ability on neurocognitive testing (McCaul et al., 2018; Poynter et al., 2019; Roberson et al., 2013).

In conclusion, while depression is associated with mild declines in select cognitive domains, these declines are generally insufficient to lead to raised false-positive rates on PVTs in patients with documented depression. PVTs may differ in sensitivity to feigned psychiatric presentations, with processing speed and visual attention/memory PVTs showing the highest true positive rates.

CASE EXAMPLES THAT HIGHLIGHT VARIOUS SVT AND PVT PATTERNS

This section presents case examples in which the differential diagnosis of actual versus feigned depression incorporated use of the MMPI-2-RF and various patterns of SVT and/or PVT failures. The data on patients with depression depicted in the graphs are drawn from Schroeder, Baade, and colleagues (2012).

Case Example 1: Identification of Credible Depression Using SVTs and PVTs

This 48-year-old White, married male physician was referred by his psychiatrist due to the patient's concern regarding his cognitive function; he was not seeking disability or other compensation for his symptoms. The patient reported a 20-year history of depression that was exacerbated when he lost his job three years prior to evaluation, at which time he began to notice cognitive problems, particularly in the area of visual memory; he provided the example of not being able to recall how to navigate between cities. He rated the current level of depression as "2½ to 3" on a 10-point severity scale. Medical history was negative except for a concussion at age 10; he had remained hospitalized for two months, but this was related to management of orthopedic injury. He reported no cognitive sequelae from the concussion or orthopedic injury. He was a good student in school and denied any history of learning problems or attention-deficit disorder. He had discontinued an antidepressant one year prior to the evaluation due to side effects, and he denied current use of prescribed medications. Family psychiatric history was positive for depression in the patient's mother, grandmother, and sister.

No obvious psychiatric or cognitive abnormalities were observed during the exam. In terms of behavioral observations, the patient expressed irritability that his copy of the Rey figure was "not precise," although he received full credit. As shown in Table 12.1, on neurocognitive testing, the patient passed performance validity indicators across 10 of

TABLE 12.1. Case Examples of Neurocognitive and Personality Test Scores

	Case 1	Case 2	Case 3	Case 4	Case 5
Dedicated PVTs					
Dot Counting Test E-score					
E-score	—	*15.5*	*28.0*	–	8
Mean grouped time	–	4.0	*6.7"*	–	1.8"
Mean ungrouped time	–	*11.5*	*14.5"*	–	6.5"
Errors	–	0	7	–	0
b Test					
E-score	–	*146*	239	273	54
Time	–	*669"*	*631"*	346"	428"
Omission errors	–	11	67	20	16
Commission errors	–	*5 (4 d's)*	*11 (2 d's)*	*13 (10 d's)*	1 (0 d's)
Warrington—Words					
Total	–	*39*	*31*	*36*	47
Time	–	*301"*	112"	147"	130"
Rey Word Recognition Test					
Total	–	3	*4*	7	9
False Positives	–	0	*4*	1	0
Rey 15-Item					
Total recall	15	*10*	*11*	–	–
Recognition	14	*8 (2FP)*	*9 (1FP)*	–	–
Combination score	29	*16*	*19*	–	–
Standard neurocognitive Tests (raw scores with the exception of WAIS-III scale scores)					
WAIS-III					
Vocabulary ACSS	12	9	–	16	–
Similarities ACSS	17	–	–	–	–
Arithmetic ACSS	16	–	–	–	–
Digit Span					
ACSS	13	7	*5*	8	10
Reliable Digit Span	12	8	*5*	8	10
3-digit time	–	1"	1.5"	1	1"
4-digit time	–	*4.5"*	*6.0"*	2.5"	2"
Information ACSS	14	–	–	–	–
Picture Completion					
ACSS	15	*4*	*4*	5	12
Most Disc. Index	6	*1*	2	*1*	6
Digit Symbol					
ACSS	13	5	–	9	7
Recognition Eq.	–	–27	–	86	86
Block Design ACSS	14	–	–	7	–
Matrix Reasoning ACSS	16	–	–	–	–
FSIQ	133	–	–	–	–
Rey Auditory Verbal Learning Test (RAVLT)					
Total	43	34	32	50	–
Trial 1	6; 41st %	4; 3rd%	6; 41st%	7; 31st%	–
Trial 5	11; 52nd%	8; <1st%	7; 3rd%	12; 30th%	–
Trial 7	9; 39th%	5; 1st%	4; 1st%	10; 14th%	–
Trial 8	9; 29th%	4; <1st%	3; 1st%	6; 1st%	–
Recognition	10	*5*	10 (2FP)	9 (2FP)	–
Effort Equation	13	*7*	*12*	*10*	–

(continued)

TABLE 12.1. *(continued)*

	Case 1	Case 2	Case 3	Case 4	Case 5
Rey–Osterrieth Complex Figure Test					
Copy	36	31.0	*19.5*	33.0	34
3-minute delay	25; 84th%	10.5; 9th%	12.0; 5th%	19.0; 18th%	19; 50th%
Recognition true positives	10	–	*4 (2FP)*	6	8
Effort Equation	66	–	*31.5*	51	58
Trail Making Test					
Part A	17″; 81st%	–	–	–	–
Part B	38″;7 0th%	–	–	–	–
Comalli Stroop					
Word Reading	51″; 8th%	–	–	–	–
Color Naming	51″; 67th%	–	–	–	–
Color Interference	96″; 63rd%	–	–	–	–
Boston Naming Test	59	–	–	–	–
Wechsler Memory Scale—3rd Edition (WMS-III)					
Logical Memory I	32; 86rd%	–	–	–	–
Logical Memory II	32; 94th%	–	–	–	–
Finger Tapping Test					
Dominant	–	*30*; 1st%	47.0; 16th%	35.0; 1st%	–
Nondominant	–	*26;* <1st%	49.3; 54th%	33.3; 2nd%	–
Controlled Oral Word Association Test (COWAT)					
FAS raw score	31; 8th%	38; 28th%	*30;* 7th%	–	
Wisconsin Card Sorting Test (WCST)					
Categories Completed	5 in 1 deck	–	–	–	–
Failure to Maintain Set	0	–	–	–	–
Other Responses	0	–	–	–	–
MMPI-2-RF (T-scores)					
Cannot Say	0	0	0	0	0
Validity Scales					
VRIN-r	48	48	48	58	39
TRIN-r	50	57	50	57F	57
F-r	61	*92*	*106*	70	*120*
Fp-r	59	68	*119*	42	59
Fs	*91*	66	58	74	*99*
FBS-r	*80*	*89*	70	*89*	*89*
RBS	*101*	*97*	*84*	71	*120*
L-r	42	62	37	57	57
K-r	35	45	31	42	31
Higher-Order Scales					
EID	79	87	83	72	93
THD	53	57	63	60	63
BXD	63	40	63	40	50
Restructured Clinical Scales					
RCd	77	85	81	69	86
RC1	74	72	63	74	97
RC2	80	95	88	76	99
RC3	49	47	83	47	61

(continued)

TABLE 12.1. *(continued)*

	Case 1	Case 2	Case 3	Case 4	Case 5
MMPI-2-RF (T-scores) *(continued)*					
Restructured Clinical Scales (continued)					
RC4	59	43	52	54	65
RC6	56	75	84	56	80
RC7	65	73	68	62	88
RC8	66	39	56	63	66
RC9	51	43	69	36	43
Somatic/Cognitive Scales					
MLS	69	87	81	81	87
GIC	64	80	46	80	88
HPC	78	72	65	72	85
NUC	70	59	53	59	80
COG	91	80	86	69	91
Internalizing Scales					
SUI	66	45	66	66	100
HLP	88	88	88	79	88
SFD	76	76	76	52	76
NFC	64	75	64	64	80
STW	73	65	73	73	81
AXY	70	91	80	59	100
ANP	80	66	80	59	66
BRF	56	63	63	63	94
MSF	46	78	59	46	46
Externalizing Scales					
JCP	57	50	40	50	57
SUB	55	41	41	50	55
AGG	61	61	79	37	51
ACT	44	39	44	39	44
Interpersonal Scales					
FML	58	58	53	84	90
IPP	68	68	34	49	74
SAV	52	80	80	70	80
SHY	66	66	66	66	66
DSF	44	58	98	58	78
PSY-5					
AGGR-r	43	45	78	41	32
PSYC-r	59	47	63	59	63
DISC-r	59	35	54	44	51
NEGE-r	73	66	73	66	84
INTR-r	67	90	87	80	90

Note. Items in **bold italic** reflect exceeded PVT and SVT cutoffs. *References for normative data:* RAVLT percentiles derived from Geffen et al. (1990); Rey-Osterrieth Complex Figure Test percentiles derived from Boone et al. (1993; for ages ≥45) or Mitrushina et al. (2005) meta-analytic norms (for ages <45); Trail Making Test percentiles derived from Mitrushina et al. (2005) meta-analytic norms; Stroop percentiles derived from Boone et al. (1990); COWAT (FAS) percentiles derived from Mitrushina et al. (2005) meta-analytic norms; Finger Tapping Test percentiles derived from Trahan et al. (1987). *PVT cutoff references:* Dot Counting Test (McCaul et al., 2018); b Test (Roberson et al., 2013); Warrington Words (M. S. Kim et al., 2010); Rey Word Recognition Test (Bell-Sprinkel et al., 2013); Rey 15-Item plus Recognition (Poynter et al., 2019); Digit Span variables (Babikian et al., 2006); Picture Completion Most Discrepant Index (Solomon et al., 2010); Digit Symbol Coding Recognition Equation (N. Kim et al., 2010); RAVLT Effort Equation (Boone et al., 2021); Rey–Osterrieth Complex Figure Test variables (Reedy et al., 2013); Trail Making Test (Iverson et al., 2002); Comalli Stroop (Arentsen et al., 2013); Boston Naming Test (Whiteside et al., 2015); Finger Tapping Test (Axelrod et al., 2014); COWAT (FAS) (Backhaus et al., 2004); WCST variables (Greve et al., 2009).

10 performance validity indicators (Rey 15-item and cutoffs applied to scores from Digit Span, Wisconsin Card Sorting Test, Trail Making Test, Stroop, FAS, Rey–Osterrieth, Picture Completion Most Discrepant Index, Boston Naming Test, and Rey Auditory Verbal Learning Test [RAVLT]). Executive skills were borderline to average; processing speed was borderline to high average; basic attention, visual memory, vocabulary, and word-retrieval were high average; visual perceptual/spatial skills were high average to superior; math computation was superior; and overall intelligence was very superior. Verbal memory was average to superior, although word list recall tended to be in the lower end of the average range.

As shown in Table 12.1 and Figure 12.1, the MMPI-2-RF validity scales revealed no significant overreport of psychiatric symptoms, with the exception of a possible overreport of memory symptoms (RBS = 84T), although the patient's score was within 4 points of the mean for patients with psychiatric conditions (RBS mean = 79.4T; Schroeder, Baade, et al., 2012). Across substantive scales, significant elevations were present on scales that measured depression (including social avoidance), stress/worry (possibly reflecting obsessive–compulsive disorder [OCD] tendencies), and some somatic (gastrointestinal, malaise) and cognitive symptoms. The depression appeared to be long-standing and characterological (INTR-r = 80T).

It was concluded that personality test responses reflected the presence of significant depression and that mild, variable weaknesses in processing speed, executive skills, and rote verbal learning/recall were consistent with expected changes found in depression. Alternatively, the relative lowering of verbal skills (verbal processing speed vs. nonverbal processing speed, timed word generation, verbal memory vs. visual memory) could reflect a premorbid weakness in language skills, not rising to the level of a learning disability, in this highly intelligent individual. It was also considered that relatively isolated lowered scores could to some extent represent normal variability. Indeed, even within very

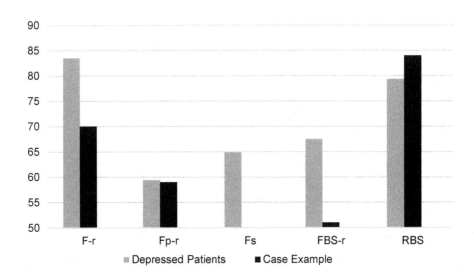

FIGURE 12.1. MMPI-2-RF overreport scale data for Case Example 1 as compared to mean scores of nonlitigating psychiatric patients primarily diagnosed with depression. Data from Schroeder, Baade, et al. (2012).

intelligent populations, scattered lowered neurocognitive scores are found (Zakzanis & Jeffay, 2011). Despite his expressed concern regarding poor visual memory, visual memory in fact appeared to be fully intact, and it is possible that his perception of visual memory difficulties was related to OCD and/or perfectionistic tendencies.

Case Example 2: Noncredible Depression Identified with PVTs and Psychiatric and Somatic/Cognitive SVTs

This 47-year-old White, married female with 17 years of education reported significant work stress over a 15-year period that involved verbal abuse and excessive workload that at times required working in excess of 60 hours per week. She applied for disability compensation and was evaluated at the request of her disability insurance carrier. Seven years prior to the evaluation, she experienced an episode in which she collapsed due to severe pain and suffered an "almost paralysis" and numbness of her legs. Emergency medical evaluation was negative, and the patient was diagnosed with anxiety/panic attacks. She declined to return to work as an engineer and was unemployed in the interim, but she did obtain a real estate license two years prior to the exam for the stated reason of saving commission fees on the sale of her home. She reported that she had also completed "a few" real estate transactions in the year prior to the exam, but that completing "all the forms caused anxiety" and her husband had to "calm me down."

At the time of the evaluation, the patient reported various physical symptoms that she judged had interfered with her employability, including chronic fatigue, feeling like she had been "hit by a truck" upon awakening in the morning, pain in her arms and legs that kept her awake at night, "numbing pain" in the back of her neck when stressed, chronic indigestion, and heart palpitations under "minimal stress." Cognitive symptoms included "limited focus," "forgetfulness," "difficulty making decisions," and "fragmented" thinking (which she described as starting to do something and soon forgetting what she was doing). Regarding current psychological symptoms, the patient reported anxiety "over little things," losing sleep due to "obsessing," anger and problems with her temper, insomnia, and depression, rated as "7" or "8" on a 10-point severity scale. She participated in psychotherapy with a psychologist two times per month and medication management with a psychiatrist every two months. The prescribed psychotropic medications included sertraline, citalopram, and zolpidem.

Medical history, earlier psychiatric history, and family psychiatric history were reported to be insignificant. Regarding additional stressors, the patient cited infertility, but she judged this as much less stressful than the work situation. She spoke English as a second language, but at the time of the exam reported speaking English 100% of the time; she had immigrated to the United States at age 12. The patient denied any history of learning problems or attention-deficit disorder; she described herself as a "mostly A" student in high school, and a B and C student in college. At the time of the exam, her daily activities involved errands, shopping, and visiting her father three times per week.

In terms of behavioral observations, no obvious cognitive or psychiatric abnormalities were noted, with the exception of some tearfulness when she described the work stress. No signs of pain or other discomfort were present (e.g., spontaneous comments regarding pain, repositioning, massaging body areas). The patient claimed to be "too tired" to complete the MMPI-2-RF on the date of the exam. She returned two days later but again left before the test was finished because she was "exhausted and nauseous"; she completed the inventory the following day.

As shown in Table 12.1, on neurocognitive testing, the patient failed performance validity indicators across 10 separate tests, including five dedicated PVTs (Dot Counting Test, b Test, Warrington Recognition Memory Test—Words, Rey Word Recognition Test, Rey 15-Item Test) and five embedded PVTs (WAIS-III Picture Completion most discrepant index, Digit Span 4-digit time, RAVLT effort equation, Digit Symbol recognition equation, and finger tapping). Of note, the patient exhibited a nonphysiological "fast–slow" tapping pattern on the finger tapping test.

The patient scored within the impaired range in finger speed; in the impaired to borderline range in verbal memory; in the impaired to low average range in visual memory, and visual perceptual/constructional skill; in the borderline range in processing speed; in the low average range in basic attention; and in the average range in vocabulary. However, given that she failed performance validity indicators associated with all of the below-average scores, those were judged to be an underestimate of her true skill level. Furthermore, impaired cognitive scores were inconsistent with normal cognitive function observed in spontaneous behaviors during the exam, and the fact that she had obtained a real estate license two years earlier and had conducted real estate transactions. In addition, she scored poorly in testing of finger speed, but no dysfunction of her fingers was reported on interview or observed in spontaneous use of her fingers during the exam (e.g., when using a pen and paper, turning booklet pages, etc.), and lowered finger speed is not found in depression (Arnold et al., 2005).

As shown in Table 12.1 and Figure 12.2, the MMPI-2-RF revealed nonplausible over-report of psychiatric, physical, and cognitive symptoms (F-r = 92T, FBS-r = 89T; RBS =

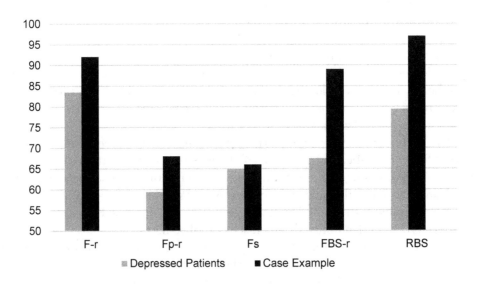

FIGURE 12.2. MMPI-2-RF overreport scale data for Case Example 2 as compared to mean scores of nonlitigating psychiatric patients primarily diagnosed with depression. Data from Schroeder, Baade, et al. (2012).

97T). The patient's responses to the MMPI-2-RF demonstrated elevations on substantive scales that reflected depression, anxiety, anger-related disorder, and persecutory ideation, but given evidence of psychiatric symptom overreport, it remained unclear to what extent she had a current psychiatric disorder. It was concluded that the patient was failing to perform to true ability on neurocognitive testing, and as such, there was no documentation of neurocognitive disorder.

Case Example 3: Noncredible Depression Identified with PVTs and Psychiatric SVTs

This 44-year-old White, married male with 15 years of education had been placed on disability for a major depressive episode that began 2 years prior to the examination; the evaluation was requested on behalf of the patient's disability carrier. The patient's claimed symptoms included feelings of inferiority and low self-esteem, decreased energy, decline in hygiene, social isolation, reduced concentration, slowed thinking, insomnia, decreased libido, eating binges, anger, compulsiveness, anxiety, and paranoia. He rated the current level of depression as 4 to 8.5 on a 10-point severity scale. Psychiatric history was noteworthy for a previous depressive episode approximately 10 years earlier in the context of financial reversals; medical history was unremarkable. Family psychiatric history was positive for an unspecified psychiatric condition in the patient's mother, and it was reported that she had engaged in physical and verbal abuse of her children, although the patient indicated that he had "blocked most of it out." The patient was an average student and may have had an attentional disorder; his son was diagnosed with attention-deficit/hyperactivity disorder (ADHD). The patient had been employed as a real estate investor/broker for the previous 18 years, and his job duties involved calling contacts, finding properties for clients to purchase, and participating in meetings. At the time of the exam, he was in treatment with a psychiatrist and psychologist, and he had been prescribed Effexor.

No obvious psychiatric or cognitive abnormalities were observed during the exam. As shown in Table 12.1 on neurocognitive testing, the patient failed performance validity indicators across nine separate tests, including five dedicated PVTs (Dot Counting Test, b Test, Warrington Recognition Memory Test—Words, Rey Word Recognition Test, Rey 15-Item Test), and four embedded PVTs (WAIS-III Picture Completion most discrepant index, and Digit Span, RAVLT, and Rey–Osterrieth variables); cutoffs applied to finger tapping and the Controlled Oral Word Association Test (COWAT-FAS) were passed. Some implausible qualitative errors were also noted in his copy of the Rey figure (e.g., four lines drawn instead of five for detail #12; three lines drawn instead of four for detail #8; omission of the "x" in detail #6).

The patient scored within the impaired range in visual perceptual/constructional skill; in the impaired to borderline range in visual and verbal memory; in the borderline range in basic attention; in the low average to average range in finger speed; and in the average range in rapid word generation. However, given that he failed performance validity indicators associated with all of the impaired to borderline skill areas, those were judged to be an underestimate of his true skill level. Furthermore, impaired cognitive scores were inconsistent with normal cognitive function observed in spontaneous behaviors during

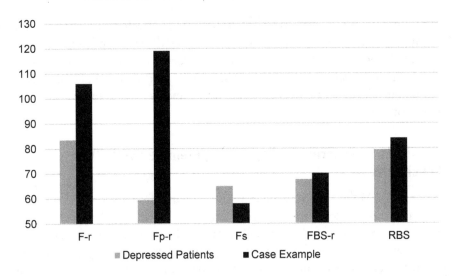

FIGURE 12.3. MMPI-2-RF overreport scale data for Case Example 3 as compared to mean scores of nonlitigating psychiatric patients primarily diagnosed with depression. Data from Schroeder, Baade, et al. (2012).

the exam. If his impaired to borderline scores in memory and visual perceptual/spatial skills were judged to be accurate, he would need to be referred for removal of his driver's license.

As shown in Table 12.1 and Figure 12.3, the MMPI-2-RF was invalid due to marked nonplausible overreport of psychiatric symptoms, including psychotic-type symptoms (F-r = 106T; Fp-r = 119T). The extreme psychiatric symptom report, including prominent paranoid ideation, was inconsistent with the patient's daily life functionality (he continued to live independently, drive, and parent). Indeed, if he truly had this level of psychiatric dysfunction, it would have been apparent in spontaneous interactions during the exam, and it would likely have required inpatient psychiatric placement and treatment.

Interestingly, despite the fact that the patient failed multiple PVTs and was clearly underperforming to true skill level on cognitive testing, he did not engage in noncredible report of physical and/or cognitive symptoms on personality testing.

It was concluded that this patient was failing to perform to true ability on neurocognitive testing and was markedly overreporting psychiatric symptoms in a nonplausible manner. Moreover, if any dysfunction was in fact present, it was not of the magnitude reflected in cognitive and psychological test scores.

Case Example 4: Likely Noncredible Depression Identified with PVTs and a Somatic/Cognitive SVT

This 31-year-old White, married female attorney had been placed on disability for a major depressive episode that began 2 years previous to the examination; the evaluation was requested on behalf of the patient's disability carrier. The patient's claimed symptoms included reduced attention span and ability to focus, forgetfulness, reduced cognitive efficiency, insomnia, feeling of being overwhelmed, "strange" anxiety attacks (feeling of near vomiting associated with becoming cold, shaky, and as if a" blanket was over her," which would lead her to get under her desk at work or to get down on the floor of her car), and eating disorder (which began in college). She rated the level of depression as a 7 on a 10-point severity scale.

The patient described several major stressors in her life in the 2 years preceding the evaluation, including abandonment by her fiancé; her subsequent pregnancy and birth of a child; relationship problems with her current boyfriend; death of a grandfather; and cancer detected in her father. The patient described herself as a high achiever at the law firm where she was employed until 15 months prior to exam, but records in fact showed that 2½ years before the exam she was reprimanded at work, and 1½ years prior to exam she had informed her family physician that she was unhappy in her occupation as an attorney and was actively seeking different employment. The initial certification of disability by the physician repeatedly cited job stress. In the same month as the neuropsychological evaluation, the patient had begun a part-time job that involved administrative work, while also caring for her infant.

Medical history was unremarkable with the exception of premature birth, and the patient denied a psychiatric history prior to 2 years before the exam. Family psychiatric history was noteworthy for eating disorders in her mother and sisters; the patient had no relationship with her biological father. There were no reported academic problems. The patient had been employed as an attorney for 3 years prior to being placed on disability. At the time of the exam, she was in treatment with a marriage and family therapist, and had been prescribed antidepressant medications by her family physician, which were discontinued at the time of her pregnancy.

No obvious psychiatric or cognitive abnormalities were observed during the exam, with the exception that the patient became tearful at times during the interview. As shown in Table 12.1, on neurocognitive testing, the patient failed performance validity indicators across five separate tests, including two dedicated PVTs (b Test, Warrington Recognition Memory Test— Words; passed the Rey Word Recognition Test) and three embedded PVTs (WAIS-III Picture Completion most discrepant index, and RAVLT and COWAT variables; Digit Span, Digit Symbol recognition, finger tapping, and Rey–Osterrieth PVT cutoffs were passed, but some implausible qualitative errors were noted in copy of the Rey figure, e.g., five lines were drawn instead of four for detail #8; six lines were drawn instead of five for detail #12).

The patient scored within the impaired range in finger speed; in the impaired to average range in verbal memory; in the borderline range in visual perceptual skill and rapid word generation; in the low average range in visual memory; in the low average to average range in constructional skill; in the lower end of average in basic attention and processing speed; and in the superior range in vocabulary range. However, given that she failed performance validity indicators associated with all of the below-average skill areas, those were judged to be an underestimate of true ability level. Her lowered cognitive scores were inconsistent with her functionality in instrumental daily life activities (working part-time as an administrator while caring for an infant). She scored poorly in testing of finger speed, but no dysfunction of her fingers was reported on interview or observed elsewhere during the exam, and lowered finger speed is not associated with depression (Arnold et al., 2005).

As shown in Table 12.1 and Figure 12.4, the MMPI-2-RF was valid, although she did obtain a moderate elevation on FBS-r (89T), which suggested that she was reporting cognitive and/or somatic dysfunction in a nonplausible manner. Her FBS-r elevation would be consistent with having failed several PVTs. Across substantive scales, the patient obtained significant elevations on characterological depression and anxiety, social discomfort leading to social avoidance and/or social phobia, family conflict, and somatization indices.

The question arose as to whether the patient had any actual depressive symptoms; that is, she did not elevate on psychiatric symptom SVTs and did elevate on depression-related substantive scales, but she failed numerous neurocognitive validity indicators. When a patient obtains generally unelevated scores on the MMPI-2-RF validity scales, it indicates that they were not overreporting symptoms in a noncredible manner, but not that they necessarily have the claimed psychiatric condition. That is, they could be reporting symptoms in a plausible manner, but not truly be experiencing the reported symptoms. For example, a patient could have experienced previous depressive episodes or observed them in family members or friends, and be well aware of depressive symptoms, and then falsely report them in the future. In this context, the failed PVTs assume critical importance because they document deliberate misrepresentation of current function. It can be argued that if the patient is feigning cognitive symptoms as part of the claimed condition, it is possible, if not likely, that the reported noncognitive (i.e., psychiatric) symptoms are falsified as well.

It was concluded that while the environmental stressors reported by the patient could reasonably be expected to have led to significant depressive and anxiety symptoms, the examiner was concerned by discrepancies between the patient report and medical records regarding previous workplace function, the unusual nature of her anxiety attacks, and the fact that the patient was not credible on neurocognitive testing. It was pointed out that

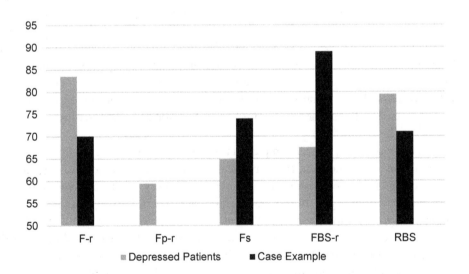

FIGURE 12.4. MMPI-2-RF overreport scale data for Case Example 4 as compared to mean scores of nonlitigating psychiatric patients primarily diagnosed with depression. Data from Schroeder, Baade, et al. (2012).

data from medical records raised clear doubts regarding the patient's motivation to return to work as an attorney.

Case Example 5: Noncredible Depression Identified with SVTs in the Context of Passed PVTs

This 51-year-old White, separated male with 18 years of education had been placed on disability for a major depressive episode with onset 12 years prior to the examination; the evaluation was requested on behalf of the patient's disability carrier. The patient's claimed symptoms included overeating and 40-pound weight gain, insomnia, isolating himself, "not caring," and panic attacks; he rated the current level of depression as 7 on a 10-point severity scale. He denied a psychiatric history prior to 12 years ago, at which time he was involved in a motor vehicle accident that resulted in a probable mild traumatic brain injury complicated by alcohol intoxication. The patient reported that subsequent to the accident, he exhibited bizarre behaviors that included using "Tourette-like" speech, saying "vulgar things," and yelling and screaming. He also described himself as an alcoholic for the past 10 years, but he characterized his current drinking as under control. Family psychiatric history was positive for MDD in a sister, father, and maternal grandfather, and bipolar disorder in another sister. The patient described himself as a B student in high school and college; he denied learning disability but reported that he was previously diagnosed with ADHD. Medical history was only significant for hypertension and gastrointestinal disease.

The patient had been employed as a manager for numerous software and communications companies but was fired from each position after 1 to 2 years for nonperformance; he had been receiving disability compensation for the 2½ years prior to the examination. He had reportedly become suicidal at the time of his exit from his last employment position, which resulted in psychiatric hospitalization for 4 days. Subsequently, he was again psychiatrically hospitalized for 3 weeks for suicidal ideation 1½ years prior to the exam, and again 3 months prior to the current exam. He described numerous stressors in the 2 years prior to exam that included being in the midst of a divorce and unable to sell his home, which necessitated that he continue to live with his wife; father with terminal cancer; death of his dog; parents' loss of home due to foreclosure and having to help financially support his parents; upcoming colon surgery; and unsuccessful job hunting.

He was in treatment with a marriage and family therapist one time per week, along with antidepressant medication management with a psychiatrist; he expressed dissatisfaction with several previous therapists. The patient indicated that he had been tried on a "dozen" combinations of psychotropic medications, which at the time of exam were vilzodone, asenapine, eszopiclone, and alprazolam. His daily activities involved transporting his daughter to and from school, supervising her homework, watching TV, and sending out resumes as part of searching for a job.

No obvious psychiatric or cognitive abnormalities were observed during the exam. As shown in Table 12.1, on neurocognitive testing, the patient passed performance validity indicators across eight separate tests, including four dedicated PVTs (Dot Counting Test, b Test, Warrington Recognition Memory Test—Words, and Rey Word Recognition Test) and four embedded PVTs (WAIS-III Picture Completion most discrepant index, Digit

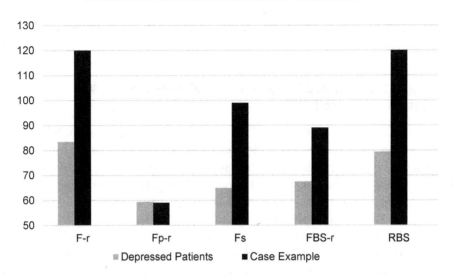

FIGURE 12.5. MPI-2-RF overreport scale data for Case Example 5 as compared to mean scores of nonlitigating psychiatric patients primarily diagnosed with depression. Data from Schroeder, Baade, et al. (2012).

Span variables, Digit Symbol recognition, and Rey–Osterrieth effort equation). On cognitive screening, the patient scored within the low average range in processing speed, in the average range in attention and visual memory, and in the high average range in visual perception.

As shown in Table 12.1 and Figure 12.5, the MMPI-2-RF was invalid due to marked nonplausible overreport of psychiatric symptoms (F-r = 120T). The extreme psychiatric symptom report was inconsistent with his daily life function functionality (he continued to live independently, drive, and parent); if he truly had this level of psychiatric dysfunction, it would have been apparent in spontaneous interactions during the exam. The patient also was markedly elevated on overreport scales assessing for credibility of physical and cognitive symptoms (RBS = 120T; Fs = 99T; FBS-r = 89T).

It was concluded that this patient was markedly overreporting psychiatric, physical, and cognitive symptoms in a nonplausible manner and that if any symptoms were in fact present, they were below the magnitude reflected in psychological test scores. It was also noted that despite a nonplausible cognitive symptom report, cognitive function on screening was within normal limits. His bizarre and dramatic symptoms postconcussion and his problematic relationship with treaters were judged to be likely reflective of a borderline personality disorder, which had also been diagnosed by previous evaluators, and that he might well also have diagnoses of ADHD and alcohol use disorder.

RECOMMENDATIONS FOR CLINICAL PRACTICE

In summary, well-validated SVTs that measure not only psychiatric, but also cognitive and physical, symptom report are critical in the differential diagnosis of actual versus feigned depression because they provide data as to whether the test taker is reporting a plausible amount and type of symptoms associated with depression. However, more research on SVTs in "real-world" credible and noncredible depression populations is needed to confirm the optimal cutoff scores. It should be kept in mind that SVTs assess for credibility of depressive symptoms, but that these scales may be ineffective in detecting individuals who report plausible symptoms that are not actually present. To the extent that test takers report credible depressive symptoms, even if they are experiencing no depressive symptoms at the time, they will not be identified as noncredible on SVTs.

PVTs are an important adjunctive technique because they assess whether the individual is misrepresenting the extent of cognitive dysfunction associated with depression. Without PVT data, evidence of falsification of depressive disorder would have been minimal in Case Example 4 and somewhat equivocal in Case Example 2. Case Examples 2 through 5 demonstrated that individuals feigning depression can differ in type and extent of noncredible cognitive dysfunction and in psychiatric, physical, and cognitive symptom overreport. These case examples highlight that there is no one noncredible depression profile. In clinical practice, it is recommended to:

1. Administer a well-validated personality inventory with comprehensive overreport validity scales that assess for veracity of self-reported psychiatric, cognitive, and physical symptoms.
2. Administer multiple performance validity indicators that encompass many neurocognitive domains to assess for veracity of reported neurocognitive complaints.
3. Consider whether reported symptoms and lowered neurocognitive scores are consistent or inconsistent with symptoms and cognitive test performance documented in depression.
4. Consider whether lowered neurocognitive scores and elevated psychological scale scores are consistent or inconsistent with evidence as to how the patient actually functions in daily life activities.

REFERENCES

American Psychiatric Association. (1994). *Diagnostic and statistical manual of mental disorders* (4th ed.). Washington, DC: Author.

Arentsen, T. J., Boone, K. B., Lo, T. T., Goldberg, H. E., Cottingham, M. E., Victor, T. L., et al. (2013). Effectiveness of the Comalli Stroop Test as a measure of negative response bias. *Clinical Neuropsychologist, 27*(6), 1060–1076.

Arnold, G., Boone, K. B., Lu, P., Dean, A., Wen, J., Nitch, S., & McPherson, S. (2005). Sensitivity and specificity of finger tapping test scores for the detection of suspect effort. *Clinical Neuropsychologist, 19*(1), 105–120.

Axelrod, B. N., Meyers, J. E., & Davis, J. J. (2014). Finger tapping test performance as a measure of performance validity. *Clinical Neuropsychologist, 28*(5), 876–888.

Babikian, T., Boone, K. B., Lu, P., & Arnold, G. (2006). Sensitivity and specificity of various digit span scores in the detection of suspect effort. *Clinical Neuropsychologist, 20*(1), 145–159.

Backhaus, S. L., Fichtenberg, N. L., & Hanks, R. A. (2004). Detection of sub-optimal performance using a floor effect strategy in patients with traumatic brain injury. *Clinical Neuropsychologist, 18*(4), 591–603.

Basso, M. R., & Bornstein, R. A. (1999). Relative memory deficits in recurrent versus first-episode major depression on a word-list learning task. *Neuropsychology, 13*(4), 557.

Bell-Sprinkel, T. L., Boone, K. B., Miora, D., Cottingham, M., Victor, T., Ziegler, E., et al. (2013). Re-examination of the Rey Word Recognition Test. *Clinical Neuropsychologist, 27*(3), 516–527.

Ben-Porath, Y. S., & Tellegen, A. (2008). *MMPI-2-RF, Minnesota Multiphasic Personality Inventory–2 Restructured Form: Manual for Administration, Scoring and Interpretation*. Minneapolis: University of Minnesota Press.

Ben-Porath, Y. S., & Tellegen, A. (2020). *Minnesota Multiphasic Personality Inventory–3 technical manual*. Minneapolis: University of Minnesota Press.

Boone, K. B. (2013). *Clinical practice of forensic neuropsychology: An evidence-based approach*. New York: Guilford Press.

Boone, K. B., Ghaffarian, S., Lesser, I. M., Hill-Gutierrez, E., & G. Berman, N. (1993). Wisconsin Card Sorting Test performance in healthy, older adults: Relationship to age, sex, education, and IQ. *Journal of Clinical Psychology, 49*(1), 54–60

Boone, K. B., Lesser, I. M., Hill-Gutierrez, E., Berman, N. G., & D'elia, L. F. (1993). Rey–Osterrieth Complex Figure performance in healthy, older adults: Relationship to age, education, sex, and IQ. *Clinical Neuropsychologist, 7*(1), 22–28.

Boone, K. B., Lesser, I. M., Miller, B. L., Wohl, M., Berman, N., Lee, A., et al. (1995). Cognitive functioning in older depressed outpatients: Relationship of presence and severity of depression to neuropsychological test scores. *Neuropsychology, 9*(3), 390.

Boone, K. B., Lesser, I. M., Miller, B. L., Wohl, M., Berman, N., Lee, A., et al. (1995). Cognitive functioning in older depressed outpatients: Relationship of presence and severity of depression to neuropsychological test scores. *Neuropsychology, 9*(3), 390.

Boone, K. B., Miller, B. L., Lesser, I. M., Hill, E., & D'Elia, L. (1990). Performance on frontal lobe tests in healthy, older individuals. *Developmental Neuropsychology, 6*(3), 215–223.

Boone, K. B., Sherman, D., Mishler, J., Daoud, G., Cottingham, M., Victor, T. L., et al. (2021). Cross-validation of RAVLT performance validity indicators and the RAVLT/RO discriminant function in a large known groups sample. *The Clinical Neuropsychologist*.

Cannizzaro, M., Reilly, N., & Snyder, P. J. (2004). Speech content analysis in feigned depression. *Journal of Psycholinguistic Research, 33*(4), 289–301.

Clegg, C., Fremouw, W., & Mogge, N. (2009). Utility of the Structured Inventory of Malingered Symptomatology (SIMS) and the Assessment of Depression Inventory (ADI) in screening for malingering among outpatients seeking to claim disability. *Journal of Forensic Psychiatry and Psychology, 20*(2), 239–254.

Dandachi-FitzGerald, B., Ponds, R. W., Peters, M. J., & Merckelbach, H. (2011). Cognitive underperformance and symptom over-reporting in a mixed psychiatric sample. *Clinical Neuropsychologist, 25*(5), 812–828.

Dunn, T. M., Shear, P. K., Howe, S., & Ris, M. D. (2003). Detecting neuropsychological malingering: Effects of coaching and information. *Archives of Clinical Neuropsychology, 18*(2), 121–134.

Forbey, J. D., Lee, T. T., Ben-Porath, Y. S., Arbisi, P. A., & Gartland, D. (2013). Associations between MMPI-2-RF validity scale scores and extra-test measures of personality and psychopathology. *Assessment, 20*(4), 448–461.

Gaasedelen, O. J., Whiteside, D. M., Altmaier, E., Welch, C., & Basso, M. R. (2019). The construction and the initial validation of the Cognitive Bias Scale for the Personality Assessment Inventory. *The Clinical Neuropsychologist, 33*(8), 1467–1484.

Geffen, G., Moar, K. J., O'hanlon, A. P., Clark, C. R., & Geffen, L. B. (1990). Performance measures of 16- to 86-year-old males and females on the auditory verbal learning test. *Clinical Neuropsychologist, 4*(1), 45–63.

Goldberg, H. E., Back-Madruga, C., & Boone, K. B. (2007). The impact of psychiatric disorders on cognitive symptom validity test scores. In K. B. Boone (Ed.), *Assessment of feigned cognitive impairment: A neuropsychological perspective* (pp. 281–309). New York: Guilford Press.

Goldberg, H. E., & Birath, J. B. (2021). The impact of psychotic, depressive, bipolar, obsessive–compulsive, and anxiety disorders on performance validity test results. In K. B. Boone (Ed.), *Assessment of feigned cognitive impairment* (pp. 387–432). New York: Guilford Press.

Greve, K. W., Heinly, M. T., Bianchini, K. J., & Love, J. M. (2009). Malingering detection with the Wisconsin Card Sorting Test in mild traumatic brain injury. *Clinical Neuropsychologist, 23*(2), 343–362.

Greve, K. W., Ord, J., Curtis, K. L., Bianchini, K. J., & Brennan, A. (2008). Detecting malingering in traumatic brain injury and chronic pain: A comparison of three forced-choice symptom validity tests. *Clinical Neuropsychologist, 22*(5), 896–918.

Iverson, G. L., Lange, R. T., Green, P., & Franzen, M. D. (2002). Detecting exaggeration and malingering with the Trail Making Test. *Clinical Neuropsychologist, 16*(3), 398–406.

Kim, M. S., Boone, K. B., Victor, T., Marion, S. D., Amano, S., Cottingham, M. E., et al. (2010). The Warrington Recognition Memory Test for words as a measure of response bias: Total score and response time cutoffs developed on "real world" credible and noncredible subjects. *Archives of Clinical Neuropsychology, 25*(1), 60–70.

Kim, N., Boone, K. B., Victor, T., Lu, P., Keatinge, C., & Mitchell, C. (2010). Sensitivity and specificity of a digit symbol recognition trial in the identification of response bias. *Archives of Clinical Neuropsychology, 25*(5), 420–428.

Lee, A., Boone, K., Lesser, I., Wohl, M., Wilkins, S., & Parks, C. (2000). Performance of older depressed patients on two cognitive malingering tests: False positive rates for the Rey 15-Item Memorization and Dot Counting Tests. *Clinical Neuropsychologist, 14*(3), 303–308.

McCaul, C., Boone, K. B., Ermshar, A., Cottingham, M., Victor, T. L., Ziegler, E., et al. (2018). Cross-validation of the Dot Counting Test in a large sample of credible and non-credible patients referred for neuropsychological testing. *Clinical Neuropsychologist, 32*(6), 1054–1067.

Merten, T., Merckelbach, H., Giger, P., & Stevens, A. (2016). The Self-Report Symptom Inventory (SRSI): A new instrument for the assessment of distorted symptom endorsement. *Psychological injury and law, 9*(2), 102–111.

Millon, T. (1996). *Millon Clinical Multiaxial Inventory: MCMI-III.* Upper Saddle River, NJ: Pearson Assessments.

Millon, T., Grossman, S., & Millon, C. (2015). *MCMI-IV.* Minneapolis: Pearson.

Mitrushina, M., Boone, K. B., Razani, J., & D'Elia, L. F. (2005). *Handbook of normative data for neuropsychological assessment.* New York: Oxford University Press.

Mittenberg, W., Patton, C. L., Canyock, E. M., & Condit, D. C. (2002). Base rates of malingering and symptom exaggeration. *Journal of Clinical and Experimental Neuropsychology, 24*(8), 1094–1102.

Mogge, N. L. (2006). The Assessment of Depression Inventory (ADI): An appraisal of validity in an inpatient sample. *Depression and Anxiety, 23*(7), 434–436.

Mogge, N. L., & LePage, J. P. (2004). The Assessment of Depression Inventory (ADI): A new instrument used to measure depression and to detect honesty of response. *Depression and Anxiety, 20*(3), 107–113.

Mogge, N. L., Lepage, J. S., Bell, T., & Ragatz, L. (2010). The negative distortion scale: A new PAI validity scale. *Journal of Forensic Psychiatry and Psychology, 21*(1), 77–90.

Mogge, N. L., Steinberg, J. S., Fremouw, W., & Messer, J. (2008). The Assessment of Depression Inventory (ADI): An appraisal of validity in an outpatient sample. *Depression and Anxiety, 25*(1), 64–68.

Monaro, M., Toncini, A., Ferracuti, S., Tessari, G., Vaccaro, M. G., De Fazio, P., et al. (2018). The detection of malingering: A new tool to identify made-up depression. *Frontiers in Psychiatry, 9*, 249.

Morey, L. C. (1991). *Personality Assessment Inventory.* Odessa, FL: Psychological Assessment Resources.

Morey, L. C. (1996). *An interpretive guide to the Personality Assessment Inventory (PAI).* Odessa, FL: Psychological Assessment Resources.

Morgan, C. D., Schoenberg, M. R., Dorr, D., & Burke, M. J. (2002). Overreport on the MCMI-III: Concurrent validation with the MMPI-2 using a psychiatric inpatient sample. *Journal of Personality Assessment, 78*(2), 288–300.

Nguyen, C. T., Green, D., & Barr, W. B. (2015). Evaluation of the MMPI-2-RF for detecting over-reported symptoms in a civil forensic and disability setting. *Clinical Neuropsychologist, 29*(2), 255–271.

Nitch, S., Boone, K. B., Wen, J., Arnold, G., & Alfano, K. (2006). The utility of the Rey Word Recognition Test in the detection of suspect effort. *Clinical Neuropsychologist, 20*(4), 873–887.

Otto, M. W., Bruder, G. E., Fava, M., Delis, D. C., Quitkin, F. M., & Rosenbaum, J. F. (1994). Norms for depressed patients for the California Verbal Learning Test: Associations with depression severity and self-report of cognitive difficulties. *Archives of Clinical Neuropsychology, 9*(1), 81–88.

Poynter, K., Boone, K. B., Ermshar, A., Miora, D., Cottingham, M., Victor, T. L., et al. (2019). Wait, there's a baby in this bath water!: Updates on quantitative and qualitative cut-offs for Rey 15-Item Recall and Recognition. *Archives of Clinical Neuropsychology, 34*(8), 1367–1380.

Reedy, S. D., Boone, K. B., Cottingham, M. E., Glaser, D. F., Lu, P. H., Victor, T. L., et al. (2013). Cross validation of the Lu and colleagues (2003). Rey-Osterrieth Complex Figure Test effort equation in a large known-group sample. *Archives of Clinical Neuropsychology, 28*(1), 30–37.

Roberson, C. J., Boone, K. B., Goldberg, H., Miora, D., Cottingham, M., Victor, T., et al. (2013). Cross validation of the b Test in a large known groups sample. *Clinical Neuropsychologist, 27*(3), 495–508.

Rogers, R., Gillard, N. D., Berry, D. T., & Granacher, R. P. (2011). Effectiveness of the MMPI-2-RF validity scales for feigned mental disorders and cognitive impairment: A known-groups study. *Journal of Psychopathology and Behavioral Assessment, 33*(3), 355–367.

Rogers, R., Sewell, K. W., Morey, L. C., & Ulstad, K. L. (1996). Detection of feigned mental disorders on the Personality Assessment Inventory: A discriminant analysis. *Journal of Personality Assessment, 67*(3), 629–640.

Root, J. C., Robbins, R. N., Chang, L., & Van Gorp, W. G. (2006). Detection of inadequate effort on the California Verbal Learning Test: Forced choice recognition and critical item analysis. *Journal of the International Neuropsychological Society, 12*(5), 688–696.

Schroeder, R. W., Baade, L. E., Peck, C. P., VonDran, E. J., Brockman, C. J., Webster, B. K., et al. (2012). Validation of MMPI-2-RF validity scales in criterion group neuropsychological samples. *Clinical Neuropsychologist, 26*(1), 129–146.

Schroeder, R. W., Twumasi-Ankrah, P., Baade, L. E., & Marshall, P. S. (2012). Reliable Digit Span: A systematic review and cross-validation study. *Assessment, 19*(1), 21–30.

Sellbom, M., & Bagby, R. M. (2008). Response styles on multiscale inventories. *Clinical Assessment of Malingering and Deception, 3*, 182–206.

Slick, D. J., Sherman, E. M., & Iverson, G. L. (1999). Diagnostic criteria for malingered neurocognitive dysfunction: Proposed standards for clinical practice and research. *Clinical Neuropsychologist, 13*(4), 545–561.

Solomon, R. E., Boone, K. B., Miora, D., Skidmore, S., Cottingham, M., Victor, T., et al. (2010). Use of the WAIS-III picture completion subtest as an embedded measure of response bias. *Clinical Neuropsychologist, 24*(7), 1243–1256.

Stevens, A., Schmidt, D., & Hautzinger, M. (2018). Major depression—a study on the validity of clinicians' diagnoses in medicolegal assessment. *Journal of Forensic Psychiatry and Psychology*, 1–16.

Sumanti, M., Boone, K. B., Savodnik, I., & Gorsuch, R. (2006). Noncredible psychiatric and cognitive symptoms in a workers' compensation "stress" claim sample. *Clinical Neuropsychologist, 20*(4), 754–765.

Tarescavage, A. M., Wygant, D. B., Gervais, R. O., & Ben-Porath, Y. S. (2013). Association between the MMPI-2 Restructured Form (MMPI-2-RF) and malingered neurocognitive dysfunction among non-head injury disability claimants. *Clinical Neuropsychologist, 27*(2), 313–335.

Tylicki, J. L., Gervais, R. O., & Ben-Porath, Y. S. (2020). Examination of the MMPI-3 over-reporting scales in a forensic disability sample. *The Clinical Neuropsychologist*.

Tylicki, J. L., Rai, J. K., Arends, P., Gervais, R. O., & Ben-Porath, Y. S. (2021). A comparison of the MMPI-2-RF and PAI overreporting indicators in a civil forensic sample with emphasis on the Response Bias Scale (RBS) and the Cognitive Bias Scale (CBS). *Psychological Assessment, 33*(1), 71.

Trahan, D. E., Patterson, J., Quintana, J., & Biron, R. (1987). The Finger Tapping Test: A re-examination of traditional hypotheses regarding normal adult performance. *Journal of Clinical and Experimental Neuropsychology, 9*(1), 52–52.

Van Dyke, S. A., Millis, S. R., Axelrod, B. N., & Hanks, R. A. (2013). Assessing effort: Differentiating performance and symptom validity. *Clinical Neuropsychologist, 27*(8), 1234–1246.

Whiteside, D. M., Kogan, J., Wardin, L., Phillips, D., Franzwa, M. G., Rice, L., et al. (2015). Language-based embedded performance validity measures in traumatic brain injury. *Journal of Clinical and Experimental Neuropsychology, 37*(2), 220–227.

Widows, M. R., & Smith, G. P. (2005). *SIMS: Structured Inventory of Malingered Symptomatology.* Odessa, FL: Psychological Assessment Resources.

Wiggins, C. W., Wygant, D. B., Hoelzle, J. B., & Gervais, R. O. (2012). The more you say the less it means: Overreporting and attenuated criterion validity in a forensic disability sample. *Psychological Injury and Law, 5*(3–4), 162–173.

Wygant, D. B., Ben-Porath, Y. S., Arbisi, P. A., Berry, D. T., Freeman, D. B., & Heilbronner, R. L. (2009). Examination of the MMPI-2 restructured form (MMPI-2-RF) validity scales in civil forensic settings: Findings from simulation and known group samples. *Archives of Clinical Neuropsychology, 24*(7), 671–680.

Zakzanis, K. K., & Jeffay, E. (2011). Neurocognitive variability in high-functioning individuals: Implications for the practice of clinical neuropsychology. *Psychological Reports, 108*(1), 290–300.

CHAPTER 13

Inclusion and Diversity

Kayla Tureson
Alaina I. Gold
April D. Thames

O ver 300 million people (4.4% of the global population) worldwide suffer from depression, an illness determined to be the leading cause of disability (World Health Organization, 2017). It is estimated that by 2030, depression will be the leading cause of disease burden globally according to the World Health Organization. Nearly half of the 300+ million people with depression live in regions of Southeast Asia and the Western Pacific, reflecting the relatively larger populations of those two regions (especially India and China). While there are some commonalities in depression statistics across countries—higher prevalence among women and peaking in older adulthood across both gender groups—regional and cultural differences exist in arguably the most critical areas, namely, the manifestation, assessment, and interpretation of symptoms. This chapter focuses on issues of inclusion and diversity that warrant attention in the diagnosis, management, and treatment of depression.

ORIGINS OF "DEPRESSION"

Culture has shaped our understanding of depression since the second millennium B.C.E. Although not initially termed *depression*, observations of symptoms and behaviors have been documented through translations of Babylonian writings (Reynolds & Wilson, 2013). Furthermore, beliefs surrounding mental illness largely centered around spiritual causes, which influenced the way people with mental illness were treated in society. However, among Ancient Greek philosophers and physicians, depression was believed to be caused by an imbalance in biological fluids (humors). Indeed, the first reference to "black bile" appeared in the *Corpus Hippocraticum* (460–370 B.C.E.). Eventually, scholars began to reject the notion of humoral theory, given the lack of etiologic evidence. Nevertheless, Galen (129–200 C.E.) revised the ancient "humoral theory" by combining Hippocrates' ideas about the four humors with Pythagorean theory of the four elements, and his own conception of the spirit (*pneuma*), separating melancholia, the illness (i.e., black bile melancholia), from melancholic temperament (i.e., yellow bile melancholia). Galen also divided melancholia into general melancholia, brain melancholia, and hypochondriacal melancholia (Garrison, 1929). In Muslim society (ninth century C.E.), mental illness was conceptualized by scholars, including the founder of modern medicine, Ibn Sina (known in the West as Avicenna), as a condition that had a physiological basis. Ishaq Ibn Imran combined the concepts of melancholia and phrenitis (inflammation) and thought that melancholy could emerge from a variety of biological and social etiologies including malfunctions of the sperm or uterus in utero, imbalance of humors (largely influenced by Galen), or improper social environments (Omrani, Holtzman, Akiskal, & Ghaemi, 2012).

The association between sadness and melancholia—which largely influenced North American views—can be traced to Freud's 1917 work "Mourning and Melancholia." In this paper, Freud emphasized melancholia as a subjective state of reliving an early loss. Adolf Meyer, a contemporary of Freud, was a Switzerland-born pathologist who influenced American psychiatry by elaborating on the definition of mental illness as "reactions" to a variety of psychobiological factors (Alarcon, 2009). His influential arguments against the use of melancholia was the catalyst for adopting the term *depression*. Meyer's views were so well received that the first *Diagnostic and Statistical Manual of Mental Disorders* (DSM-I; American Psychiatric Association, 1952) contained *depressive reaction* and DSM-II (American Psychiatric Association, 1968) *depressive neurosis*, defined as an excessive reaction to internal conflict or an identifiable event (DSM-IV-TR; American Psychiatric Association, 2000).

DEPRESSION AND CULTURE

Depression is considered a cross-cultural illness and has been linked to vulnerability factors, including lack of social support, increased stress, high unemployment, and poverty, a demanding climate, family history of depression, adverse childhood experiences, and a high level of trait neuroticism across cultural contexts (Chapman et al., 2004; Chentsova-Dutton & Tsai, 2009; Kirmayer et al., 2001; Sullivan, Neale, & Kendler, 2000). Nevertheless, cultural context impacts the way depression is *experienced and expressed* and plays a role in shaping a community's general beliefs about mental health and illness, and how treatment is approached (Chentsova-Dutton & Tsai, 2009; Ng et al., 2016).

The impact of culture on the experience and presentation of depressive symptoms has been attributed to a number of cultural differences in the conceptualization of depression. Previous research suggests that at least three cultural factors may contribute to the presentation and diagnosis of depression: cultural representations of the self, mind–body relations, and emotional regulation or expression (Tsai, Chentsova-Dutton, Freire-Bebeau, & Przymus, 2002). Across cultures, there is uniformity with regard to the tendency to provide a causal explanation of symptoms (Hagmayer & Engelmann, 2014), and the complexity of the causal belief (i.e., identifying more than one cause) tends to be similar across cultures. However, causal explanations have been found to be more difficult when depression co-occurs with psychotic symptoms (Hagmayer & Engelmann, 2014; Swami, Loo, & Furnham, 2010). Hence, as symptom presentations become more complex, cultural beliefs about mental illness become more influential in causal explanations. To illustrate, Patel (1995) found that in sub-Saharan Africa causal explanations for mental illness usually point to a cause with a greater power than the event itself, and he observed that all events with high importance or impact are also caused by an intentional agent. It is believed that spirits (ancestral and others) and witchcraft can cause or at least influence events. These beliefs may explain why sub-Saharan Africans believe that mental illnesses are caused by social, economic, and/or biological factors (proximate causes) and supernatural causes like spirits and witchcraft (ultimate causes) at the same time.

SYMPTOM MANIFESTATION BY CULTURE

In North American societies, depression is highly influenced by mainstream Western cultural values of "feeling good about the self" (Tsai et al., 2002). Hence, decreased positive affect is considered a deviation from this value and not surprisingly, a core feature of depression. In contrast, regulation of emotional expression to promote group harmony, particularly with regard to positive affect, remains an emphasis of many non-Western, collectivistic societies. Studies have found that the endorsement of positive and negative affect differs across cultures (Iwata & Buka, 2002; Iwata & Higuchi, 2000). Using the Center for Epidemiologic Studies Depression Scale in Japan, native Japanese students reported less positive affect than their White American counterparts, while their negative affect scores were comparable to those of White Americans (Iwata & Buka, 2002). Thus, while positive emotions and open expression may be encouraged and rewarded in individualistic cultures, collectivistic cultures may value an individual's balance and control of emotional expression to maintain group harmony (Markus & Kitayama, 1991). Furthermore, current depressive symptomatology in American societies has been influenced by a dualistic view of mind–body relations (Lewis-Fernandez & Kleinman, 1994), which may influence either a primary somatic and psychological presentation. In contrast, in Asian cultures, unitary beliefs about mind–body relations may influence individuals to present both somatic and psychological complaints as depressive symptoms (Cheung & Lau, 1982). Potential cultural variations in depressive symptoms are optimally captured by scales that assess several domains of depression. Cultural differences in reporting depression symptoms vary across studies and may be related to factors such as variation measurement methods (e.g., use of closed versus open-ended self-report questions to evaluate symptoms), degree of acculturation, and other sociodemographic factors (e.g., education level of participants; Loveys, Torrez, Fine, Moriarty, & Coppersmith, 2018).

Because of the variation in the cultural expression of symptoms, approximately 200 folk illnesses have been considered to be "culture-bound syndromes" (Simons & Hughes, 1986). The work of Kleinman and Good (Kleinman, 1980; Kleinman, Eisenberg, & Good, 1978) demonstrate the importance of eliciting patients' causal models in order to diagnose and develop a treatment plan. Culture-specific idioms of distress refer to the ways of talking about distress in a given culture. Most of these idioms, although they may refer to bodily distress, also imply social and interactional problems (Kirmayer, 2001). For example, *hwa-byung*, a Korean term meaning "fire-illness," refers not only to symptoms of epigastric burning and other forms of somatic distress but also to anger due to interpersonal conflict and a wider sense of collectively experienced injustice (Lee, Wachholtz, & Choi, 2014). Some of the descriptions of these culture-bound syndromes mimic some of the symptoms of what is classified as depression today. For example, in certain parts of the Philippines when a person becomes ill in a number of very different ways (fever, stomach ache, shouting during sleep, incessant crying, various skin ailments), it may be said that the individual is suffering from *lanti*. This is a way of saying that the presumed etiology of all of these complaints is caused by being shocked or startled some time before. There is no discrete *lanti* syndrome that has an identifiable cause. Instead, the illness label is used as an explanation for a variety of troubles. In Peruvian Amazon, *saladera* is also a way of explaining any of a host of misfortunes such as a persistent run of bad luck, and the cause is thought to be supernatural (Simons, 2001). In the United States, African Americans experience "falling out," a culture-bound syndrome of sudden collapse following an episode of dizziness. Sleep paralysis, which is characterized by an inability to move while awakening or falling asleep, is also sometimes observed in African Americans (Bell, Dixie-Bell, & Thompson, 1986). Importantly, culture-bound syndromes are not limited to a single culture, and similar presentations and signs of distress have been observed in multiple cultures (see Table 13.1). Culture-bound syndromes, regardless of presentation, share common features of being well known to the given culture, classified as a disease within the culture, and typically identified and treated through folk medicine with local healers (Baig, 2010).

TABLE 13.1. Selected Culture-Bound Syndromes Most Closely Related to Depression

Culture	Syndrome/term	English translation	Symptomatic features
Korea	*Hwa-byung*	Fire illness	• Epigastric burning • Other forms of somatic distress • Anger due to interpersonal conflict and a wider sense of collectively experienced injustice
Philippines	*Lanti*	A label used as an explanation for a variety of troubles	• Fever, stomach ache, shouting during sleep, incessant crying, various skin ailments • Believed to be caused by being shocked or startled some time before
Peru (Amazon)	*Saladera*	Derived from *sal*, the Spanish word for salt	• Strong lack of somatization • Anxiety response to stress • Believed to be due to bad luck or misfortune
United States (African Americans)	Falling out	N/A	Sudden collapse following an episode of dizziness
Caribbean, particularly Puerto Rico (Guarnaccia, 1993)	*Ataque de nervios*	Attack of nerves	• Triggered by personal loss or conflict • Uncontrollable trembling, shouting • Occasional aggression, collapsing, or amnesia

The implication of this cultural shaping of illness must be understood by clinicians in primary care and mental health settings. Unlike the Westernized understanding of medical illness that predominates the perception of depressive symptomatic presentation, symptoms cannot simply be interpreted as indices of disorder or disease. Instead, they must be understood as interpersonal communications between the patient and clinician as well as the patient's support group.

Linguistic Expressions

Language is a critical component in understanding cultural idioms of distress. Linguistic investigations have found differences between depressed and nondepressed people using online data (e.g., social media). Compared to nondepressed individuals, depressed individuals use language with greater self-focus (Coppersmith, Dredze, & Harman, 2014; Preoţiuc-Pietro et al., 2015), tentativeness (Coppersmith et al., 2014), general negativity (De Choudhury, Gamon, Counts, & Horvitz, 2013), anger (Coppersmith et al., 2014), interpersonal hostility (Preoţiuc-Pietro et al., 2015), and perceived hopelessness (Schwartz et al., 2014). To our knowledge, two studies have used online data to examine cultural differences in linguistic predictors of depression (De Choudhury et al., 2013; Loveys et al., 2018). De Choudhury and colleagues (2013) analyzed the Tweets of Twitter users who self-reported a diagnosis of a mental illness, including depression, or experience of suicidal ideation. Comparisons were made between Western (e.g., United States, United Kingdom) and non-Western (e.g., South Africa, India) groups with the Linguistic Inquiry and Word Count (LIWC2015) software and topic modeling. Non-Western cultural groups were less likely to express their mental illness experience online, which resulted in higher positive affect and lower negative affect, anger, anxiety, and sadness in comparison to Western cultural groups. Western groups were more likely to discuss functioning, such as social concerns, health, body, and biology, than non-Western groups. Other differences included topics of discussion. Western cultures were more likely to discuss social isolation, death, and self-destruction, whereas non-Western cultures were more likely to discuss shame from experiencing a mental illness and make confessions related to their mental health struggles. Loveys and colleagues (2018) found cultural differences in the rate of positive to negative emotion expression (which was referred to as "tone"). Specifically, Asian or Pacific Islander users showed more inhibition of negative emotion, whereas non-Hispanic White and Black or African American users expressed more negativity (in other words, they exhibited less regulation of their negative emotional state). Hispanic or Latinx users expressed a large amount of both positive and negative emotion compared to other groups. Moreover, cultural differences in cognitive categories were observed; notably, cognitive effects of depression were less evident in the language of Asian or Pacific Islander users. Additionally, discussions of functioning were impacted by culture. Non-Hispanic White users appeared to be less social and were more likely to report on health and death or self-destruction compared to other groups. Asian or Pacific Islander users were less open to discussing health or death, though social terms were more present. Black or African American users discussed social terms to a high degree and were comparatively less likely to discuss death, but they were more willing to talk about health compared to other groups. In contrast to Black or African American users, Hispanic/Latinx users with depression made few mentions of social terms and were less willing to make disclosures about death or self-destruction, religion, or health (Loveys et al., 2018).

DEPRESSION SCREENING INSTRUMENTS AND VALIDATION IN DIVERSE GROUPS

Due to their feasibility and ease of administration, screening measures are the most commonly employed method for assessing depressive symptomology in diverse groups, typically administered in primary care settings (Kerr & Kerr, 2001). The most common depression screening measures (see Pace & Husain, Chapter 10, this volume, for additional information) include the Beck Depression Inventory–II (Beck, Steer, & Brown, 1996), Patient Health Questionnaire–9 (Kroenke, Spitzer, & Williams, 2001), Hamilton Rating Scale for Depression (Hamilton, 1960), the Center for Epidemiologic Studies Depression Scale (Radloff, 1977), and the Geriatric Depression Scale (Yesavage et al., 1983). These screening measures have been adapted, translated, and validated in multiple languages, and through this adaptation process, a number of short or alternative forms have also been developed. Because of the heterogeneous presentation of depression across cultures, it cannot be assumed that a screening measure is equivalent or valid from one culture to the next (Ferrari et al., 2013; Jayawickreme, Verkuilen, Jayawickreme, Acosta, & Foa, 2017). The following section summarizes the extant literature regarding translation, adaptation, and validation of screening measures in diverse groups, in both Western and non-Western countries.

Beck Depression Inventory–II

The Beck Depression Inventory–II (BDI-II) is a commonly utilized depression screener in the United States, and its utility among diverse samples has been examined in both the United States and non-Western countries (see Table 13.2). Among a sample of low-income African American medical outpatients, the BDI-II demonstrated high internal consistency (Cronbach's $\alpha = 0.90$), and a confirmatory factor analysis revealed two first-order factors (i.e., somatic and cognitive), which together reflected a second factor order, depression, thus supporting its use within this population (Grothe et al., 2005). A study of demographic influences of the Spanish language version of the BDI-I among a sample of Hispanic/Latinx men and women of Mexican descent from border regions of Arizona and California revealed gender differences and lower mean scores than those from the normative sample of the English language BDI-I (Beck & Steer, 1987). Hispanic/Latinx women were more likely to endorse Somatic scale questions of the BDI-I than Cognitive scale questions. Across the entire sample, the most frequently endorsed items were changes in sleep patterns, loss of interest in sex, and increased guilt (Dawes et al., 2010). Another study suggested that acculturation may be a risk factor for depressive symptomatology among U.S. Hispanic/Latinx of Mexican descent, such that adaptation to U.S. mainstream cultural pressures and ideas, including socioeconomic gain, higher stress related to job pressures, and decreased familial structure, may increase depressed mood (Lewis-Fernandez, Das, Alfonso, Weissman, & Olfson, 2005).

TABLE 13.2. BDI-II Validation in Diverse Groups

	Region									
	United States			Central and South America		Europe	Asia			
	Asian American	Black/African American	Hispanic/Latinx	Brazil	Dominican Republic	Germany	Japan	Malaysia	Singapore	Turkey
Supporting studies	Jayawickreme et al. (2017)	Grothe et al. (2015)	Wiebe & Penley (2005)	Gomes-Oliveira et al. (2012)	García-Batista et al. (2018)	Kleim et al. (2014)	Kojima et al. (2002)	Wan Mahmud et al. (2004)	Nyunt et al. (2009)	Canel-Çınarbaş et al. (2011)
Study sample characteristics	Sri Lankan female trauma refugee survivors	Low-income medical outpatient clinic	Spanish-language BDI compared with English-language BDI, University of El Paso undergraduates	Medical students and community sample in São Paolo	General population and primary care clinic	German general population, used BDI-FastScreen	Primary care patients in central Japan	Malay postpartum women	Community-dwelling older adults	Turkish undergraduate students
Cronbach's α/ sensitivity and specificity (%)	Not recommended for comparison of subscales; Sri Lankan sample endorsed more somatic symptoms	α = 0.90; sensitivity and specificity not provided	α = 0.91 for Spanish version, α = 0.89 for English version	α = 0.89 student sample, α = 0.93 community sample; cutoff score of 10+; sensitivity: 70%, specificity: 84%	α = 0.89; sensitivity and specificity not provided	α = 0.84; sensitivity and specificity not provided	α = .87; sensitivity and specificity not provided	α = .89, 9.5+ cutoff score sensitivity: 100%, specificity: 98%	α = 0.80; sensitivity: 97%, specificity: 95%	α = 0.88; sensitivity and specificity not provided

(continued)

TABLE 13.2. (continued)

	Region					
	Africa					
	Kenya	Malawi	South Africa	Tanzania	Zambia	Zimbabwe
Supporting studies	Kilburn et al. (2018)		Baron, Davies, & Lund (2017)	Kilburn et al. (2018)		
Study sample characteristics	Youth samples from low-income families in Kenya	Youth samples from low-income families in Malawi	Xhosa-, Afrikaans-, and Zulu-speaking participants ages 15 years or older	Youth samples from low-income families in Tanzania	Youth samples from low-income families in Zambia	Youth samples from low-income families in Kenya, Malawi, Tanzania, Zambia, and Zimbabwe
Cronbach's α/ sensitivity and specificity	α = 0.43; sensitivity and specificity not provided	α = 0.46; sensitivity and specificity not provided	α = 0.69–0.89; sensitivity: Zulu: 71.4%, Afrikaans: 84.6%, Xhosa: 95%; specificity: Zulu: 72.6%, Afrikaans: 84.0%, Xhosa: 95%	α = 0.39; sensitivity and specificity not provided	α = 0.46; sensitivity and specificity not provided	α = 0.49; sensitivity and specificity not provided

227

In a non-Western sample of Sri Lankan refugee trauma survivors in the United States, the BDI-II was found to be roughly equivalent for assessing depression, though comparison through subscales provided by the BDI-II is not recommended (Jayawickreme et al., 2017). The Malay translation of the BDI has been validated, including in subpopulations such as Malay postpartum women (Wan Mahmud, Awang, Herman, & Mohamed, 2004). In a Sri Lankan population, the BDI-II was not found to capture functional impairment related to depression and anxiety; the authors recommended the use of local idioms of distress when adapting measures in non-Western, war-affected populations, as these are more predictive of impairment than translations of Western screening measures such as the BDI-II (Jayawickreme, Jayawickreme, Atanasov, Goonasekera, & Foa, 2012). The BDI-II Japanese translation has also been cross-culturally validated, though higher scores were observed among women compared to men (Kojima et al., 2002).

The BDI has been validated in several Central and South American countries. A confirmatory factor analysis of the BDI-II in the Dominican Republic revealed a general depression factor, and three specific factors (cognitive, affective, and somatic) best fit the data and effectively discriminated between the general and clinical population, with moderate to high internal reliability of the identified general and specific factors (García-Batista, Guerra-Peña, Cano-Vindel, Herrera-Martínez, & Medrano, 2018). The Portuguese Brazilian translation of the BDI-II has been validated in a Brazilian community sample and demonstrated a strong internal consistency, with a Cronbach's α level of 0.93 (Gomes-Oliveira, Gorenstein, Lotufo Neto, Andrade, & Wang, 2012).

Another consideration when using the BDI is the BDI-Fast Screen (BDI-FS), which measures the depression severity corresponding to nonsomatic diagnostic criteria in the measure, though it is utilized less frequently than the full BDI-II (Kleim, Mößle, Zenger, & Brähler, 2014). Somatization of distress is a common misconception about depressive symptom presentation in non-Western populations. Importantly, somatic symptoms serve as expressions of cultural idioms of distress and, upon misinterpretation by the clinician, may result in inappropriate diagnosis and treatment (Kirmayer, 2001). Therefore, a screener that takes out somatization subscales may be more appropriate in non-Western populations, though ideally a screening measure should be translated and adapted by incorporating appropriate local idioms of distress.

Patient Health Questionnaire–9

The Patient Health Questionnaire–9 (PHQ-9) is a self-administered measure that was created to be a screener of depression and other mental health disorders in a primary care setting. With only nine items, the PHQ-9 is favorable for its short length, as well as its ability to diagnose depression and grade the individual's symptom severity (Kroenke et al., 2001). This measure was originally validated with two U.S.-based studies in primary care settings, with 3,000 subjects in each study (see Table 13.3). The first of Kroenke and colleagues' (2001) studies recruited predominantly non-Hispanic White primary care patients (79% White, 13% African American, 4% Hispanic). The subsequent study, which recruited women from obstetrics-gynecology sites, was more inclusive of Hispanic/Latinx adults (39% White, 15% African American, 39% Hispanic/Latinx). From these, a screening cutoff score of 10 or greater indicates major depression, with a sensitivity of 88%, specificity of 88%, and positive likelihood of 7.1 (Kroenke et al., 2001; Kroenke & Spitzer, 2002). Kroenke and colleagues suggest the following cut points for thresholds of severity: a score of 5, 10, 15, and 20 indicates mild moderate, moderately severe, and severe depression, respectively. A meta-analysis by Manea, Gilbody, and McMillan (2015), which included studies from many countries and across many languages, recommended a cut point of 10 or higher to maximize sensitivity. The PHQ-9 has been validated in multiple languages, as detailed below.

A Chinese translation of the PHQ-9, as well as subscales PHQ-2 and PHQ-1, demonstrated reliability and validity in detecting major depressive disorder (MDD) in a sample of Taiwanese primary care patients (Liu et al., 2011). The study found that a cutoff of 10 or higher on the PHQ-9 had a sensitivity of 86% and a specificity of 93.9%, indicating an equal sensitivity to the English version of the PHQ-9, as well as a higher specificity. In this group, a one-factor structure was found with an eigenvalue of 3.78. The Thai translation of the PHQ-9 was found to have acceptable sensitivity (0.84) and specificity (0.77) as a depression screening measure, with a recommended cutoff of 9 or higher indicating depressive symptomatology (Lotrakul, Sumrithe, & Saipanish, 2008). The PHQ-9 adapted and validated in Nepal used lay Nepali terminology, thus enabling easy administration by literate individuals who may not have specialized mental health training (Kohrt, Luitel, Acharya, & Jordans, 2016). In a sample of Filipino female migrant workers living in China, a Filipino translation of the PHQ-9 and PHQ-15 was found to be better described by a two-factor model. In this model, the first factor, cognitive/affective, captures anhedonia, depressed mood, feeling of worthlessness, and thoughts of death. The second factor, somatic, is composed of sleep difficulties, fatigue, appetite changes, concentration difficulties, and psychomotor retardation (Mordeno, Carpio, Mendoza, & Hall, 2018). This finding contrasts previous findings of a one-factor model, though the authors note that emerging literature has begun to demonstrate support for a two-factor model of MDD.

The Spanish-language version of the PHQ-9 has been validated in a primary care setting in Spain (Muñoz-Navarro et al., 2017). When using the cutoff score of 10 points, the sensitivity was 0.95 and the specificity was 0.67, indicating a higher likelihood of false positives. When increasing the cutoff point to 12 points, the cutoff value of 10 points was as follows: sensitivity, 0.95; specificity, 0.67. When using a cutoff of 12 points, the sensitivity decreased slightly to 0.84 and the specificity increased to 0.78. This higher screening cutoff may be more appropriate in this population (Muñoz-Navarro et al., 2017). The Spanish version of the PHQ-9 has also been evaluated among Latinx women of predominantly Mexican origin in the United States and was found to have good internal consistency (α = 0.85) and structural validity, as well as fit the one-factor model (Merz, Malcarne, Roesch, Riley, & Sadler, 2011). In rural Mexico, the Spanish version of the PHQ-2 was found to be a good measure for screening depression, with high sensitivity (80.0%) and specificity (86.9%) at a cutoff score of 3 (Arrieta et al., 2017). Within this sample, a one-factor model of the PHQ-9 was also supported with good internal consistency. The internal consistency remained high (α = 0.80–0.90) for subgroups separated by gender, literacy, and age. In a study of the PHQ-9 in Mexican women, good internal consistency (α = 0.89) was found, and a one-factor solution was recommended (Familiar et al., 2014).

In a sample of Nigerian students, the PHQ-9 had excellent sensitivity (0.846) and specificity (0.994) in screening for MDD, with a cutoff score of 10 (Adewuya, Ola, & Afolabi,

TABLE 13.3. PHQ-9 Validation in Diverse Groups

	Region						
	United States			Central and South America			Europe
	Asian American	Black/African American	Hispanic/Latinx	Brazil	Mexico		Spain
Supporting studies	Huang et al. (2006)	Huang et al. (2006)	Merz et al., (2011)	De Lima Osório, Vilela Mendes, Crippa, & Loureiro (2009)	Familiar et al. (2014)	Arrieta et al. (2017)	Muñoz-Navarro et al. (2017)
Study sample characteristics	Chinese American primary care patients in New York City	African American primary care patients in New York City	Latinx women of predominantly Mexican origin	Brazilian women in primary health care	Mexican women	Adults in a rural community	Primary care centers
Cronbach's α/ Sensitivity & Specificity	α = 0.79, Sensitivity & Specificity not provided	α = 0.80, Sensitivity & Specificity not provided	α = 0.85, Sensitivity & Specificity not provided	Cutoff score of 10+, Sensitivity 100%, Specificity 98%	α = 0.89, Sensitivity & Specificity not provided	α = 0.8, Sensitivity: 80.5%, Specificity: 86.9%	Cutoff score of 10+, Sensitivity 95%, Specificity 67%

(continued)

TABLE 13.3. *(continued)*

	Region										
	Asia						**Africa**				
	China	Malaysia	Nepal	Taiwan	Thailand	Thailand	Ethiopia	Nigeria	South Africa	South Africa	Uganda
Supporting studies	Mordeno, Carpio, Mendoza, & Hall (2018)	Azah et al. (2005)	Kohrt, Luitel, Acharya, & Jordans (2016)	Liu et al. (2011)	Lotrakul, Sumrithe, & Saipanish (2008)	Lotrakul et al. (2008)	Gelaye et al. (2013b)	Adewuya, Ola, & Afolabi (2006)	Baron, Davies, & Lunc (2017)	Cholera et al. (2014)	Nakku et al. (2016)
Study sample characteristics	Filipino domestic workers in China	Adults attending family medicine clinics	Rural primary health care center	Taiwanese primary care patients	Family practice clinic outpatients	Family practice clinic outpatients	Ethiopian adults in outpatient clinic at a major hospital	Nigerian university students	Xhosa, Afrikaans and Zulu-speaking participants aged 15 years or older	Primary health care patients in Johannesburg	Primary care patients
Cronbach's α/ Sensitivity & Specificity	α = 0.81; Cutoff score of 10+, Sensitivity & Specificity not provided	α = 0.67; Cutoff score of 5+ Sensitivity: 69% Specificity of 60.5%	Cutoff score of 10+, Sensitivity 94%, Specificity 80%	α = .80; Cutoff score of 10+ Sensitivity 86% Specificity of 93.9%	α = .79; Cutoff score of 9+ Sensitivity: 84% Specificity of 77%	Cutoff score of 9+, Sensitivity 84%, Specificity 77%	α = 0.81; Cutoff score of 10+, Sensitivity: 86% Specificity of 67%	Cutoff score of 10+, Sensitivity 84.6%, Specificity 99.4%	Cutoff score of 8+; Sensitivity: Zulu - 66.7%, Xhose - 82.7%, Afrikaans - 81% Specificity: Zulu - 73.1%, Afrikaans - 79.1%, Xhosa - 87.2%	Cutoff score of 9+, Sensitivity 87.2%, Specificity 73.4%	Cutoff score of 5+, Sensitivity 67.4%, Specificity 78.1%

231

2006). The PHQ-9 has also been translated into isiZulu, isiXhosa, seSotho, seTswana, and English and has been administered in a primary health care setting to individuals from South Africa and Zimbabwe in Johannesburg (Cholera et al., 2014). It was found to perform modestly, with a sensitivity of 87.2% and a specificity of 73.4% for a cutoff score of 8, and a sensitivity of 78.7% and a specificity of 83.4% for a cutoff score of 10. Nakku and colleagues (2016) suggest that while the Lugandan translation was a moderately useful screening measure of depression in Uganda, revising the PHQ-9 to incorporate local Lugandan idioms of distress would improve its clinical utility.

While the PHQ-9 has been repeatedly validated in different patient samples and in different languages, few studies have examined its utility within a psychiatric population (Beard, Hsu, Rifkin, Busch, & Björgvinsson, 2016). Beard and colleagues (2016) note that this validation is necessary, for the measure may be used more frequently as a severity measure than as a screener in a psychiatric setting. Their U.S.-based study found the PHQ-9 to have a sensitivity of 0.93, a specificity of 0.52, and a positive predictive value of 0.74 at a cutoff score of 10. Of note, a two-factor structure, first cognitive and affective items followed by somatic items, was found to best fit the data, in contrast to the uni-dimensional structure found in the majority of studies in non-psychiatric samples. This study benefited from a heterogeneous psychiatric sample, which included subjects with MDD, bipolar disorder, panic disorder, posttraumatic stress disorder, and panic disorder. However, the sample was largely composed of well-educated non-Hispanic White adults. Replication studies should be conducted in more diverse samples, and further investigation in the different translated versions of the PHQ-9 in different countries is necessary to better understand the measure's utility in diverse groups.

Hamilton Depression Rating Scale

Another commonly utilized depression screening measure is the Hamilton Rating Scale for Depression (HRSD), also abbreviated as HAM-D, which has long been considered a gold-standard measure. However, more recent studies have suggested poor replication in the factor structure and content validity of the HRSD, as well as questionable utility of items among different clinical populations, such as those with terminal cancer (Bagby, Ryder, Schuller, & Marshall, 2004; Olden, Rosenfeld, Pessin, & Breitbart, 2009; see Table 13.4). A meta-analysis by Vindbjerg, Makransky, Mortensen, and Carlsson (2018) examined the cross-cultural psychometric properties of the HRSD based on 12 available studies, which included the following countries: Japan, France, Brazil, Turkey, United Arab Emirates, China, Israel, and a sample of Bedouin Arabs (Akdemir et al., 2001; Bachner, 2016; Bachner, O'Rourke, Goldfracht, Bech, & Ayalon, 2013; Fleck et al., 2004; Furukawa et al., 2005; Hamdi, Amin, & Abou-Saleh, 1997; Lee, Liu, & Hung, 2017; Lin et al., 2018). Results of a confirmatory factor analysis across all included studies identified a four- to six-item depression general factor structure of the HRSD, which included depressed mood, guilt, psychomotor slowing, and loss of interest as the four main factors. Two additional factors, suicide and anxiety, loaded to a lesser extent for the six-item general factor structure (Vindbjerg et al., 2018). However, Vindbjerg and colleagues note that a multidimensional factor scale of the HRSD across cultural adaptations was difficult, particularly since most studies included in the meta-analysis relied on exploratory factor structure. Perhaps, the

TABLE 13.4. HRSD Validation in Diverse Groups

Region

	United States			Central and South America	Europe
	Asian American	Black/African American	Hispanic/Latinx	Brazil	Spain
Supporting studies	Rao, Poland, & Lin (2012)			Fleck et al. (2004)	Ramos-Brieva & Cordero-Villafáfila (1988)
Study sample characteristics	Primarily of Chinese descent, recruited from community mental health centers in Los Angeles County	Recruited from community mental health centers in Los Angeles County	Mexican American, recruited from community mental health centers in Los Angeles County	Inpatients diagnosed with major depression	Spanish-language HDRS, inpatients in a Madrid hospital and previous participants in an antidepressant drug trial
Cronbach's α/ sensitivity and specificity (%)	No information provided, participants reported higher anxiety and somatic symptoms	No information provided, nonsignificant trend of lower scores among participants relative to other racial/ethnic groups	No information provided; participants reported higher anxiety and somatic symptoms	No information provided	α = 0.72; sensitivity and specificity not provided

Region

Asia

	China	Israel		Japan	Korea	Saudia Arabia	Thailand	Turkey	United Arab Emirates
Supporting studies	Zheng et al. (1988)	Lin et al. (2018)	Bachner (2016)	Furukawa et al. (2005)	Yi et al. (2005)	Alhadi et al. (2018)	Lotrakul et al. (1996)	Akdemir et al. (2001)	Hamdi et al. (1997)
Study sample characteristics	Urban and rural Chinese inpatients and outpatients	Adults with epilepsy	Bedouin Arabs who are primary caregivers of cancer patients	Participants in an antidepressant drug trial	Inpatients and outpatients with depressive diagnoses; Korean-language version	Community sample of medical students and outpatient; utilized Arabic translation of HAM-D 7	Inpatients and outpatients with depressive diagnoses	Sample of patients with mood disorder	Inpatient and outpatient nationals and expatriates from other Arab countries who met depressive disorder diagnostic criteria
Cronbach's α/ sensitivity and specificity (%)	α = 0.71; sensitivity and specificity not provided	α = 0.83; sensitivity: 97%, specificity: 94%	No information provided	No information provided	α = 0.71; sensitivity and specificity not provided	α = 0.641, retest α = 0.73	No information provided	α = 0.75; sensitivity and specificity not provided	α = 0.51; sensitivity and specificity not provided

authors theorized, a unidimensional factor structure would be best in the future, though this would require greater statistical rigor (Vindbjerg et al., 2018).

Center for Epidemiologic Studies Depression Scale

The Center for Epidemiologic Studies Depression Scale (CES-D), another well-known self-report depression screening measure, consists of 20 questions that are composed of somatic, affective, and psychological symptoms of depression (see Table 13.5). Patients are asked to rate the frequency of depressive symptoms in the past week on a Likert scale from 0 (rarely or none of the time, less than 1 day) to 3 (most of the time, 5–7 days) for 20 items. Consistent with other depression screening measures, higher scores indicate more severe depression symptomatology (Carleton et al., 2013). The factor structure originally proposed for the CES-D included four factors: anhedonia, depressed affect, somatic inactivity, and interpersonal challenges. However, a recent factor analysis study found that items related to interpersonal challenges (e.g., item 19, "I felt that people disliked me") are not consistent with current diagnostic criteria for depression (Carleton et al., 2013). Moreover, item 17, "I had crying spells," reflected robust sex differences, such that it may inflate scores among women. Therefore, the authors suggested the removal of this item in future use, given the implications of sex and cultural biases that may have significant social and health care implications, given the artificial inflation of depression scores among women (Carleton et al., 2013). The CES-D has been translated and adapted less frequently compared to the BDI and the PHQ-9. A study of a Greek translation of the CES-D found that the translated measure had strong internal consistency, with a Cronbach's α of 0.95 (Fountoulakis et al., 2001).

More recent studies have found mixed results with the CES-D among Latinx and African American adults. A study of urban-dwelling Hispanic/Latinx adults of predominantly Mexican origin in California found that the original four-factor model proposed for the CES-D did not fit Latinx men well, and age and acculturation significantly impacted item endorsement among Latinx women (Posner, Stewart, Marín, & Pérez-Stable, 2001). A CES-D validation study among a sample of Latinx adults of Puerto Rican origin in the Northeastern United States found that the 10-item CES-D was better than the 20-item version in this population, with a sensitivity and specificity of 84% and 64%, respectively, at the cut point of 3, which is lower than the cutoff point of 4 that is typically used (Robison, Gruman, Gaztambide, & Blank, 2002). Importantly, few studies have validated the CES-D among Latinx populations, and caution should be taken to not generalize CES-D validity from one Latinx subgroup to another, as there is great heterogeneity across Latinx subgroups.

A CES-D factor analysis study among a sample of older African Americans identified a factor structure that differed by gender; a four-factor structure was identified among African American women, but a seven-factor structure was identified for African American men (Callahan & Wolinsky, 1994). An item-level analysis of CES-D among African American, Latinx, and non-Hispanic White adults with coronary artery disease revealed that African Americans were 1.6 times more likely to have a score at or above the 16-point cutoff compared to non-Hispanic Whites. Latinx adults were three times more likely to have a score at or above the cutoff and were more likely to endorse somatic items compared

TABLE 13.5. CES-D Validation in Diverse Groups

	Region					
	United States		Europe	Asia		
	Black/African American	Hispanic/Latinx	Greece	China		Japan
Supporting studies	Boutin-Foster (2008)	Robison et al. (2002)	Fountoulakis et al. (2001)	Chin, Choi, Chan, & Wong (2015)	Cheng & Chan (2005)	Kojima et al. (2002)
Study sample characteristics	African Americans, ages 50+	Primary care patients of Puerto Rican origin, ages 50+, residing in Northeastern United States	Patients from inpatient and outpatient units, and members of the hospital staff and relatives of patients	Chinese primary care patients	Chinese elderly (ages 60+)	Visitors at a public health care center
Cronbach's α/ sensitivity and specificity	$\alpha = 0.87$; sensitivity and specificity not provided	10-item using cutoff of 3; sensitivity: 84%, specificity: 64%	$\alpha = 0.95$, CES-D level 23/24; sensitivity: 90%, specificity: 90.83%	Reliability: 0.855 (ωH), sensitivity: AUC = 0.75	Threshold of 22, sensitivity: 75%, specificity: 51%	$\alpha = 0.87$; sensitivity: 90%, specificity: 90.83%

to non-Hispanic Whites, which may reflect higher levels of stress or greater burden of medical comorbidities among Latinx participants. African American participants also endorsed the item of "people were unfriendly," which may be an indicator of higher levels of discrimination, and thus could increase stress levels and likelihood of endorsing items on the CES-D. Importantly, the authors note that the higher CES-D scores among Latinx and African American adults may be a function of lower socioeconomic status compared to non-Hispanic White adults (Boutin-Foster, 2008).

Little research on the validation of CES-D has been conducted among Asian and Asian American groups. One study of the CES-D in a sample of Koreans and Korean Americans revealed that both groups were significantly less likely to endorse positive affect items compared to non-Hispanic White participants. However, Korean Americans were more likely to endorse these items than the Korean sample. Korean Americans who were less acculturated to U.S. mainstream culture were less likely to endorse positive affect items than those who were more highly acculturated (Jang, Kwag, & Chiriboga, 2010). Another study conducted on a Chinese primary care sample found that a two-factor structure, which included somatic complaints and depressed affects, was best. The authors also noted that two items may be misinterpreted in the Hong Kong sample, with item 4 being interpreted as a comparison of general living standards, and item 11 perhaps misinterpreted as sleep deprivation due to a variety of circumstances, such as bedtime social activities, aging, or work-related stress (Chin, Choi, Chan, & Wong, 2015). Thus, these findings highlight the impact of culture on item endorsement among diverse groups, and universal cutoffs across diverse groups may not be suitable.

Although the CES-D is not as commonly translated or adapted as other depression screening measures, existing studies among diverse populations suggest that the measure should be used with caution, given the differential factor structure and higher scores among diverse groups. In particular, its somatic and interpersonal challenge factors may not be appropriate for capturing depressive symptoms in ethnically/linguistically diverse populations.

Geriatric Depression Scale

The Geriatric Depression Scale (GDS) is a depression screening measure designed for older adult populations, which features a yes/no response format ideal for use with those who may have age-related cognitive decline, as well as the exclusion of questions regarding certain somatic symptoms that may be due to comorbid medical conditions. A meta-analysis conducted by Kim, DeCoster, Huang, and Bryant (2013) investigated the influence of language among different GDS translations across 26 studies. The included studies examined Chinese, Japanese, Korean, Greek, Hindi, Portuguese, Turkish, Italian, and Iranian languages. The factorial structure of the GDS ranged from two to nine factors, with a four-factor model achieving the best fit. The most consistent factors across languages included dysphoria, social withdrawal–apathy–cognitive impairment, and positive mood, though the individual factor loadings of each within the studies were not consistent. Kim, DeCoster, and colleagues concluded that different language versions of the GDS produce significantly different and distinct factor structures due to linguistic and/or cultural factors.

TRANSLATION AND ADAPTATION OF DEPRESSION SCREENING INSTRUMENTS

The previous section raises important concerns regarding the use of depression screening instruments among culturally/linguistically diverse populations, particularly within the realm of translating and adapting existing screening measures in other languages and ensuring they are valid for use among non-Western cultures. While most studies found translated or adapted versions to be consistent with the English version, others reported that some concepts did not translate well or did not exist in the culture of interest. Thus, the inclusion of local idioms of distress more appropriately captured depressive symptoms in these populations (Kirmayer, 2001; Nakku et al., 2016). Language and culture can significantly impact item endorsement even with a well-translated measure, which in turn can affect factor loading (Huang et al., 2006; Merz, Malcarne, Roesch, Riley, & Sadler, 2011; Posner et al., 2001). Moreover, adjusting cutoff scores for different populations may yield better sensitivity and specificity scores and lead to better detection of depression.

VALIDATION AND USE OF DEPRESSION STRUCTURED CLINICAL INTERVIEWS IN DIVERSE GROUPS

Although screening measures are a fast and readily employed tool in many primary care and mental health settings, structured interviews are a tool that can be used to aid in the actual diagnosis of depression. Screening measures do not serve as diagnostic indicators, as they only provide a brief snapshot of self-reported recent depressive symptomatology. Therefore, a structured clinical interview can provide a more thorough and comprehensive means of assessing specific depressive symptoms and their duration to help clinicians determine whether a depression diagnosis should be given. Although a number of structured clinical interviews exist, for the purpose of this chapter we review the Structured Clinical Interview for DSM-IV and the Composite International Diagnostic Interview, which have been well researched and validated on many diverse groups.

Structured Clinical Interview for DSM Disorders

The Structured Clinical Interview for DSM Disorders (SCID; see Pace & Husain, Chapter 10, this volume, for additional information) was developed following the publication of DSM-III (American Psychiatric Association, 1980) and the potential limitations of using the National Institute of Mental Health Diagnostic Interview Schedule as a diagnostic assessment tool (Spitzer, Williams, Gibbon, & First, 1992). The SCID was field-tested in 1985 and has undergone several versions. Lopez and Nunez (1987) highlighted cultural limitations in interview schedules such as the SCID, which had referred to culture only once. Hence, despite attention to this problem, utilizing a cultural perspective to determine psychiatric diagnosis has been unevenly implemented across the field (Alarcón et al., 2009; Neighbors et al., 2003). Despite using structured interviews, such as the SCID, the diagnosis of MDD tends to be lower among African Americans than Whites (Barnes & Bates, 2017). In a study examining diagnostic concordance between hospital and research diagnosis using the SCID, Whites were more likely to receive a diagnosis of mood disorders than African Americans, whereas African Americans were more likely to receive a diagnosis of schizophrenia than Whites (Neighbors et al., 1999). A recent meta-analytic investigation comparing racial disparities in the diagnosis rates of schizophrenia did not find that using structured interviews attenuated racial differences in schizophrenia diagnoses compared with studies using unstructured assessments (Olbert, Nagendra, & Buck, 2018). Chasson, Williams, Davis, and Combs (2017) found poor diagnostic utility of the SCID obsessive–compulsive disorder, with 66.2% (N = 49) correctly identified and 33.8% (N = 25) incorrectly diagnosed.

Composite International Diagnostic Interview

The Composite International Diagnostic Interview (CIDI) is a fully structured diagnostic interview, developed by the World Health Organization for ready use by lay interviewers in diverse settings, maps symptoms onto DSM-IV and *International Classification of Diseases* (ICD-9) diagnostic criteria (Andrews & Peters, 1997). The instrument includes a depression and mania module that assesses first with three initial screening questions that assess for feelings of sadness/depressed mood, discouragement, and loss of interest lasting several days or more. If any of these questions are endorsed, further structured questions to address the nine symptoms of depression are subsequently generated for the examiner to ask in the interview. The interview includes questions regarding the following symptoms: dysphoric mood/anhedonia, significant weight loss/appetite disturbance, insomnia/hypersomnia, fatigue/energy loss, psychomotor retardation/agitation, feelings of excessive guilt/worthlessness, loss of ability to concentrate, and recurrent suicidal thoughts. A diagnosis is given if the examinee endorses at least five of nine symptoms persisting for 2 weeks or more. The CIDI has been translated in over 30 languages and is available for both lifetime and 12-month interview versions. A study comparing concordance between the CIDI and the SCID found that the CIDI had more conservative lifetime prevalence estimates compared to the SCID. However, 12-month CIDI estimates were more unbiased compared to the SCID (Haro et al., 2006).

Importantly, structured clinical interviews may not capture cultural differences in depressive symptom identification. Among Asian Americans, the CIDI may not be as sensitive to MDD diagnoses, for Asian Americans are less likely endorse depressed mood or sadness as their primary complaint. This may lead to less probing queries regarding other relevant depressive symptoms unrelated to sadness (Kim, Park, Storr, Tran, & Juon, 2015). Thus, a structured clinical interview is not recommended as the sole basis of making a diagnosis, but it is nonetheless a useful tool to inform diagnosis.

Several studies have examined the cultural adaptation and validity of translated versions of the CIDI. Gelaye and colleagues (2013a, 2013b) examined the Amharic version of the CIDI among a sample of participants in a diagnostic assessment study at a major hospital in Ethiopia. The Amharic version demonstrated strong internal reliability (Cronbach's α = 0.97), fair specificity (72%), but low sensitivity (51%). Gelaye and colleagues caution that using only a structured clinical interview such as the CIDI in this population may lead to underdetection of depression.

Navarro-Mateu and colleagues (2013) adapted and validated the Spanish-language CIDI for a sample in Murcia, Spain. The original Spanish-language CIDI was translated for use in Latin American Spanish-speaking countries. The authors noted that 372 questions in the interview needed to have linguistic or cultural adaptations in order to capture experiential or conceptual equivalences in Spain's dialect. This study highlights the importance of taking not only linguistic but also cultural factors into consideration when translating and adapting a structured clinical interview for use in another country, particularly Spanish-speaking countries where there is considerable heterogeneity in cultural and linguistic expressions from one country to the next.

In sum, although structured interviews were designed to reduce bias in diagnostic decisions, considerable cultural and linguistic factors have been found to reduce diagnostic accuracy. Therefore, when working with cultural and linguistically diverse groups, it is important that the examiner have an understanding of the limitations of structured interviews and take into account cultural expressions of distress.

TREATMENT AND ADHERENCE

In addition to appropriately identifying depressive symptoms among diverse populations, culturally competent treatment is another important consideration. Lo and Fung (2003) outline two distinct forms of cultural competence: generic and specific. Generic cultural competence encompasses the knowledge and skill sets needed for any cross-cultural clinical experience, whereas specific cultural competence indicates that a clinician has the knowledge necessary to effectively work with a particular ethnocultural community (Lo & Fung, 2003). Not only can depression have heterogeneous presentations in diverse groups, but also diverse views may be held about the origins of depression and its treatment, views that are rooted in the individual's health beliefs. Although the use of antidepressant medications is a common depression treatment avenue in Western countries, this may not be a preferred or efficacious treatment avenue for diverse groups, especially in non-Western populations where medication access may be particularly scarce and traditional healers may be preferred. Medication adherence is influenced both by access to health care services and by beliefs related to medications. It is crucial to take into account differing beliefs related to medications as well as existing culturally rooted treatment avenues, such as visiting local healers or using herbs, natural medicine, or home remedies when treating depression in diverse groups.

Attitudes and beliefs related to medications can significantly impact treatment of depression among diverse groups. A study of treatment attitudes and beliefs among African American and non-Hispanic White adults revealed that African American men and women expressed greater concern about antidepressant medications than their non-Hispanic White counterparts. African American men were more likely to express negative attitudes toward health care providers than African American and non-Hispanic White women. Additionally, African American women were more likely to endorse a medication other than an antidepressant as their most important medication than non-Hispanic White men and women and were also less adherent to antidepressant medications than non-Hispanic White women (Burnett-Zeigler et al., 2014).

Another study examined the utility of the CES-D in a sample of Vietnamese Americans and Latinx adults of Mexican origin with diabetes, which revealed that both groups were more likely to endorse depressive symptoms on the CES-D than non-Hispanic Whites but were less likely than non-Hispanic Whites to be diagnosed with depression. Moreover, minority patients who reported lower trust in their physician were significantly less likely to be diagnosed or treated for depression (Sorkin et al., 2011). Latinx adults with diabetes have a higher prevalence of comorbid depression than non-Hispanic Whites with diabetes, and Latinx adults are less likely to receive treatment for their depression (Li et al., 2009; Sorkin et al., 2011). A study of depression treatment attitudes among an ethnically diverse sample of African American, Asians/Pacific Islanders, and Latinx adults found that all three groups were more likely to prefer counseling to antidepressant medications, whereas non-Hispanic Whites were more likely to prefer antidepressants (Givens, Houston, Van Voorhees, Ford, & Cooper, 2007). Furthermore, ethnic minority participants were less likely to believe in the efficacy of antidepressants or a biological basis for depression, but they were more likely to believe antidepressants were addictive and to find counseling and prayer to be more efficacious treatments for depression. Further analysis revealed attitudes and beliefs somewhat attenuated the relationship between ethnicity and treatment preferences (Givens et al., 2007). Both attitudes related to medications and trust in health care providers significantly impact diagnosis and treatment outcomes in diverse groups. The physician–patient relationship, particularly trust in physicians, appears to be a salient factor among diverse groups and warrants consideration when examining depression symptomatology and treatment.

Another important consideration is access to and utilization of health care services. Underrepresented minority populations are less likely to have access to health care services, be prescribed and take newer antidepressants, and receive a nonpharmacological treatment (e.g., therapy) compared to their non-Hispanic White counterparts (Lesser et al., 2010). Financial constraints significantly impact medication adherence for diverse groups. Diverse groups are less likely to be insured and more likely to be in a lower socioeconomic position than non-Hispanic Whites. Blacks and Latinx adults are also more likely to report cost-related nonadherence to antidepressant medications than non-Hispanic Whites (Gellad, Haas, & Safran, 2007).

Latinx populations are often conceptualized as a monolithic group in research. As a result, little research has been done on potential differential treatment and health care impact, which may vary by Latinx subgroup. One study examined health care utilization (e.g., frequency of emergency room visits, number of prescription medications) among U.S. Latinx adults of Cuban, Puerto Rican, Mexican, Central American/Caribbean, and South American origin. Latinx adults of Cuban and Mexican origin were found to have fewer emergency room visits than non-Hispanic Whites, whereas Latinx adults of Puerto Rican descent were more likely to have more frequent emergency department visits. All Latinx subgroups were less likely to have prescription medications, with all Latinx adults born outside of the United States having no prescription medications (Weinick, Jacobs, Stone, Ortega, & Burstin, 2004). This study highlights the heterogeneity of Latinx groups and their diverse barriers to and utilization of health care services, all of which should be taken into consideration when treating a Latinx patient. Future research about depression screening and treatment among Latinx populations should focus on adequately characterizing different Latinx subgroups and potential cultural and linguistic variabilities that may influence depression symptom identification and treatment across different Latinx subgroups.

With regard to psychological treatment methods for depression among diverse groups, cultural adaptations of psychological treatment have been demonstrated to be efficacious. A systematic review of psychological treatments for depression found that adaptations frequently take the form of changes in language, context, and therapist delivering the treatment (Chowdary et al., 2014). As previously noted, going beyond a direct, literal translation can improve a measure or a treatment. Such changes include incorporating idioms relevant to the target culture, replacing technical terms with colloquial expressions, and using metaphors to increase relevance (Chowdary et al., 2014). Adaptations of treatment to fit into the patient's social context include reducing barriers to treatment, improving access, and enhancing feasibility and acceptability. Changes in psychological treatments may also be used for different cultural groups, such as simplifying the steps of the overall treatment and reducing elements of treatment that require literacy (Chowdary et al., 2014).

CONCLUSION

To conclude, culture is a critical lens to assess and interpret symptoms of depression. This chapter has reviewed a variety of cultural considerations when using common depression assessment measures as well as treatment recommendations. Future work in this area should include examination of the moderating effect of the clinician's cultural competency on diagnostic ratings—even when using measures with known limitations. Further training in this area is sorely needed, particularly in community-based settings that often serve as a medical hub for treatment among culturally and linguistically diverse groups. It is important that diagnostic formulations and treatment recommendations take into account the individual's social context, health beliefs, and prior history of treatment fidelity.

CLINICAL CONSIDERATIONS

• Evaluate one's competency as a clinician to work with a patient from a diverse background, particularly if the patient is a linguistic minority. It is advised to consult or refer to a clinician with appropriate expertise, cultural competency, and linguistic fluency to screen the patient for depression.

• Utilize the best available screening measure that has been validated and determined to be appropriate for use with your patient's racial/ethnic/linguistic background

• Do not use screening tools as diagnostic indicators; these only indicate depressive symptomatology, largely from a Western perspective. A comprehensive clinical interview with a thorough assessment of the patient's sociocultural context should be conducted when assessing depression in diverse groups.

- Consider the potential influence on acculturation on depression presentation. Patients who are less acculturated to the United States may present with symptoms that may be characteristic of depressive symptoms in their primary culture of origin.

- Avoid translating measures either orally or by hand, regardless of whether a clinician is fluent in the language. Provide a measure only if it has been validated for use in the language of interest and if it is administered by a clinician with adequate linguistic fluency.

REFERENCES

Adewuya, A. O., Ola, B. A., & Afolabi, O. O. (2006). Validity of the patient health questionnaire (PHQ-9) as a screening tool for depression amongst Nigerian university students. *Journal of Affective Disorders, 96*, 89–93.

Akdemir, A., Türkçapar, M. H., Orsel, S. D., Demiurgi, N., Dag, I., & Ozbay, M. H. (2001). Reliability and validity of the Turkish version of the Hamilton Depression Rating Scale. *Comprehensive Psychiatry, 42*, 161–165.

Alarcón, R. D. (2009). Culture, cultural factors and psychiatric diagnosis: Review and projections. *World Psychiatry, 8*, 131–139.

Alarcón, R. D., Becker, A. E., Lewis-Fernandez, R., Like, R. C., Desai, P., Foulks, E., et al. (2009). Issues for DSM-V: the role of culture in psychiatric diagnosis. *Journal of Nervous and Mental Disease, 197*, 559–560.

Alhadi, A. N., Alarabi, M. A., Alshomrani, A. T., Shuqdar, R. M., Alsuwaidan, M. T., & McIntyre, R. S. (2018). Arabic translation, validation and cultural adaptation of the 7-Item Hamilton Depression Rating Scale in two community samples. *Sultan Qaboos University Medical Journal, 18*, e167–e172.

American Psychiatric Association. (1952). *Diagnostic and statistical manual of mental disorders* (1st ed.). Washington, DC: Author.

American Psychiatric Association. (1968). *Diagnostic and statistical manual of mental disorders* (2nd ed.). Washington, DC: Author.

American Psychiatric Association. (1980). *Diagnostic and statistical manual of mental disorders* (3rd ed.). Washington, DC: Author.

American Psychiatric Association. (2000). *Diagnostic and statistical manual of mental disorders* (4th ed., text rev.). Washington, DC: Author.

Andrews, G., & Peters, L. (1997). The psychometric properties of the Composite International Diagnostic Interview. *Social Psychiatry and Psychiatric Epidemiology, 33*, 80–88.

Arrieta, J., Aguerrebere, M., Raviola, G., Flores, H., Elliott, P., Espinosa, A., et al. (2017). Validity and utility of the Patient Health Questionnaire (PHQ)-2 and PHQ-9 for screening and diagnosis of depression in rural Chiapas, Mexico: A cross-sectional study. *Journal of Clinical Psychology, 73*, 1076–1090.

Azah, M. N. N., Shah, M. E. M., Juwita, S., Bahri, I. S., Rushidi, W. M. W., & Jamil, Y. M. (2005). Validation of the Malay Version Brief Patient Health Questionnaire (PHQ-9) among adults attending family medicine clinics. *International Medical Journal, 12*, 259–264.

Bachner, Y. G. (2016). Psychometric properties of responses to an Arabic version of the Hamilton Depression Rating Scale (HAM-D6). *Journal of the American Psychiatric Nurses Association, 22*, 27–30.

Bachner, Y. G., O'Rourke, N., Goldfracht, M., Bech, P., & Ayalon, L. (2013). Psychometric properties of responses by clinicians and older adults to a 6-item Hebrew version of the Hamilton Depression Rating Scale (HAM-D6). *BMC Psychiatry, 13*, 2.

Bagby, R. M., Ryder, A. G., Schuller, D. R. & Marshall, M. B. (2004). The Hamilton Depression Rating Scale: Has the gold standard become a lead weight? *American Journal of Psychiatry, 161*, 2163–2177.

Baig, B. J. (2010). Social and transcultural aspects of psychiatry. In E. C. Johnstone (Ed.), *Companion to Psychiatric Studies* (8th ed., pp. 109–119). London: Churchill Livingstone.

Barnes, D. M., & Bates, L. M. (2017). Do racial patterns in psychological distress shed light on the Black-White depression paradox?: A systematic review. *Social Psychiatry and Psychiatric Epidemiology, 52,* 913–928.

Baron, E. C., Davies, T., & Lund, C. (2017). Validation of the 10-item Centre for Epidemiological Studies Depression Scale (CES-D-10) in Zulu, Xhosa and Afrikaans populations in South Africa. *BMC Psychiatry, 17,* 6.

Beard, C., Hsu, K. J., Rifkin, L. S., Busch, A. B., & Björgvinsson, T. (2016). Validation of the PHQ-9 in a psychiatric sample. *Journal of Affective Disorders, 193,* 267–273.

Beck A., & Steer R. A. (1987). *Beck Depression Inventory manual.* San Antonio, TX: The Psychological Corporation.

Beck, A. T., Steer, R. A., & Brown, G. K. (1996). *Manual for the Beck Depression Inventory–II.* San Antonio, TX: Psychological Corporation.

Bell, C. C., Dixie-Bell, D. D., & Thompson, B. (1986). Panic attacks: Relationship to isolated sleep paralysis. *American Journal of Psychiatry, 143,* 1484.

Boutin-Foster, C. (2008). An item-level analysis of the Center for Epidemiologic Studies Depression Scale (CES-D) by race and ethnicity in patients with coronary artery disease. *International Journal of Geriatric Psychiatry, 23,* 1034–1039.

Burnett-Zeigler, I., Kim, H. M., Chiang, C., Kavanagh, J., Zivin, K., Rockefeller K., et al. (2014). The association between race and gender, treatment attitudes, and antidepressant treatment adherence. *International Journal of Geriatric Psychiatry, 29,* 16–77.

Callahan, C. M., & Wolinsky, F. D. (1994). The effect of gender and race on the measurement properties of the CES-D in older adults. *Medical Care, 32,* 341–356.

Canel-Çınarbaş, D., Cui, Y., & Lauridsen, E. (2011). Cross-cultural validation of the Beck Depression Inventory–II across U.S. and Turkish samples. *Measurement and Evaluation in Counseling and Development, 44,* 77–91.

Carleton, R. N., Thibodeau, M. A., Teale, M. J., Welch, P. G., Abrams, M. P., Robinson, T., et al. (2013). The Center for Epidemiologic Studies Depression Scale: A review with a theoretical and empirical examination of item content and factor structure. *PLOS ONE, 8,* e58067.

Chan, A. C. (1996). Clinical validation of the Geriatric Depression Scale (GDS): Chinese version. *Journal of Aging and Health, 8,* 238–253.

Chapman, D. P., Whitfield, C. L., Felitti, V. J., Dube, S. R., Edwards, V. J., & Anda, R. F. (2004). Adverse childhood experiences and the risk of depressive disorders in adulthood. *Journal of Affective Disorders, 82,* 217–225.

Chasson, G., Williams, M. T., Davis, D. M., & Combs, J. Y. (2017). Missed diagnosis in African Americans with obsessive compulsive disorder: The Structured Interview for DSM-IV Axis I Disorders (SCID-I). *BMC Psychiatry, 17,* 258.

Cheng, S. T., & Chan, A. C. (2005). The Center for Epidemiologic Studies Depression Scale in older Chinese: Thresholds for long and short forms. *International Journal of Geriatric Psychiatry, 20,* 465–470.

Chentsova-Dutton, Y. E., & Tsai, J. L. (2009). Understanding depression across cultures. In I. H. Gotlib & C. L. Hammen (Eds.), *Handbook of depression* (pp. 363–385). New York: Guilford Press.

Cheung, F. M., and Lau, B. W. K. (1982) Situational variations of help-seeking behavior among Chinese patients. *Comprehensive Psychiatry, 23,* 252–262.

Chin, W. Y., Choi, E. P. H., Chan, K. T. Y., & Wong, C. K. H. (2015). The psychometric properties of the Center for Epidemiologic Studies Depression Scale in Chinese primary care patients: Factor structure, construct validity, reliability, sensitivity and responsiveness. *PLoS One, 10,* e0135131.

Cholera, R., Gaynes, B. N., Pence, B. W., Bassett, J., Qangule, N., Macphail, C., et al. (2014). Validity of the Patient Health Questionnaire-9 to screen for depression in a high-HIV burden primary health-care clinic in Johannesburg, South Africa. *Journal of Affective Disorders, 167,* 160–166.

Chowdary, N., Jotheeswaran, A. T., Nadkarni, A., Hollon, S. D., King, M., Jordans, M. J. D., et al. (2014).

The methods and outcomes of cultural adaptations of psychological treatments for depressive disorders: A systematic review. *Psychological Medicine, 44*, 1131–1146.

Coppersmith, G., Dredze, M., & Harman, C. (2014). Quantifying mental health signals in Twitter. *Proceedings of the Workshop on Computational Linguistics and Clinical Psychology: From Linguistic Signal to Clinical Reality*, pp. 51–60.

Dawes, S. E., Suarez, P., Vaida, F., Marcotte, T. D., Atkinson, J. H., Grant, I., et al. (2010). Demographic influences and suggested cut-scores for the Beck Depression Inventory in a non-clinical Spanish speaking population from the US-Mexico border region. *International Journal of Culture and Mental Health, 3*, 34–42.

De Choudary, M., Gamon, M., Counts, S., & Horvitz, E. (2013). Predicting depression via social media. *International AAAI Conference on Web and Social Media, 13*, 1–10.

De Lima Osório, F., Vilela Mendes, A., Crippa, J. A., & Loureiro, S. R. (2009). Study of the Discriminative Validity of the PHQ-9 and PHQ-2 in a Sample of Brazilian Women in the Context of Primary Health Care. *Perspectives in Psychiatric Care, 45*, 216–227.

Ertan, T., and Eker, E. (2000). Reliability, validity, and factor structure of the Geriatric Depression Scale in Turkish elderly: Are there different factor structures for different cultures? *International Psychogeriatrics, 12*, 163–172.

Familiar, I., Ortiz-Panozo, E., Hall, B., Vieitez, I., Romieu, I., Lopez-Ridaura, R., et al. (2014). Factor structure of the Spanish version of the Patient Health Questionnaire-9 in Mexican women. *International Journal of Methods in Psychiatric Research, 24*, 74–82.

Ferrari, A. J., Charlson, F. J., Norman, R. E., Patten, S. B., Freedman, G., Murray, C. J., et al. (2013). Burden of depressive disorders by country, sex, age, and year: Findings from the global burden of disease study 2010. *PLoS Medicine, 10*(11), e1001547.

Fleck, M. P., Chaves M. L., Poirier-Littre, M. F., Bourdel, M. C., & Loo, H., & Guelfi, J. D. (2004). Depression in France and Brazil: Factorial structure of the 17-item Hamilton Depression Scale in inpatients. *Journal of Nervous and Mental Disease, 192*, 103–110.

Fountoulakis, K., Iacovides, A., Kleanthous, S., Samolis, S., Kaprinis, S. G., Sitzoglou, K., et al. (2001). Reliability, validity and psychometric properties of the Greek translation of the Center for Epidemiological Studies-Depression (CES-D) Scale. *BMC Psychiatry, 1*, 3.

Freud, S. (1957). Mourning and melancholia. In J. Strachey (Ed. and Trans.), *Standard edition of the complete psychological works of Sigmund Freud* (Vol. 14). London: Hogarth Press. (Original work published 1917)

Furukawa, T. A., Streiner, D. L, Azuma, H., Higuchi, T., Kamijima, K., Kanba, S., et al. (2005). Cross-cultural equivalence in depression assessment: Japan–Europe–North American study. *Acta Psychiatrica Scandinavica 112*, 279–285.

García-Batista, Z. E., Guerra-Peña, K., Cano-Vindel, A., Herrera-Martínez, S. X., & Medrano, L. A. (2018). Validity and reliability of the Beck Depression Inventory (BDI-II) in general and hospital population of Dominican Republic. *PLoS One, 13*, e0199750.

Garrison, F. H. (1929). *An introduction to the history of medicine* (4th ed.). Philadelphia: Saunders.

Gelaye, B., Williams, M. A., Lemma, S., Deyessa, N., Bahretibeb, Y., Shibre, T., et al. (2013a). Diagnostic validity of the composite international diagnostic interview (CIDI) depression module in an East African population. *International Journal of Psychiatry in Medicine, 46*, 387–405.

Gelaye, B., Williams, M. A., Lemma, S., Deyessa, N., Bahretibeb, Y., Shibre, T., et al. (2013b). Validity of the Patient Health Questionnaire-9 for depression screening and diagnosis in East Africa. *Psychiatry Research, 210*, 653–661.

Gellad, W. F., Haas, J. S., & Safran, D. G. (2007). Race/ethnicity and nonadherence to prescription medications among seniors: Results of a national study. *Journal of General Internal Medicine, 22*, 1572–1578.

Givens, J. L., Houston, T. K., Van Voorhees, B. W., Ford, D. E., & Cooper, L. A. (2007). Ethnicity and preferences for depression treatment. *General Hospital Psychiatry, 29*, 182–191.

Gomes-Oliveira, M. H., Gorenstein, C., Lotufo Neto, F., Andrade, L. H., & Wang, Y. P. (2012). Validation of the Brazilian Portuguese version of the Beck Depression Inventory-II in a community sample. *Revista Brasileira de Psiquiatria, 34*, 389–394.

Grothe, K. B., Dutton, G. R., Jones, G. N., Bodenlos, J., Ancona, M., & Brantley, P. J. (2005). Validation of the Beck Depression Inventory-II in a low-income African American sample of medical outpatients. *Psychological Assessment, 17*, 110–114.

Guarnaccia, P. J. (1993). Ataques de nervios in Puerto Rico: culture-bound syndrome or popular illness? *Medical Anthropology, 15*, 157–170.

Hagmayer, Y., & Engelmann, N. (2014). Causal beliefs about depression in different cultural groups— what do cognitive psychological theories of causal learning and reasoning predict? *Frontiers in Psychology, 5*, 1303.

Hamdi, E., Amin, Y., & Abou-Saleh, M. T. (1997). Performance of the Hamilton Depression Rating Scale in depressed patients in the United Arab Emirates. *Acta Psychiatrica Scandinavica, 96*, 416–423.

Hamilton, M. (1960). A rating scale for depression. *Journal of Neurology, Neurosurgery, and Psychiatry, 23*, 56–62.

Haro, J. M., Arbabzadeh-Bouchez, S., Brugha, T. S., de Girolamo, G., Guyer, M. E., Jin, R., et al. (2006). Concordance of the Composite International Diagnostic Interview Version 3.0 (CIDI 3.0) with standardized clinical assessments in the WHO World Mental Health surveys. *International Journal of Methods in Psychiatric Research, 15*, 167–180.

Huang, F. Y., Chung, H., Kroenke, K., Delucchi, K. L., & Spitzer, R. L. (2006). Using the Patient Health Questionnaire-9 to measure depression among racially and ethnically diverse primary care patients. *Journal of General Internal Medicine, 21*, 547–552.

Iwata, N., & Buka, S. (2002). Race/ethnicity and depressive symptoms: A cross-cultural/ethnic comparison among university students in East Asia, North and South America. *Social Science and Medicine, 55*, 2243–2252.

Iwata, N., & Higuchi, H. R. (2000). Responses of Japanese and American university students to the STAI items that assess the presence or absence of anxiety. *Journal of Personality Assessment, 74*(1), 48–62.

Jang, Y., Kwag, K. H., & Chiriboga, D. A. (2010). Not saying I am happy does not mean I am not: Cultural influences on responses to positive affect items in the CES-D. *Journal of Gerontology: Psychological Sciences, 65B*, 684–690.

Jayawickreme, N., Jayawickreme, E., Atanasov, P., Goonasekera, M. A., & Foa, F. B. (2012). Are culturally specific measures of trauma-related anxiety and depression needed?: The case of Sri Lanka. *Psychological Assessment, 24*, 791–800.

Jayawickreme, N., Verkuilen, J., Jayawickreme, E., Acosta, K., & Foa, E. B. (2017). Measuring depression in a non-Western war-affected displaced population: Measurement equivalence of the Beck Depression Inventory. *Frontiers in Psychology, 8*, 1670.

Kerr, L. K., & Kerr, L. D. (2001). Screening tools for depression in primary care: The effects of culture, gender, and somatic symptoms on the detection of depression. *Western Journal of Medicine, 175*, 349–352.

Kilburn, K., Prencipe, L., Hjelm, L., Peterman, A., Handa, S., & Palermo, T. (2018). Examination of performance of the Center for Epidemiologic Studies Depression Scale Short Form 10 among African youth in poor, rural households. *BMC Psychiatry, 18*, 201.

Kim, G., Decoster, J., Huang, C-H., & Bryant, A. N. (2013). A meta-analysis of the factor structure of the Geriatric Depression Scale (GDS): The effects of language. *International Psychogeriatric, 25*, 71–81.

Kim, H. J., Park, E., Storr, C. L., Tran, K., & Juon, H.-S. (2015). Depression among Asian-American adults in the community: Systematic review and meta-analysis. *PLoS One, 10*, e0127760.

Kirmayer, L. J. (2001). Cultural variations in the clinical presentation of depression and anxiety: implications for diagnosis and treatment. *Journal of Clinical Psychiatry, 62*, 22–28.

Kleim, S., Mößle, T., Zenger, M., & Brähler, E. (2014). Reliability and validity of the Beck Depression Inventory-Fast Screen for medical patients in the general German population. *Journal of Affective Disorders, 156*, 236–239.

Kleinman, A. M. (1980). Healers in the context of culture. Berkeley: University of California Press.

Kleinman, A., Eisenberg, L, & Good, B. (1978). Culture, illness, and care: Clinical lessons from anthropologic and cross-cultural research. *Annals of Internal Medicine, 88*, 251–258.

Kohrt, B. A., Luitel, N. P., Acharya, P., & Jordans, M. J. (2016). Detection of depression in low resource settings: Validation of the Patient Health Questionnaire (PHQ-9) and cultural concepts of distress in Nepal. *BMC Psychiatry, 16,* 58.

Kojima, M., Furukawa, T. A., Takahashi, H., Kawai, M., Nagaya, T., & Tokudome, S. (2002). Cross-cultural validation of the Beck Depression Inventory-II in Japan. *Psychiatry Research, 110,* 291–299.

Kroenke, K., & Spitzer, R. L. (2002). The PHQ-9: A new depression diagnostic and severity measure. *Psychiatric Annals, 32,* 509–515.

Kroenke, K., Spitzer, R. L., & Williams, J. B. (2001). The PHQ-9: Validity of a brief depression severity measure. *Journal of General Internal Medicine, 16,* 606–613.

Lee, C. P., Liu, C. Y., & Hung, C. I. (2017). Psychometric evaluation of a 6-item Chinese version of the Hamilton Depression Rating Scale: Mokken scaling and item analysis. *Asia-Pacific Psychiatry, 9,* 1–3.

Lee, J., Wachholtz, A., & Choi, K. H. (2014). A Review of the Korean cultural syndrome Hwa Byung: Suggestions for theory and intervention. *Asia T'aep'yongyang sangdam yon'gu, 4,* 49.

Lesser, I. M., Myers, H. F., Lin, K. M., Bingham Mira, C., Joseph, N. T., Olmos, N. T., Schettino, J., et al. (2010). Ethnic differences in antidepressant response: A prospective multi-site clinical trial. *Depression and Anxiety, 27,* 56–62.

Lewis-Fernandez, R., Das, A. K., Alfonso, C., Weissman, M., & Olfson, M. (2005). Depression in US Hispanics: Diagnostic and management considerations in family practice. *Journal of the American Board Family Practice, 18,* 282–296.

Lewis-Fernandez, R. & Kleinman, A. (1994). Culture, personality, and psychopathology. *Journal of Abnormal Psychology, 103,* 67–71.

Li, C., Ford, E. S., Zhao, G., Ahluwalia, I. B., Pearson, W. S., & Mokdad, A. H. (2009). Prevalence and correlates of undiagnosed depression among U.S. adults with diabetes: The Behavioral Risk Factor Surveillance System, 2006. *Diabetes Research and Clinical Practice, 83,* 268–279.

Lin, J., Wang, X., Dong, F., Du, Y., Shen, J., Ding, S., et al. (2018). Validation of the Chinese version of the Hamilton Rating Scale for Depression in adults with epilepsy. *Epilepsy and Behavior, 89,* 148–152.

Liu, S., Yeh, Z., Huang, H., Sun, F., Tjung, J., Hwang, L., et al. (2011). Validation of Patient Health Questionnaire for depression screening among primary care patients in Taiwan. *Comprehensive Psychiatry, 52,* 96–101.

Lo, H. T., & Fung, K. P. (2003). Culturally competent psychotherapy. *Canadian Journal of Psychiatry, 18,* 161–170.

Lopez, S. R., & Nunez, J. A. (1987). Cultural factors considered in selected diagnostic criteria and interview schedules. *Journal of Abnormal Psychology, 96,* 270–272.

Lotrakul, M., Sukanit, P., & Sukying, C. (1996). The validity and reliability of the Hamilton Rating scale for depression, Thai version. *Journal of the Psychiatric Association of Thailand, 41,* 235–246.

Lotrakul, M., Sumrithe, S., & Saipanish, S. (2008). Reliability and validity of the Thai version of the PHQ-9. *BMC Psychiatry, 8,* 46.

Lotufo Neto, F., Andrade, L. H., & Wang, Y. P. (2012). Validation of the Brazilian Portuguese version of the Beck Depression Inventory-II in a community sample. *Revista Brasileira de Psiquiatria, 34,* 389–394.

Loveys, K., Torrez, J., Fine, A., Moriarty, G., & Coppersmith, G. (2018). Cross-cultural differences in language markers of depression online. In *Proceedings of the Fifth Workshop on Computational Linguistics and Clinical Psychology: From Keyboard to Clinic,* pp. 78–87.

Manea, L., Gilbody, S., & McMillan, D. (2015). A diagnostic meta-analysis of the Patient Health Questionnaire-9 (PHQ-9) algorithm scoring method as a screen for depression. *General Hospital Psychiatry, 37*(1), 67–75.

Markus, H. R., & Kitayama, S. (1991). Culture and the self: Implications for cognition, emotion, and motivation. *Psychological Review, 98,* 224–253.

Merz, E. L., Malcarne, V. L., Roesch, S. C., Riley, N., & Sadler, G. R. (2011). A multigroup confirmatory factor analysis of the Patient Health Questionnaire-9 among English- and Spanish-speaking Latinas. *Cultural Diversity and Ethnic Minority Psychology, 17*, 309–316.

Mordeno, I. G., Carpio, J. G. E., Mendoza, N. B., & Hall, B. J. (2018). The latent structure of major depressive symptoms and its relationship with somatic disorder symptoms among Filipino female domestic workers in China. *Psychiatry Research, 270*, 587–594.

Muñoz-Navarro, R., Cano-Vindel, A., Medrano, L. A., Schmitz, F., Ruiz-Rodríguez, P., Abellán-Maeso, C., et al. (2017). Utility of the PHQ-9 to identify major depressive disorder in adult patients in Spanish primary care centres. *BMC Psychiatry, 17*, 291.

Nakku, J., Rathod, S., Kizza, D., Breuer, E., Mutyaba, K., Baron, E., et al. (2016). Validity and diagnostic accuracy of the Luganda version of the 9-item and 2-item Patient Health Questionnaire for detecting major depressive disorder in rural Uganda. *Global Mental Health, 3*, E20.

Navarro-Mateu F., Morán-Sánchez, I., Alonso, J., Tormo, M. J., Pujalte, M. L., Garriga, A., et al. (2013). Cultural adaptation of the Latin American version of the World Health Organization Composite International Diagnostic Interview (WHO-CIDI) (v 3.0) for use in Spain. *Gaceta Sanitaria, 27*, 325–331.

Neighbors, H. W., Trierweiler, S. J., Ford, B. C., & Muroff, J. R. (2003). Racial differences in DSM diagnosis using a semi-structured instrument: The importance of clinical judgment in the diagnosis of African Americans. *Journal of Health and Social Behavior, 44*, 237–256.

Neighbors, H. W., Trierweiler, S. J., Munday, C., Thompson, E. E., Jackson, J. S., Binion, V. J., et al. (1999). Psychiatric diagnosis of African Americans: Diagnostic divergence in clinician structured and semistructured interviewing conditions. *Journal of the National Medical Association, 91*, 601–612.

Ng, L. C., Magidson, J. F., Hock, R. S., Joska, J. A., Fekadu, A., Hanlon, C., et al. (2016). Proposed training areas for global mental health researchers. *Academic Psychiatry, 40*, 679–685.

Nyunt, M. S., Fones, C., Niti, M., & Ng, T. P. (2009). Criterion-based validity and reliability of the Geriatric Depression Screening Scale (GDS-15) in a large validation sample of community-living Asian older adults. *Aging and Mental Health, 13*(3), 376–382.

Olbert, C. M., Nagendra, A., & Buck, B. (2018). Meta-analysis of Black vs. White racial disparity in schizophrenia diagnosis in the United States: Do structured assessments attenuate racial disparities? *Journal of Abnormal Psychology, 127*, 104–115.

Olden, M., Rosenfeld, B., Pessin, H., & Breitbart, W. (2009). Measuring depression at the end of life: Is the Hamilton Depression Rating Scale a valid instrument? *Assessment, 16*, 43–54.

Omrani, A., Holtzman, N. S., Akiskal, H. S., & Ghaemi, S. N. (2012). Ibn Imran's 10th century treatise on melancholy. *Journal of Affective Disorders. 141*, 116–119.

Patel, V. (1995). Explanatory models of mental illness in sub-Saharan Africa. *Social Science and Medicine, 40*, 1291–1298.

Posner, S. F., Stewart, A. L., Marín, G., & Pérez-Stable, E. J. (2001). Factor variability of the Center for Epidemiological Studies Depression Scale (CES-D) among urban Latinos. *Ethnicity and Health, 6*, 137–144.

Preoţiuc-Pietro, J. D., Eichstaedt, J., Park, G., Sap, M., Smith, L., Tobolsky, V., et al. (2015). The role of personality, age, and gender in tweeting about mental illness. *Proceedings of the 2nd Workshop on Computational Linguistics and Clinical Psychology: From Linguistic Signal to Clinical Reality*, pp. 21–30.

Radloff, L. S. (1977). The CES-D scale: A self report depression scale for research in the general population. *Applied Psychological Measurements, 1*, 385–401.

Ramos-Brieva, J. A., & Cordero-Villafafila, A. (1988). A new validation of the Hamilton Rating Scale for depression. *Journal of Psychiatric Research, 22*, 21–28.

Rao, U., Poland, R. E., & Lin, K. M. (2012). Comparison of symptoms in African-American, Asian-American, Mexican-American and Non-Hispanic White patients with major depressive disorder. *Asian Journal of Psychiatry, 5*, 28–33.

Reynolds, E. H., & Wilson, J. V. (2013). Depression and anxiety in Babylon. *Journal of the Royal Society of Medicine, 106*, 478–481.

Robison, J., Gruman, C., Gaztambide, S., & Blank, K. (2002). Screening for depression in middle-aged and older Puerto Rican primary care patients. *Journals of Gerontology. Series A, Biological Sciences and Medical Sciences, 57,* M308–314.

Schwartz, H., Eichstaedt, J., Kern, M., Park, G., Sap, M., Stillwell, D., et al. (2014, June). Towards assessing changes in degree of depression through Facebook. *Proceedings of the Workshop on Computational Linguistics and Clinical Psychology: From Linguistic Signal to Clinical Reality,* pp. 118–125.

Simons, R. (2001). Introduction to culture bound syndromes. *Psychiatric Times, 18,* 1–3.

Simons, R. C., & Hughes, C. C. (1986). *The culture-bound syndromes: Folk illnesses of psychiatric and anthropological interest.* Boston: Reidel.

Sorkin, D. H., Ngo-Metzger, Q., Billimek, J., August, K. J., Greenfield, S., & Kaplan, S. H. (2011). Underdiagnosed and undertreated depression among racially/ethnically diverse patients with type 2 diabetes. *Diabetes Care, 34,* 598–600.

Spitzer, R. L., Williams, J. B., Gibbon, M., & First, M. B. (1992). The Structured Clinical Interview for DSM-III-R (SCID) I: History rationale and description. *Archives of General Psychiatry, 49,* 624–649.

Sullivan, P. F., Neale, M. C. & Kendler, K. S. (2000). Genetic epidemiology of major depression: Review and metaanalysis. *American Journal of Psychiatry, 157,* 1552–1562.

Swami, V., Loo, P., & Furnham, A. (2010). Public knowledge and beliefs about depression among urban and rural Malays in Malaysia. *International Journal of Social Psychiatry 56,* 480–498.

Tsai J. L., Chentsova-Dutton, Y., Freire-Bebeau, L., & Przymus, D. E. (2002). Emotional expression and physiology in European Americans and Hmong Americans. *Emotion, 2,* 380–397.

Vindbjerg, E., Makransky, G., Mortensen, E. L., & Carlsson, J. (2018). Cross-cultural psychometric properties of the Hamilton Depression Rating Scale. *Canadian Journal of Psychiatry,* 1–18.

Wan Mahmud, W. M., Awang, A., Herman, I., & Mohamed, M. N. (2004). Analysis of the psychometric properties of the Malay version of Beck Depression Inventory II (BDI-II) among postpartum women in Kedah, north west of peninsular Malaysia. *Malaysian Journal of Medical Sciences, 11,* 19–25.

Weinick, R. M., Jacobs, E. A., Stone, L. C., Ortega, A. N., & Burstin, H. (2004). Hispanic healthcare disparities: Challenging the myth of a monolithic Hispanic population. *Medical Care, 42,* 313–320.

Wiebe, J. S., & Penley, J. A. (2005). A psychometric comparison of the Beck Depression Inventory–II in English and Spanish. *Psychological Assessment, 17,* 481–485.

World Health Organization. (2017). *Depression and Other Common Mental Disorders: Global Health Estimates.* Geneva: World Health Organization.

Yesavage, J. A., Brink, T. L., Rose, T. L., Lum, O., Huang, V., Adey, M., et al. (1983). Development and validation of a geriatric depression screening scale: A preliminary report. *Journal of Psychiatric Research, 17,* 37–49.

Yi, J. S, Bae, S. O., Ahn, Y. M., Park, D. B., Noh, K. S., Shin, H. K., et al. (2005). Validity and reliability of the Korean version of the Hamilton Depression Rating Scale (K-HDRS) *Journal of Korean Neuropsychiatric Association, 44,* 456–465.

Zheng, Y. P., Zhao, J. P., Phillips, M., Liu, J. B., Cai, M. F., Sun, S. Q., et al. (1988). Validity and reliability of the Chinese Hamilton Depression Rating Scale. *British Journal of Psychiatry, 152,* 660–664.

CHAPTER 14

Using Motivational Interviewing to Enhance Neuropsychological Practice for Adults with Depression and Neurocognitive Difficulties

Mariann Suarez
Valeria Martinez-Kaigi

Motivational interviewing (MI) was first introduced in 1983 and has become an internationally utilized and empirically supported clinical application centered on helping people reduce their ambivalence, while simultaneously increasing their internal motivation to make positive changes in behavior (Miller & Rollnick, 2013). Proven efficacious to facilitate changes in a plethora of clinical settings and a span of populations, MI offers emerging evidence of potential clinical utility for practitioners working with persons diagnosed with psychiatric disorders, and neurocognitive difficulties (Miller & Rollnick, 2013).

In this chapter, we present an overview of MI, followed by a review of emerging MI research applications for patients with depressive disorders and neurocognitive difficulties. Core foundational elements of MI, including the four-processes model (Miller & Rollnick, 2013); highlights of several person-centered core interviewing and goal-oriented skills; as well as practical clinical considerations and key tips, will underscore how clinical neuropsychological providers can incorporate MI to enhance their consultation, assessment, and feedback practices with patients coping with depression.

A BRIEF OVERVIEW OF MI

While a comprehensive review of MI is beyond the scope of this chapter, we primarily focus on the key components and skills that are relevant to clinical neuropsychological assessment and feedback practices of adults with depression and neurocognitive difficulties. (Interested readers can access a more comprehensive review of topics ranging from adolescents and young adults [Naar & Suarez, 2021] to adults [Miller & Rollnick, 2013] via the *Applications of Motivational Interviewing* series published by The Guilford Press.) MI is a collaborative, goal-oriented style of communication, with particular attention to the language of change, designed to strengthen personal motivation for commitment to a specific goal by eliciting and exploring the person's own reasons for change within an atmosphere of acceptance and compassion (Miller & Rollnick, 2013). Empirically supported and atheoretically based, MI honors a person's autonomy and embodies a collaborative approach to addressing motivation to change, while concurrently maintaining a goal-oriented focus. Practitioners new to MI often have misperceptions of how it is applied in practice (Miller & Rose, 2009). For instance, MI is not "trickery" that is done "to" a patient. Rather, it is an active collaboration with a person and/or family that can be useful in addressing the ambivalence that often arises during the clinical neuropsychological assessment. It can also help to facilitate discussions to enhance internal motivation for change during therapeutic feedback visits and during consultation with other health care team members (Miller & Rollnick, 2013).

EMERGING MI RESEARCH APPLICATIONS FOR ADULTS WITH DEPRESSION AND NEUROCOGNITIVE DIFFICULTIES

The efficacy of MI has and continues to emerge in the area of neurocognitive rehabilitation for persons with associated psychiatric disorders, including depression, as well as their families (Miller & Rollnick, 2013; Schoenberg & Scott, 2011; Suarez, 2011). Highlights of recent evidence, presented in the next section, have demonstrated how MI can be applied to enhance clinical neuropsychological diagnostic assessment and feedback purposes, as well as complex and comprehensive cognitive remediation and rehabilitation interventions with this population.

MI has been found to enhance services for persons and families with neuropsychiatric and neurodegenerative disorders, including Alzheimer's disease, traumatic brain injury, and stroke (Bell et al., 2005; Bombardier et al., 2009; Byers, Lamanna, & Rosenberg, 2010; Choi & Twamley, 2013; Watkins et al., 2007, 2011). Further evidence suggests that MI is an effectively adapted intervention for persons with cognitive impairment and associated generalized psychiatric disorders. For example, in a randomized controlled trial, adaptations of MI cognitive rehabilitation interventions relative to sham interventions for persons diagnosed with comorbid cognitive disorder and schizophrenia based on diagnostic criteria in the fifth edition of the *Diagnostic and Statistical Manual of Mental Disorders* (American Psychiatric Association, 2013), have shown more improvements in task-specific motivation, attendance, and compliance rates (Fiszdon, Kurtz, Choi, Bell, & Martino, 2016). Furthermore, large-scale clinical trials indicate MI's superior efficacy, compared to intensive and structured treatments, in individuals with depression, anxiety, clinically significant cognitive impairment, and lower conceptual levels of cognitive functioning (Chien, Mui, Gray, & Cheung, 2016; Ponsford et al., 2016). Specific to depression and medical illnesses, randomized clinical trials have suggested that the application of MI as a stand-alone and augmentation strategy for patient care is efficacious. This effect has been evidenced in patients with major depressive disorder, postpartum depression and anxiety, and depression secondary to cardiac disease, who after receiving an

MI intervention showed decreased depressive symptoms, and better treatment-seeking and adherence behaviors (Holt, Milgrom, & Gemmill, 2017; Keeley et al., 2014, 2016; Navidian, Mobaraki, & Shakiba, 2017). Both MI and cognitive-behavioral therapy have proven efficacious in a variety of comorbid psychiatric and mental health related areas (Naar & Safren, 2017). Overall, these studies provide evidence that MI can enhance the practice of clinical neuropsychology that branches out beyond traditional assessment and diagnostic practices. Indeed, MI has great potential to positively impact a broader scope of cognitive rehabilitation interventions that are effective in patients with both psychiatric and neurocognitive disorders.

INCORPORATING MI INTO CLINICAL NEUROPSYCHOLOGICAL PRACTICE

In 2013, Miller and Rollnick incorporated and updated MI to include the four-processes model, which involves engaging, focusing, evoking, and planning. The model offers a guide for practitioners to strategically enhance the use of person-centered core-interviewing and goal-oriented skills in MI within each of the processes. We next present the fundamental skills of MI, along with an overview of the processes and clinical examples that illuminate the differences between typical practice versus MI responses. The chapter ends with a summary and a brief list of resources designed to enhance skills in MI.

THE SPIRIT OF MI: MAINTAIN PACE

MI entails the incorporation of a person-centered spirit that is termed PACE (Partnership, Acceptance, Compassion, and Evocation). Within this framework, the clinician will convey a partnership, acceptance, compassion, and evocative stance in all aspects of the assessment and feedback process. While working with highly complex persons with comorbid depression and neurocognitive difficulties (who often present with difficulties in completing a basic testing battery due to cognitive fatigue and other factors), coupled with limited time demands faced in daily practice, clinicians will find that maintaining the spirit can sometimes be overlooked and/or inconsistently applied. As such, it is essential for them to maintain a PACE (see Table 14.1) and recognize how it can enhance patient outcomes.

TABLE 14.1. An Overview of PACE

Partnership: Collaboration among two experts; specifically, the practitioner as a clinical expert and the patient as an expert of him- or herself

Acceptance: Regardless of professional agreement, the clinician supports the patients' liberty to make decisions (or not).

Compassion: The clinician deliberately commits to actively promote the patient's and family's well-being and needs.

Evocation: The clinician plans, guides, and tailors the therapeutic responses to facilitate internal motivation and activate action in the change process.

PERSON-CENTERED CORE INTERVIEWING SKILLS: USING OARS + I

A core component of MI entails the use of several person-centered and core-interviewing skills, termed *OARS + I.* These skills specifically include open-ended questions, affirmations, reflections, summaries and information, and advice giving. As there are a multitude of variants for how the overarching umbrella of OARS + I skills can be applied, a brief synopsis of these fundamental MI skills and examples are highlighted. Akin to the MI spirit, these person-centered skills will undoubtedly resonate with clinicians. However, *how* these skills are strategically applied, in tandem with goal-oriented skills (described below), offers a unique clinical utility, specific only to MI.

1. *Open-ended question:* A question that does not elicit a one-word or yes/no response.
   - *Example:* "Sometimes you forget, get distracted, and then get bummed out— it's like a vicious cycle. What are your thoughts about how you could better remember to . . . ?"

2. *Affirmation:* Validating, confirming, and positively stating what the person has said using the stem of "you" and excluding the practitioner's use of "I" language.
   - *Example:* "Despite all the inconveniences, you knew how important it is for you and our team to arrive on time today and bring all of your paperwork. You are invested in feeling better."

3. *Reflections:* Restating the message heard; incorporates change-talk language.
   - *Example:* "You want to plan better and know what will work for you."

4. *Summaries:* Pulling together relevant topics in a concise manner; aids in shifting focus and can be followed up with a transitional open-ended question to shift gears in the content of the conversation.
   - *Example:* "Despite the annoyances of being distracted, you were able to come prepared today and have ideas about how to use these assessment results to plan for your next steps. Tell me what you think would help next. . . ."

5. *Information and advice—ask–tell–ask:* Providing information and advice is a necessity in assessment practice, particularly when cognitive challenges are present that can impede clear communication. The ask–tell–ask strategy, adapted from Miller and Rollnick (2013) and Naar and Safren (2017), offers a unique strategy that maintains PACE skills while conveniently allowing the clinician to assess the patient's knowledge, offer information as needed, and facilitate both the assessment and treatment planning process in an efficient manner.
   a. *Ask:* Permission to discuss and clarify needed information.
      - *Example:* "If it's all right, I'd like to discuss next what your cognitive assessment results mean and how you can use some different strategies to help you better remember things."
   b. *Tell:* Information, results, concerns, and/or feedback recommendations using brief (five to seven words) and understandable language.
      - *Example:* "Your results confirm that you have memory difficulties. This means

that when you are trying to remember information, you will benefit from repetition of the information and writing down what you want to remember."

c. *Ask:* Ask for the patient's interpretation and understanding of the information, followed by a reflection of the response.

  * *Example:* "What do you know about memory problems?," "What are some things that you have tried that help you remember better?." "Would it be OK if we discussed some strategies that can help some people with memory problems improve memory?"

GOAL-ORIENTED SKILLS: THE IMPORTANCE OF CHANGE TALK AND COMMITMENT LANGUAGE

For adults with depression and neurocognitive difficulties, clinical neuropsychological assessment guided and tailored recommendations can help improve functional abilities, instrumental activities of daily living, and quality of life. While discussions tailored to goal setting are common in these practices, issues related to nonadherence to treatment-planning recommendations are common. A complicating factor for adherence and non-adherence of the patient is the impact of the practitioner's use of prescriptive method for advice giving. For example, when parlaying treatment recommendations, we have found in our practice that many practitioners were trained to use a predominantly prescriptive advice-giving feedback style. While this type of interaction can work quite well for patients who actively seek advice and are adherent to recommendations and treatment, it has little to no utility for patients who are ambivalent about making a change (i.e., approximately 80% of patients in the general population; Miller, & Rollnick, 2013).

A fundamental component of MI that differentiates it from other therapeutic interventions and feedback modalities is its focus on how practitioners can help reduce ambivalence in patients by both achieving and sustaining desired outcomes. This approach is based on how the practitioners guide the conversation to elicit and strengthen the patient's own internal motivation for change. Of the over 1,000 clinical trials to date, MI has proven efficacious in showing that when a person is ambivalent and/or experiencing challenges in sustaining new (and often difficult) changes in their behavioral repertoire, the most predictive measure of change involves actively voicing "change talk" and "commitment language" (Miller & Rollnick, 2013). Specifically, change talk entails the person actively voicing statements in favor of change or against sustaining current behaviors. These change-talk statements indicate a desire, reason, ability, and/or need for change and have been proven to predict a person's commitment (the strongest level of change talk) to make actual changes. Commitment language entails a person "committing" to a change and is typified by the use of statements such as "I will."

CHANGE TALK AND COMMITMENT LANGUAGE: DARN-C

Based on empirical support of change processes in MI, change talk and commitment language are recognized in the encounter when a person specifically expresses certain statements about change. These statements center on the use of language that reflects a person's: desire, ability, reason, and need, and these statements are clinically predictive of their making a commitment to change. The following highlight samples of change talk and commitment language, which is typically referred to as "DARN-C."

1. *Desire language:* Want, prefer, wish.
   - *Example:* "I have too many difficulties even remembering the simplest of things like I used to since I have felt depressed. I really *wish* I could feel better."
   - *Reflective desire response:* "Part of you knows life could be easier and you *want* to do something different that will help you feel better regarding feeling depressed."

2. *Ability language:* Able, can, could, possible.
   - *Example:* "I maybe *could* do it. I used to be really on top of going to my rehab appointments. It's just sometimes I forget. All these stupid appointments they have me scheduled for all of the time—it's nonstop. No one knows how hard it is to keep track of everything, and then I end up getting mad at myself for missing and not going to appointments."
   - *Reflective ability response:* "You know you have the ability to make the appointments and *can* do it."

3. *Reason language:* Specific arguments and reasons for change.
   - *Example:* "There's just one reason, Doc. I need to get off disability and return back to work. I'm over it. I'm over the meds, talking to weird therapists like you and this depression stuff that everyone keeps telling me that I have."
   - *Reflective reason response:* "You feel like you are wasting your time and money, and you are *ready* to get back to working."

4. *Need language:* Important, have to, got to
   - *Example:* "I really can't keep coming to these appointments and spending a wasted day like today for people like you to ask me questions, make me do all this stuff with blocks and repeating stuff I could care less about. Your questions after questions, they are really getting on my nerves. I'm tired and *have to* take a break."
   - *Reflective need response:* "These tests are long and tedious and you are tired of them. If it's OK, let's talk next about how these tests we are doing next are *important* and could help."

5. *Commitment language:* Going to, will.
   - *Example:* "OK, I *will* make the appointment with that other doctor if you think it will help."
   - *Reflective commitment language response:* "Great. Continuing with recommended treatment can be one of the first steps you can take to start to feel better. With our time that's left for our feedback session today, would it be OK if I offer you a menu of some other things you may or may not find of interest? I could help you plan for how to go about making your appointments for rehabilitation, talk more about how you could communicate better with your other health care providers, something else on the treatment plan or other ideas that you'd like to pursue. For now, what is *going to* suit you best?"

THE FOUR PROCESSES AND NEUROPSYCHOLOGICAL APPLICATIONS

As previously noted, Miller and Rollnick incorporated and updated MI to include the four-processes model, which involves engaging, focusing, evoking, and planning. The model offers a guide for practitioners to strategically enhance the use of person-centered core-interviewing and goal-oriented skills in MI within each of the processes (see Table 14.2).

Engaging: The Relational Foundation

Engaging the patient during clinical neuropsychological evaluation and feedback sessions sets the stage for establishing a collaborative discussion and provides a clinical environment tailored to supporting the therapeutic relationship and feeling of being understood. Engaging is extremely important during the initial evaluation and assessment sessions because patients may already be hesitant and avoidant to disclose their potentially disturbing private events and/or changes in their lifestyle to the practitioner. Paired with this, a patient's depressive symptoms (e.g., pessimistic thoughts, decreased self-esteem, irrational guilt) can similarly impact a patient's willingness to engage with the clinician. Furthermore, patients arriving at the initial clinical neuropsychological evaluation may not yet have an official diagnosis, and the many fast-paced assessment-driven questions from an essentially unknown practitioner can be intimidating and anxiety provoking for patients. Thus, it is important for the practitioner to continue engaging with patients and families in a collaborative manner by incorporating clinical expertise and recognizing the expertise of the patients and families.

MI Tips for Working with Adults with Depression and Neurocognitive Difficulties

- As the patient is depressed and may have difficulties in understanding abstract questions due to limitations in executive functions (e.g., cognitive flexibility), tailor language accordingly to the patient.

- Avoid disengagement traps such as using several closed-ended questions in a row, maintaining an expert only role, prematurely focusing on a behavior change plan, and engaging in idle conversation when the patient may need a break from the lengthy assessment process.

TABLE 14.2. An Overview of the Four-Processes Model

Engaging: The relational foundation

Focusing: The strategic direction

Evoking: Preparation for change

Planning: The bridge to change

Motivational Interviewing Practitioner Considerations

- How am I adapting to the patient's and family's limitations and cognitive needs in my communication style?
- How does my use of more concrete or abstract language enhance or, conversely, diminish the patient's engagement?
- How am I helping to make the patient/family feel comfortable?
- Given the cognitive impairments and psychiatric symptoms of the patient, what am I saying to facilitate a collaborative and supportive conversation?

Focusing: The Strategic Direction

Developing and maintaining a *focused* and *strategic direction* about change is integral to any clinical neuropsychological intervention as patients with depression and comorbid neurocognitive difficulties often present with a complex list of change priorities they may want to address. However, those change priorities may be different from what the practitioner deems to be of most importance. The importance of being mindful of the patient's goals for change and how the practitioner might develop a collaborative plan in a clear and focused manner cannot be underestimated. For example, clinicians are aware of time limitations faced in daily practice to complete a thorough assessment to determine the patients' cognitive strengths and weaknesses, which can often fuel discord in the clinician, maintaining a strategic and planful focus on the specific direction of what is most relevant to the patient and their family.

MI Tips for Working with Adults with Depression and Neurocognitive Difficulties

- Clinical symptom presentations typical of this population can include broad and common cognitive difficulties, including slower processing speed, compromised attentional processes, executive dysfunction, and poor short-term memory.
- Usually, there are multiple and sometimes competing goals, and maintaining a strategic focus on one or two goals can facilitate small changes that can lead to larger and durable positive health-related improvements.
- Listen, ask, and inform in a relatively equal balance (ask–tell–ask).
- If difficulties in selecting a focus arise, consider whether the patient is actually engaged. If so, help with the use of a summary statement and ask permission to offer a short menu of options, such as those in the treatment planning recommendations.

MI Practitioner Considerations

- What, if any, are the patient's actual goals for change (i.e., relief from depression, better management of neurocognitive difficulties, both, or something else)?

● How is my use of a guiding style and the specific language used during the assessment and breaks helping to maintain a strategic focus on change ideas and goals offered by the patient and family?

Evoking: Preparing for Change

Practitioners who provide clinical neuropsychological evaluations bring a unique clinical opportunity to the integrated health care team by offering patients the opportunity to disclose both abilities and functionally objective skills that are quantitatively definable during an assessment, as well as during the more qualitatively therapeutic feedback session. Akin to adolescents and young adults, practitioner efforts to carefully evoke change talk and commitment language, particularly with persons experiencing neurocognitive difficulties, can offer new opportunities within the field. The incorporation of evoking processes in MI in patients with depression and cognitive difficulties can be viewed as an active process in change. This process is often overlooked when typical advice giving and general recommendations in clinical practice fail to correspond with the clinical and/or practical life outcomes sought by patients/families in the treatment quest.

MI Tips for Working with Adults with Depression and Neurocognitive Difficulties

● Evoking internal motivation for change is central to MI, and it is imperative to evoke, listen, and reinforce any change talk.

● Impairments in higher-order cognitive functioning (e.g., planning, problem solving, cognitive flexibility) can sometimes impede the patient's ability to offer unsolicited ideas about change and/or change talk. Incorporating direct questions that elicit change talk can help maximize the patient's confidence in discussing what they deem to be important to change and to enhance engagement.

● When ambivalence is strong, the use of direct questions may be too overwhelming for the patient and can result in disengagement. In these situations, both the patient and the clinician may become frustrated, particularly given the time limitations and significant amount of feedback that needs to be covered, discussed, and processed during feedback sessions. The use of imagining questions to look in the future or past and discuss how life would be different if changes or more compliance with treatment recommendations were made can help to reduce frustrations. Also, questions tailored to how changes would benefit the patient's interpersonal relationships can help to minimize frustration and facilitate engagement.

● While persons with depression and neurocognitive difficulties may need the assistance of the integrated health care team after the clinical neuropsychological evaluation is completed, inquiring about personal values and how their efforts to change and/or comply with recommendations can help them lead a more productive life and offer a sense of hope that change can occur and quality of life will improve.

MI Practitioner Considerations

- What are the person's own reasons for change and/or for adherence to treatment planning recommendations?
- What change-talk language am I hearing, and how am I responding to it?
- If I am becoming frustrated with the person's ambivalence or lack of responding during the assessment or feedback session, how can I adjust my responses? Am I being overly prescriptive and how can I alter my responses to elicit and facilitate more engagement?

Planning: The Bridge for Change

On the one hand, clinicians conducting clinical neuropsychological evaluations face specific practice challenges, namely, time limitations and the termination of the professional relationship once feedback is provided to patients and their families. On the other hand, clinicians have a unique opportunity to facilitate focused and goal-oriented discussions about change planning. This last of the four processes, planning, focuses on collaboratively guiding the discussion to help the patient to commit to a change in behavior and activate a concrete, behaviorally based plan of action. The planning process allows each patient and clinician to maintain their own expertise (i.e., the patient is an expert of themselves and the practitioner is an expert in clinical neuropsychological practice) while maintaining engagement to collaboratively develop plans for embarking on small changes that are feasible, achievable, and, hopefully, sustainable such that these gains will lead to further positive changes in overall health.

MI Tips for Working with Adults with Depression and Neurocognitive Difficulties

- MI emphasizes the formation of a change plan that includes sufficient detail to increase the likelihood of success while continuing to evoke and ensure the presence of motivation. Common issues of cognitive fatigue can impact motivation and adherence to the testing demands; thus, monitoring fatigue is imperative.
- When higher-order executive functioning skills (e.g., cognitive flexibility, organization, self-monitoring) are compromised, patients may offer change talk and ideas about goals that are in contrast to what the evaluating clinician and treatment team are recommending. Although it may be tempting to ignore such statements by the patient and compromise engagement, the continued use of reflections that reinforce any change-talk language, along with a summary that synthesizes ambivalence (if present), can facilitate the transition to discuss assessment results, treatment planning, and recommendations.
- Independent ideas about planning may be particularly difficult for the patient in the context of their depressive symptoms. Adjusting your responses by making more concrete reflections and offering more tailored, yet open-ended, questions and/or multiple-choice questions can help guide the patient and promote planning.

- Maintaining a guiding stance is imperative. Use of MI skills such as asking open-ended questions that directly elicit language about commitment and taking steps, asking for elaboration, reinforcing and reflecting any change talk, incorporating the ask–tell–ask strategy to provide information, and including advice or a menu of options for change can all help the patient delineate steps to increase the likelihood of adherence with treatment planning recommendations.

- Adults with depression and neurocognitive difficulties may have had prior difficulties with successfully sustaining change. As a result, identifying barriers to overcome potential challenges in the treatment planning recommendations and knowing what to do about them are essential. Using clinician expertise (with permission) and offering options about ideas to overcome potential barriers can be facilitated by using the ask–tell–ask strategy.

- Recognizing and discussing with the patient that change planning may need to be revisited with others in the integrated health care team can facilitate a sense of hope in the patient, particularly if the patient is concurrently completing other medical or psychiatric evaluations and treatments.

- Commitment language, stated by the patient, indicates the likelihood of engaging in a behavioral change. It is important to reinforce and reflect such language, as such language is most predictive of the patient engaging in actual change (Miller & Rollnick, 2013).

MI Practitioner Considerations

- How are both the development of a commitment to change and formulation of a concrete plan of action being conveyed, incorporating the patient's neurocognitive difficulties and needs as well as the needs of the family?

- How am I offering needed advice or information with permission, and how is my approach different from that of other practitioners the patient has seen?

- As the patient has likely been involved in other treatment settings by the time a clinical neuropsychological evaluation is made, consider how am I using evocation versus a prescriptive planning stance to elicit change talk in treatment planning?

- When I hear commitment language, how am I reinforcing it or negating it by taking a prescriptive stance?

SUMMARY

Motivational interviewing has emerged as a promising empirically supported, evidence-based intervention that can enhance clinical neuropsychological practice, including diagnostic assessment, therapeutic feedback, and cognitive rehabilitation interventions. MI can assist with optimizing the therapeutic alliance as well as offer an ever growing body of translational applications to help adults with depression and neurocognitive difficulties make difficult changes that optimize treatment outcomes and maximize their full potential (Miller & Rollnick, 2013; Naar & Suarez, 2021; Steinberg & Miller, 2015; Suarez & Mullins, 2008). MI can help establish patient-centered and goal-oriented approaches that focus on the patient's language and commitment to change during the assessment and feedback processes, as well as strengthen engagement and compliance with treatment recommendations to improve clinical, neurocognitive, functional, and quality-of-life outcomes (Suarez, 2011).

REFERENCES

American Psychiatric Association. (2013). *Diagnostic and statistical manual of mental disorders* (5th ed.). Arlington, VA: Author.

Bell, K. R., Temkin, N. R., Esselman, P. C., Doctor, J. N., Bombardier, C. H., Fraser, R. T., et al. (2005). The effect of a scheduled telephone intervention on outcome after moderate to severe traumatic brain injury: A randomized trial. *Archives of Physical Medicine and Rehabilitation, 86*(5), 851–856.

Bombardier, C. H., Bell, K. R., Temkin, N. R., Fann, J. R., Hoffman, J., & Dikmen, S. (2009). The efficacy of a scheduled telephone intervention for ameliorating depressive symptoms during the first year after traumatic brain injury. *Journal of Head Trauma Rehabilitation, 24*(4), 230–238.

Byers, A. M., Lamanna, L., & Rosenberg, A. (2010). The effect of motivational interviewing after ischemic stroke on patient knowledge and patient satisfaction with care: A pilot study. *Journal of Neuroscience Nursing, 42*(6), 312–322.

Chien, W. T., Mui, J., Gray, R., & Cheung, E. (2016). Adherence therapy versus routine psychiatric care for people with schizophrenia spectrum disorders: A randomised controlled trial. *BMC Psychiatry, 16*, 42.

Choi, J., & Twamley, E. W. (2013). Cognitive rehabilitation therapies for Alzheimer's disease: A review of methods to improve treatment engagement and self-efficacy. *Neuropsychology Review, 23*(1), 48–62.

Fiszdon, J. M., Kurtz, M. M., Choi, J., Bell, M. D., & Martino, S. (2016). Motivational interviewing to increase cognitive rehabilitation adherence in schizophrenia. *Schizophrenia Bulletin, 42*(2), 327–334.

Holt, C., Milgrom, J., & Gemmill, A. W. (2017). Improving help-seeking for postnatal depression and anxiety: A cluster randomised controlled trial of motivational interviewing. *Archives of Women's Mental Health, 20*(6), 791–801.

Keeley, R. D., Brody, D. S., Engel, M., Burke, B. L., Nordstrom, K., Moralez, E., et al. (2016). Motivational interviewing improves depression outcome in primary care: A cluster randomized trial. *Journal of Consulting and Clinical Psychology, 84*(11), 993–1007.

Keeley, R. D., Burke, B. L., Brody, D., Dimidjian, S., Engel, M., Emsermann, C., et al. (2014). Training to use motivational interviewing techniques for depression: A cluster randomized trial. *Journal of the American Board of Family Medicine, 27*(5), 621–636.

Miller, W. R., & Rollnick, S. R. (2013). *Motivational interviewing: Helping people change* (3rd ed.). New York: Guilford Press.

Miller, W. R., & Rose, G. S. (2009). Toward a theory of motivational interviewing. *American Psychologist, 64*(6), 527–537.

Naar, S., & Safren, S. A. (2017). *Motivational interviewing and CBT: Combining strategies for maximun effectiveness.* New York: Guilford Press.

Naar, S., & Suarez, M. (2021). *Motivational interviewing with adolescents and young adults* (2nd ed.). New York: Guilford Press.

Navidian, A., Mobaraki, H., & Shakiba, M. (2017). The effect of education through motivational interviewing compared with conventional education on self-care behaviors in heart failure patients with depression. *Patient Education and Counseling, 100*(8), 1499–1504.

Ponsford, J., Lee, N. K., Wong, D., McKay, A., Haines, K., Alway, Y., et al. (2016). Efficacy of motivational interviewing and cognitive behavioral therapy for anxiety and depression symptoms following traumatic brain injury. *Psychological Medicine, 46*(5), 1079–1090.

Schoenberg, M. R., & Scott, J. G. (Eds.). (2011). *The little black book of neuropsychology: A syndrome-based approach*. New York: Springer.

Steinberg, M., Miller, W. R. (2015). *Motivational interviewing in diabetes care*. New York: Guilford Press.

Suarez, M., (2011). Application of Motivational Interviewing to neuropsychology practice: A new frontier for evaluations and rehabilitation. In M. R. Schoenberg & J. G. Scott (Eds.), *The little black book of neuropsychology: A syndrome-based approach* (pp. 863–-871). New York: Springer.

Suarez, M., & Mullins, S. (2008). Motivational interviewing and pediatric health behavior interventions. *Journal of Developmental and Behavioral Pediatrics, 29*(5), 417–428.

Watkins, C. L., Auton, M. F., Deans, C. F., Dickinson, H. A., Jack, C. I., Lightbody, C. E., et al. (2007). Motivational interviewing early after acute stroke: A randomized, controlled trial. *Stroke, 38*(3), 1004–1009.

Watkins, C. L., Wathan, J. V., Leathley, M. J., Auton, M. F., Deans, C. F., Dickinson, H. A., et al. (2011). The 12-month effects of early motivational interviewing after acute stroke: A randomized controlled trial. *Stroke, 42*(7), 1956–1961.

PART IV

NEUROPSYCHOLOGICAL EFFECTS OF ANTIDEPRESSANT TREATMENT

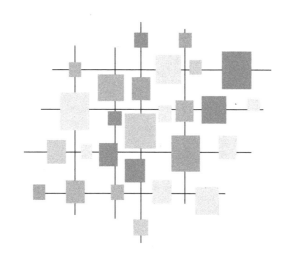

CHAPTER 15

Psychotropic Medications

Joshua Rosenblat

Psychotropic medications are frequently used in the treatment of mental illness (Kantor, Rehm, Haas, Chan, & Giovannucci, 2015; Ohayon & Lader, 2002). Both psychotropic and nonpsychotropic medications may have diverse effects on neurocognition, with potentially positive, negative, or neutral effects on cognitive function, depending on the specific medication and dose (Berg & Dellasega, 1996; Brooks & Hoblyn, 2007; Sole, Jimenez, Martinez-Aran, & Vieta, 2015). Additionally, cognitive effects of medications vary by disorder (e.g., the same medication may be pro-cognitive in one disorder while having no effect in another because of the varied pathophysiology of cognitive dysfunction); no medication has demonstrated robust transdiagnostic pro-cognitive effects (Sole et al., 2015). Rather, the cognitive effects of most psychotropics are specific to the disorder being treated, with additional individual patient factors varying the cognitive response to a given medication, even when being used at the same dose for the same indication (McIntyre, 2014). With regards to major depressive disorder (MDD), the cognitive effects of antidepressants are of great interest and the focus of the current chapter.

Antidepressants are frequently used in the treatment of moderate to severe MDD. As a class, antidepressants have been demonstrated by hundreds of randomized clinical trials (RCTs) to be generally effective, significantly reducing the depressive symptom burden for most patients (Cipriani et al., 2018). Achieving remission of depressive symptoms (typically defined by depression scores returning within normal range) may have variable effects on the individual symptoms of depression (McClintock et al., 2011; Rock, Roiser, Riedel, & Blackwell, 2014). In recent years, MDD symptom domains have been recognized as having both distinct and overlapping pathophysiology with other symptom domains (Insel et al., 2010). Accordingly, specific interventions, such as antidepressants, may differentially impact various symptoms of depression (McClintock et al., 2011). Therefore, the impact of specific MDD treatments on cognitive function may differ compared to the overall antidepressant efficacy of these interventions.

Specifically with antidepressants, replicated clinical trial and real-world effectiveness evidence has demonstrated that some symptoms more commonly persist with treatment after achieving an antidepressant response (e.g., greater than 50% reduction in depressive symptoms). According to the Sequenced Treatment Alternatives to Relieve Depression (STAR*D) trial, sleep difficulties and cognitive dysfunction have been identified as key symptom domains that often persist with first-line antidepressant treatments (Gaynes et al., 2009; McClintock et al., 2011). Persistence of cognitive dysfunction with antidepressant treatment is of particular concern, for cognitive function is strongly associated with overall function in MDD, with significant social and occupational disability caused by cognitive impairment (Woo, Rosenblat, Kakar, Bahk, & McIntyre, 2016). Cognitive dysfunction is recognized as a key feature of the syndrome of depression, being one of the nine symptom criteria of MDD in the fifth edition of the *Diagnostic and Statistical Manual of Mental Disorders* (American Psychiatric Association, 2013). However, the pathophysiology, and thus required interventions, are both overlapping and independent from the other domains of depression. Therefore, the objectives of the current chapter are the following: (1) summarize the effects of antidepressants, as a group, on cognitive function, (2) compare and contrast the cognitive effects of specific antidepressants, and (3) discuss new and emerging pharmacological treatments targeting cognition in MDD. Practical clinical implications of the presented evidence are also discussed, followed by a discussion of future directions for improving cognitive function in MDD using pharmacological interventions.

CLASS EFFECT OF ANTIDEPRESSANTS ON COGNITIVE FUNCTION

While the cognitive effects of antidepressants remain understudied, several trends have emerged to suggest that antidepressants may have both positive and negative effects on cognitive function. The *net effect* may be positive, negative, or neutral on overall cognitive function, as illustrated by Figure 15.1. Pro-cognitive effects of antidepressant may be mood-dependent, with cognitive function improving in a colinear fashion, along with the improvement of other depressive symptoms. Alternatively, antidepressants may have pro-cognitive effects through distinct mechanisms that are independent of improvement in mood symptoms (e.g., cognitive improvements observed, regardless of the presence of an antidepressant response). Antidepressants with pro-cognitive effects via one or both of these pathways may also have negative effects on cognition through off-target effects (e.g., sedative effects, anticholinergic and antihistaminergic effects). The "balance" of these effects determines the *net effect* on cognitive function. Additionally, effects may either be cognitive domain specific (e.g., working memory, processing speed) or global (e.g., improving all cognitive domains at a similar magnitude).

Several meta-analyses assessing the effects of antidepressants (as a group) on cognitive function have been completed, with converging evidence to suggest that antidepressants have minimal effects on cognitive function in both depressed and nondepressed samples (Keefe et al., 2014; Prado, Watt, & Crowe, 2018; Rock et al., 2014; Rosenblat, Kakar, & McIntyre, 2015). Rock and colleagues (2014) examined the cognitive function of patients with MDD, also including patients who were not taking medications, to broadly assess the cognitive function of patients with MDD during acute depressive episodes and when remitted from depression. While the meta-analysis was not limited to patients using antidepressants, the majority of included studies used antidepressants, suggesting that the

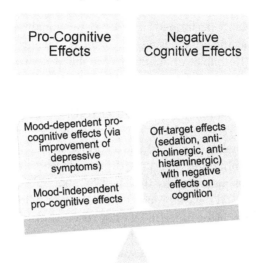

| Pro-Cognitive Effects | Negative Cognitive Effects |

Mood-dependent pro-cognitive effects (via improvement of depressive symptoms)

Mood-independent pro-cognitive effects

Off-target effects (sedation, anti-cholinergic, anti-histaminergic) with negative effects on cognition

FIGURE 15.1. Net effect of psychotropic medications on cognition. Medications may have both positive and negative effects on cognitive function via different mechanisms, leading to an overall net positive, neutral, or negative effect.

results were likely also applicable to antidepressant treatment. In Rock and colleagues' analysis, moderate cognitive deficits in executive function, memory, and attention were observed in MDD patients relative to controls (Cohen's d effect sizes ranging from –0.34 to –0.65). Statistically significant moderate deficits in executive function and attention (d ranging from –0.52 to –0.61) and nonsignificant small to moderate deficits in memory (d ranging from –0.22 to –0.54) were found to persist in patients whose depressive symptoms had remitted, indicating that treatments of depression, including antidepressants, are fairly ineffective at improving MDD-related cognitive dysfunction, even when other symptoms of depression remit.

Keefe and colleagues (2014) performed a systematic review and meta-analysis more specifically analyzing the cognitive effects of pharmacotherapy (e.g., not including the effects of nonpharmacological interventions) in the acute treatment of MDD. The authors identified a total of 43 studies, 31 of which were with antidepressant monotherapy (8 placebo-controlled, 11 active-comparator, 12 open-label) and 12 of which used augmentation pharmacotherapy (7 placebo-controlled, 5 open-label). Given the significant heterogeneity in study design, sample types, medications, and cognitive tests used, the authors emphasized the difficulty, and uncertainty, of pooling these studies together. Nevertheless, most individual studies reported small effect sizes in favor of improving overall cognition with pharmacotherapy. While no specific cognitive domains were reliably improved, pooled effect sizes revealed two significant positive effects of pharmacotherapy: verbal memory improved with antidepressant monotherapy ($d = 0.10$; 95% confidence interval [CI] = 0.091 to 0.117], and visual memory improved with augmentation therapy ($d = 0.44$; 95% CI = 0.436 to 0.452). Notably, antidepressant monotherapy was associated with worsening processing speed, and augmentation was associated with worsening attention, verbal fluency and memory compared to placebo.

Our group subsequently performed an updated meta-analysis on the cognitive effects of pharmacotherapy, specifically focusing on cognitive changes associated with antidepressant monotherapy (Rosenblat et al., 2015). Notably, this was the first meta-analysis to include studies using vortioxetine, a recently approved novel multimodal antidepressant; numerous studies have evaluated its cognitive effects, compared to other antidepressants. In this meta-analysis, nine placebo-controlled RCTs (2,550 participants) evaluating the cognitive effects of vortioxetine ($n = 728$), duloxetine ($n = 714$), paroxetine ($n = 23$), citalopram ($n = 84$), phenelzine ($n = 28$), nortryptiline ($n = 32$), and sertraline ($n = 49$) were included. Overall, antidepressants, compared to placebo, had a pooled positive effect on psychomotor speed, as measured by the Digit Symbol Substitution Test (DSST) ($d = 0.16$; 95% CI 0.05–0.27) and delayed recall ($d = 0.24$; 95% CI 0.15–0.34). The effect on cognitive control and executive function did not reach statistical significance. Of note, after removal of vortioxetine studies from the analysis, statistical significance was lost for psychomotor speed. An additional analysis was performed assessing trials comparing the cognitive effects of different antidepressants. Eight head-to-head RCTs comparing the effects of selective serotonin reuptake inhibitors (SSRIs) ($n = 371$), selective serotonin–norepinephrine reuptake inhibitors (SNRIs) ($n = 25$), tricyclic antidepressants (TCAs) ($n = 138$), and norepinephrine–dopamine reuptake inhibitors (NDRIs) ($n = 46$) were identified. No statistically significant difference in cognitive effects was found when results were pooled from head-to-head trials of SSRIs, SNRIs, TCAs, and NDRIs. This analysis had several important limitations, including the heterogeneity of results, limited number of studies, and small sample sizes.

More recently, Baune, Brignone, and Larsen (2018) performed a network meta-analysis specifically assessing the effects of antidepressants on executive function, as measured by the DSST in MDD, including 12 RCTs assessing the effects of SSRIs, SNRIs, and other nonselective serotonin reuptake inhibitors/serotonin–norepinephrine reuptake inhibitors. The network meta-analysis showed that vortioxetine was the only antidepressant that improved cognitive dysfunction on the DSST compared to placebo ($d = 0.325$; 95% CI $= 0.120$ to 0.529). Compared with other antidepressants, vortioxetine was statistically more efficacious on the DSST versus escitalopram, nortriptyline, and the SSRI and TCA classes. While this analysis had similar limitations to the previous meta-analyses, it provided further evidence that, in general, there does not appear to be a "class effect" of antidepressants improving cognitive function. Conversely, specific antidepressants, such as vortioxetine, may improve cognitive function in MDD.

One of the largest studies to date that was not included in the above meta-analyses was conducted by Shilyansky and colleagues (2016). The authors performed a randomized longitudinal study, as part of the International Study to Predict Optimized Treatment in Depression (iSPOT-D) trial, to assess the effects of antidepressant treatment in a large patient population ($n = 1,008$), across clinical remission outcomes, on a range of cognitive domains: attention, response inhibition, executive function during visuospatial navigation, cognitive flexibility, verbal memory, working memory, decision speed, information-processing speed, and psychomotor response speed. The authors enrolled a large population of medication-free (i.e., untreated) outpatients in a major depressive episode (MDE) and assessed them for cognitive function at enrollment (pretreatment), and again after 8 weeks of treatment with one of three antidepressant drugs (escitalopram, sertraline, or venlafaxine extended-release; three commonly prescribed first-line antidepressants known to have strong efficacy among antidepressants). Patients were randomly assigned (1:1:1). As a comparison group, they also simultaneously enrolled matched healthy participants. Healthy participants received no medication or intervention but were assessed for change in cognitive and clinical measures during the same interval and testing protocol. Therefore, this group acts as a test–retest control for the primary outcome measure examined in this study: change in cognitive measures over 8 weeks of treatment in depressed patients. Impairment in five domains, namely, attention, response inhibition, verbal memory, decision speed, and information processing, showed no relative improvement with acute treatment (controlling for time or repeated testing), irrespective of antidepressant treatment group, even in patients whose depression remitted acutely according to clinical measures. As such, the authors concluded that MDD is associated with impairments in higher-order cognitive functions and information processing, which persist independently of clinical symptom change with treatment. They identified no difference between the three antidepressants tested, with none of them showing efficacy for these impairments. Although the 8-week treatment period limits interpretation to acute treatment effects, it does highlight cognitive impairment as an untargeted contributor to incomplete treatment success.

In addition, the long-term effects of antidepressants on cognitive function, and risk of dementia has remained controversial (Wang et al., 2018). More specifically, some have questioned the possible role of antidepressants in increasing or decreasing the risk of dementia. However, previous studies have shown that SSRIs may decrease amyloid-beta generation and plaque load (Byers & Yaffe, 2011). Furthermore, in a recent study, Bartels and colleagues (2018) evaluated the impact of SSRIs treatment on biomarkers and progression from mild cognitive impairment (MCI) to Alzheimer's dementia. Datasets from 755 currently nondepressed participants from the longitudinal Alzheimer's Disease Neuroimaging Initiative were evaluated. In MCI patients with a history of depression, long-term SSRI treatment (greater than 4 years) was significantly associated with a *delayed* progression to Alzheimer's dementia by approximately 3 years, compared with short-term SSRI treatment, treatment with other antidepressants, or no treatment and compared with MCI patients without a history of depression. No differences in biomarker levels were observed between treatment groups. These results suggest that SSRIs might have protective effects, rather than deleterious effects, on cognition and risk of dementia in the long term, when used appropriately. These effects likely relate to the neurodegenerative and neurotoxic effects of untreated depression that might be prevented, or decreased, by effective treatment leading to remission (Brown, McIntyre, Rosenblat, & Hardeland, 2018).

Taken together, the pro-cognitive effects of antidepressants, as a group, are minimal in the acute treatment of MDEs. However, the long-term effects of antidepressants on cognition remain relatively unclear, as improvement in cognitive function might be much later than observed improvements in other depressive symptoms. Thus, these effects may be "missed" by 8- to 12-week RCTs. While the pooled "class effect" of antidepressants for improving cognitive function is small, significant differences have been identified between specific antidepressants (Baune et al., 2018). As such, answering the question "Do antidepressants improve cognitive function?" is likely less relevant compared to understanding which *specific* antidepressants improve cognitive function. Moreover, understanding the cognitive domain specific effects and magnitude of these effects is also of great importance.

MEDICATION-SPECIFIC EFFECTS ON COGNITIVE FUNCTION

The previous section described the effects of antidepressants, as a group, on cognitive function, suggesting that overall antidepressants have a neutral to slightly positive effect on cognitive function in MDD, even when other depressive symptoms have remitted. However, the meta-analyses discussed also suggested that there are likely differences between the effects of specific antidepressants. As such, the current section discusses the effects of specific antidepressants. Notably, the evidence base for cognitive effects of antidepressants is still limited, for cognitive function in MDD has been historically understudied and identifying statistically significant changes in cognitive testing often requires much larger sample sizes, compared to testing for changes in overall depressive symptoms (Kaser, Zaman, & Sahakian, 2017; Keefe et al., 2014; Szabo et al., 2015). As such, there is also concern that many negative studies (e.g., studies showing neutral effects of antidepressants on cognitive function) may have been underpowered, resulting in a type II error (i.e., false negative). Nevertheless, the currently available evidence, along with clinical experience, suggests that vortioxetine has the strongest pro-cognitive effects, bupropion likely has some pro-cognitive effects, SSRIs and SNRIs have variable, but mostly minimal effects; while antidepressants with off-target sedating effects likely have negative effects on cognition (e.g., mirtazapine, fluvoxamine, sedating tricyclics). Based on the available evidence, clinical experience, and pharmacodynamic profile, the relative cognitive effects of antidepressants are summarized in Figure 15.2, showing the spectrum negative, neutral or positive effects of various antidepressants. The limited evidence is summarized herein.

Selective Serotonin Reuptake Inhibitors

The class of selective serotonin reuptake inhibitors (SSRIs) includes sertraline, citalopram, escitalopram, fluvoxamine, paroxetine, and fluoxetine. Sertraline, citalorpram, and escitalopram are often considered the "cleanest" SSRIs (i.e., they target the serotonin transporter with fewest off-target effects) and are also the most commonly prescribed due to strong evidence for antidepressant efficacy with good overall tolerability, compared to older agents (Stahl, 1998). However, all three of these commonly prescribed SSRIs have failed to demonstrate pro-cognitive effects compared to placebo in the treatment of MDD. In the previously described iSPOT-D trial ($n = 1,008$), sertraline and escitalopram failed to demonstrate pro-cognitive effects in the acute treatment of MDD. Additionally, in another SSRI trial assessing cognition, a group of older adults with MDD received either placebo ($n = 90$) or citalopram ($n = 84$) during an 8-week RCT. While citalopram demonstrated antidepressant efficacy, there was no significant between-group differences on any cognitive domains, as tested by objective and validated cognitive measures (Culang et al., 2009). However, a small subset of participants had improvements in cognitive function, which was partly dependent on antidepressant response.

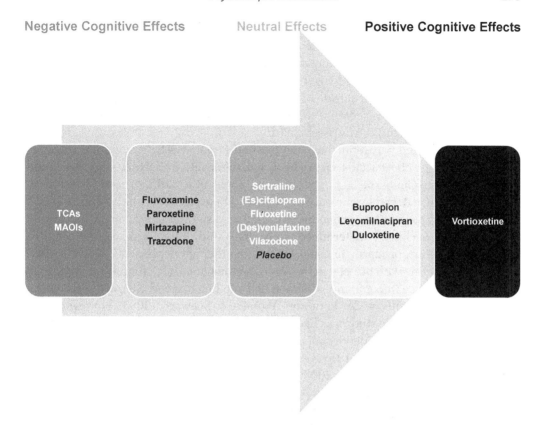

FIGURE 15.2. Relative effects of antidepressants on cognitive function. Illustrated spectrum of effects based on limited available evidence, clinical experience, and pharmacodynamic profiles of specific medications (e.g., effects of medications on receptors, neurotransmitters). Placebo is placed in neutral category as a point of reference.

In a separate placebo-controlled RCT, sertraline ($n = 49$) failed to demonstrate superiority for improved cognitive function as compared to placebo ($n = 49$) in all cognitive domains tested after 16 weeks of treatment. This trial was twice the length of typical acute MDE trials (e.g., usually 8 weeks), which provided evidence against the previous hypothesis that antidepressants might have delayed pro-cognitive effects missed by 8-week trials (Hoffman et al., 2008). While sertraline failed to outperform placebo, several trials have demonstrated that sertraline is associated with improved cognitive function (primarily improved processing speed and overall executive function) compared to TCAs (nortriptyline and desipramine; Bondareff et al., 2000; Culang-Reinlieb, Sneed, Keilp, & Roose, 2012) and another SSRI (fluoxetine; Newhouse et al., 2000). Fluoxetine was also superior to desipramine on measures of executive function (Levkovitz, Caftori, Avital, & Richter-Levin, 2002).

While all six antidepressants are categorized as SSRIs, their relative effects on serotonin transporters (e.g., relative inhibition of transporters), other monoamine transporters (e.g., norepinephrine and dopamine), along with off-target effects (e.g., GABA-ergic, histaminergic, and cholinergic effects), vary greatly, leading to potentially different net effects on cognitive function. The effects of serotonin signaling may vary depending on brain region and serotonin receptor, with 5-HT7 antagonism likely having the greatest pro-cognitive effects (Baune & Renger, 2014). Additionally, medications with significant off-target effects (e.g., acting outside of serotonin), namely, anticholinergic and antihistaminergic effects leading to sedating effects, often negatively affect cognition (Stahl, Lee-Zimmerman, Cartwright, & Morrissette, 2013).

Fluvoxamine and paroxetine have the most off-target effects (e.g., antihistaminergic and anticholinergic effects) and thus are likely to have negative effects on cognition (Stahl, 1998; Stahl, Lee-Zimmerman, Cartwright, & Morrissette, 2013). These pharmacodynamic effects are matched by clinical observations. However, the cognitive effects of both fluvoxamine and paroxetine remain understudied, and so their effects on cognitive function cannot be conclusively determined. Only small studies have assessed the cognitive effects of paroxetine, primarily in comparison with other antidepressants. Only one RCT compared paroxetine with placebo in the acute treatment of MDD, finding no statistically significant difference in continuity attention and combined speed comparing paroxetine ($n = 23$) with placebo ($n = 26$; Ferguson, Wesnes, & Schwartz, 2003). However, given the small sample size, the study was likely underpowered. In other clinical trials comparing paroxetine to other antidepressants, no significant differences were identified in any domain, or global cognitive function between groups, including bupropion (Gorlyn et al., 2015), nortriptyline (Nebes et al., 2003), and tianeptine (Nickel et al., 2003). In these trials, patients achieving remission with paroxetine continued to have cognitive impairment compared to healthy controls. This finding suggests that the negative off-target effects may be outweighing any mood-dependent pro-cognitive effects (conceptually shown in Figure 15.1).

Taken together, there is a lack of evidence to support improvements in cognition with SSRIs in the acute treatment of MDD. However, there are likely important differences within the class of SSRIs, with some evidence suggesting that "cleaner" SSRIs (e.g., agents with less off-target effects, such as sertraline) have better cognitive outcomes compared to other SSRIs. Furthermore, SSRIs with significant off-target effects, such as paroxetine and fluvoxamine, likely have negative effects on cognitive function. However, clinical trials are still needed to determine the relative positive and negative cognitive effects of these agents. Results regarding the influence of antidepressant response on cognitive function with SSRIs (e.g., mood-dependent versus mood-independent effects leading to improved cognition) are mixed.

Selective Serotonin–Norepinephrine Reuptake Inhibitors

Selective serotonin–norepinephrine reuptake inhibitors (SNRIs) are also commonly prescribed for MDD and include venlafaxine, desvenlafaxine, duloxetine, and levomilnacipran. SNRIs may theoretically have pro-cognitive effects given the important role of norepinephrine in the prefrontal cortex in higher-order cognitive tasks (e.g., executive function; Sole et al., 2015). However, clinical data has revealed mixed results. The effects of duloxetine have been most studied with four larger phase III placebo-controlled RCTs (Katona, Hansen, & Olsen, 2012; Mahableshwarkar, Zajecka, Jacobson, Chen, & Keefe,

2015; Oakes et al., 2012; Raskin et al., 2007; Robinson et al., 2014). In adult MDD patients (ages 18–65), duloxetine ($n = 187$) compared to placebo ($n = 167$) only led to improvement in subjective cognitive function based on the perceived deficits questionnaire (PDQ), while there was no statistically significant difference on objective cognitive testing scores by the end of the 8-week trial.

Three additional trials were conducted in older adults. In MDD participants over the age of 65, Robinson and colleagues (2014) found no between-group differences in cognitive function after 24 weeks of duloxetine ($n = 180$) versus placebo ($n = 87$). Conversely, Katona and colleagues (2012) evaluated the effects of duloxetine in older MDD patients (age over 65), demonstrating small, but statistically significant, improvements in the Rey Auditory Verbal Learning Test (RAVLT) acquisition and RAVLT delayed recall measures, with no significant difference on the DSST comparing 8 weeks of duloxetine ($n = 151$) to placebo ($n = 145$). Similarly, Raskin and colleagues (2007) demonstrated improvements in delayed recall but not in processing speed, with duloxetine ($n = 196$) compared to placebo ($n = 99$) in older adults. Taken together, duloxetine appears to have some small benefits for subjective cognition and delayed recall.

Venlafaxine and its metabolite, desvenlafaxine, have been inadequately studied. Early phase II studies have failed to demonstrate significant improvements in cognitive function with venlafaxine, but these studies were likely underpowered (Trick, Stanley, Rigney, & Hindmarch, 2004). Similar to the other antidepressants in the iSPOT-D trials, the venlafaxine group failed to demonstrate significant improvements in cognition, even in participants achieving an antidepressant response/remission (Shilyansky et al., 2016). Similarly, desvenlafaxine has minimal benefits compared to placebo in cognitive outcomes. In a 12-week RCT, only a small improvement with desvenlafaxine 50 mg/day ($n = 52$) compared with placebo ($n = 29$) was observed on the quality of working memory measure. Improvement in speed of working memory and attention was significant for desvenlafaxine and for placebo, but no significant between-group differences were found (Reddy, Fayyad, Edgar, Guico-Pabia, & Wesnes, 2016).

The most recently approved SNRI, levomilnacipran, shows promise for potential pro-cognitive effects based on a post-hoc analysis of a large phase III MDD trial. In this post-hoc analysis, levomilnacipran demonstrated greater improvements in power and continuity of attention from baseline compared to placebo (Wesnes et al., 2017). The subgroup of participants with impaired attention at baseline had greater cognitive benefits with levomilnacipran, which was also associated with improved overall function. Although interpretation of this data is limited by the post-hoc design, the potential pro-cognitive effects of levomilnacipran are still promising.

In summary, while SNRIs are conceptually and mechanistically promising for having pro-cognitive effects, clinical trials assessing cognition have yielded mixed results. Only duloxetine has been adequately studied, with results suggesting potential improvements only in delayed recall in older adults and only subjective cognitive improvements in adults ages 18–65, without evidence of objective improvements. It also remains unclear whether cognitive improvements with SNRIs are dependent on antidepressant response. The preponderance of the evidence suggests that improvements in cognition are mostly independent of SSRIs or SNRI antidepressant response (Herrera-Guzman, Gudayol-Ferre, et al., 2010; Herrera-Guzman et al., 2009; Herrera-Guzman, Herrera-Abarca, et al., 2010).

Norepinephrine–Dopamine Reuptake Inhibitors

The only NDRI that is indicated as a first-line monotherapy treatment for MDD is bupropion. Given the similar mechanism of action as stimulants and benefits in attention-deficit/hyperactivity disorder (ADHD), NDRIs also have theoretical pharmacodynamic reasons for having pro-cognitive effects, but this treatment has been understudied. While there have been no placebo-controlled RCTs, two small phase II studies demonstrated minor improvements with bupropion over an 8-week course of treatment, with improvements in memory, attention, and processing speed (Gorlyn et al., 2015; Soczynska et al., 2014). These early findings, in addition to the positive effects of bupropion in ADHD (Verbeeck, Bekkering, Van den Noortgate, & Kramers, 2017), show promise for the pro-cognitive effects of bupropion in MDD. However, adequately powered RCTs are still required to demonstrate potential pro-cognitive effects.

Noradrenergic and Specific Serotonergic Antidepressants

Mianserin and mirtazapine are noradrenergic and specific serotonergic antidepressants (NaSSAs) indicated for the treatment of MDD with a novel mechanism of action, increasing the transmission of serotonin and norepinephrine via alpha-2 antagonism. Additionally, NaSSAs specifically antagonize specific serotonin receptors to theoretically improve positive effects and decrease adverse effects. Mirtazapine is the most commonly used NaSSA and has grown in popularity, likely because of its strong antidepressant and anxiolytic efficacy and sedating effects, as insomnia often persists during euthymia with other antidepressants (Soehner, Kaplan, & Harvey, 2013). Mirtazapine does not inhibit monoamine reuptake. Rather, it antagonizes alpha-2, histamine 1 (H1), 5-HT2A/C, and 5-HT3 receptors. The H1 blockade is the strongest, with mirtazapine exerting potent H1 blockade at low doses and thus is associated with hypnotic/sedating effects even at subtherapeutic doses (Anttila & Leinonen, 2001). As such, mirtazapine is at times used off-label as a sleep aid at low doses. Given its sedating antihistaminergic effects, however, mirtazapine may have negative effects on cognition. While this treatment has been inadequately studied, preliminary studies have suggested negative effects on cognition, leading to functional impairments, such as hampering reaction times and the ability to drive, even 8 hours after a single dose (Iwamoto et al., 2013). However, given the tolerance associated with chronic H1-antagonism, some evidence suggests that the negative cognitive effects may decrease with time (Borkowska, Drpzdz, Ziółkowska-Kochan, & Rybakowski, 2007; Sasada et al., 2013). Furthermore, some studies hypothesize that mirtazapine may have longer-term benefits for cognition, given the cognitive benefits of improved sleep (Borkowska et al., 2007; Yaffe, Falvey, & Hoang, 2014).

Serotonin Modulators and Stimulators

As the newest class of antidepressants, serotonin modulators and stimulators (SMSs) both exert serotonin reuptake inhibition (similar to SSRIs) and modulate specific serotonin receptors, in an attempt to increase efficacy and decrease adverse effects related to specific receptor antagonism/agonism. Vortioxetine and vilazodone are approved SMS antidepressants for the acute treatment of MDD, demonstrating efficacy comparable to SSRIs and SNRIs (Cipriani et al., 2018). The cognitive effects of vilazodone have yet to be studied (McIntyre, 2017). Conversely, vortioxetine was developed and tested for improving cognition in MDD. The precise mechanism of action remains unclear and is likely multifactorial, given the multiple targets of vortioxetine. However, antagonism of 5-HT7 and glutamate modulation are likely key targets (McIntyre, Harrison, Loft, Jacobson, & Olsen, 2016).

Vortioxetine is the most studied antidepressant for its effects on cognition with several phase III RCTs demonstrating improvements in cognitive function with moderate effect sizes (McIntyre et al., 2016). Indeed, several large prospective RCTs and post-hoc analyses have consistently demonstrated clinically and statistically significant improvements in cognition. Path analysis has suggested that improvements in cognition are both mood-independent (e.g., improvements with or without antidepressant response) and mood-dependent (e.g., improvements associated with antidepressant response; Harrison, Lophaven, & Olsen, 2016; McIntyre, 2017; McIntyre et al., 2016). Pro-cognitive effects have been demonstrated in large phase III trials with adults (ages 18–65; Mahableshwarkar et al., 2015; McIntyre et al., 2016; McIntyre, Lophaven, & Olsen, 2014) and older adults (over age 65; Katona et al., 2012) with MDD. There were consistent improvements in validated objective measures of executive function, processing speed, delayed recall, and global cognitive function with medium effect sizes, along with substantial improvements in subjective cognitive function. As discussed previously, a recent network meta-analysis of the effects of antidepressants on the DSST (processing speed and executive function) revealed vortioxetine's significant superiority for improving DSST compared to all other agents (e.g., SSRIs, SNRIs, TCAs, monoamine oxidase inhibitors [MAOIs]). It was also the only agent to improve DSST scores compared to placebo (Baune et al., 2018).

TCAs and MAOIs

While TCAs and MAOIs are less frequently used currently, with the advent of SSRIs and SNRIs, TCAs and MAOIs are highly effective antidepressants that are often used for treatment-resistant and treatment-refractory MDD. Both TCAs and MAOIs are less commonly used owing to their poor safety and adverse effect profiles secondary to numerous off-target effects (e.g., anticholinergic and antihistaminergic effects; risk of death with overdose). These off-target effects may also lead to worsening cognitive impairment, even while improving mood symptoms. Of the TCAs, sedating TCAs with high anticholinergic burden, such as imipramine, amitriptyline, and clomipramine, likely have the most adverse effects on cognitive function, based on known anticholinergic effects and clinical experience. However, the cognitive effects of TCAs remain understudied by clinical trials. Furthermore, given the currently infrequent use of TCAs, the cognitive effects of TCAs are unlikely to be studied further. Nevertheless, several small studies have demonstrated the neutral to negative effects of TCAs (Bondareff et al., 2000; Georgotas et al., 1986, 1989; Levkovitz et al., 2002; Nebes et al., 2003; Uher et al., 2009).

MAOIs are prescribed even less often than TCAs, given the significant safety concerns regarding risk of serotonin syndrome and hypertensive crisis (Stahl et al., 2013). However, MAOIs are efficacious treatments for treatment-refractory MDD and are still being used in these cases. The cognitive effects of MAOIs have been inadequately studied, and similar to TCAs, it is unlikely that prospective MAOI trials will be conducted in the future, given the availability of safer treatment alternatives (e.g., SSRIs). The limited available evidence suggests that MAOIs have negative effects on global cognitive function, especially negatively impacting executive function (Georgotas et al., 1986).

TARGETING COGNITION WITH OTHER PSYCHOTROPIC MEDICATIONS

Medications outside of antidepressants may potentially be "repurposed" to target cognition in MDD. Both psychotropic and nonpsychotropic medications are being investigated for potential pro-cognitive effects in MDD, as summarized in Figure 15.3. Given the limited pro-cognitive effects of antidepressants, numerous investigators have evaluated the potential pro-cognitive effects of other psychotropic agents that have demonstrated cognitive benefits in non-MDD samples. The main classes of psychotropic agents investigated include psychostimulants (indicated for ADHD), wake-promoting agents (indicated for narcolepsy), acetylcholinesterase inhibitors (indicated for dementia), and glutamate

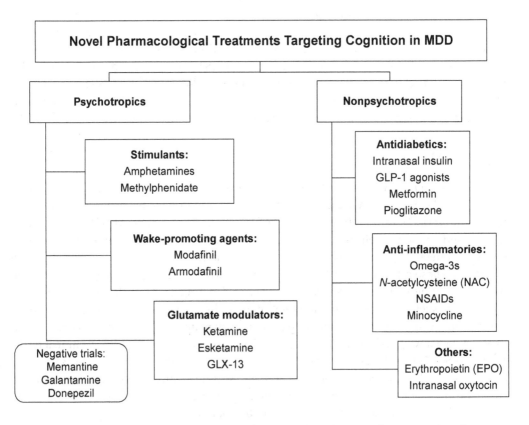

FIGURE 15.3. Novel pharmacological treatments (e.g., other than antidepressants) under investigation to target cognition in MDD. NSAIDs, nonsteroidal anti-inflammatory drugs.

modulators (indicated for schizophrenia). Conceptually, the pro-cognitive effects might be translatable into MDD samples. However, given the differences in pathophysiology of cognitive dysfunction between disorders, it should not be assumed that these agents would have pro-cognitive effect in MDD and still require rigorous clinical trials to prove, or disprove, this hypothesis.

Psychostimulants (e.g., amphetamines and methylphenidate) show promise for potential pro-cognitive effects in MDD, but they remain understudied. Psychostimulants are recommended off-label as second- or third-line MDD augmenting treatments, with some evidence for antidepressant efficacy (Kennedy et al., 2016; McIntyre et al., 2017). Madhoo and colleagues (2014) demonstrated significant improvements in executive function in partially remitted MDD with lisdexamfetamine ($n = 60$) versus placebo ($n = 59$) augmentation. While the pro-cognitive effects of lisdexamfetamine in MDD have been studied in an RCT, demonstrating positive effects, other psychostimulants have primarily been studied in open-label studies and retrospectively (Keefe et al., 2014). It remains unclear if there is a "class effect" whereby all psychostimulants have pro-cognitive effects in MDD or if these effects are agent specific.

Modafinil, a wake-promoting agent indicated in the treatment of narcolepsy, has also demonstrated promising preliminary results for pro-cognitive effects in MDD. In a study of 31 partially remitted MDD patients, modafinil was associated with significant improvements in validated measures of executive function after 4 weeks of treatment (Debattista, Lembke, Solvason, Ghebremichael, & Poirier, 2004). Modafinil has also demonstrated antidepressant effects as an augmenting agent and is recommended in some MDD treatment guidelines (DeBattista, Doghramji, Menza, Rosenthal, & Fieve, 2003; Fava, Thase, & DeBattista, 2005; Minzenberg & Carter, 2008).

Cognitive enhancers used in the treatment of major neurocognitive disorders (e.g., dementia) have also been evaluated in MDD. Unfortunately, a small number of proof-of-concepts studies have failed to demonstrate pro-cognitive effects in MDD with acetylcholine esterase inhibitors, such as galantamine (Elgamal & Macqueen, 2008; Holtzheimer et al., 2008) and donepezil (Pelton et al., 2008; Reynolds et al., 2011). Furthermore, these trials did not demonstrate antidepressant effects with these agents; therefore, cognitive enhancers are not currently prescribed as augmenting agents in MDD. While interest in acetylcholine esterase inhibitors for MDD has almost completely diminished given these negative trials, it is notable that these studies were underpowered, as more recent study design conventions for cognitive outcomes have suggested that larger sample sizes are required to be adequately powered (Kaser et al., 2017).

The rapid and robust antidepressant effects of ketamine (an *N*-methyl-D-aspartate [NMDA] antagonist approved as an anesthetic agent) have been established over the last decade, drawing attention to targeting the glutamate system in mood disorders (Caddy et al., 2015). The potential pro-cognitive effects of ketamine and other glutamate modulators in MDD are also of interest (Lener, Kadriu, & Zarate, 2017). Although further study is still required, initial results suggest that ketamine is associated with transient (minutes to hours) worsening of cognition followed by improvements in executive function and memory, with these pro-cognitive effects potentially facilitating the anti-suicidal effects observed with ketamine (Lee et al., 2016). Other glutamate modulators, such as GLY-13 and memantine, are also of interest. However, memantine (an NMDA antagonist indicated for dementia) has failed to demonstrate antidepressant or pro-cognitive effects in MDD (Smith et al., 2013; Sole et al., 2015; Zarate et al., 2006).

Taken together, several psychotropic medications (outside of antidepressants) show promise for improving cognitive outcomes in MDD, with lisdexamfetamine and modafinil having the strongest evidence currently as augmenting agents for partially or fully remitted MDD with persistent cognitive impairment. Cognitive enhancers indicated for dementia have failed to demonstrate benefits. Other glutamate modulators, such as ketamine and GLYX-13, require further investigation.

NONPSYCHOTROPIC AGENTS UNDER INVESTIGATION TO TARGET COGNITION

Aside from repurposing psychotropic agents with pro-cognitive effects in other disorders, numerous other agents are being investigated that are not traditionally considered "pro-cognitive." These agents target various aspects of the pathophysiology of MDD-related cognitive impairment, as described in other chapters of this volume. Most notably, targeting the immune and insulin-signaling systems that are hypothesized to play a role in cognitive dysfunction in mood disorders has been investigated with preliminary proof-of-concept studies.

Immune dysfunction has been implicated as a key pathophysiological process underlying mood and cognitive symptoms of mood disorders. Therefore, numerous anti-inflammatories have been evaluated in the treatment of MDD (Husain, Strawbridge, Stokes, & Young, 2017; Rosenblat, Cha, Mansur, & McIntyre, 2014). More recently, the role of anti-inflammatories in targeting cognition has been investigated. For example, omega-3s (naturally occurring anti-inflammatories) have been evaluated by two proof-of-concept trials, with one RCT showing no effects on cognitive function compared to placebo (Rogers et al., 2008) and the other RCT demonstrating benefits only in emotional decision making, but not other domains of cognition (Antypa, Smelt, Strengholt, & Van der Does, 2012). More recently, however, the benefits of omega-3s in MDD have been shown to be helpful for only a subset of patients with evidence of elevated inflammatory markers. As such, it is still possible that omega-3s, and anti-inflammatories in general, may possess pro-cognitive effects in the subgroup of "inflammatory-MDD" (Bloch & Hannestad, 2012; Rapaport et al., 2016). Similarly, N-acetylcysteine shows promise as an agent with anti-inflammatory and anti-oxidant properties that may have trans-iagnostic pro-cognitive effects (Berk, Malhi, Gray, & Dean, 2013; Fernandes, Dean, Dodd, Malhi, & Berk, 2015; Skvarc et al., 2017). Minocycline, an antibiotic with anti-inflammatory properties, has also demonstrated promising results for potential pro-cognitive effects, However, results need to be replicated in rigorously designed RCTs, preferably stratified by inflammatory markers (Nakasujja et al., 2013; Rosenblat & McIntyre, 2018; L. Zhang et al., 2006).

Insulin resistance has also been implicated in the pathophysiology of cognitive dysfunction, MDD, and dementia (Awad, Gagnon, & Messier, 2004; Bourdel-Marchasson, Mouries, & Helmer, 2010; Brietzke et al., 2018; Brown et al., 2018; Rosenblat, McIntyre,

Alves, Fountoulakis, & Carvalho, 2015). Indeed, insulin resistance may directly impair neuroplasticity in key brain regions subserving cognitive function, such as the hippocampus and prefrontal cortex (Artola, Kamal, Ramakers, Biessels, & Gispen, 2005; Fotuhi, Do, & Jack, 2012). As such, the potential antidepressant and pro-cognitive effects of intranasal insulin, GLP-1 agonists, metformin, and pioglitazone are currently being investigated with promising preliminary results (Banks, Owen, & Erickson, 2012; Kashani et al., 2013; McIntyre et al., 2013; Ying et al., 2014). As all studies have been small proof-of-concepts trials, along with preclinical studies (e.g., animal models), these results cannot yet be translated into clinical practice. They do, however, merit further investigation.

Taken together, targeting insulin signaling and the immune system presents as promising to improve cognitive function in MDD, but further study is still required to determine the clinical utility of these agents. Of note, the potential pro-cognitive effects of oxytocin and erythropoietin (EPO) have also been evaluated, with promising preliminary results (Bakermans-Kranenburg & van IJzendoorn, 2013; Miskowiak et al., 2010, 2014; Miskowiak, Vinberg, Harmer, Ehrenreich, & Kessing, 2012). Nonpharmacological interventions that improve insulin sensitivity, such as exercise, are also being investigated for antidepressant and pro-cognitive effects with promising results (Cooney et al., 2013).

TREATMENT IMPLICATIONS

Given the problematic persistence of cognitive dysfunction in MDD, targeted approaches are required to specifically improve cognition (see Table 15.1 for a summary of these

TABLE 15.1. Strategies for Targeting Cognitive Function in MDD

Strategies to target cognitive function	Comments
Measurement-based care	Use of validated subjective and objective cognitive measures at initial assessment and throughout treatment
Removing medications with negative effects on cognition	Removal of sedating and anticholinergic agents such as benzodiazepine, hypnotics, and sedating antipsychotics (if negative cognitive effects outweigh clinical benefits, e.g., anxiolysis)
Preferentially selecting antidepressants with pro-cognitive effects	Use of agents with evidence for pro-cognitive effects, such as vortioxetine
Pharmacological augmenting strategies with pro-cognitive effects	Use of stimulants (e.g., lisdexamfetamine) and wake-promoting agents (e.g., modafinil)—off-label use
Use of nonpharmacological strategies to improve cognition	Simultaneous use of pharmacological and nonpharmacological strategies to improve cognitive function

approaches). As part of measurement-based care (Trivedi & Daly, 2007), effective assessment of the cognitive function at baseline and throughout treatment is of great importance, so that cognitive impairment is not 'missed' when focusing solely on overall depressive symptom severity scores. Both subjective and objective measures of cognition should be evaluated at baseline and with any treatment changes (Kaser et al., 2017). Evidence-based, validated scales of cognition should be utilized, as described in other chapters of this volume, as part of gold-standard-measurement-based care. If cognitive dysfunction is detected, appropriate interventions should be pursued.

In addressing cognitive impairment, removal of medications with potential negative effects on cognition should be considered. Polypharmacy (e.g., prescription of numerous medications to a single patient) is common practice in MDD, given its high rates of comorbidity with other psychiatric disorders and treatment resistance, which require additional psychotropic medications to adequately alleviate symptoms (Basso et al., 2007; Baune, McAfoose, Leach, Quirk, & Mitchell, 2009; Rittmannsberger et al., 1999). Unfortunately, however, many of these medications have potential negative effects on cognitive function. Of particular concern are sedating medications that have negative effects on processing speed and working memory (Baune et al., 2009; Stranks & Crowe, 2014). Commonly co-prescribed medications (e.g., in addition to antidepressants) in MDD (particularly with comorbid anxiety) that may have negative effects on cognition include benzodiazepine (e.g., clonazepam, lorazepam), GABA-ergic anxiolytics (e.g., pregabalin, gabapentin), "z-drug" hypnotics (e.g., zopiclone, zolpidem), and sedating antipsychotics (e.g., olanzapine, quetiapine; Golombok, Moodley, & Lader, 1988; Hill, Bishop, Palumbo, & Sweeney, 2010; Stewart, 2005; Stranks & Crowe, 2014; Zhang, Zhou, Meranus, Wang, & Kukull, 2016). Symptoms of anxiety are the most common comorbid symptoms of MDD, with over 80% of MDD patients having anxious distress and/or a comorbid anxiety disorder (Fava et al., 2008; Kessler et al., 2003). While antidepressants remain the first-line treatment of anxiety disorders, many of the aforementioned sedating medications are prescribed in MDD to alleviate comorbid symptoms of anxiety. While these agents are effective in relieving symptoms of anxiety, along with targeting a subset of symptoms of MDD (e.g., insomnia), these medications may worsen cognitive function. As such, a careful assessment of cognitive risks versus other clinical benefits should be discussed with the patient in deciding to continue, discontinue, or decrease the dose of these medications.

In addition to removing medications with negative cognitive effects, prioritizing the use of antidepressants with greater pro-cognitive effects should also be considered. As discussed, vortioxetine has shown the strongest evidence for pro-cognitive effects, with a spectrum of effects on cognition associated with other antidepressants as shown in Figure 15.2. The off-label use of augmenting agents with pro-cognitive effects should also be considered if cognitive symptoms do not remit with antidepressant monotherapy. Although stimulants (e.g., lisdexamfetamine) and wake-promoting agents (e.g., modafinil) may be helpful, they are not approved for the treatment of MDD, requiring adequate informed consent for off-label use. Additionally, use of nonpharmacological interventions to improve cognition should also be considered, as discussed in other chapters of this volume (Baune & Renger, 2014).

CONCLUSIONS AND FUTURE DIRECTIONS

Cognitive dysfunction is a common and disabling problem associated with MDD. Unfortunately, the majority of currently available antidepressants have minimal effects on improving cognitive function; MDD patients frequently experience persistent cognitive dysfunction, even after achieving remission of depressive symptoms. Based on meta-analytic level evidence, as a group, antidepressants have failed to demonstrate pro-cognitive effects compared to placebo. However, significant variability exists among antidepressants, suggesting that improved cognition is not only a product of antidepressant response. Only vortioxetine has demonstrated robust and replicated benefits for improving executive function, memory, and global cognitive function with medium effect sizes. Other antidepressants remain understudied. SSRIs and SNRIs, as a group, appear to have mostly neutral effects on cognition, with some specific agents potentially have small pro-cognitive effects (e.g., levomilnacipram, duloxetine) while others might having small negative effects (e.g., paroxetine, fluvoxamine) due to off-target antihistaminergic and anticholinergic effects. The NDRI bupropion also has promising results for potential pro-cognitive effects, but it requires further study. Older antidepressants, such as TCAs and MAOIs, appear to have small to moderate negative effects on cognition, due to their numerous off-target effects. Numerous psychotropics used for augmentation and/or for treatment of comorbid disorders (e.g., antipsychotics, sleep aids, anxiolytics) may also have negative effects on cognition.

Several other psychotropic agents that have been evaluated in MDD have demonstrated pro-cognitive effects in other disorders (e.g., cognitive benefits in ADHD, dementia). Psychostimulants (e.g., lisdexamfetamine) show the most promise among these agents, with some promising results for wake-promoting agents (e.g., modafinil) as well. Cognitive enhancers indicated for dementia have not been found to improve cognition compared to placebo in MDD, but studies may have been underpowered. Repurposing nonpsychotropic medications has also provided additional agents of interest targeting the immune, insulin, EPO and oxytocin systems, with promising preliminary results requiring further study.

REFERENCES

American Psychiatric Association. (2013). *Diagnostic and statistical manual of mental disorders* (5th ed.). Arlington, VA: Author.

Anttila, S. A. K., & Leinonen, E. V. J. (2001). A review of the pharmacological and clinical profile of mirtazapine. *CNS Drug Reviews, 7*(3), 249–264.

Antypa, N., Smelt, A. H. M., Strengholt, A., & Van der Does, A. J. W. (2012). Effects of omega-3 fatty acid supplementation on mood and emotional information processing in recovered depressed individuals. *Journal of Psychopharmacology, 26*(5), 738–743.

Artola, A., Kamal, A., Ramakers, G. M., Biessels, G. J., & Gispen, W. H. (2005). Diabetes mellitus concomitantly facilitates the induction of long-term depression and inhibits that of long-term potentiation in hippocampus. *European Journal of Neuroscience, 22*, 169–178.

Awad, N., Gagnon, M., & Messier, C. (2004). The relationship between impaired glucose tolerance, type 2 diabetes, and cognitive function. *Journal of Clinical and Experimental Neuropsychology, 26*, 1044–1080.

Bakermans-Kranenburg, M. J., & van IJzendoorn, M. H. (2013). Sniffing around oxytocin: Review and meta-analyses of trials in healthy and clinical groups with implications for pharmacotherapy. *Translational Psychiatry, 3*(5), e258.

Banks, W. A., Owen, J. B., & Erickson, M. A. (2012). Insulin in the brain: There and back again. *Pharmacology and Therapeutics, 136*, 82–93.

Bartels, C., Wagner, M., Wolfsgruber, S., Ehrenreich, H., Schneider, A., & Alzheimer's Disease Neuroimaging Initiative. (2018). Impact of SSRI therapy on risk of conversion from mild cognitive impairment to Alzheimer's dementia in individuals with previous depression. *American Journal of Psychiatry, 175*(3), 232–241.

Basso, M. R., Lowery, N., Ghormley, C., Combs, D., Purdie, R., Neel, J., et al. (2007). Comorbid anxiety corresponds with neuropsychological dysfunction in unipolar depression. *Cognitive Neuropsychiatry, 12*, 437–456.

Baune, B. T., Brignone, M., & Larsen, K. G. (2018). A network meta-analysis comparing effects of various antidepressant classes on the digit symbol substitution Test (DSST) as a measure of cognitive dysfunction in patients with major depressive disorder. *International Journal of Neuropsychopharmacology, 21*(2), 97–107.

Baune, B. T., McAfoose, J., Leach, G., Quirk, F., & Mitchell, D. (2009). Impact of psychiatric and medical comorbidity on cognitive function in depression. *Psychiatry and Clinical Neuroscience, 63*, 392–400.

Baune, B. T., & Renger, L. (2014). Pharmacological and non-pharmacological interventions to improve cognitive dysfunction and functional ability in clinical depression—A systematic review. *Psychiatry Research, 219*, 25–50.

Berg, S., & Dellasega, C. (1996). The use of psychoactive medications and cognitive function in older adults. *Journal of Aging and Health, 8*(1), 136–149.

Berk, M., Malhi, G. S., Gray, L. J., & Dean, O. M. (2013). The promise of N-acetylcysteine in neuropsychiatry. *Trends in Pharmacological Sciences, 34*, 167–177.

Bloch, M. H., & Hannestad, J. (2012). Omega-3 fatty acids for the treatment of depression: Systematic review and meta-analysis. *Molecular Psychiatry, 17*, 1272–1282.

Bondareff, W., Alpert, M., Friedhoff, A. J., Richter, E. M., Clary, C. M., & Batzar, E. (2000). Comparison of sertraline and nortriptyline in the treatment of major depressive disorder in late life. *American Journal of Psychiatry, 157*, 729–736.

Borkowska, A., Drozdz, W., Ziółkowska-Kochan, M., & Rybakowski, J. (2007). Enhancing effect of mirtazapine on cognitive functions associated with prefrontal cortex in patients with recurrent depression. *Neuropsychopharmacologia Hungarica, 9*(3), 131–136.

Bourdel-Marchasson, I., Mouries, A., & Helmer, C. (2010). Hyperglycaemia, microangiopathy, diabetes and dementia risk. *Diabetes and Metabolism, 36*(Suppl. 3), S112–S118.

Brietzke, E., Mansur, R. B., Subramaniapillai, M., Balanzá-Martínez, V., Vinberg, M., González-Pinto, A., et al. (2018). Ketogenic diet as a metabolic therapy for mood disorders: Evidence and developments. *Neuroscience and Biobehavioral Reviews, 94*, 11–16.

Brooks, J. O., & Hoblyn, J. C. (2007). Neurocognitive costs and benefits of psychotropic medications in older adults. *Journal of Geriatric Psychiatry and Neurology, 20*(4), 199–214.

Brown, G. M., McIntyre, R. S., Rosenblat, J., & Hardeland, R. (2018). Depressive disorders: Processes leading to neurogeneration and potential novel treatments. *Progress in Neuro-psychopharmacology and Biological Psychiatry, 80*, 189–204.

Byers, A. L., & Yaffe, K. (2011). Depression and risk of developing dementia. *Nature Reviews Neurology, 7*, 323–331.

Caddy, C., Amit, B. H., McCloud, T. L., Rendell, J. M., Furukawa, T. A., McShane, R., et al. (2015). Ketamine and other glutamate receptor modulators for depression in adults. *Cochrane Database of Systematic Reviews*, CD011612.

Cipriani, A., Furukawa, T. A., Salanti, G., Chaimani, A., Atkinson, L. Z., Ogawa, Y., et al. (2018). Comparative efficacy and acceptability of 21 antidepressant drugs for the acute treatment of adults with major depressive disorder: A systematic review and network meta-analysis. *Lancet, 391*, 1357–1366.

Cooney, G. M., Dwan, K., Greig, C. A., Lawlor, D. A., Rimer, J., Waugh, F. R., et al. (2013). Exercise for depression. *Cochrane Database of Systematic Reviews, 9,* CD004366.

Culang, M. E., Sneed, J. R., Keilp, J. G., Rutherford, B. R., Pelton, G. H., Devanand, D. P., et al. (2009). Change in cognitive functioning following acute antidepressant treatment in late-life depression. *American Journal of Geriatric Psychiatry, 17,* 881–888.

Culang-Reinlieb, M. E., Sneed, J. R., Keilp, J. G., & Roose, S. P. (2012). Change in cognitive functioning in depressed older adults following treatment with sertraline or nortriptyline. *International Journal of Geriatric Psychiatry, 27,* 777–784.

DeBattista, C., Doghramji, K., Menza, M. A., Rosenthal, M. H., & Fieve, R. R. (2003). Adjunct modafinil for the short-term treatment of fatigue and sleepiness in patients with major depressive disorder: A preliminary double-blind, placebo-controlled study. *Journal of Clinical Psychiatry, 64,* 1057–1064.

Debattista, C., Lembke, A., Solvason, H. B., Ghebremichael, R., & Poirier, J. (2004). A prospective trial of modafinil as an adjunctive treatment of major depression. *Journal of Clinical Psychopharmacology, 24*(1), 87–90.

Elgamal, S., & Macqueen, G. (2008). Galantamine as an adjunctive treatment in major depression. *Journal of Clinical Psychopharmacology, 28*(3), 357–359.

Fava, M., Rush, A. J., Alpert, J. E., Balasubramani, G. K., Wisniewski, S. R., Carmin, C. N., et al. (2008). Difference in treatment outcome in outpatients with anxious versus nonanxious depression: A STAR*D report. *American Journal of Psychiatry, 165,* 342–351.

Fava, M., Thase, M. E., & DeBattista, C. (2005). A multicenter, placebo-controlled study of modafinil augmentation in partial responders to selective serotonin reuptake inhibitors with persistent fatigue and sleepiness. *Journal of Clinical Psychiatry, 66,* 85–93.

Ferguson, J. M., Wesnes, K. A., & Schwartz, G. E. (2003). Reboxetine versus paroxetine versus placebo: Effects on cognitive functioning in depressed patients. *International Clinical Psychopharmacology, 18,* 9–14.

Fernandes, B., Dean, O., Dodd, S., Malhi, G. S., & Berk, M. (2015). N-acetylcysteine in depressive symptoms and functionality: A systematic review and meta-analysis. *Journal of Clinical Psychiatry, 7*(4), e457–466.

Fotuhi, M., Do, D., & Jack, C. (2012). Modifiable factors that alter the size of the hippocampus with ageing. *Nature Reviews Neurology, 8,* 189–202.

Gaynes, B. N., Warden, D., Trivedi, M. H., Wisniewski, S. R., Fava, M., & Rush, A. J. (2009). What did STAR*D teach us?: Results from a large-scale, practical, clinical trial for patients with depression. *Psychiatric Services, 60,* 1439–1445.

Georgotas, A., McCue, R. E., Reisberg, B., Ferris, S. H., Nagachandran, N., Chang, I., et al. (1989). The effects of mood changes and antidepressants on the cognitive capacity of elderly depressed patients. *International Psychogeriatrics/IPA, 1,* 135–143.

Georgotas, A., McCue, R. E., Worth, W. H., Friedman, E., Kim, O. M., Welkowitz, J., et al. (1986). Comparative efficacy and safety of MAOIs versus TCAs in treating depression in the elderly. *Biological Psychiatry, 21*(12), 1155–1166.

Golombok, S., Moodley, P., & Lader, M. (1988). Cognitive impairment in long-term benzodiazepine users. *Psychological Medicine, 18*(2), 365–374.

Gorlyn, M., Keilp, J., Burke, A., Oquendo, M., Mann, J. J., & Grunebaum, M. (2015). Treatment-related improvement in neuropsychological functioning in suicidal depressed patients: Paroxetine vs. Bupropion. *Psychiatry Research, 225,* 407–412.

Harrison, J. E., Lophaven, S., & Olsen, C. K. (2016). Which cognitive domains are improved by treatment with vortioxetine? *International Journal of Neuropsychopharmacology, 19*(10), 1–6.

Herrera-Guzman, I., Gudayol-Ferre, E., Herrera-Abarca, J. E., Herrera-Guzman, D., Montelongo-Pedraza, P., Padros Blazquez, F., et al. (2010). Major depressive disorder in recovery and neuropsychological functioning: Effects of selective serotonin reuptake inhibitor and dual inhibitor depression treatments on residual cognitive deficits in patients with major depressive disorder in recovery. *Journal of Affective Disorders, 123,* 341–350.

Herrera-Guzman, I., Gudayol-Ferre, E., Herrera-Guzman, D., Guardia-Olmos, J., Hinojosa-Calvo, E., & Herrera-Abarca, J. E. (2009). Effects of selective serotonin reuptake and dual serotonergic-noradrenergic reuptake treatments on memory and mental processing speed in patients with major depressive disorder. *Journal of Psychiatric Research, 43,* 855–863.

Herrera-Guzman, I., Herrera-Abarca, J. E., Gudayol-Ferre, E., Herrera-Guzman, D., Gomez-Carbajal, L., Pena-Olvira, M., et al. (2010). Effects of selective serotonin reuptake and dual serotonergic-noradrenergic reuptake treatments on attention and executive functions in patients with major depressive disorder. *Psychiatry Research, 177,* 323–329.

Hill, S. K., Bishop, J. R., Palumbo, D., & Sweeney, J. A. (2010). Effect of second-generation antipsychotics on cognition: Current issues and future challenges. *Expert Review of Neurotherapeutics, 10*(1), 43–57.

Hoffman, B. M., Blumenthal, J. A., Babyak, M. A., Smith, P. J., Rogers, S. D., Doraiswamy, P. M., et al. (2008). Exercise fails to improve neurocognition in depressed middle-aged and older adults. *Medicine and Science in Sports and Exercise, 40,* 1344–1352.

Holtzheimer, P. E., Meeks, T. W., Kelley, M. E., Mufti, M., Young, R., McWhorter, K., et al. (2008). A double blind, placebo-controlled pilot study of galantamine augmentation of antidepressant treatment in older adults with major depression. *International Journal of Geriatric Psychiatry, 23*(6), 625–631.

Husain, M. I., Strawbridge, R., Stokes, P. R., & Young, A. H. (2017). Anti-inflammatory treatments for mood disorders: Systematic review and meta-analysis. *Journal of Psychopharmacology, 31*(9), 1137–1148.

Insel, T., Cuthbert, B., Garvey, M., Heinssen, R., Pine, D. S., Quinn, K., et al. (2010). Research Domain Criteria (RDoC): Toward a new classification framework for research on mental disorders. *American Journal of Psychiatry, 167*(7), 748–751.

Iwamoto, K., Kawano, N., Sasada, K., Kohmura, K., Yamamoto, M., Ebe, K., et al. (2013). Effects of low-dose mirtazapine on driving performance in healthy volunteers. *Human Psychopharmacology, 28*(5), 523–528.

Kantor, E. D., Rehm, C. D., Haas, J. S., Chan, A. T., & Giovannucci, E. L. (2015). Trends in prescription drug use among adults in the United States from 1999–2012. *JAMA, 314*(17), 1818–1830.

Kaser, M., Zaman, R., & Sahakian, B. J. (2017). Cognition as a treatment target in depression. *Psychological Medicine, 47*(6), 987–989.

Kashani, L., Omidvar, T., Farazmand, B., Modabbernia, A., Ramzanzadeh, F., Tehraninejad, E. S., et al. (2013). Does pioglitazone improve depression through insulin-sensitization?: Results of a randomized double-blind metformin-controlled trial in patients with polycystic ovarian syndrome and comorbid depression. *Psychoneuroendocrinology, 38,* 767–776.

Katona, C., Hansen, T., & Olsen, C. K. (2012). A randomized, double-blind, placebo-controlled, duloxetine-referenced, fixed-dose study comparing the efficacy and safety of Lu AA21004 in elderly patients with major depressive disorder. *International Clinical Psychopharmacology, 27,* 215–223.

Keefe, R. S., McClintock, S. M., Roth, R. M., Doraiswamy, P. M., Tiger, S., & Madhoo, M. (2014). Cognitive effects of pharmacotherapy for major depressive disorder: A systematic review. *Journal of Clinical Psychiatry, 75,* 864–876.

Kennedy, S. H., Lam, R. W., McIntyre, R. S., Tourjman, S. V., Bhat, V., Blier, P., et al. (2016). Canadian Network for Mood and Anxiety Treatments (CANMAT) 2016 Clinical Guidelines for the Management of Adults with Major Depressive Disorder: Section 3. Pharmacological Treatments. *Canadian Journal of Psychiatry, 61,* 540–560.

Kessler, R. C., Berglund, P., Demler, O., Jin, R., Koretz, D., Merikangas, K. R., et al. (2003). The epidemiology of major depressive disorder: Results from the National Comorbidity Survey Replication (NCS-R). *JAMA, 289,* 3095–3105.

Lee, Y., Syeda, K., Maruschak, N. A., Cha, D. S., Mansur, R. B., Wium-Andersen, I. K., et al. (2016). A new perspective on the anti-suicide effects with ketamine treatment: A procognitive effect. *Journal of Clinical Psychopharmacology, 36*(1), 50–56.

Lener, M. S., Kadriu, B., & Zarate, C. A. (2017). Ketamine and beyond: Investigations into the potential of glutamatergic agents to treat depression. *Drugs, 77,* 381–401.

Levkovitz, Y., Caftori, R., Avital, A., & Richter-Levin, G. (2002). The SSRIs drug fluoxetine, but not the noradrenergic tricyclic drug desipramine, improves memory performance during acute major depression. *Brain Research Bulletin, 58*, 345–350.

Madhoo, M., Keefe, R. S., Roth, R. M., Sambunaris, A., Wu, J., Trivedi, M. H., et al. (2014). Lisdexamfetamine dimesylate augmentation in adults with persistent executive dysfunction after partial or full remission of major depressive disorder. *Neuropsychopharmacology, 39*(6), 1388–1398.

Mahableshwarkar, A. R., Zajecka, J., Jacobson, W., Chen, Y., & Keefe, R. S. (2015). A randomized, placebo-controlled, active-reference, double-blind, flexible-dose study of the efficacy of vortioxetine on cognitive function in major depressive disorder. *Neuropsychopharmacology, 40*(8), 2025–2037.

McClintock, S. M., Husain, M. M., Wisniewski, S. R., Nierenberg, A. A., Stewart, J. W., Trivedi, M. H., et al. (2011). Residual symptoms in depressed outpatients who respond by 50% but do not remit to antidepressant medication. *Journal of Clinical Psychopharmacology, 31*(2), 180–186.

McIntyre, R. S. (2014). A vision for drug discovery and development: Novel targets and multilateral partnerships. *Advances in Therapy, 31*, 245–246.

McIntyre, R. S. (2017). The role of new antidepressants in clinical practice in Canada: A brief review of vortioxetine, levomilnacipran ER, and vilazodone. *Neuropsychiatric Disease and Treatment, 13*, 2913–2919.

McIntyre, R. S., Harrison, J., Loft, H., Jacobson, W., & Olsen, C. K. (2016). The effects of vortioxetine on cognitive function in patients with major depressive disorder: A meta-analysis of three randomized controlled trials. *International Journal of Neuropsychopharmacology, 19*(10), pyw055.

McIntyre, R. S., Lee, Y., Zhou, A. J., Rosenblat, J. D., Peters, E. M., Lam, R. W., et al. (2017). The efficacy of psychostimulants in major depressive episodes: A systematic review and meta-analysis. *Journal of Clinical Psychopharmacology, 37*(4), 412–418.

McIntyre, R. S., Lophaven, S., & Olsen, C. K. (2014). A randomized, double-blind, placebo-controlled study of vortioxetine on cognitive function in depressed adults. *International Journal of Neuropsychopharmacology, 17*, 1557–1567.

McIntyre, R. S., Powell, A. M., Kaidanovich-Beilin, O., Soczynska, J. K., Alsuwaidan, M., Woldeyohannes, H. O., et al. (2013). The neuroprotective effects of GLP-1: Possible treatments for cognitive deficits in individuals with mood disorders. *Behavioural Brain Research, 237*, 164–171.

Minzenberg, M. J., & Carter, C. S. (2008). Modafinil: A review of neurochemical actions and effects on cognition. *Neuropsychopharmacology, 33*, 1477–1502.

Miskowiak, K. W., Favaron, E., Hafizi, S., Inkster, B., Goodwin, G. M., Cowen, P. J., & Harmer, C. J. (2010). Erythropoietin modulates neural and cognitive processing of emotional information in biomarker models of antidepressant drug action in depressed patients. *Psychopharmacology, 210*(3), 419–428.

Miskowiak, K. W., Vinberg, M., Christensen, E. M., Bukh, J. D., Harmer, C. J., Ehrenreich, H., et al. (2014). Recombinant human erythropoietin for treating treatment-resistant depression: A double-blind, randomized, placebo-controlled phase 2 trial. *Neuropsychopharmacology, 39*, 1399–1408.

Miskowiak, K. W., Vinberg, M., Harmer, C. J., Ehrenreich, H., & Kessing, L. V. (2012). Erythropoietin: A candidate treatment for mood symptoms and memory dysfunction in depression. *Psychopharmacology, 219*, 687–698.

Nakasujja, N., Miyahara, S., Evans, S., Lee, A., Musisi, S., Katabira, E., et al. (2013). Randomized trial of minocycline in the treatment of HIV-associated cognitive impairment. *Neurology, 80*, 196–202.

Nebes, R. D., Pollock, B. G., Houck, P. R., Butters, M. A., Mulsant, B. H., Zmuda, M. D., et al. (2003). Persistence of cognitive impairment in geriatric patients following antidepressant treatment: A randomized, double-blind clinical trial with nortriptyline and paroxetine. *Journal of Psychiatric Research, 37*, 99–108.

Newhouse, P. A., Krishnan, K. R., Doraiswamy, P. M., Richter, E. M., Batzar, E. D., & Clary, C. M. (2000). A double-blind comparison of sertraline and fluoxetine in depressed elderly outpatients. *Journal of Clinical Psychiatry, 61*, 559–568.

Nickel, T., Sonntag, A., Schill, J., Zobel, A. W., Ackl, N., Brunnauer, A., et al. (2003). Clinical and neurobiological effects of tianeptine and paroxetine in major depression. *Journal of Clinical Psychopharmacology, 23*, 155–168.

Oakes, T. M., Myers, A. L., Marangell, L. B., Ahl, J., Prakash, A., Thase, M. E., et al. (2012). Assessment of depressive symptoms and functional outcomes in patients with major depressive disorder treated with duloxetine versus placebo: Primary outcomes from two trials conducted under the same protocol. *Human Psychopharmacology, 27*, 47–56.

Ohayon, M. M., & Lader, M. H. (2002). Use of psychotropic medication in the general population of France, Germany, Italy, and the United Kingdom. *Journal of Clinical Psychiatry, 63*(9), 817–825.

Pelton, G. H., Harper, O. L., Tabert, M. H., Sackeim, H. A., Scarmeas, N., Roose, S. P., et al. (2008). Randomized double-blind placebo-controlled donepezil augmentation in antidepressant-treated elderly patients with depression and cognitive impairment: A pilot study. *International Journal of Geriatric Psychiatry, 23*(7), 670–676.

Prado, C. E., Watt, S., & Crowe, S. F. (2018). A meta-analysis of the effects of antidepressants on cognitive functioning in depressed and non-depressed samples. *Neuropsychology Review, 28*(1), 32–72.

Rapaport, M. H., Nierenberg, A. A., Schettler, P. J., Kinkead, B., Cardoos, A., Walker, R., et al. (2016). Inflammation as a predictive biomarker for response to omega-3 fatty acids in major depressive disorder: A proof-of-concept study. *Molecular Psychiatry, 21*, 71–79.

Raskin, J., Wiltse, C. G., Siegal, A., Sheikh, J., Xu, J., Dinkel, J. J., et al. (2007). Efficacy of duloxetine on cognition, depression, and pain in elderly patients with major depressive disorder: An 8-week, double-blind, placebo-controlled trial. *American Journal of Psychiatry, 164*, 900–909.

Reddy, S., Fayyad, R., Edgar, C. J., Guico-Pabia, C. J., & Wesnes, K. (2016). The effect of desvenlafaxine on cognitive functioning in employed outpatients with major depressive disorder: A substudy of a randomized, double-blind, placebo-controlled trial. *Journal of Psychopharmacology (Oxford, England), 30*(6), 559–567.

Reynolds, C. F., Butters, M. A., Lopez, O., Pollock, B. G., Dew, M. A., Mulsant, B. H., et al. (2011). Maintenance treatment of depression in old age: A randomized, double-blind, placebo-controlled evaluation of the efficacy and safety of donepezil combined with antidepressant pharmacotherapy. *Archives of General Psychiatry, 68*(1), 51–60.

Rittmannsberger, H., Meise, U., Schauflinger, K., Horvath, E., Donat, H., & Hinterhuber, H. (1999). Polypharmacy in psychiatric treatment. Patterns of psychotropic drug use in Austrian psychiatric clinics. *European Psychiatry, 14*(1), 33–40.

Robinson, M., Oakes, T. M., Raskin, J., Liu, P., Shoemaker, S., & Nelson, J. C. (2014). Acute and long-term treatment of late-life major depressive disorder: Duloxetine versus placebo. *American Journal of Geriatric Psychiatry, 22*, 34–45.

Rock, P. L., Roiser, J. P., Riedel, W. J., & Blackwell, A. D. (2014). Cognitive impairment in depression: A systematic review and meta-analysis. *Psychological Medicine, 44*(10), 2029–2040.

Rogers, P. J., Appleton, K. M., Kessler, D., Peters, T. J., Gunnell, D., Hayward, R. C., et al. (2008). No effect of n-3 long-chain polyunsaturated fatty acid (EPA and DHA) supplementation on depressed mood and cognitive function: A randomised controlled trial. *British Journal of Nutrition, 99*(2), 421–431.

Rosenblat, J. D., Cha, D. S., Mansur, R. B., & McIntyre, R. S. (2014). Inflamed moods: A review of the interactions between inflammation and mood disorders. *Progress in Neuropsychopharmacology and Biological Psychiatry, 53*, 23–34.

Rosenblat, J. D., Kakar, R., & McIntyre, R. S. (2015). The cognitive effects of antidepressants in major depressive disorder: A systematic review and meta-analysis of randomized clinical trials. *International Journal of Neuropsychopharmacology, 19*(2), pyv082.

Rosenblat, J. D., & McIntyre, R. S. (2018). Efficacy and tolerability of minocycline for depression: A systematic review and meta-analysis of clinical trials. *Journal of Affective Disorders, 227*, 219–225.

Rosenblat, J. D., McIntyre, R. S., Alves, G. S., Fountoulakis, K. N., & Carvalho, A. F. (2015). Beyond monoamines-novel targets for treatment-resistant depression: A comprehensive review. *Current Neuropharmacology, 13*(5), 636–655.

Sasada, K., Iwamoto, K., Kawano, N., Kohmura, K., Yamamoto, M., Aleksic, B., et al. (2013). Effects of repeated dosing with mirtazapine, trazodone, or placebo on driving performance and cognitive function in healthy volunteers. *Human Psychopharmacology, 28*(3), 281–286.

Shilyansky, C., Williams, L. M., Gyurak, A., Harris, A., Usherwood, T., & Etkin, A. (2016). Effect of antidepressant treatment on cognitive impairments associated with depression: A randomised longitudinal study. *Lancet. Psychiatry, 3*(5), 425–435.

Skvarc, D. R., Dean, O. M., Byrne, L. K., Gray, L., Lane, S., Lewis, M., et al. (2017). The effect of N-acetylcysteine (NAC) on human cognition—A systematic review. *Neuroscience and Biobehavioral Reviews, 78,* 44–56.

Smith, E. G., Deligiannidis, K. M., Ulbricht, C. M., Landolin, C. S., Patel, J. K., & Rothschild, A. J. (2013). Antidepressant augmentation using the N-methyl-D-aspartate antagonist memantine: A randomized, double-blind, placebo-controlled trial. *Journal of Clinical Psychiatry, 74,* 966–973.

Soczynska, J. K., Ravindran, L. N., Styra, R., McIntyre, R. S., Cyriac, A., Manierka, M. S., et al. (2014). The effect of bupropion XL and escitalopram on memory and functional outcomes in adults with major depressive disorder: Results from a randomized controlled trial. *Psychiatry Research, 220,* 245–250.

Soehner, A. M., Kaplan, K. A., & Harvey, A. G. (2013). Insomnia comorbid to severe psychiatric illness. *Sleep Medicine Clinics, 8,* 361–371.

Sole, B., Jimenez, E., Martinez-Aran, A., & Vieta, E. (2015). Cognition as a target in major depression: New developments. *European Neuropsychopharmacology, 25,* 231–247.

Stahl, S. M. (1998). Mechanism of action of serotonin selective reuptake inhibitors. Serotonin receptors and pathways mediate therapeutic effects and side effects. *Journal of Affective Disorders, 51,* 215–235.

Stahl, S. M., Lee-Zimmerman, C., Cartwright, S., & Morrissette, D. A. (2013). Serotonergic drugs for depression and beyond. *Current Drug Targets, 14,* 578–585.

Stewart, S. A. (2005). The effects of benzodiazepines on cognition. *Journal of Clinical Psychiatry, 66*(Suppl. 2), 9–13.

Stranks, E. K., & Crowe, S. F. (2014). The acute cognitive effects of zopiclone, zolpidem, zaleplon, and eszopiclone: A systematic review and meta-analysis. *Journal of Clinical and Experimental Neuropsychology, 36*(7), 691–700.

Szabo, S. T., Kinon, B. J., Brannan, S. K., Krystal, A. K., van Gerven, J. M. A., Mahableshwarkar, A., et al. (2015). Lessons learned and potentials for improvement in CNS drug development: ISCTM section on designing the right series of experiments. *Innovations in Clinical Neuroscience, 12*(3–4), 11S–25S.

Trick, L., Stanley, N., Rigney, U., & Hindmarch, I. (2004). A double-blind, randomized, 26-week study comparing the cognitive and psychomotor effects and efficacy of 75 mg (37.5 mg b.i.d.) venlafaxine and 75 mg (25 mg mane, 50 mg nocte) dothiepin in elderly patients with moderate major depression being treated in general practice. *Journal of Psychopharmacology, 18,* 205–214.

Trivedi, M. H., & Daly, E. J. (2007). Measurement-based care for refractory depression: A clinical decision support model for clinical research and practice. *Drug and Alcohol Dependence, 88,* S61–S71.

Uher, R., Maier, W., Hauser, J., Marusic, A., Schmael, C., Mors, O., et al. (2009). Differential efficacy of escitalopram and nortriptyline on dimensional measures of depression. *British Journal of Psychiatry, 194,* 252–259.

Verbeeck, W., Bekkering, G. E., Van den Noortgate, W., & Kramers, C. (2017). Bupropion for attention deficit hyperactivity disorder (ADHD) in adults. *Cochrane Database of Systematic Reviews, 10,* CD009504.

Wang, Y.-C., Tai, P.-A., Poly, T. N., Islam, M. M., Yang, H.-C., Wu, C.-C., et al. (2018). Increased risk of dementia in patients with antidepressants: A meta-analysis of observational studies. *Behavioural Neurology, 2018,* 5315098.

Wesnes, K. A., Gommoll, C., Chen, C., Sambunaris, A., McIntyre, R. S., & Harvey, P. D. (2017). Effects of levomilnacipran extended-release on major depressive disorder patients with cognitive impairments: Post-hoc analysis of a phase III study. *International Clinical Psychopharmacology, 32*(2), 72–79.

Woo, Y. S., Rosenblat, J. D., Kakar, R., Bahk, W.-M., & McIntyre, R. S. (2016). Cognitive deficits as a mediator of poor occupational function in remitted major depressive disorder patients. *Clinical Psychopharmacology and Neuroscience, 14*(1), 1–16.

Yaffe, K., Falvey, C. M., & Hoang, T. (2014). Connections between sleep and cognition in older adults. *Lancet Neurology, 13,* 1017–1028.

Ying, M. A., Maruschak, N., Mansur, R., Carvalho, A. F., Cha, D. S., & McIntyre, R. S. (2014). Metformin: Repurposing opportunities for cognitive and mood dysfunction. *CNS and Neurological Disorders Drug Targets, 13*(10), 1836–1845.

Zarate, C. A., Singh, J. B., Quiroz, J. A., De Jesus, G., Denicoff, K. K., Luckenbaugh, D. A., et al. (2006). A double-blind, placebo-controlled study of memantine in the treatment of major depression. *American Journal of Psychiatry, 163,* 153–155.

Zhang, L., Kitaichi, K., Fujimoto, Y., Nakayama, H., Shimizu, E., Iyo, M., et al. (2006). Protective effects of minocycline on behavioral changes and neurotoxicity in mice after administration of methamphetamine. *Progress in Neuropsychopharmacology and Biological Psychiatry, 30,* 1381–1393.

Zhang, Y., Zhou, X.-H., Meranus, D. H., Wang, L., & Kukull, W. A. (2016). Benzodiazepine use and cognitive decline in elderly with normal cognition. *Alzheimer Disease and Associated Disorders, 30*(2), 113–117.

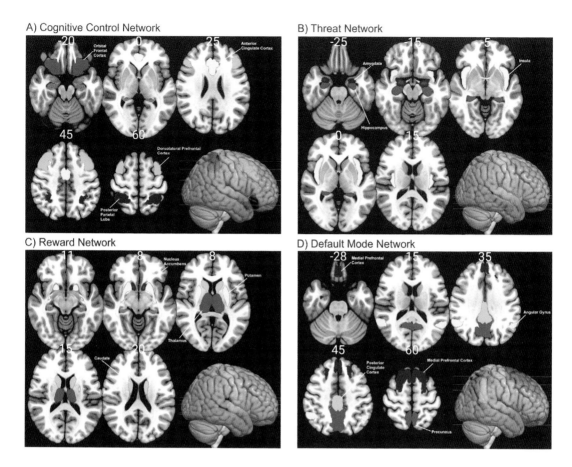

PLATE 2.1. Neural networks in depression. Images indicate key regions of (A) the cognitive control network, (B) the threat network, (C) the reward network, and (D) the default mode network. MRIcron and the Harvard–Oxford Cortical and Subcortical Structural Atlases were used to create these images.

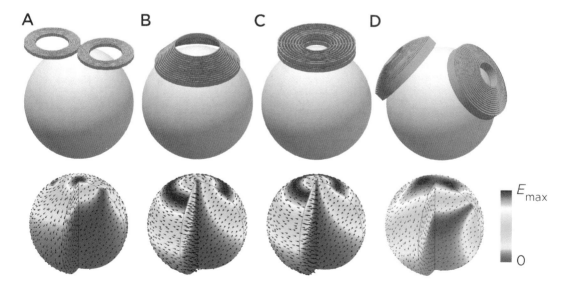

PLATE 21.1. MST coil configurations and electrical field distribution. The figure shows four unique MST coil configurations—(A) 70-mm figure-8 coil; (B) cap coil; (C) circular coil; and (D) twin coil—with corresponding electric field distribution on a spherical head model.

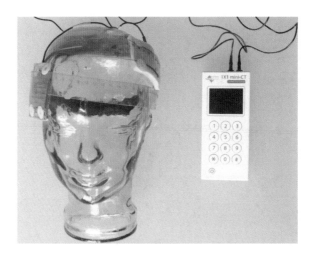

PLATE 24.1. tDCS device.

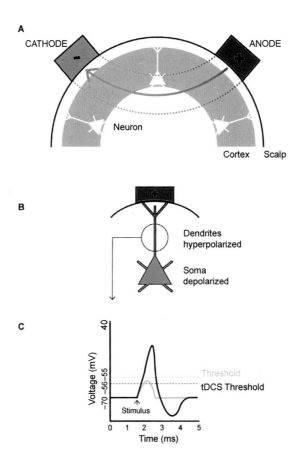

PLATE 24.2. Mechanisms of action of tDCS. (A) A unidirectional current flows between the electrodes from the positively charged anode to the negatively charged cathode. The current passes through the intervening tissue, with some shunting of current across the scalp. (B) tDCS polarizes the compartments of a neuron and alters the resting membrane potential. Positive charge partially depolarizes the resting membrane potential of the soma, whereas negative charge hyperpolarizes it. (C) By altering the resting membrane potential of the soma, tDCS alters the likelihood that a neuron will propagate an incoming signal and generate a subsequent action potential. Anodal tDCS partially depolarizes cell membranes, thereby facilitating the propagation of action potentials and increasing neuronal excitability.

CHAPTER 16

Nutraceuticals

Julia Browne
David Mischoulon
Jerome Sarris

Major depressive disorder (MDD) is a serious mental illness affecting over 300 million people worldwide (World Health Organization [WHO], 2017). Its symptoms include low mood, loss of interest/pleasure in activities, changes in weight and/or appetite, changes in sleep, psychomotor agitation/retardation, lack of energy, feelings of worthlessness or guilt, difficulty concentrating, and thoughts of death or suicide (American Psychiatric Association, 2013). Because of its negative impact on educational, vocational, and social functioning, MDD is considered "the single largest contributor to global disability" (WHO, 2017, p. 5). Although antidepressants (typically selective serotonin reuptake inhibitors [SSRIs] or serotonin–norepinephrine reuptake inhibitors) are considered first-line medications for MDD, they do not provide remission for approximately two-thirds of individuals (Rush, 2007). Furthermore, multiple medication trials can be burdensome and do not guarantee eventual remission (Warden et al., 2007). As such, there remains a need for continued research into more effective treatments for MDD.

An emerging approach to improve non- or partial response to antidepressants is the use of adjunctive nutraceuticals, a term that refers to nutrient-based products (and sometimes herbal medicines) that are prepared and formulated for potential medical benefits (Sarris et al., 2016). The use of adjunctive nutraceuticals may augment the clinical effect of antidepressants by addressing several key neurobiological abnormalities underpinning the disorder, including monoamine impairment, neuroendocrinological changes, reduced brain-derived neurotrophic factor, and cytokine alterations (Papakostas & Ionescu, 2015). In addition to their impact on depressive symptoms, nutraceuticals have been shown to be beneficial for cognition (Mathias & Mischoulon, 2015). Thus, nutraceuticals might be particularly valuable as a treatment option, given that cognitive impairment and depression often co-occur, especially in elderly adults (Panza et al., 2010). Unfortunately, despite evidence demonstrating the value in nutraceuticals, many practitioners in the field are not familiar with these products or their impact on mood or cognitive symptoms. Therefore, this chapter provides a summary of the main evidence for application of selected nutrient and herbal medicines in treating MDD and improving cognition.

CURRENT EVIDENCE FOR DEPRESSION TREATMENTS

Nutrient-Based Medicines

Among nutritional supplements, the most robust literature base exists for the impact of omega-3, one-carbon-cycle nutrients (e.g., S-adenosylmethionine [SAMe], methylfolate, folic acid, folinic acid, and vitamins B6 and B12), and tryptophan (and 5-hydroxytryptophan [5-HTP]) on depression. A smaller number of studies have examined zinc, vitamins C and D, creatine, inositol, and certain amino acid combinations. In their review and meta-analysis of 40 studies, Sarris and colleagues (2016) concluded that SAMe, methylfolate, omega-3, and vitamin D have the most positive support for their use in combination with antidepressants to reduce depressive symptoms. Yet, given the significant heterogeneity in study methodology, as well as the dearth of rigorous studies of some nutrients, a closer examination of the existing research is of value.

Omega-3 Fatty Acids

Clinical trials of omega-3 fatty acids for treating depression have typically involved eicosapentaenoic acid (EPA) or a combination of EPA and docosahexaenoic acid. Due to methodological differences among studies (e.g., preparation, dose, and duration), a clear consensus regarding the most effective administration of omega-3s has not yet occurred. Nonetheless, a number of studies, with varying methodological characteristics, have illustrated the benefits of omega-3s on depressive symptoms when utilized as an adjunct to antidepressant medications. Specifically, omega-3s have been shown to be superior to placebo in double-blind trials ranging from 4 to 12 weeks and in combination with several antidepressants (Sarris et al., 2016). These supplements may be more effective for individuals who are overweight and/or who have high levels of inflammatory markers (Rapaport et al., 2016).

Omega-3s also tend to have low risk for serious side effects, with gastrointestinal problems being most commonly reported. There have been concerns, however, regarding cycling to mania in individuals with bipolar disorder; in such cases, coadministration with a mood stabilizer is recommended (Mischoulon, 2018). The mechanism of action is not fully understood; however, membrane stabilization, anti-inflammatory effects, and inhibiting G-protein signal transduction have been proposed (Mischoulon, 2018). Despite the heterogeneity of studies and limited understanding of the mechanisms, the evidence illustrates value in utilizing omega-3 supplements as an adjunct to antidepressant treatment.

One-Carbon-Cycle Nutrients

Of the one-carbon-cycle nutrients, SAMe has been most extensively examined in the context of clinical trials for depression, with a recent review citing the existence of over 50 clinical trials (19 randomized controlled trials [RCTs]; Mischoulon, 2018). The majority of studies compared the efficacy of SAMe to placebo and/or tricyclic antidepressants (TCAs) and found that it is superior to placebo and equivalent to such antidepressants. An early meta-analysis by Hardy and colleagues (2002), covering 28 selected studies, supports these conclusions. A recent systematic review (Sharma et al., 2017) generally agreed with previous meta-analyses. However, it is interesting to note that in the first and only study to independently compare SAMe to an SSRI (escitalopram) in a 12-week double-blind, randomized, placebo-controlled clinical trial of 189 outpatients, Mischoulon and colleagues (2014) found that 1,600–3,200 mg/day of SAMe did not significantly differ from 10–20 mg/day of escitalopram in the effect on depression when compared to each other and to placebo. Sarris and colleagues' (2016) review provided additional evidence for the benefits of SAMe as an adjunctive agent to antidepressants for treatment-resistant individuals.

Overall, the evidence suggests that SAMe may be equivalent to TCAs and may serve as an effective augmenting agent for a variety of antidepressants. However, a recent 8-week double-blind RCT of 107 outpatients found that due to the high placebo-response rate, SAMe given adjunctively to antidepressants in adults with nonremittent MDD was not more effective than placebo (Sarris et al., 2018). Regardless, SAMe is considered safe, with the most common side effect being gastrointestinal distress and no serious drug–drug interactions (Mischoulon, 2018).

In addition to SAMe, folic acid and methylfolate have been evaluated as an adjunct to antidepressant treatment. Overall, the results for folic acid appear to be more mixed than those for methylfolate. Specifically, Sarris and colleagues (2016) identified five studies that examined the effect of folic acid on depressive symptoms with three of the five reporting significant results. Yet, when meta-analyzed, there was a nonsignificant effect of folic acid over placebo (Sarris et al., 2016). All three studies that examined folinic acid or methylfolate reported primarily significant effects on depressive symptoms (Alpert et al., 2002; Godfrey et al., 1990; Papakostas et al., 2012), which suggest promise for its use as an adjunctive treatment. Finally, when meta-analyzed as a single class, the one-carbon-cycle intermediates (SAMe, folic acid, folinic acid, methylfolate, B_6, and B_{12}) were shown to be superior to placebo and to result in improvements from baseline in treatment-resistant depression (Sarris et al., 2016).

Tryptophan and 5-Hydroxytryptophan

A considerable number of studies have examined the effects of tryptophan and 5-HTP on symptoms of depression, the vast majority of which were conducted prior to 2000. Iovieno, Dalton, Fava, and Mischoulon (2011) purported that the once heightened interest in examining this nutrient significantly diminished around 1987, when the first SSRI was approved in the United States. Yet, in light of early promising evidence and the growing literature on natural medicines, consideration of its value in treating depression may be warranted.

Tryptophan and 5-HTP are thought to impact depression through serotonergic mechanisms. Specifically, tryptophan is converted into 5-HTP and subsequently into serotonin (Iovieno et al., 2011). Although individuals typically consume a small amount of tryptophan in their diet, ingesting additional amounts is thought to result in an increased production of serotonin (although conversion into serotonin is rate-limited), which consequently modulates mood effects. In terms of published efficacy studies, 5-HTP was shown to be more effective than placebo in 7 out of 11 studies (Iovieno et al., 2011), whereas tryptophan (or L-tryptophan or DL-tryptophan) was shown to be more effective than placebo in four out of seven studies (Sarris et al., 2016).

Although the most common side effects include nausea, vomiting, and diarrhea, the potential for developing eosinophilia–myalgia syndrome (EMS) was previously a grave concern, given the documented history. Iovieno and colleagues (2011) explained that between 1989 and 1990 over 1,500 people became infected with EMS after consuming contaminated tryptophan, with approximately 38 deaths ensuing. Tryptophan was banned, and it was later determined that faulty production, rather than specific qualities of the nutrient, was responsible for contamination (Iovieno et al., 2011). Nevertheless, this history likely continues to worry potential prescribers and consumers. Another serious side effect is the potential for the development of serotonin syndrome, given that 5-HTP is thought to result in an increase of serotonin. Yet, research has not formally implicated 5-HTP in the development of this syndrome when administered on its own or in combination with another antidepressant (Iovieno et al., 2011). This is more likely to be a potential issue with 5-HTP (the precursor of serotonin) rather than the amino acid L-tryptophan. All in all, promising early findings suggest that 5-HTP might be beneficial in treating depression. Yet, the significant methodological concerns of published trials in combination with limited contemporary research and the potential for serious side effects limit firm conclusions.

Additional Nutrients

Several other nutrients, including zinc, vitamins C and D, creatine, inositol, and amino acids, have been considered as potentially valuable augmenting agents to antidepressants. As described in Sarris and colleagues' (2016) review and meta-analysis, there appears to be preliminary support for the use of vitamin D, creatine, and amino acid. However, the limited number of existing studies should be considered. Results for the use of zinc and vitamin C were mixed, and the two studies examining inositol as an adjunct did not demonstrate effects for its use over placebo (Sarris et al., 2016). It should be noted, however, that there is very modest evidence that inositol may outperform antidepressants when administered on its own (Levine et al., 1995; Mukai, Kishi, Matsuda, & Iwata, 2014). Taken together, this limited body of research suggests the need for further examination of nutrients such as adjunctive agents and/or as monotherapy in the treatment of depression.

Herbal Medicines

Among herbal medicines, *Hypericum perforatum* (St. John's wort), *Crocus sativus* (saffron), and *Curcuma longa* (turmeric) have the strongest research base (Mischoulon, 2018; Sarris, 2018). Additionally, some encouraging evidence supports use of *Rhodiola rosea* (roseroot) for treating depression (Iovieno et al., 2011). As such, an understanding of effective uses of these herbal medicines would be valuable.

Hypericum perforatum (St. John's Wort)

St. John's wort (SJW) is one of the most extensively examined nutraceuticals for depression, with over 40 published clinical trials. Evidence from recent studies suggests that SJW leads to higher remission rates and may be more effective for individuals with mild depression (Mischoulon, 2018; Sarris, 2018). Given the significant number of studies examining the effect of SJW on depression, numerous meta-analyses and reviews have summarized the findings. For example, Linde and Kriston (2008) reviewed 29 trials and found that SJW was superior to placebo and equivalent to standard antidepressants. Furthermore, Ng, Koh, Chan, and Ho (2017) examined 27 clinical trials and found that SJW and SSRIs did not differ in response and remission rates; however, SJW had significantly lower discontinuation rates. Finally, in the largest review, that of 35 studies, SJW was associated with more treatment responders than placebo and did not differ in response rates against antidepressants (Apaydin et al., 2016).

In terms of the mechanism of action for SJW's effect on depression, it has been proposed that it involves in part an interaction with the hypothalamus–pituitary–adrenal axis that leads to decreased cortisol (Mischoulon, 2018). SJW has also been shown in preclinical studies to have an antidepressant action that involves nonselective inhibition of reuptake of several neurotransmitters (e.g., serotonin, dopamine, norepinephrine, gamma-aminobutyric acid), decreased degradation of neurochemicals, and a sensitization of and increased binding to certain receptors (Sarris, 2018). There is some doubt, however, as to whether these *in vitro* assay results are generalizable to human neurobiological effects, which are subject to neurochemical bioavailability. The most common side effects are mild (e.g., dizziness, dry mouth, constipation), with phototoxicity being uncommon. The potential for drug–drug interactions via the liver enzyme CYP-450-3A4 from SJW formulas rich in hyperforin is extensive and includes a wide range of medications such as warfarin, cyclosporin, oral contraceptives, theophylline, fenprocoumon, digoxin camptosar, indinavir, zolpidem, irinotecam, and olanzapine (Mischoulon, 2018). Other concerns include cycling to mania in cases of bipolar disorder, and serotonin syndrome when SJW is combined with SSRIs (Mischoulon, 2018). Use of SJW should therefore be carefully considered, especially for individuals who may be receiving medication/treatment for bipolar illness and/or comorbid medical conditions (e.g., HIV, cancer, and status posttransplant). Despite these caveats, the evidence as a whole suggests that SJW may be effective and mostly safe for treating depression, in particular mild to moderate cases (Mischoulon, 2018).

Crocus sativus (Saffron)

With its traditional use in Persian medicine, saffron has continued to be the subject of evaluation as a therapeutic option for depression (Sarris, 2018). A meta-analysis of five RCTs demonstrated that saffron treatment was superior to placebo and not significantly different from antidepressant treatment in terms of its effect on depressive symptoms (Hausenblas, Saha, Dubyak, & Anton, 2013). As such, these results suggest that saffron performed similarly to antidepressant medications in terms of reducing depressive symptoms. Two specific studies are worthy of mention. One showed that 30 mg/day of saffron was similarly effective to 40 mg/day of fluoxetine in a 6-week randomized double-blind parallel-group trial of 40 participants with mild-moderate depression who underwent percutaneous coronary intervention (Shahmansouri et al., 2014). Another study showed that the addition of 30 mg of saffron to 20 mg of fluoxetine showed no superiority over 20 mg of fluoxetine plus placebo in a 4-week double blind trial of 40 participants with MDD (Sahraian, Jelodar, Javid, Mowla, & Ahmadzadeh, 2016). Nonetheless, it must be cautioned that both trials had relatively small samples ($n = 40$) as well as very short durations (4–6 weeks). The high monetary cost of Saffron may be a barrier for consistent use. Overall, there appears to be promising evidence for using saffron in the treatment of depression.

Curcuma longa (Turmeric)

Turmeric's main active ingredient is curcumin, which is involved in anti-inflammatory (reducing C-reactive protein and interleukin-6 and 1b), antioxidant, neuroprotective, and monoaminergic (serotonergic and dopaminergic) modulatory activities. It has been proposed that Turmeric may be effective in alleviating depressive symptoms due to its anti-inflammatory capabilities. Emerging human clinical trial evidence supports curcumin as an antidepressant. For example, a 6-week randomized, double-blind, placebo-controlled study of 108 male participants experiencing an episode of major depression found that 1000 mg/day of curcumin was an effective adjunct to 5–15 mg/day of escitalopram (Yu et al., 2015). In respect to studies assessing curcumin versus placebo, a meta-analysis of six studies illustrates turmeric's significant effects over placebo in terms of reducing depressive symptoms (Ng et al., 2017). An additional meta-analysis of the data from an overall sample of six clinical trials revealed a significant effect in favor of the herbal agent over placebo (Al-Karawi, Al Mamoori, & Tayyar, 2016). Heterogeneity was very low, with sample sizes being between 30 and 111, trial lengths between 4 and 8 weeks, and doses of 500 mg–1 g of curcumin (commonly 1 g/day), either with the addition of piperine or prepared via a formulation designed to enhance bioavailability. This is a common strategy to circumvent the poor bioavailability of raw curcumin.

Rhodiola rosea (Roseroot)

Rhodiola rosea, a plant that has been extensively examined in Russia and Scandinavia, is known for stimulating the nervous system, preventing altitude sickness, enhancing physical and mental performance, and helping to alleviate depression, stress, and fatigue (Iovieno et al., 2011). The capabilities of this plant have led it to be classified as an "adaptogen, a substance that nonspecifically increases the resistance of an organism to a variety of chemical, biological, and physical stressors" (Iovieno et al., 2011, p. 344). Studies show the apparent promise of *Rhodiola rosea* in stimulating antidepressant activity (Iovieno et al., 2011). For example, Darbinyan and colleagues (2007) found that individuals with mild to moderate depression who received either 340 or 680 mg/day of *Rhodiola rosea* experienced greater reductions in depressive symptoms than those who received placebo in a 6-week double blind trial of 89 participants with MDD. *Rhodiola rosea* also appears to improve physical fitness, fatigue, and mental performance in healthy individuals. A more robust study of 57 participants compared 340 mg of the plant to 50 mg of sertraline and placebo over 12 weeks and found modest (though not statistically significant) reductions in depressive symptoms for sertraline over the other treatment groups (Mao et al., 2015). Mao and colleagues (2015) also noted that more participants in the sertraline group reported adverse events as compared to those in the plant or placebo group. Taken together, *Rhodiola rosea* appears to have some potential benefits. Moreover, it is reported to be quite safe, with the potential for mild (albeit rare) side effects and no known serious drug–drug interactions (Iovieno et al., 2011).

CURRENT EVIDENCE FOR COGNITION

Ginkgo biloba

A significant literature base exists for the impact of *Ginkgo biloba* on cognition. The most recent Cochrane review and meta-analysis included 36 trials and noted unreliable and inconsistent results for the effect of leaf-based extracts from the tree on cognition (Birks & Evans, 2009). Yet, several studies conducted after this Cochrane review have reported positive effects on various cognitive outcomes. For example, a 24-week double-blind RCT with 410 outpatients illustrated that once daily *Ginkgo biloba* (240 mg of EGb 761 preparation) resulted in greater improvements, as compared to placebo among those with dementia (Herrschaft et al., 2012; Ihl et al., 2011). Additionally, Canevelli and colleagues (2014) found that the addition of *Ginkgo biloba* (EGb 761 preparation) to cholinesterase inhibitors resulted in cognitive benefits for individuals with Alzheimer's disease (AD) at 12-month follow-up in their cohort study of 828 participants. A 2015 meta-analysis of nine studies showed that *Ginkgo biloba* could aid in stabilizing or slowing decline in cognition for those with cognitive impairment and dementia (Tan et al., 2015). Finally, in a study of 136 elderly individuals with depression, Dai, Hu, Shang, and Xie (2018) found that 20 mg/day of citalopram with 19.2 mg of adjunctive *Ginkgo biloba* (EGb tablets) three times a day resulted in improved depressive symptoms and reduced expression of serum S100B (a marker of brain injury). Regardless, the data are not fully supportive of a preventative effect on dementia, with large studies showing that, compared with placebo, 120 mg of *Ginkgo biloba* (EGb 761 preparation) 2x/day did not lead to reduced cognitive decline or reduced progression to AD in an RCT of 3,069 participants (Snitz et al., 2009) or in an RCT of 2,854 participants (Vellas et al., 2012). Nevertheless, more recent evidence shows that *Ginkgo biloba* is associated with the enhancement of some cognitive domains (Canevelli et al., 2014; Herrschaft et al., 2012; Ihl et al., 2011). Moreover, given the relative safety and tolerability of *Ginkgo biloba* (Mathias & Mischoulon, 2015), continued examination of its value in the treatment of individuals with cognitive concerns is warranted.

Other Herbal and Nutritional Agents

Though far fewer studies have been conducted on other agents such as phosphatidylserine (PS) as compared to *Gingko biloba*, the results of existing studies suggest promise for this agent in preventing and treating cognitive decline (Mathias & Mischoulon, 2015). Specifically, Vakhapova and colleagues (2010) examined the effects of a novel preparation of PS (containing polyunsaturated fatty acids; referred to as PS-DHA) on the cognitive functioning of 157 elderly individuals with memory concerns but not dementia, and found benefits (particularly in immediate verbal recall) for those randomized to receive PS-DHA over placebo for the 15-week trial duration. Participants with higher cognitive functioning at baseline experienced the greatest improvements. Vakhapova and colleagues (2014) extended their work by conducting a 15-week open-label trial of PS-DHA at the completion of the 2010 randomized trial. Results of the open label trial with 122 participants showed that those who continued receiving PS-DHA maintained their cognitive abilities and those in the treatment naïve group experienced significant improvements in attention and memory recognition. Finally, Richter, Herzog, Cohen, and Steinhart (2010) reported the benefits of PS-containing omega-3 long chain polyunsaturated fatty acid on memory in a small 6-week pilot study of eight elderly participants. None of these studies reported serious adverse effects, suggesting that this may be both a promising and safe agent for use in treating cognitive impairments. Nonetheless, given the few studies conducted to date, continued study of PS is critical.

In addition to PS, other herbal and nutritional medicines have been explored in terms of their impact on cognition, including *Panax ginseng* (Asian and Korean ginseng), *Melissa officinalis* (lemon balm), *Salvia officinalis* (sage), *salvia lavandulaefolia* (Spanish sage), vitamins, and omega-3s. In terms of herbal medicines, there have been some positive findings from RCTs illustrating that 300–800 mg/day of Korean ginseng were associated with improvements in healthy volunteers in areas such as abstract thinking (Sorensen & Sonne, 1996) and accuracy and working memory (Reay, Scholey, & Kennedy, 2010). Additionally, some studies have focused on the use of lemon balm in individuals with AD and dementia. For example, a placebo-controlled RCT of 71 participants with dementia and agitation found that after 4 weeks, those who received the lemon balm aromatherapy experienced significant reductions in agitation and improvements in quality of life (Ballard et al., 2002). Moreover, lemon balm aromatherapy was found to result in improvements in cognition as well as reduced agitation compared to placebo in a 4-month RCT of 42 patients with AD (Akhondzadeh et al., 2003). Lastly, sage has been examined as an herbal medicine with cognitive enhancement properties. Four double-blind RCT crossover studies of healthy adults revealed the superiority of Spanish sage (doses ranging from 50–150 ml to 167–1,332 mg) in promoting improved cognitive functioning (Kennedy et al., 2011; Scholey et al., 2008; Tildesley et al., 2005).

In terms of nutritional medicines, there is limited evidence in favor of omega-3s, with one double-blind RCT of 204 patients with AD reporting no differences in the rate of cognitive decline between those randomized to receive omega-3 fatty acids (1.7 g of docosahexaenoic acid and 0.6g of eicosapentaenoic acid) as compared to placebo at 6 months (Freund-Levi et al., 2006). The impact of vitamins on cognition has also been explored, with a cross-sectional and prospective study of dementia reporting that vitamin E and C supplements were associated with reduced prevalence and incidence of AD (Zandi et al., 2004). Moreover, Grima, Pase, Macpherson, and Pipingas (2012) reported on 10 RCTs in their systematic review and meta-analysis and concluded that multivitamins were effective in improving immediate free recall memory. Taken together, there appear to be several promising herbal and nutritional medicines worthy of continued study in the area of cognition.

SUMMARY

This chapter provides a brief overview of current evidence for the use of nutrient-based and herbal medicines in the treatment of depression and cognition. In terms of nutrient-based medicines for depression, the most favorable support exists for omega-3, vitamin D, and, to some extent, tryptophan and 5-HTP, particularly as adjuncts to standard antidepressant treatment. There also appears to be promising support for the use of amino acids and creatine as adjunctive agents, mixed evidence for SAMe, and tentative evidence for inositol as monotherapy. Among herbal medicines for depression, research generally supports the value of SJW, saffron, and turmeric, and, though less extensively studied, *Rhodiola rosea*. In terms of cognition, the most significant literature base exists for *Ginkgo biloba*, with many of the earlier studies report mixed and unreliable results, or being negative. More recent studies, however, suggest that this agent may be valuable in the treatment of general cognitive impairments (Mathias & Mischoulon, 2015). Research from three studies over the past decade provides initial encouraging support for the use of PS in treatment of dementia and cognitive issues (Richter et al., 2010; Vakhapova et al., 2010, 2014).

Although the most common side effects are mild, nutraceuticals are not without the potential to produce significant adverse effects, most notably with tryptophan and 5-HTP as well as SJW. As a result, careful administration and monitoring of such medicines, particularly when combined with other medications, is strongly advised. Care should also be taken in treating individuals with bipolar depression, so as to prevent cycling to mania. Typically, co-administration with mood stabilizers is a good preventive strategy that can be used with any natural antidepressants (Mischoulon & Iovieno, 2019).

Many intriguing future directions exist in the field of nutraceuticals for depression and cognition. First, as noted throughout this chapter, there have been a limited number of contemporary studies of several nutrient-based medicines (e.g., 5-HTP and tryptophan as well as vitamins C and D, creatine, and amino acids) and herbal medicines (e.g., *Rhodiola rosea*) for depression as well as agents for cognition (e.g., PS). As such, methodologically rigorous examination of such medicines could prove beneficial. Second, future work should consider examining the effects of nutraceuticals on different severity levels of depression. As Sarris and colleagues (2016) suggested, it may behoove prescribers to consider whether the potential risks outweigh the benefits of nutraceuticals for those with mild depression. Moreover, it may be valuable to examine the extent to which nutraceuticals may augment the nonpharmacological types of treatments for those with depression and cognitive concerns (e.g., psychological treatments). In sum, there appears to be valuable existing work on the use of nutraceuticals for depression and on the potential for continued development and growth.

REFERENCES

Akhondzadeh, S., Noroozian, M., Mohammadi, M., Ohadinia, S., Jamshidi, A. H., & Khani, M. (2003). *Melissa officinalis* extract in the treatment of patients with mild to moderate Alzheimer's disease: A double blind, randomised, placebo controlled trial. *Journal of Neurology, Neurosurgery and Psychiatry, 74*(7), 863–866.

Al-Karawi, D., Al Mamoori, D. A., & Tayyar, Y. (2016). The role of curcumin administration in patients with major depressive disorder: Mini meta-analysis of clinical trials. *Phytotherapy Research, 30*(2), 175–183.

Alpert, J. E., Mischoulon, D., Rubenstein, G. E., Bottonari, K., Nierenberg, A. A., & Fava, M. (2002). Folinic acid (Leucovorin) as an adjunctive treatment for SSRI-refractory depression. *Annals of Clinical Psychiatry, 14*(1), 33–38.

American Psychiatric Association. (2013). *Diagnostic and statistical manual of mental disorders* (5th ed.). Arlington, VA: Author.

Apaydin, E. A., Maher, A. R., Shanman, R., Booth, M. S., Miles, J. N., Sorbero, M. E., et al. (2016). A systematic review of St. John's wort for major depressive disorder. *Systematic Reviews, 5*(1), 148.

Ballard, C. G., O'Brien, J. T., Reichelt, K., & Perry, E. K. (2002). Aromatherapy as a safe and effective treatment for the management of agitation in severe dementia: The results of a double-blind, placebo-controlled trial with Melissa. *Journal of Clinical Psychiatry, 63*(7), 553–558.

Birks, J., & Evans, J. G. (2009). *Ginkgo biloba* for cognitive impairment and dementia. *Cochrane Database of Systematic Reviews*, Issue 2, CD003120.

Canevelli, M., Adali, N., Kelaiditi, E., Cantet, C., Ousset, P. J., & Cesari, M. (2014). Effects of *Gingko biloba* supplementation in Alzheimer's disease patients receiving cholinesterase inhibitors: Data from the ICTUS study. *Phytomedicine, 21*(6), 888–892.

Dai, C. X., Hu, C. C., Shang, Y. S., & Xie, J. (2018). Role of *Ginkgo biloba* extract as an adjunctive treatment of elderly patients with depression and on the expression of serum S100B. *Medicine, 97*(39), e12421.

Darbinyan, V., Aslanyan, G., Amroyan, E., Gabrielyan, E., Malmström, C., Panossian, A. (2007). Clinical trial of *Rhodiola rosea L.* extract SHR-5 in the treatment of mild to moderate depression. *Nordic Journal of Psychiatry, 61*(5), 343–348.

Freund-Levi, Y., Eriksdotter-Jönhagen, M., Cederholm, T., Basun, H., Faxen-Irving, G., Garlind, A., et al. (2006). Omega-3 fatty acid treatment in 174 patients with mild to moderate Alzheimer disease: OmegAD study: a randomized double-blind trial. *Archives of Neurology, 63*, 1402–1408.

Godfrey, P. S. A., Toone, B. K., Bottiglien, T., Laundy, M., Reynolds, E. H., Carney, M. W. P., et al. (1990). Enhancement of recovery from psychiatric illness by methylfolate. *Lancet, 336*(8712), 392–395.

Grima N. A., Pase, M. P., Macpherson, H., & Pipingas, A. (2012). The effects of multivitamins on cognitive performance: A systematic review and meta-analysis. *Journal of Alzheimer's Disease, 29*(3), 561–569.

Hardy, M. L., Coulter, I., Morton, S. C., Favreau, J., Venuturupalli, S., Chiappeli, F., et al. (2002). *S-adenosyl-L-methionine for treatment of depression, osteoarthritis, and liver disease* (Evidence Reports/Technology Assessments, 64). Rockville, MD: Agency for Healthcare Research and Quality.

Hausenblas, H. A., Saha, D., Dubyak, P. J., & Anton, S. D. (2013). Saffron (*Crocus sativus L.*) and major depressive disorder: A meta-analysis of randomized clinical trials. *Journal of Integrative Medicine, 11*, 377–383.

Herrschaft, H., Nacu, A., Likhachev, S., Sholomov, I., Hoerr, R., & Schlaefke, S. (2012). *Ginkgo biloba* extract EGb 761® in dementia with neuropsychiatric features: A randomised, placebo-controlled trial to confirm the efficacy and safety of a daily dose of 240 mg. *Journal of Psychiatric Research, 46*(6), 716–723.

Ihl, R., Bachinskaya, N., Korczyn, A. D., Vakhapova, V., Tribanek, M., Hoerr, R., et al. (2011). Efficacy and safety of a once-daily formulation of *Ginkgo biloba* extract EGb 761 in dementia with neuropsychiatric features: A randomized controlled trial. *International Journal of Geriatric Psychiatry, 26*(11), 1186–1194.

Iovieno, N., Dalton, E. D., Fava, M., & Mischoulon, D. (2011). Second-tier natural antidepressants: Review and critique. *Journal of Affective Disorders, 130*(3), 343–357.

Kennedy, D. O., Dodd, F. L., Robertson, B. C., Okello, E. J., Reay, J. L., Scholey, A. B., et al. (2011). Monoterpenoid extract of sage (*Salvia lavandulaefolia*) with cholinesterase inhibiting properties improves cognitive performance and mood in healthy adults. *Journal of Psychopharmacology, 25*(8), 1088–1100.

Levine, J., Barak, Y., Gonzalves, M., Szor, H., Elizur, A., Kofman, O., et al. (1995). Double-blind, controlled trial of inositol treatment of depression. *American Journal of Psychiatry, 152*(5), 792–793.

Linde, K., Berner, M. M., & Kriston L. (2008). St John's wort for major depression. *Cochrane Database of Systematic Reviews,* Issue 4, CD000448.

Mao, J. J., Xie, S. X., Zee, J., Soeller, I., Li, Q. S., Rockwell, K., et al. (2015). *Rhodiola rosea* versus sertraline for major depressive disorder: A randomized placebo-controlled trial. *Phytomedicine, 22*(3), 394–399.

Mathias, I. S., & Mischoulon, D. (2015). Natural remedies for mental health and aging. In H. Lavretsky, M. Sajatovic, & C. Reynolds III (Eds.), *Complementary and integrative therapies for mental health and aging.* New York: Oxford University Press.

Mischoulon, D. (2018). Popular herbal and natural remedies used in psychiatry. *Focus, 16*(1), 2–11.

Mischoulon, D., & Iovieno, N. (2019). Supplements and natural remedies for depression. In B. Shapero, D. Mischoulon, & C. Cusin (Eds.), *The Massachusetts General Hospital guide to depression—new treatment insights and options* (pp. 195–209). New York: Springer.

Mischoulon, D., Price, L. H., Carpenter, L. L., Tyrka, A. R., Papakostas, G. I., Baer, L., et al. (2014). A double-blind, randomized, placebo-controlled clinical trial of S-adenosyl-l-methionine (SAMe) vs. escitalopram in major depressive disorder. *Journal of Clinical Psychiatry, 75*(4), 370–376.

Mukai, T., Kishi, T., Matsuda, Y., & Iwata, N. (2014). A meta-analysis of inositol for depression and anxiety disorders. *Human Psychopharmacology: Clinical and Experimental, 29*(1), 55–63.

Ng, Q. X., Koh, S. S. H., Chan, H. W. & Ho, C. Y. X. (2017). Clinical use of curcumin in depression: A meta-analysis. *Journal of the American Medical Directors Association, 18,* 503–508.

Panza, F., Frisardi, V., Capurso, C., D'introno, A., Colacicco, A. M., Imbimbo, B. P., et al. (2010). Late-life depression, mild cognitive impairment, and dementia: possible continuum? *American Journal of Geriatric Psychiatry, 18*(2), 98–116.

Papakostas, G. I., & Ionescu, D. F. (2015). Towards new mechanisms: An update on therapeutics for treatment-resistant major depressive disorder. *Molecular Psychiatry, 20*(10), 1142–1150.

Papakostas, G. I., Shelton, R. C., Zajecka, J. M., Etemad, B., Rickels, K., Clain, A., et al. (2012). L-methylfolate as adjunctive therapy for SSRI-resistant major depression: Results of two randomized, double-blind, parallel-sequential trials. *American Journal of Psychiatry, 169*(12), 1267–1274.

Rapaport, M. H., Nierenberg, A. A., Schettler, P. J., Kinkead, B., Cardoos, A., Walker, R., et al. (2016). Inflammation as a predictive biomarker for response to omega-3 fatty acids in major depressive disorder: A proof-of-concept study. *Molecular Psychiatry, 21*(1), 71–79.

Reay J. L., Scholey, A. B., & Kennedy, D. O. (2010). *Panax ginseng* (G115) improves aspects of working memory performance and subjective ratings of calmness in healthy young adults. *Human Psychopharmacology, 25*(6), 467–471.

Richter, Y., Herzog, Y., Cohen, T., & Steinhart, Y. (2010). The effect of phosphatidylserine-containing omega-3 fatty acids on memory abilities in subjects with subjective memory complaints: A pilot study. *Clinical Interventions in Aging, 5,* 313–316.

Rush, A. J. (2007). STAR*D: what have we learned? *American Journal of Psychiatry, 164*(2), 201–204.

Sahraian, A., Jelodar, S., Javid, Z., Mowla, A., & Ahmadzadeh, L. (2016). Study the effects of saffron on depression and lipid profiles: A double blind comparative study. *Asian Journal of Psychiatry, 22,* 174–176.

Sarris, J. (2018). Herbal medicines in the treatment of psychiatric disorders: 10-year updated review. *Phytotherapy Research, 32*(7), 1147–1162.

Sarris, J., Byrne, G. J., Bousman, C., Stough, C., Murphy, J., MacDonald, P., et al. (2018). Adjunctive S-adenosylmethionine (SAMe) in treating non-remittent major depressive disorder: An 8-week double-blind, randomized, controlled trial. *European Neuropsychopharmacology, 28*(10), 1126–1136.

Sarris, J., Murphy, J., Mischoulon, D., Papakostas, G. I., Fava, M., Berk, M., et al. (2016). Adjunctive nutraceuticals for depression: A systematic review and meta-analyses. *American Journal of Psychiatry, 173*(6), 575–587.

Scholey, A. B., Tildesley, N. T., Ballard, C. G., Wesnes, K. A., Tasker, A., Perry, E. K., et al. (2008). An extract of *Salvia* (sage) with anticholinesterase properties improves memory and attention in healthy older volunteers. *Psychopharmacology, 198*(1), 127–139.

Shahmansouri, N., Farokhnia, M., Abbasi, S. H., Kassaian, S. E., Tafti, A. A. N., Gougol, A., et al. (2014). A randomized, double-blind, clinical trial comparing the efficacy and safety of Crocus sativus L. with fluoxetine for improving mild to moderate depression in post percutaneous coronary intervention patients. *Journal of Affective Disorders, 155*, 216–222.

Sharma, A., Gerbarg, P., Bottiglieri, T., Massoumi, L., Carpenter, L. L., Lavretsky, H., et al. (2017). S-Adenosylmethionine (SAMe) for neuropsychiatric disorders: A clinician-oriented review of research. *Journal of Clinical Psychiatry, 78*(6), e656–e667.

Snitz, B. E., O'meara, E. S., Carlson, M. C., Arnold, A. M., Ives, D. G., Rapp, S. R., et al. (2009). *Ginkgo biloba* for preventing cognitive decline in older adults: A randomized trial. *JAMA, 302*(24), 2663–2670.

Sorensen, H. S., & Sonne, J. (1996). A double-masked study of the effects of ginseng on cognitive functions. *Current Therapeutic Research, 57*, 959–968.

Tan, M. S., Yu, J. T., Tan, C. C., Wang, H. F., Meng, X. F., Wang, C., et al. (2015). Efficacy and adverse effects of ginkgo biloba for cognitive impairment and dementia: A systematic review and meta-analysis. *Journal of Alzheimer's Disease, 43*(2), 589–603.

Tildesley, N. T. J., Kennedy, D. O., Perry, E. K., Ballard, C. G., Wesnes, K. A., & Scholey, A. B. (2005). Positive modulation of mood and cognitive performance following administration of acute doses of *Salvia lavandulaefolia* essential oil to healthy young volunteers. *Physiology and Behavior, 83*(5), 699–709.

Vakhapova, V., Cohen, T., Richter, Y., Herzog, Y., & Korczyn, A. D. (2010). Phosphatidylserine containing ω-3 fatty acids may improve memory abilities in non-demented elderly with memory complaints: A double-blind placebo-controlled trial. *Dementia and Geriatric Cognitive Disorders, 29*(5), 467–474.

Vakhapova, V., Cohen, T., Richter, Y., Herzog, Y., Kam, Y., & Korczyn, A. D. (2014). Phosphatidylserine containing omega-3 Fatty acids may improve memory abilities in nondemented elderly individuals with memory complaints: Results from an open-label extension study. *Dementia and Geriatric Cognitive Disorders, 38*(1–2), 39–45.

Vellas, B., Coley, N., Ousset, P. J., Berrut, G., Dartigues, J. F., Dubois, B., et al. (2012). Long-term use of standardised *Ginkgo biloba* extract for the prevention of Alzheimer's disease (GuidAge): A randomised placebo-controlled trial. *Lancet Neurology, 11*(10), 851–859.

Warden, D., Rush, A. J., Trivedi, M. H., Fava, M., & Wisniewski, S. R. (2007). The STAR*D Project results: A comprehensive review of findings. *Current Psychiatry Reports, 9*(6), 449–459.

World Health Organization. (2017). *Depression and other common mental disorders: Global health estimates*. Geneva: Author.

Yu, J. J., Pei, L. B., Zhang, Y., Wen, Z. Y., & Yang, J. L. (2015). Chronic supplementation of curcumin enhances the efficacy of antidepressants in major depressive disorder: A randomized, double-blind, placebo-controlled pilot study. *Journal of Clinical Psychopharmacology, 35*(4), 406–410.

Zandi, P. P., Anthony, J. C., Khachaturian, A. S., Stone, S. V., Gustafson, D., Tschanz, J. T., et al. (2004). Reduced risk of Alzheimer disease in users of antioxidant vitamin supplements: The Cache County Study. *Archives of Neurology, 61*(1), 82–88.

CHAPTER 17

Evidence-Based
Psychotherapeutic Treatments
Adaptations for Neurocognitive Impairments

Melissa Milanovic
Heather McNeely
Aamna Qureshi
Margaret C. McKinnon
Katherine Holshausen

The past few decades have seen a rapid increase in the development of psychotherapies for major depressive disorder (MDD). The fast-paced evolution of this field may pose a challenge to clinicians, making it difficult to navigate which therapies to select for our patients. A guiding principle in the practice of clinical psychology is to use evidence-based practices when selecting treatment for patients. In basic terms, *evidence-based* refers to the fact that empirical studies used to examine the treatment have demonstrated that the treatment is effective (i.e., reduces symptoms). As such, evidence-based treatments (EBTs) are considered frontline treatments as they are supported by scientific evidence in their ability to reduce the severity of psychiatric symptoms. The use of EBTs is considered the best standard offered to patients as we can be sure the interventions are likely to alleviate their symptomology and improve their suffering. In this chapter, we outline an introduction to understanding EBTs and discuss several EBTs for depression. Furthermore, this chapter emphasizes how these therapies may be modified to better support clients with MDD who have neurocognitive deficits (see Bowie, Best, Tran, & Boyd, Chapter 18, this volume, for a detailed description of neurocognitive deficits in MDD). We also briefly comment on the role of medications as they affect neurocognition and the way in which these effects may impact psychotherapy. The goal of this chapter is to leave you with a nuanced understanding of different EBTs for MDD and how to adapt them in light of known neurocognitive deficits associated with MDD.

WHAT IS EVIDENCE-BASED PRACTICE AND WHY IS IT IMPORTANT?

Evidence-based practice (EBP) exists for the simple purpose of assisting with clinical decision making to improve patient well-being. EBP can perhaps be most clearly linked to a well-known definition by David Sackett: the "explicit and conscientious attempt to find the best available research evidence to assist health professionals to make the best decisions for their patients" (Sackett, Rosenberg, Gray, Haynes, & Richardson, 1996). As such, the pursuit of EBP entails an intentional effort to synthesize information from a number of sources to enable a thorough understanding of different practices and how they may inform our clinical practice both generally and on a case-by-case basis. This understanding allows for a true integration of clinical expertise with scientific evidence. Interestingly, one criticism of EBP is that it obscures the inherent complexity of clinical practice to a rule-based one-size-fits-all approach to psychotherapy; however, the intention of EBP is neither so grandiose nor so narrow. The goal of EBP is simply to advance the notion that clinicians ought to pause to consider how science can inform their practice to promote better outcomes for patients. The true utility of EBP is to bolster and harness the intersection of clinical expertise, professional training, science, and compassion to make informed decisions to optimize patient outcome. As such, this chapter reviews empirical findings for the purpose of providing scientific evidence to inform decision making.

A Primer on How to Evaluate Evidence

Anyone can learn to do EBP, although, like any skill, the ability to engage in it does need to be learned, practiced, and honed over time. Here we provide a brief overview of the mechanisms of the spirit of inquiry that forms the basis of EBP. Borrowing from the framework established for the teaching and learning of EBP (see Hoffmann, Bennett, & Del Mar, 2013), the steps can be distilled to those seen in Table 17.1.

EBTs FOR MDD

This chapter provides an overview of EBTs that have been scientifically evaluated and found to be effective in reducing symptoms of depression among individuals who have MDD. We focus on the EBTs with the most consistent and robust evidence base, including cognitive-behavioral therapy (CBT), problem-solving therapy (PST), behavioral activation (BA), mindfulness-based cognitive therapy (MBCT), brief psychodynamic therapy (BPT), and interpersonal psychotherapy (IPT). These therapies are also the first- and second-line psychotherapies advocated for use by international medical agencies, including the American Psychiatric Association, the Canadian Psychological Association, and the National Institute for Health and Care Excellence.

Cognitive-Behavioral Therapy

Cognitive-behavioral therapy has developed into the therapy of choice for many psychological disorders. It is based on both cognitive and behavioral theories in psychology,

TABLE 17.1. Steps to Critically Evaluate Scientific Evidence

Step 1 *Convert your information needs into an answerable clinical question (i.e., ask a question).*

- This step entails turning whatever it is you want to know into a specific question. The broader the question, the more information there will be to sort through to find your answer. In general, it is helpful to find a balance between being general and specific.
- *Too broad:* "Does cognitive-behavioral therapy decrease psychiatric symptoms?"
- *Too specific:* "In older adults living in the U.S. state of Michigan, with depression, what improvement in symptoms is expected after six sessions of cognitive-behavioral therapy?"
- *Just right:* "In adults with depression, when do symptoms start to remit while engaged in cognitive-behavioral therapy?"

Step 2 *Find the best evidence to answer your clinical question (i.e., access the information).*

The most efficient way to access evidence is by using online search engines that specifically include scientific material. For example, using a general search engine like Google would not return evidence-based results, whereas Google Scholar would. There are also several other scientific platforms that permit searching through online evidence-based resources (e.g., PsycINFO, Medline). This search can be a skill unto itself, and many libraries (public and academic) offer support to patrons to help with searching online databases.

Step 3 *Critically appraise the evidence for its validity, impact, and applicability (i.e., appraise the articles found).*

Once you've found evidence, you need to examine it to ensure its findings can be trusted, have clinical relevance, and can be applied to your patient. It is not safe to assume that all published studies are of equal quality (Antonakis, 2017; Ioannidis, 2005, 2016). According to Hoffman and colleagues (2013), this step can be attained by considering these aspects:

- *Internal validity:* Are the findings trustworthy? Can you believe them? If you consider the methods of the study, do they seem to reasonably capture the research question under study? Are the findings interpreted in a way that is consistent with the results in the context of the study?
- *Impact:* Are the findings clinically important? Generally, scientific research relies on statistics to examine numerical findings. It is important to note that statistically significant findings are not the same as clinically significant findings. There can be instances wherein a finding may be statistically significant but not clinically significant (e.g., a [fictional] study may find that drinking 20 glasses of water per day for 60 days decreases depressive symptoms by .00001%. In a large sample size, this may be a statistically significant finding but may not be clinically significant. At this point, you may wish to consider alternative treatments that are more effective and less of a nuisance to the patient).
- *Applicability:* Are the findings directly relevant to your patient, or is your patient so different (e.g., diagnosis, age, gender) that the findings cannot reasonably be applied to your patient?

Step 4 *Integrate the evidence with clinical expertise; the patient's values, preferences, and circumstances; and information from the practice context (i.e., apply the information).*

Synthesize your clinical knowledge, patient-specific variables (e.g., values, preferences, past experiences), the clinical context (e.g., hospital policies), and the evidence you have found to arrive at an evidence-based decision.

Step 5 *Evaluate the effectiveness and efficiency with which Steps 1–4 were carried out, and consider different ways to improve performance over time (i.e., audit).*

The final step entails reflecting on the search and integration process, and considering how to improve and make changes in the future as you hone your skill of engaging in EBP. You may reflect on various aspects of the process, asking yourself questions such as:

- "Am I using the most effective search terms?"
- "Is there a different way to phrase my initial question? Is it too broad or too narrow?"
- "Am I evaluating whether my new practices are impacting patient care in some measurable way?"

targeting cognitions that influence how one feels and behaves, and external contingencies that shape behavior (Beck, Rush, Shaw, & Emery, 1979; Early & Grady, 2017). As a feature of treatment, patients are often given homework assignments to complete throughout the course of therapy to practice skills related to their treatment (Tredget, 2001). The essential notion behind homework is to generalize skills learned in therapy to the patient's daily life.

The basic cognitive model posits that dysfunctional thinking underlies psychological difficulties. In other words, emotional problems do not persist on their own; they are maintained by the cognitions (thoughts) and actions (behaviors) linked to them (Beck, 2011; Beck et al., 1979). As people learn to evaluate their thinking and frame perceptions and beliefs in a more realistic manner, they experience improvement in their mood and associated behaviors. An essential point of psychoeducation in CBT is to learn that thoughts are not facts and that thoughts are malleable in the face of evidence (both internally, such as memories and experiences, and externally, such as one's environment). Depending on the context, patient needs, and clinical judgment, deeper processing of cognitions may also be indicated in order to promote longer-term improvements in mood and behavior. The focus of this work is often based on the Beck cognitive triad (or negative triad) including irrational beliefs about the self, others, and the world. Modification of these core beliefs tends to promote more enduring change because the distorted infrastructure of beliefs that underlie inaccurate automatic thoughts shift and allow for change in one's overall experience of being oneself, interacting with others, and navigating the world (Beck, 2011).

Bieling, McCabe, and Antony (2006) outlined a comprehensive 17-session group CBT protocol derived from a combination of sources, including Beck and colleagues' (1979) influential work and Greenberger and Padesky's (1995) *Mind over Mood*, which is often recommended to patients as a companion manual the group. This protocol includes behavioral intervention via modification of activities to improve mood, as well as cognitive work at basic and deeper (i.e., core belief) levels of thought. Meta-analysis suggests that a varied number of group sessions are used in intervention work (e.g., Okumuru & Ichikura, 2014).

With regard to individual CBT, uncomplicated presentations of depression may be treated in only 6 to 14 sessions; 7 to 12 sessions appear to optimize effectiveness and to minimize dropout rates (Pinquart, Duberstein, & Lyness, 2007). However, some patients require 1 or 2 years of therapy to modify very rigid dysfunctional beliefs and patterns of behavior that contribute to their depression (Beck, 2011). For patients requiring longer-term therapy, often simply challenging automatic thoughts is insufficient to cause change in depressive symptoms. Such patients often have rigid and inflexibly held core beliefs that require longer-term CBT in order to achieve symptom improvement.

Problem-Solving Therapy

Problem-solving therapy is a CBT-informed treatment with a focus on training in constructive problem-solving skills and attitudes (D'Zurilla & Nezu, 2010). The aim of PST is to enhance the patient's ability to cope more effectively with stress-inducing problems in daily life. Effective coping may involve improving the situation (e.g., resolving a conflict or eliminating unpleasant conditions) and/or lessening emotional distress generated by a situation (e.g., acceptance, finding the silver lining in the problem, reducing physical tension; D'Zurilla & Nezu, 2010). The PST approach emphasizes training in a positive problem orientation and in four major problem-solving skills (i.e., problem definition and formulation, generation of alternative solutions, decision making, and implementation and verification of solutions; D'Zurilla & Nezu, 2010).

Effectiveness of CBT

Since the initial outcome study published in 1977 (Rush, Beck, Kovacs, & Hollon, 1977), CBT has undergone notable empirical testing and is undeniably considered to be an EBT. Indeed, a conservative estimate from 2011 suggested that CBT had over 500 outcome studies demonstrating its effectiveness (Beck, 2011). CBT is the most researched treatment for depression (Cuijpers et al., 2013). Initial meta-analyses demonstrated that CBT was superior to no treatment for individuals with depression (Dobson, 1989; Miller & Berman, 1983), and this continues to be true concerning control groups (Cuijpers et al., 2013). Interestingly, there also does not appear to be any outcome differences based on format (individual, group, guided self-help) or definition of depression (diagnostic interview or self-report). A related and not surprising consideration is that dropout rates may be higher for group relative to individual therapy (Pinquart et al., 2007). CBT appears to be equally effective for younger people, adults, and older adults (Dobson, 1989; Kingdon & Dimech, 2008) and may be especially well suited to populations where antidepressants would not be best practice (e.g., children and adolescents; Maneeton, 2012).

Over time, while some studies have found that CBT is superior to other psychotherapies (e.g., see a review by Kingdon & Dimech, 2008), recent meta-analyses suggest that the effects of CBT are comparable to BA, IPT, and PST (Cuijpers et al., 2013). However, there may be reason to believe that CBT is superior to nondirective supportive therapy and psychodynamic therapy when there is close adherence to Beck's procedures (Cuijpers et al., 2013). Concerning its relation with pharmacology, there are conflicting findings of the efficacy of CBT over antidepressants (Butler, Chapman, Forman, & Beck, 2006). Some meta-analyses have found that CBT and pharmacology are equally efficacious (Cuijpers et al., 2013; DeRubeis, Gelfand, Tang, & Simons, 1999), whereas previous meta-analyses found CBT to be more effective than antidepressants (Dobson, 1989; Gloaguen, Cottraux, Cucherat, & Blackburn, 1998). A clear finding is that the combination of CBT *and* pharmacotherapy is superior to pharmacotherapy alone (Cuijpers, van Straten, Warmerdam, & Andersson, 2009) and that CBT appears to be more effective for longer-term outcomes than antidepressants (Dobson et al., 2008; Vittengl, Clark, Dunn, & Jarrett, 2007). Indeed, Zhang, Zhang, Zhang, Jin, and Jhang (2018) observe that employment of CBT when in a remitted state appears to reduce risk of relapse. This is an especially important consideration given evidence that patients have a strong preference for psychotherapy over continual antidepressants (Kocsis et al., 2009; Raue, Schulberg, Heo, Klimstra, & Bruce, 2009).

Given the relative success of CBT as an EBT coupled with evidence demonstrating its cost-effectiveness (Brettschneider et al., 2015), there has been a proliferation of CBT in different settings and platforms. Much of the evidence on the effectiveness of CBT has taken place in specialized settings, and a recent meta-analysis demonstrated similar findings in primary care settings (Twomey, O'Reilly, & Byrne, 2015). Adaptations to online platforms are an attempt to offset known accessibility-based barriers (Kessler, 2012). Therapist-delivered online CBT has been shown to be superior to treatment as usual in reducing depressive symptoms (Andersson, 2010; Gerhards et al., 2010). Similarly, self-help, telephone, computerized, and mobile app formats of CBT have also shown prom-ise (Andrews, Cuijpers, Craske, McEvoy, & Titov, 2010; Bower, Richards, & Lovell, 2001; Mohr, Vella, Hart, Heckman, & Simon, 2008; Watts et al., 2013). These findings suggest that CBT has robust and reliable effects in improving depressive symptomatology across a vast number of settings and platforms.

Meta-analyses provide support of the efficacy of PST in reducing depressive symp-tomatology (Bell & D'Zurilla, 2009; Cuijpers, van Straten, & Warmerdam, 2007), with effect sizes comparable to those found for other psychological treatments of depression (Cuijpers, de Wit, Kleiboer, Karyotaki, & Ebert, 2018).

Does Engagement in CBT Affect Neurocognition?

Due to the nature of the approach, CBT is thought to rely on certain top-down cognitive skills for accurate appraisal and modification of thoughts (i.e., metacognition) and behav-ior throughout treatment. As such, executive functioning (e.g., inhibitory control, emo-tion regulation) and attention are considered to be the primary neurocognitive domains related to CBT (Groves et al., 2015). Executive functioning skills are also employed in CBT as patients can be required to monitor their physiological, behavioral, and cognitive symptoms. Despite this theoretically grounded rationale for possible change in neuro-cognition, limited evidence exists to support neuropsychological changes following CBT. Indeed, a major criticism of current psychotherapies for depression suggests that they do not adequately address neuropsychological impairment (Porter et al., 2014).

The limited studies addressing this gap in knowledge are discussed here. Groves and colleagues (2015) found no improvement in executive functioning or attention following 12 weeks of CBT in a depressed sample, though they did observe decreases in depres-sive symptomatology. Furthermore, by extension, changes in symptoms were unrelated to changes in neurocognition. Similar findings were reported in a study examining the effects of CBT and schema therapy on neurocognition, whereby depressive symptoms were significantly reduced, but there were no notable changes in neuropsychological impairment (Porter et al., 2016). These findings are somewhat perplexing as metacognition is related to executive functioning (Kraft, Jonassen, Stiles, & Landrø, 2017), and so one might anticipate changes following CBT. In a similar vein, a recent randomized controlled trial (RCT) failed to find improvements in verbal learning and memory following random-ization to 16 weeks of CBT-C (emphasizing pleasurable low-energy exercise during BA), CBT-E (emphasizing exercise), or a passive wait-list control group (Dannehl, Rief, & Eute-neuer, 2019). In contrast to the nonsignificant theme of the aforementioned findings, one study found improvements in attentional biases following 10 sessions of CBT or a positive psychology intervention (Vazquez et al., 2018). Differences in attention were captured via eye-tracking equipment whereby both groups demonstrated a significant reduction in the total time of fixations looking at negative information (i.e., sad/angry faces) and a signifi-cant increase in the total time of fixations viewing positive information (i.e., happy faces).

Problem-solving approaches in combination with compensatory strategies and care-giver participation have been shown to be helpful for significantly cognitively impaired older adults with depression (Kiosses et al., 2015). PST helps patients engage in the thoughtful process of identifying goals, considering alternative strategies toward achiev-ing goals, and weighing the potential benefits of different strategies (Nezu & Perri, 1989).

A recent investigation by Mackin and colleagues (2014) found improved performance on a task of executive functioning, with a significant information-processing speed component in older adults with late-life depression following PST, though the effects of PST on cognition were no different from those observed following supportive therapy. Taken together, these findings suggest that there is limited concrete evidence that CBT incites change in neurocognition. They also indicate that future studies ought to continue to examine this line of inquiry and consider using behavioral indicators of neurocognitive change (e.g., attentional changes evident via eye tracking).

Behavioral Activation

Behavioral activation is a structured treatment for depression, with the general aim of assisting patients to approach, rather than avoid, activities in daily life. The main tenet of BA is that what patients do has a positive impact on their feelings (Veale, 2008). Therefore, avoidant behavior leads to a significant reduction in adaptive activities that can produce a sense of gratification for the individual and would otherwise reinforce engagement in these activities. Based on the premise that increasing one's activity can lead to positive affect and a decrease in depressive symptoms, the fundamental goal in BA is to increase the patients' activation, and thereby the likelihood and frequency of positive experiences in their lives (Martell, Addis, & Jacobson, 2001). Throughout the duration of BA, the patient and therapist focus on processes that are inhibiting the patient's activation in daily life, such as escape and avoidance behaviors.

Unlike CBT, the behavioral approach directs attention to the functional analysis of the patient's behavior (to identify the antecedents and consequences of their behavioral responses) and to the techniques for addressing avoidance. Hence, the principal strategy of change in BA involves working with patients to identify avoidance patterns, developing a functional analytic style of understanding one's own behavior, and taking an action-based approach to foster changes in overt behavior (Hopko, Lejuez, Ruggiero, & Eifert, 2003). Through behavioral change, patients gain improvements in mood and often in their cognitions as well.

As with other psychotherapies, BA is highly idiographic. Throughout BA, the therapist assists the patient in planning steps toward activation until the patient can become their own coach, identifying avoidance behaviors and adapting daily life toward approach behaviors. For patients who may be fairly active in daily life but experience great difficulty with ruminative thinking, BA can focus on structuring time around pleasurable activities and focusing one's attention away from ruminative thoughts and instead, toward the experience of enjoyable activities. BA as a protocolized approach was introduced by Martell and colleagues (2001), typically following a 20- to 24-session protocol. BA exists as a stand-alone treatment, though the techniques of this therapy are also incorporated into CBT for depression.

Effectiveness of BA

Behavioral activation emerged from the behaviorist perspective on treatment. Lewinsohn, Biglan, and Zeiss (1976) developed the first behavioral treatment for depression. While several promising trials were initially conducted, in the 1980s, cognitive therapy (CT) developed by Beck and his colleagues dominated the research landscape on therapies for depression. In an attempt to determine the value of components of cognitive therapy, Jacobson and colleagues (1996) conducted a study wherein they randomized patients with depression into three groups: activity scheduling (a primary component of BA); activity scheduling with cognitive challenges to automatic thoughts; and activity scheduling with cognitive challenges to automatic thoughts, core beliefs and assumptions (full CT). The authors found no statistically significant differences between the groups, either in acute treatment of depression or in prevention of relapse across 2-year follow-up (Gortner, Gollan, Dobson, & Jacobson, 1998; Jacobson et al., 1996; Martell, Dimidjian, & Herman-Dunn, 2013). Despite opposition to the findings, in particular, concerns regarding the quality of the CT condition and the lack of a control condition (Jacobson & Gortner, 2000), this investigation revitalized interest in the behavioral approach and the need to replicate findings.

In 2006, Dimidjian and colleagues published a study comparing BA to CT and antidepressants (paroxetine). In the BA group, therapists used techniques similar to those by Jacobson and colleagues (1996) in addition to assessing and treating avoidance behaviors, establishing regularized routine, and implementing behavioral strategies to distract from rumination. For people with severe depression, BA was found to be as effective as antidepressants and significantly more effective than CT at reducing depressive symptoms. For those with lower severity depression, there were no differences among treatments to treat depressive symptoms. BA was superior to medication in keeping patients longer in treatment. Those who responded to antidepressants relapsed at a greater rate when withdrawn from medications than those who had BA or CT (Dimidjian et al., 2006; Dobson et al., 2008).

A number of early meta-analyses conducted on BA suggest the comparable effectiveness of BA to CT and CBT (Cuijpers et al., 2007; Cuijpers, van Straten, Andersson, & van Oppen, 2008; Ekers, Richards, & Gilbody, 2008; Mazzucchelli, Kane, & Rees, 2009). A recent meta-analysis by Ekers and colleagues (2014) found that BA was superior to controls and antidepressant medication. Evidence for the effectiveness of BA extend to group-based administration, with Chan and colleagues' (2017) meta-analysis including seven randomized control trials finding evidence of relieving depressive symptoms for moderate to severe depression from group-based BA. While the collective results indicate the effectiveness of BA, limitations cited in these studies include generally small sample sizes, constraints with control groups, short follow-up times, and heterogeneity in intervention length and course outlines across investigations. Still needed in the BA literature are dismantling studies to better isolate intervention components of BA to determine active ingredients that drive depressive symptom change, and follow-up studies to assess duration effects of this treatment. Additionally, greater homogeneity in BA trials will enhance the robustness of the meta-analyses conducted.

Does Engagement in BA Affect Neurocognition?

The effects of BA on neurocognitive functioning is rather sparse. It has been found that following BA, the prefrontal regions in the brain of individuals with depression may become more efficient in recruiting cognitive resources in order to disengage from sad stimuli (Dichter, Felder, & Smoski, 2010). The authors' findings support the hypothesis that symptom remission due to BA can accompany a concomitant decrease in the magnitude of prefrontal activation needed to successfully respond to cognitive control stimuli in sad contexts. A brief course of BA has also resulted in functional changes in brain structures that mediate responses to reward both during reward anticipation and reward feedback (Dichter et al., 2009).

Physical exercise, a type of activity often considered in BA, has increasingly become recognized as an effective strategy for reducing depressive symptoms (Rethorst, Wipfli, & Landers, 2009; Rimer et al., 2012; Trivedi et al., 2011). Aerobic fitness is thought to impact neurocognition by altering brain structure and function (Dishman et al., 2006). Initial evidence in depression, though limited by small sample size, suggests acute improvement in attention and inhibitory control after one session of moderate intensity exercise in depressed patients (Kubesch et al., 2003; Vasques, Moraes, Silveira, Deslandes, & Laks, 2011). In contrast, Hoffman and colleagues (2008) did not find benefits on neuropsychological tests (executive function, verbal memory, verbal fluency, and working memory) of exercise compared to placebo after 4 months of treatment in depressed patients. However, exercise participants did perform better than those assigned to an antidepressant (sertraline) on tests of executive functioning. Khatri and colleagues (2001) saw exercise-related changes for memory and executive functioning, but not attention/concentration or psychomotor speed following 4 months of aerobic exercise among depressed older adults. Greer, Grannemann, Chansard, Karim, and Trivedi (2015) found a dose-dependent effect of exercise among depressed individuals who reported cognitive impairment following only a partial response to initial treatment with a selective serotonin reuptake inhibitor. After 12 weeks of treatment, a high dose of exercise (16 kilocalories per kilogram of body weight per week) yielded improved spatial working memory, while decreased spatial working memory and set-shifting outcomes were observed in low-dose exercisers (4 kilocalories per kilogram of body weight per week). Both high- and low-dose exercisers demonstrated improved psychomotor speed, attention, visual memory and spatial planning.

BA might be particularly amenable to neurocognitively impaired individuals with depression, as techniques are largely action-based as opposed to cognitively focused as in other treatments such as CT and CBT. Thus, BA may be less taxing and more palpable for those who experience neurocognitive impairment, though this has yet to be empirically determined.

Mindfulness-Based Cognitive Therapy

Mindfulness-based cognitive therapy is a variation of CBT and entails a psychosocial group-based relapse prevention program designed for patients in remission but at high risk for depressive relapse or recurrence (Segal, Williams, & Teasdale, 2002). MBCT is based on empirical and theoretical work showing that depressive relapse is associated with the recurrence of maladaptive thinking, feeling, and behaving (e.g., avoidance behaviors and self-criticism), which can perpetuate and maintain relapse of depression.

The underlying model of MBCT specifies that previously depressed patients have greater vulnerability to states of low mood and reactivation of negative and ruminative thinking that is similar to those of prior episodes. Such reactivation can cause depression to reoccur (Segal et al., 2006; Segal, Williams, Teasdale, & Gemar, 1996; Teasdale, 1988; Teasdale, Segal, & Williams, 1995). Risk of relapse in recurrent MDD has been found to be reduced if patients can learn to be aware of their negative thinking patterns reactivated by negative mood state, and in turn, adaptively disengage from depressive rumination (Nolen-Hoeksema, 1991). MBCT was developed to address vulnerability to depression relapse by changing the patient's relationship with negative thinking patterns, mood shifts, and attitudes.

MBCT is an eight-session weekly program, involving up to 12 recovered recurrently depressed patients per group. In MBCT, Kabat-Zinn's (1990) mindfulness-based stress reduction is combined with components of Beck's CBT (Beck et al., 1979). Unlike CBT, MCBT does not emphasize changing thought content or identifying assumptions and core beliefs related to depression. Rather, MBCT takes a preventive symptom recurrence approach (Teasdale et al., 1995), and patients learn to distance themselves from the thoughts, feelings, and physical sensations they experience. In doing so, MBCT encourages attention to a specific present moment experience without critical analysis or judgment (Heeren, Van Broeck, & Philippot, 2009).

To target cognitive reactivation, in MBCT, mindfulness skills are used as a means for the patient to note distressing thoughts and feelings, and to cultivate acceptance and self-compassion to offset relapse risk (Segal, Williams, & Teasdale, 2002). Patients learn to adjust from a "doing mode" (i.e., thinking about the past and future and using these thoughts to guide efforts toward lessening discrepancies between current state and desired state) to a "being mode" (i.e., being fully present in the moment and accepting thoughts as mental events rather than factual information or directive). MBCT involves meditative practice during which patterns of thought (e.g., intrusive, negative) and associated judgments (e.g., "I should be better at this, I'll never learn") are highlighted. MBCT teaches the patient to give less authority and weight to self-judgment and blame, as perseveration on this can perpetuate depressive thinking. Instead, MBCT encourages responding in a compassionate way, observing the thinking pattern rather than having a reaction to it, thereby disengaging from unhelpful patterns of thinking (Feldman & Kuyken, 2011).

Effectiveness of MBCT

MBCT has been clinically shown to bolster recovery from depression and prevent relapse (Segal et al., 2002). Accumulating evidence suggests that MBCT yields additional benefit over treatment as usual or placebo for those who are vulnerable to relapse, including those with three or more prior episodes, those with earlier onset (Ma & Teasdale, 2004; Teasdale et al., 2000), those unable to achieve stable remission (Segal et al., 2010), those with a history of abuse or adversity (Ma & Teasdale, 2004), and those with a history of childhood trauma (Williams et al., 2014).

A systematic review and meta-analysis by Piet and Hougaard (2011) found that MBCT was associated with significant reduction in rates of depression relapse/recurrence compared with treatment as usual or placebo controls. A subanalysis in this investigation discovered that there was not a risk reduction for participants with only two episodes. Thus, MBCT was favored for only those who are at greatest risk of relapse as defined by three or more previous episodes. Similarly, a second systematic review and meta-analysis by Galante, Iribarren, and Pearce (2013) indicated that after 1 year of follow-up, patients with three or more previous episodes of depression treated with additive MBCT had on average 40% fewer relapses than patients receiving treatment as usual.

Investigations have also begun to show that MBCT may be effective not only for those in remission, but also for those currently experiencing symptomatic depression (Barnhofer et al., 2009; Eisendrath et al., 2008; Kenny & Williams, 2007; van Aalderen et al., 2012). MBCT has also been shown to reduce passive suicidal ideation among individuals with residual depressive symptoms (Forkmann et al., 2014). An adapted version of MBCT that combined traditional MBCT and Safety Planning Intervention (Stanley & Brown, 2012) demonstrated significant reductions in depressive symptoms as well as suicidal ideation among high suicide-risk psychiatric outpatients. Some studies have also shown that MBCT leads to relapse/recurrence rates comparable or superior to rates for patients with maintenance antidepressant medication. This suggests that MBCT could be an alternative course of maintenance to pharmacotherapy (Kuyken et al., 2008, 2015; Segal et al., 2010).

Does Engagement in MBCT Affect Neurocognition?

In MBCT, patients learn to challenge rumination through disengagement from thoughts, and there is evidence that development of metacognitive skills may facilitate this process. Teasdale and colleagues (2002) found that MBCT reduced relapse to major depression and resulted in a changed relationship to negative thoughts. In particular, the authors observed increased accessibility of metacognitive sets to negative thoughts and feelings in MBCT compared to treatment as usual. Hargus, Crane, Barnhofer, and Williams (2010) demonstrated that MBCT improved memory specificity and levels of meta-awareness compared to treatment as usual, both of which are modes of processing suggested to be maladaptive and linked to the relapse and persistence of depressive symptoms. The authors explain that these results suggest that mindfulness training allows patients to look back on memories of previous crises in a decentered and more detailed way, thereby permitting them to relate to these experiences more adaptively.

Van den Hurk and colleagues (2012) investigated the role of attention in the efficacy of MBCT through a RCT comparing MBCT to wait-list control patients. Despite clinical improvements in depressive symptoms, ruminative thinking, and mindfulness skills after MBCT, they found no improvements in specific components of attentional processing, which included alerting (achieving and maintaining an alert state), orienting (selecting information from sensory input), and executive attention (resolving conflict among responses; Fan, McCandliss, Sommer, Raz, & Posner, 2002). The authors suggested that clinical improvements seen after MBCT for recurrently depressed patients might not be primarily mediated through improved self-regulation of attention, but rather through the cultivation of an attitude characterized by openness and acceptance. Indeed, formerly depressed individuals show significant attentional bias for negative information and inhibition of positive information compared to controls (De Raedt et al., 2012). De Raedt and colleagues (2012) found that this pattern was altered following MBCT, wherein individuals showed reduced facilitation of attention for negative information and reduced inhibition of attention for positive information following treatment. They concluded that this finding was indicative of more open attention to all emotional information rather than selective attention to negative material and thoughts following MBCT.

Depressed individuals tend to recall overgeneralized autobiographical memories, which reinforces depressive rumination (van Vreeswijk & de Wilde, 2004). The effects of MBCT on autobiographical memory has been studied in two RCTs with depressed individuals to assess participants' recall of self-relevant past events following mindfulness treatment (Jermann et al., 2013; Williams, Teasdale, Segal, & Soulsby, 2000). While Jermann and colleagues (2013) did not find any differences in memory specificity following MBCT for patients with at least two previous episodes, Williams and colleagues (2000) reported that the treatment group showed a significantly reduced number of generic memories. It is possible that the sample reported upon in Jermann and colleagues did not observe differences in memory specificity as a result of the sample having not shown the expected relapse prevention effect (Bondolfi et al., 2010). Authors of a recent systematic review (Lao, Kissane, & Meadows, 2016) consider Williams and colleagues' study more robust. Thus, they concluded that evidence supports MBCT for improving memory specificity.

Cognitive flexibility was investigated by Jermann and colleagues (2013), who did not find differences in mental set shifting following MBCT versus treatment as usual groups. This finding contrasts with that of Shapero, Greenberg, Pedrelli, de Jong, and Desbordes (2018), who examined the effects of MBCT on subjective measures of cognitive flexibility, the ability to switch cognitive sets to adapt to changing demands in the environment (Dennis & Vander Wal, 2010), and cognitive impairment. They found that those who participated in MBCT exhibited improvements in overall self-reported cognitive flexibility and reduced cognitive deficits compared to those on a wait list. The cognitive improvements were related to reductions in depressive symptomatology. However, these findings are limited by small sample size limiting statistical power, lack of an active comparison group, utilization of subjective measures of cognition, and a subset of the sample having not met the full criteria for MDD.

The preponderance of research to date indicates the efficacy of MBCT for those at the greatest risk of relapse (i.e., those having had three or more previous episodes). In the remission phase, neurocognitive impairments persist (Hasselbalch, Knorr, & Kessing, 2011), and findings suggest that the neurocognitive function in patients with recurrent depression declines with each successive episode of depression (Basso & Bornstein, 1999; Stordal et al., 2004). Furthermore, neurocognitive impairment during depression is one of the factors predicting relapse or recurrence of MDD (Majer et al., 2004). Thus, MBCT delivered as a relapse management treatment should consider the possible effects on treatment and should plan for the presence of neurocognitive impairment, when working with clients, particularly those with greater recurrence of episodes.

Brief Psychodynamic Therapy

Brief psychodynamic therapy (also referred to as short-term psychodynamic therapy or brief dynamic therapy) focuses on identifying conflicts and unresolved issues related to dependence and independence, exploration of unconscious processes especially as these may emerge in the therapeutic relationship, and facilitation of insight for the patient

(Horowitz & Kaltreider, 1979; Rose & DelMaestro, 1990). While there are differences in the specific focus and content of BPT, common themes across formats typically include how predisposing experiences affect current well-being, the expression and resolution of emotional states, exploration of topics that patients may avoid (i.e., defenses), and creating conditions in which the patient develops insight (Gabbard & Bennet, 2006; Lewis, Dennerstein, & Gibbs, 2008; Luyten & Blatt, 2012). These aims are achieved by identifying patterns of conflict in past and current relationships and via the therapeutic relationship (Blagys & Hilsenroth, 2000; Cuijpers et al., 2008). While there is certainly some overlap with other psychotherapies, therapist competencies specific to psychodynamic therapy include one's ability to work with transference and countertransference, and the identification and skillset to work with defenses (Lemma, Roth, & Pilling, 2009).

Psychodynamic therapy is considered a "global therapy" because it considers the patient from a holistic perspective. This is unlike CBT approaches, which are considered to be "problem-based." Problem-based therapies hone in on reductions or elimination of specific symptoms of disorders, whereas global therapies, specifically psychodynamic therapy, aim to explore patients' needs, desires, and urges. The inherent assumption of psychodynamic therapy is predicated on psychodynamic theory, which suggests that psychiatric problems are rooted in unconscious patterns that began in childhood (Gabbard, 2009) and need to be identified and processed to allow resolution. Psychodynamic therapy has several components that define its utility in the treatment of MDD. According to Luyten, Mayes, Target, and Fonagy (2012), these specific elements include (1) a focus on the depressed patient's misrepresentations or cognitive affective schemas of self and others that influence misperceptions, thoughts, feelings, and actions, with an emphasis on the role of unconscious motivations and how these inadvertently maintain depressive symptoms; (2) an emphasis on the importance of a developmental perspective or analysis of developmental antecedents (Lemma et al., 2009), which promotes insight into the past by changing attitudes and emotions in the present; and (3) a person-centered (or "global") approach whereby depression is not viewed as inherently pathological in nature or distinct from other psychiatric disorders; depression is simply considered an indicator of a mismatch between a "wished-for state and an actual state of the self" (Luyten & Blatt, 2012, p. 114). Concerning duration, while the length of psychodynamic therapy has a wide range, meta-analyses and reviews evaluating BPT define it as ranging from 7 to 40 sessions (Abbass, Hancock, Henderson, & Kisely, 2006; Leichsenring, Rabung, & Leibing, 2004; Lewis et al., 2008). As such, BPT is an adapted shorter version of PT, focusing on similar goals and processes, whereby the outcome is concerned with the development of a more integrated whole that naturally alleviates depressive symptoms rather than directly targeting symptom relief.

Effectiveness of BPT

Numerous studies have demonstrated the effectiveness of psychodynamic therapy for depression (Abbass, Nowoweiski, Berneir, Tarzwell, & Beutel, 2014; Anderson & Lambert, 1995; Driessen et al., 2010; Gaston, Thompson, Gallagher, Cournoyer, & Gagnon, 1998; Shapiro et al., 1995). Several studies specifically focus on brief or short-term forms of psychodynamic therapy (Bressi, Porcellana, Marinaccio, Nocito, & Magri, 2010; Hilsenroth,

Defife, Blagys, & Ackerman, 2006). Meta-analyses demonstrate a significant initial reduction in depressive symptoms and maintenance of symptom alleviation at a 1-year-follow-up (Driessen et al., 2010; Luyten & Blatt, 2012; Shedler, 2010). Relative to other psychotherapies, evidence suggests that BPT has comparable outcomes. Most meta-analyses conclude that outcomes in MDD following BPT are on par with CBT (Barth et al., 2013; Cuijpers et al., 2008; Goldstone, 2017; Leichsenring, 2001; Leichsenring, Kruse, & Rabung, 2015), whereas a few (older) reviews demonstrate that BPT is inferior to CBT and behavioral activation (Dobson, 1989; Gloaguen et al., 1998). A consistent finding is that BPT is significantly better than treatment as usual and placebo/waitlist controls (Barth et al., 2013; Cuijpers et al., 2008; Maina, Forner, & Bogetto, 2005). In a review, Luyten and Blatt (2012) conclude that a substantial portion of individuals with depressive disorders do not improve following BPT, a portion size reported to be on par with other short-term/brief therapies (Koppers, Peen, Niekerken, Van, & Dekker, 2011). Luyten and Blatt also suggest that BPT is well suited to treating uncomplicated MDD, whereas complex mood disturbances coupled with personality disorders may be better served by long-term psychodynamic therapy or psychoanalysis.

Overall, there is a relatively contentious battle over whether psychodynamic therapy (and, by proxy, BPT) may be considered to be evidence-based. Critical reviews of the literature demonstrate that there are several notable criticisms of reviews and meta-analyses that pit psychodynamic therapy and CBT against one another. Taken together, both appear to be highly viable, reliable, and effective treatments for MDD. It would be of great benefit for future studies to more carefully examine which psychotherapies are most suited to different manifestations of MDD and the extent to which integrative practices using evidence-based modalities may suit clients based on idiographic case conceptualizations. Indeed, studies examining an integrative approach of CBT techniques with psychodynamic therapy have better patient-reported agreement on goals, tasks, and confident collaboration (Goldman, Hilsenroth, Owen, & Gold, 2013) and are associated with greater improvements in global symptomatology (Goldman, Hilsenroth, Gold, Owen, & Levy, 2018). These findings were recently replicated (Katz et al., 2019), suggesting a step in the right direction to identifying active ingredients across treatment modalities.

Does Engagement in BPT Affect Neurocognition?

The literature is somewhat sparse concerning the effects of BPT or psychodynamic therapy in inciting neurocognitive changes. Ajilchi, Nejati, Town, Wilson, and Abbass (2016) found that an intensive short-term dynamic psychotherapy (15 sessions on average) for depression resulted in significant improvements in executive functioning. These differences were relative to a wait-list control group and were evident immediately following completion of the intervention. While reductions in depressive symptoms were sustained 12 months posttreatment, the authors did not reassess executive functioning at the follow-up. It is therefore not known whether these changes resulted in long-term improvements in neurocognitive functioning. Another study examining the effects of long-term psychodynamic therapy on neurocognition found that depressed young adults demonstrated greater improvements on measures of working memory, processing speed, and executive functioning after 24 months of psychodynamic therapy (Bastos, Guimarães, & Trentini, 2013). Similarly, Yazigi and colleagues (2011) observed enhanced attention and processing speed at 1- and 2-year time points of a 2-year long-term psychodynamic therapy study. Taken together, the limited studies on psychodynamic therapy suggest that it may be associated with neurocognitive improvements, but more studies are needed, especially in the context of BPT, in order to expand upon the current studies outlined above.

Interpersonal Psychotherapy

Interpersoanl psychotherapy is a psychosocial treatment with an acute phase lasting 12–16 weeks. IPT builds on interpersonal theory and psychosocial research on depression (Klerman, Weissman, Rounsaville, & Chevron, 1984), establishing a practical link between the patient's mood and distressing life events that either trigger or follow from the onset of their mood disorder (Markowitz & Weissman, 2004). This therapy is based on the premise that depression often follows a disturbing change in one's interpersonal environment such as death of a loved one, struggles with a significant other, a geographic or career move, or physical illness. Furthermore, IPT acknowledges that regardless of cause, depression is always expressed within interpersonal relationships; thus, these relationships are crucial to explore in order to achieve symptom reduction. The role of IPT is to resolve disturbing life events, build social skills, and help organize the patient's life (Markowitz & Weissman, 2004). The solution of life problems provides a means of affecting change in depressive symptoms within the patient's interpersonal relationships.

In the initial phase of IPT, the therapist will elicit an "interpersonal inventory" through review of the patient's patterns in relationships, degree of intimacy capacity, as well as an evaluation of the patient's current state of relationships (Markowitz & Weissman, 2004). A formulation is generated using this information, and the therapist will work with the patient to draw links between the patient's experience of depression and their interpersonal issues, identifying areas wherein solving interpersonal problems might lead to improved mood. It is common in IPT to address the patient's assertiveness skills in relationships, as well as to encourage efficient expression of emotions and taking appropriate social risks (Markowitz & Weissman, 2004).

Effectiveness of IPT

Effectiveness of IPT for depression has been found since early investigations, such as that of Elkin and colleagues (1989) who found IPT to be statistically comparable to imipramine and better than placebo for severely depressed patients. In this study, IPT was compared to CBT, providing an initial suggestion of potential differential predictors of treatment outcome (Sotsky et al., 2006). Cuijpers and colleagues (2011) conducted a meta-analysis of 38 randomized trials of patients with depression and found a moderate to large effect of IPT in acute treatment of depression. They did not find that IPT had greater efficacy than other psychotherapies, including CBT, though the number of studies was too limited, and thus, definitive conclusions could not be drawn. Cuijpers and colleagues found some indications that maintenance IPT in combination with pharmacotherapy reduced the relapse rate considerably compared to pharmacotherapy alone. In a more recent meta-analysis of seven trials, Jakobsen, Hansen, Simonsen, Simonsen, and Gluud (2012) showed no significant differences in posttreatment depression severity scores between CT and IPT. However, studies included in this analysis were discovered to have a high risk of bias, and none included data after treatment termination which resulted in unknown long-term effects (Lemmens et al., 2015). Lemmens and colleagues (2015) randomized depressed adults to either CT, IPT, or a wait-list control. They found that while there were no differential effects between CT and IPT, both treatments exceeded the wait-list condition and led to considerable improvement in depression symptom severity, which was sustained up to 1 year. It is apparent that more randomized trials with low risk of bias are needed to better assess differential effects, though cumulative findings to date suggest that CT and IPT do not seem to significantly differ regarding effects on depressive symptoms, and IPT is an effective psychotherapy for depression.

Does Engagement in IPT Affect Neurocognition?

A literature basis for the effects of engagement in IPT on neurocognitive functioning has yet to emerge. However, an existing adaptation of IPT has been developed for depressed elderly individuals with significant neurocognitive impairment such as mild cognitive impairment or dementia, called IPT-CI (Miller & Reynolds, 2007). IPT-CI integrates the caregiver into the patient's treatment. This combined approach includes psychoeducation for both the patient and caregiver, problem solving for each individually, and the opportunity to have role dispute resolution in joint meetings. In IPT-CI, the caregiver has regular input into the IPT process to assist in the patient's progress in spite of neurocognitive decline. This provides much assistance to patients who may struggle largely with insight and retention of material discussed due to significant neurocognitive decline. Miller and Reynolds (2007) have written about their need to be more flexible in allowing joint sessions to problem solve, model understanding for caregivers that benefit the patient's neurocognitive ability, and sometimes suggest that the caregiver reinforce gains made in treatment session between visits. While it is currently unknown to what extent IPT may affect neurocognitive skills in depression, the development of IPT-CI signifies recognition that IPT may need adaptation when working with elderly depressed patients with significant neurocognitive impairment. It is hoped that investigations of the effects of IPT on neurocognition will emerge in the future.

WHEN NEUROCOGNITIVE DEFICITS GET IN THE WAY OF PSYCHOTHERAPY

There are already a multitude of factors to keep in mind in the provision of therapy, and given the known common neurocognitive impairments in MDD, it is important to also consider these aspects as they might impact the process of therapy. In Table 17.2 we have identified common barriers to therapy that may arise when clients have neurocognitive deficits. Alongside the barriers are possible strategies to adapt therapy to support clients with these difficulties.

TABLE 17.2. Possible Barriers Related to Specific Neurocognitive Domains and Suggested Clinical Strategies to Use in Therapy to Manage These Difficulties

Barriers	Clinical strategies
Executive functioning (including inhibitory control, problem solving)	
Impulsivity and lack of insight into recurring cognitive, behavioral, and physiological patterns.	• Work with the patient to recognize the consequences of impulsivity and the benefits of intentionality when faced with a task requiring attention skills. • Increase core mindfulness; highlight impulsive and habitual patterns of thinking that may be present and associated aversion to negative mind states and judgments. An emphasis on the benefits and consequences of impulsive versus slowed and thoughtful ways of thinking is warranted when aiming to develop intentional attention.
Perseveration and deficits in a patient's ability to solve problems and generate multiple options may thwart therapeutic gains.	• Break problems down with the patient into smaller components or steps. • Ask the patient to reflect back their understanding of the problem to identify where reasoning gaps may persist. • Emphasize to the patient that while a course of action may have had a positive outcome at one time, it is important to consider alternative courses of action if the usual response does not result in the desired outcome. • Review with the patient that in the future, when a similar situation in the environment arises, what alternative responses could be generated. In doing so, the patient is encouraged to come up with several possible behavioral approaches, weigh the consequences of each, decide on a course of action, and reflect on the outcome. Through these approaches, the flexibility skills of the patient are exercised, and learning occurs through the determination of effective strategies to select given the current situation.
Patient has difficulty in session because they are not following instructions for medication usage, or because other vulnerability factors are not appropriately managed (e.g., sleep schedule, eating habits) due to struggles with planning.	• Assist the patient in creating routines and habits—for example, always taking medication at the same time of day, having a bedtime routine, eating meals at regular times, and exercising at the same time each day. • Pairing new habits with existing ones is a good strategy—for example, where possible pair medications with a routine activity such as brushing teeth or having breakfast. • Assist the patient to create a visual summary of their daily routine, such as a chart or white board. • Suggest the use of alarms and reminders programmed into a smart phone or other device.
Difficulties in collaborative problem solving, which can be especially important in planning in advance for courses of action should an obstacle arise in the environment when the patient endeavors to complete home practice.	• Encourage the identification of multiple possible courses of action if faced with a challenge rather than just one course of action, and have the patient reflect on the outcome of the action selected. • With the patient, write down steps to complete home practice that the patient can refer to in the moment; this may include different courses of action depending on the anticipated environmental factors (e.g., family members/roommates are being loud: go to bedroom for personal space, put on headphone to enhance ability to concentrate).

(continued)

TABLE 17.2. *(continued)*

Barriers	Clinical strategies
	Memory

Poor memory to initiate or complete homework may pose barriers to completing home practice in therapies that require a significant homework component (CBT, MBCT, BA).	• Compensatory strategies to cue engagement in activation exercises may be particularly useful for patients who experience neurocognitive difficulties. Some examples include:
	  ○ Set reminder alarms with a descriptive label
	  ○ Encourage patients to inform family members or friends about planned activities in order to generate accountability and the potential for extra external reminders to engage.
	  ○ Create a daily routine or schedule for completing homework.
	  ○ Write down time to complete homework on calendar or white board.

Forgetting in-session material. To some extent, all therapies rely on a patient's ability to retain material discussed during session. Failure to do so will likely limit therapeutic gains and limit success in homework completion.	• Patients should try to get a good night's sleep before coming to therapy so that they are feeling most mentally refreshed. • Patients would likely benefit from avoiding substance use prior to sessions that may impair attention (e.g., cannabis, opioids, benzodiazepines). • Patients may benefit from note-taking and headlining of important points discussed in session to provide reminder cues for discussed material which they can use during at-home practice. • To reduce memory load, patients can be encouraged to keep a means of recording on hand so that they do not need to retrospectively recall when completing exercises (e.g., activity monitoring in BA). • Audio-record sessions so that patients have access to material outside of session to review as needed.
Forgetting or misplacing therapy-related notes/ handouts/homework.	• Encourage the patient to write all important information down in one place. • Leave materials in the therapy office and only leave with the necessary materials for that week. • Provide or encourage patient to purchase a binder for storage of information in one place. • Scan documents and provide them electronically to patient for use between sessions. • Encourage the patient to keep therapy items in the same location in their home at all times. "A place for everything, and everything in its place." • The night before therapy, set out items needed where they will be seen—for example, put the therapy binder by one's purse or by the door. • Have the patient use a sticky note on their door to remind them to bring the binder.

(continued)

TABLE 17.2. *(continued)*

Barriers	Clinical strategies

Attention

Struggling to hold their focus on tasks.

- Consider shortening the therapy session or meeting for two shorter appointments per week instead of one longer appointment. This may be especially valuable in the early stages of treatment, when building rapport and the patient is getting used to the process and structure of a therapy session.
- Consider length of homework practices based on the patient's attention capacity. For instance, for patients engaging in MBCT, the therapist should take a collaborative stance to determining appropriate and manageable duration of mindfulness exercises. Exercises prescribed and utilized in MBCT might be halved initially, and sessions shortened with greater frequency or longer duration of treatment.
- Reinforce that it's OK if the mind wanders.
- Take breaks in session if needed.

Processing speed

Taking a long time to answer questions in session

- As hard as it can be at times, patience goes a long way here. Allow time for the patient to consider information and arrive at an answer.
- Reduce the amount of information you relay and simplify language. If a patient is getting lost because you provide extensive information about psychoeducation or speak for long periods of time reflecting on what the patient has said, break down the information into smaller chunks. Check that the patient is following and understands.

Patient reports feeling confused or lost in session (related to session content).

- Intentionally focus on doing one thing at a time and avoid multitasking in-session. This may also be carried through to homework assignments.
- Ask the patient to reflect back to you the information that you have conveyed. This allows the therapist to assess how much the patient is comprehending and taking in and also allows the therapist to correct or reinforce certain concepts earlier.

Related issues

Self-defeating beliefs related to the patient's own neurocognitive skills. This may be particularly highlighted in MBCT as the focus is largely on attentional ability. May also present when patient is aware of own deficits and they become fearful or frustrated with themselves. Or in IPT, neurocognitive decline may affect self-perception of ability to adapt in interpersonal relationships and roles.

- Teach self-compassion to reframe the personal narrative. Instead of symptomatology being seen as personal failures and inadequacies, patients gradually discover how to embrace themselves with kindness and generosity. Instead of depression being seen as a personal description of failure and met with blame, it can become an experience met with kindness and curiosity.
- Remind the patient of abilities that remain intact and that can be further developed or enhanced to help compensate for abilities that are reduced (Miller et al., 2006).
- Normalization of neurocognitive weaknesses. Everyone has their own profile of neurocognitive strengths and weaknesses. Learning to identify your own is empowering.
- Normalization of age-related neurocognitive changes. After age 50, neurocognitive changes such as slowed information-processing speed, word finding, and memory retrieval are normal and not pathological. Reinforce the fact that the patient's peers are likely experiencing similar changes.

(continued)

TABLE 17.2. *(continued)*

Barriers	Clinical strategies

Relates issues (continued)

Barriers	Clinical strategies
Others becoming frustrated with the patient because of memory/attentional/planning difficulties, thereby creating interpersonal difficulties and relational strife. They may also attribute neurocognitive lapses to intentional avoidance or laziness.	• Assessing the influence of neurocognitive impairment on relationships is warranted. While neurocognitive impairments experienced in depression are not necessarily as extreme as those experienced by elderly depressed patients, adaptations used in IPT-CI may be beneficial across the lifespan. In particular, IPT for depressed individuals with neurocognitive impairment might consider bringing one's partner in for a psychoeducational session regarding the effects of depression on neurocognitive ability. This may enhance the partner's understanding of the patient's abilities, and thereby lessen interpersonal disputes in daily life, though this has yet to be empirically investigated.
Fear of making mistakes.	• It is crucial for the therapist to create a space that fosters trial-and-error and "mistakes" as part of the process of learning in therapy. For patients who experience neurocognitive impairment and have limited opportunities to exercise their neurocognitive skills, not exercising those skills may have an inadvertent negative effect. • Again, normalizing neurocognitive slips as part of depression and/or part of normal aging may be of assistance here. The therapist may offer examples of situations where they made some neurocognitive slips or mistakes as a means of normalizing this experience.
Avoidance of neurocognitive activities. For example, the patient may feel a reduction in self-efficacy to perform behaviors necessary for neurocognitively complex activities (e.g., patients who think they cannot maintain their attention long enough to read a book any more), fear of negative outcome and aversive emotions and thoughts (e.g., patients who think that if they cannot finish a book like they used to will not be able to tolerate how terribly they feel about themselves) or persistent withdrawal from neurocognitively challenging behaviors resulting in a lack of opportunity over time (for example, patients who have been unable to work for years).	• The Cognitive-Behavioral Avoidance Scale (Ottenbreit & Dobson, 2004) is often used in BA to aid therapists and patients in the discovery of domains of avoidance in life. Taking a specific approach to the identification of neurocognitive avoidance, the therapist and patient might utilize a measure that gauges the approach of neurocognitively challenging activities, such as the Need for Cognition Scale (Cacioppo & Petty, 1982), to identify those neurocognitive activities that are favorably approached versus avoided in daily life. • It is important for the therapist to validate the natural tendency to avoid neurocognitive challenge (e.g., not needing to face negative emotions if the approach fails; not needing to use neurocognitive skills that may not be as strong as they once were). The therapist will be both validating and also curious to try new behaviors and encourage a safe space to experience "failure" as a means of exploring new outcomes of the tried behavioral approach. • The patient should be encouraged to engage in smaller activities that are still neurocognitively engaging, or to break larger activities down into smaller parts. For example, if reading a lengthy novel feels overwhelming, encourage the patient to read a short story or newspaper article. Or suggest that the patient read four pages of a lengthy novel in one sitting rather than an entire chapter. Encourage the patient to take a break to refresh neurocognitively and then read another four pages. Advise the patient to use strategies to help focus attention during completion of the task, such as underlining key points or making notes in the margin. • The patient should be encouraged to positively reinforce or reward themselves for small accomplishments in previously avoided neurocognitive activities.

MEDICATION AND NEUROCOGNITION

In addition to the baseline neurocognitive difficulties that are often associated with depression, medications used to treat depression and prevent relapse may also have a negative impact on neurocognitive functioning. It is important for clinicians engaged in psychotherapy interventions to be aware of which medications their patients are prescribed in order to adjust for potential neurocognitive impairments, provide psychoeducation to patients, and/or provide feedback to the prescribing provider if medication side effects appear to be in excess of those typically observed. (For a detailed discussion of psychotropic medication in depression, please see Rosenblat, Chapter 15, this volume.)

Tricyclic antidepressants (TCAs), such as amitriptyline or nortriptyline, have been shown to have detrimental effects on attention, memory, psychomotor speed, and dexterity relative to both newer antidepressants and compared to placebo (e.g., Curran, Sakulsriprong, & Lader, 1988; Levkovitz, Caftori, Avital, & Richter-Levin, 2002; Nagane et al., 2014). However, this class of antidepressant medications is less frequently used due to the anticholinergic side effect profile, which many patients find difficult to tolerate (e.g., dry mouth, blurred vision, constipation, sexual side effects), as well as the potential for cardiac complications (Trindade, Menon, Topfer, & Coloma, 1998).

Compared to the TCAs, monoamine oxidase inhibitors (MAOIs), such as phenelzine or selegiline, have been shown to be less detrimental to neurocognitive processes such as memory. Most investigations have found MAOIs to be relatively benign in regard to neurocognition (e.g., Nolen, Haffmans, Bouvy, & Duivenvoorden, 1993). However, their tendency to induce drowsiness as a side effect can then have downstream negative effects on neurocognition. That said, clinicians today will be less likely to encounter MAOIs due to the risk of dangerous health consequences associated with the interaction of MAOIs and a number of common food groups.

The selective serotonin reuptake inhibitors (SSRIs) revolutionized pharmacological treatment of depression and remain among the most commonly used class of antidepressant medications. Medications such as fluoxetine, sertraline, and citalopram are considered safer in terms of both systemic side effect profiles and neurocognitive functioning compared to the TCAs and MAOIs. Recent studies have confirmed that there are minimal neurocognitive consequences associated with SSRIs versus various control conditions (e.g., Almeida, Glahn, Argyropoulos, & Frangou, 2010; Culang et al., 2009; Hinkelmann et al., 2012). While some studies have suggested that SSRIs give rise to improvements in neurocognition, this is more likely secondary to improved mood and amelioration of the neurocognitive deficits associated with the depressive episode (e.g., Knorr et al., 2011). However, a recent study by Kennedy and colleagues (Soczynska et al., 2014) compared the impact of bupropion XL and escitalopram on neuropsychological functioning in 36 adults assessed both pre- and posttreatment. They found that both medications improved verbal and nonverbal memory, global function, and work productivity with no significant between-group differences, and that the improvements were not solely attributable to improvements in mood. Despite largely favorable findings and widespread prescription usage, a small number of studies have suggested that SSRIs may have some detrimental effects on neurocognition, including episodic memory (e.g., Wadsworth, Moss, Simpson, & Smith, 2005), or other, more subtle neurocognitive effects such as delayed generalization of learning (e.g., Herzallah, Moustafa, Natsheh, Danoun, et al., 2013) or decreased ability to learn from negative feedback (Herzallah, Moustafa, Natsheh, Abdel-latif, et al., 2013). In most studies where neurocognitive impairment in patients treated with an SSRI was noted, this was often associated with low mood/treatment nonresponse (Talarowska, Zboralski, & Gałecki, 2013).

Despite a relatively benign neurocognitive impact, some rare but potentially life-threatening side effects are associated with use of SSRIs which may present as neuro-cognitive changes. These side effects include risk of akathisia, serotonin syndrome, and risk of discontinuation syndrome if medications are stopped abruptly. Akathisia presents as a feeling of severe inner restlessness, which patients may describe as difficulty focus-ing. This feeling is often mistaken for increased anxiety and responds to decreased dose. Serotonin syndrome is rare; however, it can be fatal. This syndrome may present similarly to delirium, with disorientation, confusion, and ataxia. It, too, responds to reductions in dose. Discontinuation syndrome is a risk given the apparent "safety" of SSRIs compared to their predecessors. Patients often stop taking their SSRI without medical advice. SSRI discontinuation syndrome may yield cognitive side effects, including confusion, dizzi-ness, and unusual sensations patients have described as "brain zaps" or "brain shocks." If patients report such symptoms in therapy, inquiring if they have made any changes to their medications would be advised, and if so, patients should be referred back to their prescriber for medical follow-up.

The most recent antidepressant medications are the selective serotonin–norepin-ephrine reuptake inhibitors (SNRIs) such as duloxetine and venlafaxine. The side-effect profile of SNRIs is similar to or better than that of SSRIs (e.g., Herrera-Guzmán et al., 2009). As with SSRIs, there is a risk of discontinuation syndrome. And again, as with SSRIs, it is particularly important for the psychotherapist to be aware of discontinuation, as clients benefiting from therapy may elect to stop taking their SSRI or SNRI without first consulting their prescriber.

Individuals with depression often suffer from comorbid anxiety and/or sleep distur-bance. As such, additional medications are often prescribed which may impair neurocog-nition. The most common class of medications used as needed to treat anxiety and sleep difficulty in this population would be benzodiazepines, such as diazepam, lorazepam, and clonazepam. While the different benzodiazepines do differ in terms of their half-life and degree of impact on neurocognition, the class in general is associated with detri-mental effects on psychomotor speed and dexterity, attention/concentration, learning, and memory (Buffett-Jerrott & Stewart, 2002). These effects are generally temporary during the period of medication use, but they can often be alarming to patients who may report unexplained "memory gaps." Inquiring about benzodiazepine use and, if relevant, provid-ing psychoeducation regarding neurocognition can be reassuring to patients.

Newer sleep aids such as the "z drugs," including zopiclone and zolpidem, are consid-ered safe for short-term use for infrequent sleep difficulty. However, patients with comor-bid mental health disorders often use these sleep medications over an extended period of time and often at higher doses than suggested on product monographs, which can lead to prolonged neurocognitive impairments. For example, in a group of long-term users of this class of sleep aid, Puustinen and colleagues (2014) found prolonged impairment of atten-tion and psychomotor function that persisted up to 6 months after discontinuation. If taken as prescribed, however, patients should not experience significant impairment of neurocognition as a consequence. Cognitive effects, including slowed information-processing speed, poor divided attention, and poor spatial memory, generally resolve 8 hours postingestion (e.g., Kuitunen, Mattila, Seppälä, Aranko, & Mattila, 1990; Wilkinson, 1995). However, at least one more recent study tested 30 healthy adults the morning after taking either Ramelteon (8 mg), Zopiclone (7.5 mg), or placebo, and found that participants who had been administered a sleep aid demonstrated significant impairments of reaction time, complex attention and delayed recall versus those given placebo. As such, long-term use may impact attention, and even short-term use may produce some residual neurocognitive impairment on the morning following use. Such neurocognitive effects could interfere with engagement in therapy or homework completed during this time window.

SUMMARY

A number of psychotherapies for MDD are available to clinicians. In this chapter, we provide a primer on how to critically evaluate the scientific literature when engaging in clinical decision making, and we review several psychotherapies for MDD that have an established evidence base. Current psychotherapies for depression have been criticized for not adequately addressing known neurocognitive deficits associated with this condition. A limited body of research exists which examines the effects of psychotherapy on neurocognition in depression. We comprehensively review these scientific findings, briefly comment on the role of medications for MDD and their effects on neurocognition, and suggest trans-therapeutic clinical adaptations to address possible barriers related to neurocognitive domains (i.e., executive functioning, memory, attention, processing speed) that may emerge in therapy. The effect of psychological intervention on neurocognitive impairment in MDD remains an important line of inquiry. Given the finite degree of published studies to date, it will be important for future work to add to this knowledge base, furthering our understanding of neurocognitive deficits in MDD.

REFERENCES

Abbass, A. A., Hancock, J. T., Henderson, J., & Kisely, S. R. (2006). Short-term psychodynamic psychotherapies for common mental disorders. *Cochrane Database of Systematic Reviews, 18*(4), 1–56.

Abbass, A. A., Nowoweiski, S. J., Bernier, D., Tarzwell, R., & Beutel, M. E. (2014). Review of psychodynamic psychotherapy neuroimaging studies. *Psychotherapy and Psychosomatics, 83*(3), 142–147.

Ajilchi, B., Nejati, V., Town, J. M., Wilson, R., & Abbass, A. (2016). Effects of intensive short-term dynamic psychotherapy on depressive symptoms and executive functioning in major depression. *Journal of Nervous and Mental Disease, 204*(7), 500–505.

Almeida, S., Glahn, D. C., Argyropoulos, S. V., & Frangou, S. (2010). Acute citalopram administration may disrupt contextual information processing in healthy males. *European Psychiatry, 25*(2), 87–91.

Anderson, E. M., & Lambert, M. J. (1995). Short-term dynamically oriented psychotherapy: A review and meta-analysis. *Clinical Psychology Review, 15*(6), 503–514.

Andersson, G. (2010). Online cognitive behavioural therapy is effective for depression in primary care. *Evidence-Based Mental Health, 13*(2), 50.

Andrews, G., Cuijpers, P., Craske, M. G., McEvoy, P., & Titov, N. (2010). Computer therapy for the anxiety and depressive disorders is effective, acceptable and practical health care: A meta-analysis. *PloS One, 5*(10), e13196.

Antonakis, J. (2017). On doing better science: From thrill of discovery to policy implications. *The Leadership Quarterly, 28*(1), 5–21.

Barnhofer, T., Crane, C., Hargus, E., Amarasinghe, M., Winder, R., & Williams, J. M. G. (2009). Mindfulness-based cognitive therapy as a treatment for chronic depression: A preliminary study. *Behaviour Research and Therapy, 47*(5), 366–373.

Barth, J., Munder, T., Gerger, H., Nüesch, E., Trelle, S., Znoj, H., et al. (2013). Comparative efficacy of seven psychotherapeutic interventions for patients with depression: A network meta-analysis. *PLOS Medicine, 10*(5), e1001454.

Basso, M. R., & Bornstein, R. A. (1999). Relative memory deficits in recurrent versus first-episode major depression on a word-list learning task. *Neuropsychology, 13*(4), 557–563.

Bastos, A. G., Guimarães, L. S. P., & Trentini, C. M. (2013). Neurocognitive changes in depressed patients in psychodynamic psychotherapy, therapy with fluoxetine and combination therapy. *Journal of Affective Disorders, 151*(3), 1066–1075.

Beck, A. T., Rush, A. J., Shaw, B. F., & Emery, G. (1979). *Cognitive therapy of depression.* New York: Guilford Press.

Beck, J. S. (2011). *Cognitive behavior therapy: Basics and Beyond* (2nd ed.). New York: Guilford Press.

Bell, A. C., & D'Zurilla, T. J. (2009). Problem-solving therapy for depression: A meta-analysis. *Clinical Psychology Review, 29*(4), 348–353.

Bieling, P. J., McCabe, R. E., & Antony, M. M. (2006). Depression. In *Cognitive-behavioral therapy in groups* (pp. 216–238). New York: Guilford Press.

Blagys, M. D., & Hilsenroth, M. J. (2000). Distinctive features of short term psychodynamic-interpersonal psychotherapy: A review of the comparative psychotherapy process literature. *Clinical Psychology: Science and Practice, 7*(2), 167–188.

Bondolfi, G., Jermann, F., Van der Linden, M., Gex-Fabry, M., Bizzini, L., Rouget, B. W., et al. (2010). Depression relapse prophylaxis with mindfulness-based cognitive therapy: Replication and extension in the Swiss health care system. *Journal of Affective Disorders, 122*(3), 224–231.

Bower, P., Richards, D., & Lovell, K. (2001). The clinical and cost-effectiveness of self-help treatments for anxiety and depressive disorders in primary care: A systematic review. *British Journal of General Practice, 51*(471), 838–845.

Bressi, C., Porcellana, M., Marinaccio, P. M., Nocito, E. P., & Magri, L. (2010). Short-term psychodynamic psychotherapy versus treatment as usual for depressive and anxiety disorders: A randomized clinical trial of efficacy. *Journal of Nervous and Mental Disease, 198*(9), 647–652.

Brettschneider, C., Djadran, H., Härter, M., Löwe, B., Riedel-Heller, S., & König, H. H. (2015). Cost-utility analyses of cognitive-behavioural therapy of depression: A systematic review. *Psychotherapy and Psychosomatics, 84*(1), 6–21.

Buffett-Jerrott, S. E., & Stewart, S. H. (2002). Cognitive and sedative effects of benzodiazepine use. *Current Pharmaceutical Design, 8*(1), 45–58.

Butler, A. C., Chapman, J. E., Forman, E. M., & Beck, A. T. (2006). The empirical status of cognitive-behavioral therapy: A review of meta-analyses. *Clinical Psychology Review, 26*(1), 17–31.

Cacioppo, J. T., & Petty, R. E. (1982). The need for cognition. *Journal of Personality and Social Psychology, 42*(1), 116–131.

Chan, A. T. Y., Sun, G. Y. Y., Tam, W. W. S., Tsoi, K. K. F., & Wong, S. Y. S. (2017). The effectiveness of group-based behavioral activation in the treatment of depression: An updated meta-analysis of randomized controlled trial. *Journal of Affective Disorders, 208*, 345–354.

Cuijpers, P., Berking, M., Andersson, G., Quigley, L., Kleiboer, A., & Dobson, K. S. (2013). A meta-analysis of cognitive-behavioural therapy for adult depression, alone and in comparison with other treatments. *Canadian Journal of Psychiatry, 58*(7), 376–385.

Cuijpers, P., de Wit, L., Kleiboer, A., Karyotaki, E., & Ebert, D. D. (2018). Problem-solving therapy for adult depression: An updated meta-analysis. *European Psychiatry, 48*, 27–37.

Cuijpers, P., Geraedts, A. S., van Oppen, P., Andersson, G., Markowitz, J. C., & van Straten, A. (2011).

Interpersonal psychotherapy for depression: A meta-analysis. *American Journal of Psychiatry,* *168*(6), 581–592.

Cuijpers, P., van Straten, A., Andersson, G., & van Oppen, P. (2008). Psychotherapy for depression in adults: A meta-analysis of comparative outcome studies. *Journal of Consulting and Clinical Psychology, 76*(6), 909–922.

Cuijpers, P., van Straten, A., & Warmerdam, L. (2007). Behavioural activation treatments of depression: A meta-analysis. *Clinical Psychology Review, 27*(3), 318–326.

Cuijpers, P., van Straten, A., Warmerdam, L., & Andersson, G. (2009). Psychotherapy versus the combination of psychotherapy and pharmacotherapy in the treatment of depression: A meta-analysis. *Depression and Anxiety, 26*(3), 279–288.

Culang, M. E., Sneed, J. R., Keilp, J. G., Rutherford, B. R., Pelton, G. H., Devanand, D. P., et al. (2009). Change in cognitive functioning following acute antidepressant treatment in late-life depression. *American Journal of Geriatric Psychiatry, 17*(10), 881–888.

Curran, H. V., Sakulsriprong, M., & Lader, M. (1988). Antidepressants and human memory: An investigation of four drugs with different sedative and anticholinergic profiles. *Psychopharmacology, 95*(4), 520–527.

Dannehl, K., Rief, W., & Euteneuer, F. (2019). Effects of cognitive behavioral therapy on verbal learning and memory in major depression: Results of a randomized controlled trial. *Clinical Psychology and Psychotherapy, 26*(3), 291–297.

Dennis, J. P., & Vander Wal, J. S. (2010). The Cognitive Flexibility Inventory: Instrument development and estimates of reliability and validity. *Cognitive Therapy and Research, 34*(3), 241–253.

De Raedt, R., Baert, S., Demeyer, I., Goeleven, E., Raes, A., Visser, A., et al. (2012). Changes in attentional processing of emotional information following mindfulness-based cognitive therapy in people with a history of depression: Towards an open attention for all emotional experiences. *Cognitive Therapy and Research, 36*(6), 612–620.

DeRubeis, R. J., Gelfand, L. A., Tang, T. Z., & Simons, A. D. (1999). Medications versus cognitive behavior therapy for severely depressed outpatients: Mega-analysis of four randomized comparisons. *American Journal of Psychiatry, 156*(7), 1007–1013.

Dichter, G. S., Felder, J. N., Petty, C., Bizzell, J., Ernst, M., & Smoski, M. J. (2009). The effects of psychotherapy on neural responses to rewards in major depression. *Biological Psychiatry, 66*(9), 886–897.

Dichter, G. S., Felder, J. N., & Smoski, M. J., (2010). The effects of brief behavioural activation therapy for depression on cognitive control in affective contexts: An fMRI investigation. *Journal of Affective Disorders, 126*(1–2), 236–244.

Dimidjian, S., Hollon, S. D., Dobson, K. S., Schmaling, K. B., Kohlenberg, R. J., Addis, M. E., et al. (2006). Randomized trial of behavioral activation, cognitive therapy, and antidepressant medication in the acute treatment of adults with major depression. *Journal of Counseling and Clinical Psychology, 74*(4), 658–670.

Dishman, R. K., Berthoud, H. R., Booth, F. W., Cotman, C. W., Edgerton, V. R., Fleshner, M. R., et al. (2006). Neurobiology of exercise. *Obesity, 14*(3), 345–356.

Dobson, K. S. (1989). A meta-analysis of the efficacy of cognitive therapy of depression. *Journal of Consulting and Clinical Psychology, 57*(3), 414–419.

Dobson, K. S., Hollon, S. D., Dimidjian, S., Schmaling, K. B., Kohlenberg, R. J., Gallop, R., et al. (2008). Randomized trial of behavioural activation, cognitive therapy, and antidepressant medication in the prevention of relapse and recurrence in major depression. *Journal of Consulting and Clinical Psychology, 76*(3), 468–477.

Driessen, E., Cuijpers, P., de Maat, S. C. M., Abbass, A. A., de Jonghe, F., & Dekker, J. J. M. (2010). The efficacy of short-term psychodynamic psychotherapy for depression: A meta-analysis. *Clinical Psychology Review, 30*(1), 25–36.

D'Zurilla, T. J., & Nezu, A. M. (2010). Problem-solving therapy. In K. S. Dobson (Ed.), *Handbook of cognitive-behavioral therapies* (pp. 197–225). New York: Guilford Press.

Early, B. P., & Grady, M. D. (2017). Embracing the contribution of both behavioural and cognitive theories to cognitive behavioural therapy: Maximizing the richness. *Clinical Social Work Journal, 45*(1), 39–48.

Eisendrath, S. J., Delucchi, K., Bitner, R., Fenimore, P., Smit, M., & McLane, M. (2008). Mindfulness-based cognitive therapy for treatment-resistant depression: A pilot study. *Psychotherapy and Psychosomatics, 77*(5), 319–320.

Ekers, D., Richards, D., & Gilbody, S. (2008). A meta-analysis of randomized trials of behavioural treatment of depression. *Psychological Medicine, 38*(5), 611–623.

Ekers, D., Webster, L., Van Straten, A., Cuijpers, P., Richards, D., & Gilbody, S. (2014). Behavioural activation for depression: An update of meta-analysis of effectiveness and subgroup analysis. *PLoS One, 9*(6), e100100.

Elkin, I., Shea, M. T., Watkins, J. T., Imber, S. D., Sotsky, S. M., Collins, J. F., et al. (1989). National Institute of Mental Health treatment of depression collaborative research program: General effectiveness of treatments. *Archives of General Psychiatry, 46*(11), 971–982.

Fan, J., McCandliss, B. D., Sommer, T., Raz, A., & Posner, M. I. (2002). Testing the efficiency and independence of attentional networks. *Journal of Cognitive Neuroscience, 14*(3), 340–347.

Feldman, C., & Kuyken, W. (2011). Compassion in the landscape of suffering. *Contemporary Buddhism, 12*(1), 143–155.

Forkmann, T., Wichers, M., Geschwind, N., Peeters, F., van Os, J., Mainz, V., et al. (2014). Effects of mindfulness-based cognitive therapy on self-reported suicidal ideation: Results from a randomised controlled trial in patients with residual depressive symptoms. *Comprehensive Psychiatry, 55*(8), 1883–1890.

Gabbard, G. O. (2009). Techniques of psychodynamic psychotherapy. In G. O. Gabbard (Ed.), *Textbook of psychotherapeutic treatments* (pp. 43–67). Arlington, VA: American Psychiatric Publishing.

Gabbard, G. O., & Bennett, T. J. (2006). Psychoanalytic and psychodynamic psychotherapy for depression and dysthymia. In D. J. Stein, D. J. Kupfer, and A. F. Schatzberg (Eds.), *Textbook of mood disorders*. Washington, DC: American Psychiatric Publishing.

Galante, J., Iribarren, S. J., & Pearce, P. F. (2013). Effects of mindfulness-based cognitive therapy on mental disorders: A systematic review and meta-analysis of randomised controlled trials. *Journal of Research in Nursing, 18*(2), 133–155.

Gaston, L., Thompson, L., Gallagher, D., Cournoyer, L., & Gagnon, R. (1998). Alliance, technique, and their interactions in predicting outcome of behavioral, cognitive, and brief dynamic therapy. *Psychotherapy Research, 8*(2), 190–209.

Gerhards, S. A. H., de Graaf, L. E., Jacobs, L. E., Severens, J. L., Huibers, M. J. H., Arntz, A., et al. (2010). Economic evaluation of online computerised cognitive-behavioural therapy without support for depression in primary care: Randomised trial. *British Journal of Psychiatry, 196*(4), 310–318.

Gloaguen, V., Cottraux, J., Cucherat, M., & Blackburn, I. M. (1998). A meta-analysis of the effects of cognitive therapy in depressed patients. *Journal of Affective Disorders, 49*(1), 59–72.

Goldman, R. E., Hilsenroth, M. J., Gold, J. R., Owen, J. J., & Levy, S. R. (2018). Psychotherapy integration and alliance: An examination across treatment outcomes. *Journal of Psychotherapy Integration, 28*(1), 14–30.

Goldman, R. E., Hilsenroth, M. J., Owen, J. J., & Gold, J. R. (2013). Psychotherapy integration and alliance: Use of cognitive-behavioral techniques within a short-term psychodynamic treatment model. *Journal of Psychotherapy Integration, 23*(4), 373–385.

Goldstone, D. (2017). Cognitive-behavioural therapy versus psychodynamic psychotherapy for the treatment of depression: A critical review of evidence and current issues. *South African Journal of Psychology, 47*(1), 84–96.

Gortner, E. T., Gollan, J. K., Dobson, K. S., & Jacobson, N. S. (1998). Cognitive-behavioral treatment for depression: Relapse prevention. *Journal of Consulting and Clinical Psychology, 66*(2), 377–384.

Greenberger, D., & Padesky, C. A. (1995). *Mind over mood: Change how you feel by changing the way you think.* New York: Guilford Press.

Greer, T. L., Grannemann, B. D., Chansard, M., Karim, A. I., & Trivedi, M. H. (2015). Dose-dependent changes in cognitive function with exercise augmentation for major depression: Results from the TREAD study. *European Neuropsychopharmacology, 25*(2), 248–256.

Groves, S. J., Porter, R. J., Jordan, J., Knight, R., Carter, J. D., McIntosh, V. V. W., et al. (2015). Changes in neuropsychological function after treatment with metacognitive therapy or cognitive behavior therapy for depression. *Depression and Anxiety, 32*(6), 437–444.

Hargus, E., Crane, C., Barnhofer, T., & Williams, J. M. G. (2010). Effects of mindfulness on meta-awareness and specificity of describing prodromal symptoms in suicidal depression. *Emotion, 10*(1), 34–42.

Hasselbalch, B. J., Knorr, U., & Kessing, L. V. (2011). Cognitive impairment in the remitted state of unipolar depressive disorder: A systematic review. *Journal of Affective Disorders, 134*(1–3), 20–31.

Heeren, A., Van Broeck, N., & Philippot, P. (2009). The effects of mindfulness on executive processes and autobiographical memory specificity. *Behaviour Research and Therapy, 47*(5), 403–409.

Herrera-Guzmán, I., Gudayol-Ferré, E., Herrera-Abarca, J. E., Herrera-Guzmán, D., Montelongo-Pedraza, P., Blázquez, F. P., et al. (2009). Major depressive disorder in recovery and neuropsychological functioning: Effects of selective serotonin reuptake inhibitor and dual inhibitor depression treatments on residual cognitive deficits in patients with major depressive disorder in recovery. *Journal of Affective Disorders, 123*(1–3), 341–350.

Herzallah, M. M., Moustafa, A. A., Natsheh, J. Y., Abdellatif, S. M., Taha, M. B., Tayem, Y. I., et al. (2013). Learning from negative feedback in patients with major depressive disorder is attenuated by SSRI antidepressants. *Frontiers in Integrative Neuroscience, 7*(67), 1–9.

Herzallah, M. M., Moustafa, A. A., Natsheh, J. Y., Danoun, O. A., Simon, J. R., Tayem, Y. I., et al. (2013). Depression impairs learning, whereas the selective serotonin reuptake inhibitor, paroxetine, impairs generalization in patients with major depressive disorder. *Journal of Affective Disorders, 151*(2), 484–492.

Hilsenroth, M. J., Defife, J. A., Blagys, M. D., & Ackerman, S. J. (2006). Effects of training in short-term psychodynamic psychotherapy: Changes in graduate clinician technique. *Psychotherapy Research, 16*(3), 293–305.

Hinkelmann, K., Moritz, S., Botzenhardt, J., Muhtz, C., Wiedemann, K., Kellner, M., et al. (2012). Changes in cortisol secretion during antidepressive treatment and cognitive improvement in patients with major depression: A longitudinal study. *Psychoneuroendocrinology, 37*(5), 685–692.

Hoffman, B. M., Blumenthal, J. A., Babyak, M. A., Smith, P. J., Rogers, S. D., Doraiswamy, P. M., et al. (2008). Exercise fails to improve neurocognition in depressed middle-aged and older adults. *Medicine and Science in Sports and Exercise, 40*(7), 1344–1352.

Hoffmann, T., Bennett, S., & Del Mar, C. (2013). *Evidence-based practice across the health professions—E-book* (2nd ed.). Sydney: Elsevier.

Hopko, D. R., Lejuez, C. W., Ruggiero, K. J., & Eifert, G. H. (2003). Contemporary behavioral activation treatments for depression: Procedures, principles, and progress. *Clinical Psychology Review, 23*(5), 669–717.

Horowitz, M. J., & Kaltreider, N. B. (1979). Brief therapy of the stress response syndrome. *Psychiatric Clinics of North America, 2*(2), 365–377.

Ioannidis, J. P. A. (2005). Why most published research findings are false. *PLoS Medicine, 2*(8), e124.

Ioannidis, J. P. A. (2016). Why most clinical research is not useful. *PLoS Medicine, 13*(6), e1002049.

Jacobson, N. S., Dobson, K. S., Truax, P. A., Addis, M. E., Koerner, K., Gollan, J. K., et al. (1996). A component analysis of cognitive-behavioural treatment for depression. *Journal of Consulting and Clinical Psychology, 64*(2), 295–304.

Jacobson, N. S., & Gortner, E. T. (2000). Can depression be de-medicalized in the 21st century: Scientific revolutions, counter-revolutions and the magnetic field of normal science. *Behaviour Research and Therapy, 38*(2), 103–117.

Jakobsen, J. C., Hansen, J. L., Simonsen, S., Simonsen, E., & Gluud, C. (2012). Effects of cognitive therapy versus interpersonal psychotherapy in patients with major depressive disorder: A systematic review of randomized clinical trials with meta-analyses and trial sequential analyses. *Psychological Medicine, 42*(7), 1343–1357.

Jermann, F., Van der Linden, M., Gex-Fabry, M., Guarin, A., Kosel, M., Bertschy, G., et al. (2013). Cognitive functioning in patients remitted from recurrent depression: Comparison with acutely depressed patients and controls and follow-up of a mindfulness-based cognitive therapy trial. *Cognitive Therapy and Research, 37*(5), 1004–1014.

Kabat-Zinn, J. (1990). *Full catastrophe living: Using the wisdom of your body and mind to face stress, pain, and illness.* New York: Delacorte.

Katz, M., Hilsenroth, M. J., Gold, J. R., Moore, M., Pitman, S. R., Levy, S. R., et al. (2019). Adherence, flexibility, and outcome in psychodynamic treatment of depression. *Journal of Counseling Psychology, 66*(1), 94–103.

Kenny, M. A., & Williams, J. M. G. (2007). Treatment-resistant depressed patients show a good response to mindfulness-based cognitive therapy. *Behaviour Research and Therapy, 45*(3), 617–625.

Kessler, R. C. (2012). The costs of depression. *Psychiatric Clinics of North America, 35*(1), 1–14.

Khatri, P., Blumenthal, J. A., Babyak, M. A., Craighead, W. E., Herman, S., Baldewicz, T., et al. (2001). Effects of exercise training on cognitive functioning among depressed older men and women. *Journal of Aging and Physical Activity, 9*(1), 43–57.

Kingdon, D., & Dimech, A. (2008). Cognitive and behavioural therapies: The state of the art. *Psychiatry, 7*(5), 217–220.

Kiosses, D. N., Ravdin, L. D., Gross, J. J., Raue, P., Kotbi, N., & Alexopoulos, G. S. (2015). Problem adaptation therapy for older adults with major depression and cognitive impairment: A randomized clinical trial. *JAMA Psychiatry, 72*(1), 22–30.

Klerman, G. L., Weissman, M. M., Rounsaville, B. J., & Chevron, E. S. (1984). *Interpersonal psychotherapy of depression.* New York: Basic Books.

Knorr, U., Vinberg, M., Gade, A., Winkel, P., Gluud, C., Wetterslev, J., et al. (2011). A randomized trial of the effect of escitalopram versus placebo on cognitive function in healthy first-degree relatives of patients with depression. *Therapeutic Advances in Psychopharmacology, 1*(5), 133–144.

Kocsis, J. H., Leon, A. C., Markowitz, J. C., Manber, R., Arnow, B., Klein, D. N., et al. (2009). Patient preference as a moderator of outcome for chronic forms of major depressive disorder treated with nefazodone, cognitive behavioral analysis system of psychotherapy, or their combination. *Journal of Clinical Psychiatry, 70*(3), 354–361.

Koppers, D., Peen, J., Niekerken, S., Van, R., & Dekker, J. (2011). Prevalence and risk factors for recurrence of depression five years after short term psychodynamic therapy. *Journal of Affective Disorders, 134*(1–3), 468–472.

Kraft, B., Jonassen, R., Stiles, T. C., & Landrø, N. I. (2017). Dysfunctional metacognitive beliefs are associated with decreased executive control. *Frontiers in Psychology, 8,* 593.

Kubesch, S., Bretschneider, V., Freudenmann, R., Weidenhammer, N., Lehmann, M., Spitzer, M., et al. (2003). Aerobic endurance exercise improves executive functions in depressed patients. *Journal of Clinical Psychiatry, 64*(9), 1005–1012.

Kuitunen, T., Mattila, M. J., Seppälä, T., Aranko, K., & Mattila, M. E. (1990). Actions of zopiclone and carbamazepine, alone and in combination, on human skilled performance in laboratory and clinical tests. *British Journal of Clinical Pharmacology, 30*(3), 453–461.

Kuyken, W., Byford, S., Taylor, R. S., Watkins, E., Holden, E., White, K., et al. (2008). Mindfulness-based cognitive therapy to prevent relapse in recurrent depression. *Journal of Consulting and Clinical Psychology, 76*(6), 966.

Kuyken, W., Hayes, R., Barrett B., Byng, R., Dalgleish, T., Kessler, D., et al. (2015) Effectiveness and cost-effectiveness of mindfulness-based cognitive therapy compared with maintenance antidepressant treatment in the prevention of depressive relapse or recurrence (PREVENT): A randomised controlled trial. *Lancet, 386,* 63–73.

Lao, S. A., Kissane, D., & Meadows, G. (2016). Cognitive effects of MBSR/MBCT: A systematic review of neuropsychological outcomes. *Consciousness and Cognition, 45,* 109–123.

Leichsenring, F. (2001). Comparative effects of short-term psychodynamic psychotherapy and cognitive-behavioral therapy in depression: A meta-analytic approach. *Clinical Psychology Review, 21*(3), 401–419.

Leichsenring, F., Kruse, J., & Rabung, S. (2015). Efficacy of psychodynamic psychotherapy in specific mental disorders: An update. In P. Luyten, L. C. Mayes, P. Fonagy, M. Target, & S. J. Blatt (Eds.),

Handbook of psychodynamic approaches to psychopathology (pp. 485–511). New York: Guilford Press.

Leichsenring, F., Rabung, S., & Leibing, E. (2004). The efficacy of psychodynamic psychotherapy in specific psychiatric disorders: A meta-analysis. *Archives of General Psychiatry, 61*(12), 1208–1216.

Lemma, A., Roth, A. D., & Pilling, S. (2009). *The competencies required to deliver effective psychoanalytic/psychodynamic therapy.* London: Research Department of Clinical, Educational and Health Psychology, University College London.

Lemmens, L. H. J. M., Arntz, A., Peeters, F., Hollon, S. D., Roefs, A., & Huibers, M. J. H. (2015). Clinical effectiveness of cognitive therapy v. interpersonal psychotherapy for depression: Results of a randomized controlled trial. *Psychological Medicine, 45*(10), 2095–2110.

Levkovitz, Y., Caftori, R., Avital, A. & Richter-Levin, G. (2002). The SSRIs drug fluoxetine, but not the noradrenergic tricyclic drug desipramine, improves memory performance during acute major depression. *Brain Research Bulletin, 58*(4), 345–350.

Lewinsohn, P. M., Biglan, A., & Zeiss, A. S. (1976). Behavioural treatment of depression. In P. O. Davidson (Ed.), *The behavioural management of anxiety, depression and pain* (pp. 91–146). New York: Brunner/Mazel.

Lewis, A. J., Dennerstein, M., & Gibbs, P. M. (2008). Short-term psychodynamic psychotherapy: Review of recent process and outcome studies. *Australian and New Zealand Journal of Psychiatry, 42*(6), 445–455.

Luyten, P., & Blatt, S. J. (2012). Psychodynamic treatment of depression. *Psychiatric Clinics of North America, 35*(1), 111–129.

Luyten, P., Mayes, L. C., Target, M., & Fonagy, P. (2012). Developmental research. In G. O. Gabbard, B. E. Litowitz, & P. Williams (Eds). *The textbook of psychoanalysis* (pp. 423–443). Washington, DC: American Psychiatric Press.

Ma, S. H., & Teasdale, J. D. (2004). Mindfulness-based cognitive therapy for depression: Replication and exploration of differential relapse prevention effects. *Journal of Consulting and Clinical Psychology, 72*(1), 31–40.

Mackin, R. S., Nelson, J. C., Delucchi, K., Raue, P., Byers, A., Barnes, D., et al. (2014). Cognitive outcomes after psychotherapeutic interventions for major depression in older adults with executive dysfunction. *American Journal of Geriatric Psychiatry, 22*(12), 1496–1503.

Maina, G., Forner, F., & Bogetto, F. (2005). Randomized controlled trial comparing brief dynamic and supportive therapy with waiting list condition in minor depressive disorders. *Psychotherapy and Psychosomatics, 74*(1), 43–50.

Majer, M., Ising, M., Künzel, H., Binder, E. B., Holsboer, F., Modell, S., et al. (2004). Impaired divided attention predicts delayed response and risk to relapse in subjects with depressive disorders. *Psychological Medicine, 34*(8), 1453–1463.

Maneeton, N. (2012). Cognitive-behavioural therapy combined with antidepressants for major depressive disorder. In L. L'Abate (Ed.), *Mental illnesses—evaluation, treatments and implications.* London: InTech.

Markowitz, J. C., & Weissman, M. M. (2004). Interpersonal psychotherapy: Principles and applications. *World Psychiatry, 3*(3), 136–139.

Martell, C. R., Addis, M. E., & Jacobson, N. S. (2001). *Depression in context: Strategies for guided action.* New York: Norton.

Martell, C. R., Dimidjian, S., & Herman-Dunn, R. (2013). *Behavioral activation for depression: A clinician's guide.* New York: Guilford Press.

Mazzucchelli, T., Kane, R., & Rees, C. (2009). Behavioral activation treatments for depression in adults: A meta-analysis and review. *Clinical Psychology: Science and Practice, 16*(4), 383–411.

Miller, M. D., & Reynolds III, C. F. (2007). Expanding the usefulness of Interpersonal Psychotherapy (IPT) for depressed elders with co-morbid cognitive impairment. *International Journal of Geriatric Psychiatry, 22*(2), 101–105.

Miller, M. D., Richards, V., Zuckoff, A., Martire, L. M., Morse, J., Frank, E., et al. (2006). A model for modifying interpersonal psychotherapy (IPT) for depressed elders with cognitive impairment. *Clinical Gerontologist, 30*(2), 79–101.

Miller, R. C., & Berman, J. S. (1983). The efficacy of cognitive behavior therapies: A quantitative review of research evidence. *Psychological Bulletin, 94*(1), 39–53.

Mohr, D. C., Vella, L., Hart, S., Heckman, T., & Simon, G. (2008). The effect of telephone-administered psychotherapy on symptoms of depression and attrition: A meta-analysis. *Clinical Psychology: Science and Practice, 15*(3), 243–253.

Nagane, A., Baba, H., Nakano, Y., Maeshima, H., Hukatsu, M., Ozawa, K., et al. (2014). Comparative study of cognitive impairment between medicated and medication-free patients with remitted major depression: Class-specific influence by tricyclic antidepressants and newer antidepressants. *Psychiatry Research, 218*(1–2), 101–105.

Nezu, A. M., & Perri, M. G. (1989). Social problem-solving therapy for unipolar depression: An initial dismantling investigation. *Journal of Consulting and Clinical Psychology, 57*(3), 408–413.

Nolen, W. A., Haffmans, P. M., Bouvy, P. F., & Duivenvoorden, H. J. (1993). Monoamine oxidase inhibitors in resistant major depression. A double-blind comparison of brofaromine and tranylcypromine in patients resistant to tricyclic antidepressants. *Journal of Affective Disorders, 28*(3), 189–197.

Nolen-Hoeksema, S. (1991). Responses to depression and their effects on the duration of depressive episodes. *Journal of Abnormal Psychology, 100*(4), 569–582.

Okumuru, Y., & Ichikura, K. (2014). Efficacy and acceptability of group cognitive behavioral therapy for depression: A systematic review and meta-analysis. *Journal of Affective Disorders, 164*, 155–164.

Ottenbreit, N. D., & Dobson, K. S. (2004). Avoidance and depression: The construction of the cognitive-behavioural avoidance scale. *Behaviour Research and Therapy, 42*(3), 293–313.

Piet, J., & Hougaard, E. (2011). The effect of mindfulness-based cognitive therapy for prevention of relapse in recurrent major depressive disorder: A systematic review and meta-analysis. *Clinical Psychology Review, 31*(6), 1032–1040.

Pinquart, M., Duberstein, P. R., & Lyness, J. M. (2007). Effects of psychotherapy and other behavioral interventions on clinically depressed older adults: A meta-analysis. *Aging and Mental Health, 11*(6), 645–657.

Porter, R. J., Bourke, C., Carter, J. D., Douglas, K. M., McIntosh, V. V. W., Jordan, J., et al. (2016). No change in neuropsychological dysfunction or emotional processing during treatment of major depression with cognitive–behaviour therapy or schema therapy. *Psychological Medicine, 46*(2), 393–404.

Porter, R. J., Douglas, K., Jordan, J., Bowie, C. R., Roiser, J., & Malhi, G. S. (2014). Psychological treatments for cognitive dysfunction in major depressive disorder: Current evidence and perspectives. *CNS and Neurological Disorders—Drug Targets, 13*(10), 1677–1692.

Puustinen, J., Lähteenmäki, R., Polo-Kantola, P., Salo, P., Vahlberg, T., Lyles, A., et al. (2014). Effect of withdrawal from long-term use of temazepam, zopiclone, or zolpidem as hypnotic agents on cognition in older adults. *European Journal of Clinical Pharmacology, 70*(3), 319–329.

Raue, P. J., Schulberg, H. C., Heo, M., Klimstra, S., & Bruce, M. L. (2009). Patients' depression treatment preferences and initiation, adherence, and outcome: A randomized primary care study. *Psychiatric Services, 60*(3), 337–343.

Rethorst, C. D., Wipfli, B. M., & Landers, D. M. (2009). The anti-depressive effects of exercise: A meta-analysis of randomized trials. *Sports Medicine, 39*(6), 491–511.

Rimer, J., Dwan, K., Lawlor, D. A., Greig, C. A., McMurdo, M., Morley, W., et al. (2012). Exercise for depression. *Cochrane Database of Systematic Reviews, 7*, CD004366.

Rose, J. M., & DelMaestro, S. G. (1990). Separation-individuation conflict as a model for understanding distressed caregivers: Psychodynamic and cognitive case studies. *Gerontologist, 30*(5), 693–697.

Rush, A. J., Beck, A. T., Kovacs, M., & Hollon, S. (1977). Comparative efficacy of cognitive therapy and pharmacotherapy in the treatment of depressed outpatients. *Cognitive Therapy and Research, 1*(1), 17–37.

Sackett, D. L., Rosenberg, W. M. C., Gray, J. A. M., Haynes, R. B., & Richardson, W. S. (1996). Evidence based medicine: What it is and what it isn't. *British Medical Journal, 312*, 71–72.

Segal, Z. V., Bieling, P., Young, T., MacQueen, G., Cooke, R., Martin, L., et al. (2010). Antidepressant monotherapy vs. sequential pharmacotherapy and mindfulness-based cognitive therapy, or placebo, for relapse prophylaxis in recurrent depression. *Archives of General Psychiatry, 67*(12), 1256–1264.

Segal, Z. V., Kennedy, S., Gemar, M., Hood, K., Pedersen, R., & Buis, T. (2006). Cognitive reactivity to sad mood provocation and the prediction of depressive relapse. *Archives of General Psychiatry, 63*(7), 749–755.

Segal, Z. V., Williams, J. M. G., & Teasdale, J. D. (2002). *Mindfulness-based cognitive therapy for depression: A new approach to preventing relapse.* New York: Guilford Press.

Segal, Z. V., Williams, J. M. G., Teasdale, J. D., & Gemar, M. (1996). A cognitive science perspective on kindling and episode sensitization in recurrent affective disorder. *Psychological Medicine, 26*(2), 371–380.

Shapero, B. G., Greenberg, J., Pedrelli, P., de Jong, M., & Desbordes, G. (2018). Mindfulness-based interventions in psychiatry. *Focus, 16*(1), 32–39.

Shapiro, D. A., Rees, A., Barkham, M., Hardy, G., Reynolds, S., & Startup, M. (1995). Effects of treatment duration and severity of depression on the maintenance of gains after cognitive-behavioral and psychodynamic-interpersonal psychotherapy. *Journal of Consulting and Clinical Psychology, 63*(3), 378–387.

Shedler, J. (2010). The efficacy of psychodynamic psychotherapy. *American Psychologist, 65*(2), 98–109.

Soczynska, J. K., Ravindran, L. N., Styra, R., McIntyre, R. S., Cyriac, A., Manierka, M. S., et al. (2014). The effect of bupropion XL and escitalopram on memory and functional outcomes in adults with major depressive disorder: Results from a randomized controlled trial. *Psychiatry Research, 220*(1–2), 245–250.

Sotsky, S. M., Glass, D. R., Shea, M. T., Pilkonis, P. A., Collins, F., Elkin, I., et al. (2006). Patient predictors of response to psychotherapy and pharmacotherapy: Findings in the NIMH Treatment of Depression Collaborative Research Program. *Focus, 4*(2), 278–290.

Stanley, B., & Brown, G. K. (2012). Safety planning intervention: A brief intervention to mitigate suicide risk. *Cognitive and Behavioural Practice, 19*(2), 256–264.

Stordal, K. I., Lundervold, A. J., Egeland, J., Mykletun, A., Asbjørnsen, A., Landrø, N. I., et al. (2004). Impairment across executive functions in recurrent major depression. *Nordic Journal of Psychiatry, 58*(1), 41–47.

Talarowska, M., Zboralski, K., & Gałecki, P. (2013). Correlations between working memory effectiveness and depression levels after pharmacological therapy. *Psychiatria Polska, 47*(2), 255–267.

Teasdale, J. D. (1988). Cognitive vulnerability to persistent depression. *Cognition and Emotion, 2*(3), 247–274.

Teasdale, J. D., Moore, R. G., Hayhurst, H., Pope, M., Williams, S., & Segal, Z. V. (2002). Metacognitive awareness and prevention of relapse in depression: Empirical evidence. *Journal of Consulting and Clinical Psychology, 70*(2), 275–287.

Teasdale, J. D., Segal, Z., & Williams, J. M. G. (1995). How does cognitive therapy prevent depressive relapse and why should attentional control (mindfulness) training help? *Behaviour Research and Therapy, 33*(1), 25–39.

Teasdale, J. D., Segal, Z. V., Williams, J. M., Ridgeway, V. A., Soulsby, J. M., & Lau, M. A. (2000). Prevention of relapse/recurrence in major depression by mindfulness-based cognitive therapy. *Journal of Consulting and Clinical Psychology, 68*(4), 615–623.

Tredget, J. (2001). Introducing and explaining CBT. *Mental Health Nursing, 21*(6), 8–13.

Trindade, E., Menon, D., Topfer, L. A., & Coloma, C. (1998). Adverse effects associated with selective serotonin reuptake inhibitors and tricyclic antidepressants: A meta-analysis. *Canadian Medical Association Journal, 159*(10), 1245–1252.

Trivedi, M. H., Greer, T. L., Church, T. S., Carmody, T. J., Grannemann, B. D., Galper, D. I., et al. (2011). Exercise as an augmentation treatment for nonremitted major depressive disorder: A randomized, parallel dose comparison. *Journal of Clinical Psychiatry, 72*(5), 677–684.

Twomey, C., O'Reilly, G., & Byrne, M. (2015). Effectiveness of cognitive behavioural therapy for anxiety and depression in primary care: A meta-analysis. *Family Practice, 32*(1), 3–15.

van Aalderen, J. R., Donders, A. R. T., Giommi, F., Spinhoven, P., Barendregt, H. P., & Speckens, A. E.

M. (2012). The efficacy of mindfulness-based cognitive therapy in recurrent depressed patients with and without a current depressive episode: A randomized controlled trial. *Psychological Medicine, 42*(5), 989–1001.

van den Hurk, P. A. M., van Aalderen, J. R., Giommi, F., Donders, R. A. R. T., Barendregt, H. P., & Speckens, A. E. M. (2012). An investigation of the role of attention in mindfulness-based cognitive therapy for recurrently depressed patients. *Journal of Experimental Psychopathology, 3*(1), 103–120.

van Vreeswijk, M. F., & de Wilde, E. J. (2004). Autobiographical memory specificity, psychopathology, depressed mood and the use of the Autobiographical Memory Test: A meta-analysis. *Behaviour Research and Therapy, 42*(6), 731–743.

Vasques, P. E., Moraes, H., Silveira, H., Deslandes, A. C., & Laks, J. (2011). Acute exercise improves cognition in the depressed elderly: The effect of dual-tasks. *Clinics, 66*(9), 1553–1557.

Vazquez, C., Duque, A., Blanco, I., Pascual, T., Poyato, N., Lopez-Gomez, I., et al. (2018). CBT and positive psychology interventions for clinical depression promote healthy attentional biases: An eye-tracking study. *Depression and Anxiety, 35*(10), 966–973.

Veale, D. (2008). Behavioural activation for depression. *Advances in Psychiatric Treatment, 14*, 29–36.

Vittengl, J. R., Clark, L. A., Dunn, T. W., & Jarrett, R. B. (2007). Reducing relapse and recurrence in unipolar depression: A comparative meta-analysis of cognitive-behavioral therapy's effects. *Journal of Consulting and Clinical Psychology, 75*(3), 475–488.

Wadsworth, E. J. K., Moss, S. C., Simpson, S. A., & Smith, A. P. (2005). SSRIs and cognitive performance in a working sample. *Human Psychopharmacology: Clinical and Experimental, 20*(8), 561–572.

Watts, S., Mackenzie, A., Thomas, C., Griskaitis, A., Mewton, L., Williams, A., et al. (2013). CBT for depression: A pilot RCT comparing mobile phone vs. computer. *BMC Psychiatry, 13*(1), 49.

Wilkinson, C. J. (1995). The acute effects of zolpidem, administered alone and with alcohol, on cognitive and psychomotor function. *Journal of Clinical Psychiatry, 56*(7), 309–318.

Williams, J. M., Crane, C., Barnhofer, T., Brennan, K., Duggan, D. S., Fennell, M. J. V., et al. (2014). Mindfulness-based cognitive therapy for preventing relapse in recurrent depression: A randomized dismantling trial. *Journal of Consulting and Clinical Psychology, 82*(2), 275–286.

Williams, J. M., Teasdale, J. D., Segal, Z. V., & Soulsby, J. (2000). Mindfulness-based cognitive therapy reduces overgeneral autobiographical memory in formerly depressed patients. *Journal of Abnormal Psychology, 109*(1), 150–155.

Yazigi, L., Semer, N. L., Amaro, T. D., Fiore, M. L. D., da Silva, J. F. R., & Botelho, N. L. P. (2011). Rorschach and the WAIS-III after one and two years of psychotherapy. *Psicologia: Reflexão e Crítica, 24*(1), 10–18.

Zhang, Z., Zhang, L., Zhang, G., Jin, J., & Zheng, Z. (2018). The effect of CBT and its modifications for relapse prevention in major depressive disorder: A systematic review and meta-analysis. *BMC Psychiatry, 18*(1), 50–64.

CHAPTER 18

Cognitive Remediation

Christopher R. Bowie
Michael W. Best
Tanya Tran
Jenna E. Boyd

*C*ognitive remediation (CR) refers to behavioral, learning-based interventions aimed at improving cognitive processes with a goal that these changes will be durable and generalizable to real-world functioning (Barlati, Deste, De Peri, Ariu, & Vita, 2013; Bowie et al., 2020). CR can be broadly categorized into two therapeutic approaches: (1) compensatory strategies, which refer to alternative strategies for identified areas of weakness that rely on a patient's strengths, and (2) restorative-based treatment, focused on "rebuilding" dysfunctional systems (Podd, 2011). Compensatory approaches might focus on modification of the individual's living environment to minimize how cognitive issues limit functioning and provide strategies for problem solving in daily life (Twamley, Savla, Zurhellen, Heaton, & Jeste, 2008). Restorative-based approaches can be further categorized as "bottom-up" or "top-down" (Best & Bowie, 2017). Bottom-up approaches begin with remediation of basic skills, such as attention (e.g., via skill-drill exercises), advancing to more complex skills, while top-down approaches begin with remediation of complex skills (e.g., problem solving) with the aim of improving more basic skills via downstream effects (Barlati et al., 2013). To date, studies of CR in mood disorders have focused mostly on restorative approaches.

CR emerged out of the traumatic brain injury literature, with the first reports of attempted rehabilitation of brain-injured patients emerging after World War II (Podd, 2011). More systematic attempts were made to study CR in the late 1970s and early 1980s when early proponents described strategies that included adapting games to help brain-damaged patients improve their cognitive functioning and that later evolved into computerized cognitive training (CCT). CR gained recognition by the National Institutes of Health in 1999 and was described as an effective treatment tool. Cicerone and colleagues (2005) conducted a systematic review of CR studies for individuals with brain injury and stroke, concluding that CR, particularly programs that focused on compensatory strategies, was significantly beneficial in comparison to alternative treatments (e.g., conventional rehabilitation, psychosocial treatments) for deficits in attention, memory, and self-regulation. Despite the early traction of CR, more randomized controlled trials in different clinical populations were necessary if it were to become part of gold-standard intervention for cognitive impairments (Podd, 2011).

Since the recognition of CR techniques as effective interventions for neurological populations, CR has been extended to improve cognitive and functional outcomes among individuals with serious mental illness, with most of the work focusing on schizophrenia-spectrum illness (Medalia & Choi, 2009; Wykes, Huddy, Cellard, McGurk, & Czobor, 2011). Individuals with schizophrenia demonstrate cognitive deficits across multiple domains, including attention, verbal memory, and executive functioning. Cognitive deficits are related to worse functional outcome and impaired ability to benefit from psychosocial rehabilitation (Medalia & Choi, 2009). As reviewed in a 2011 meta-analysis, over 40 clinical trials of CR interventions had been completed among individuals with schizophrenia-spectrum illnesses, where small to moderate effects of CR were found at posttreatment and follow-up across cognitive domains (Wykes et al., 2011). However, cognitive gains from traditional CR alone often did not transfer to improvements in real-world functioning.

The next wave of CR studies took on a restorative approach, with both cognitive and functional recovery aims. Studies supplemented the CR curriculum with some form of functional skills training that was more likely to produce positive changes in functional competence and real-world behaviors (i.e., Bowie, McGurk, Mausbach, Patterson, & Harvey, 2012). As follows, the core elements of the restorative approach to cognitive remediation that focus on skills development include (1) drill-and-practice CCT exercises, (2) strategy monitoring, and (3) activities that aid in the transfer of cognitive gains from training to real-world functional contexts. Delivery of these treatment elements can range from independent administration to therapist facilitation, with the latter typically associated with sustainable treatment effects.

Drill-and-practice CCT exercises are designed to improve specific cognitive skills via the principles of neuroplasticity. Much as certain gym equipment can be used to train a muscle group, patients repeatedly complete trials of computerized exercises that stimulate and strengthen the neural connections underlying targeted domains of cognitive functioning. Indeed, drill-and-practice CCT exercises have been found to result in physiological adaptations in the brain in parallel with enhanced processing and learning (Best, Gale, Tran, Haque, & Bowie, 2019; Best, Milanovic, Iftene, & Bowie, 2019; Eack et al., 2010; Subramaniam et al., 2012; Wykes et al., 2002).

While a number of CCT programs are on the market, most feature game design elements. These often include real-time and posttrial performance feedback, freedom to select from multiple exercises that address a broad range of cognitive domains, and systematic advancement to a higher difficulty level after the individual maintains high levels of accurate performance (typically 80% accuracy for the CCT programs used in research settings for depressed groups). Parameters of exercises are carefully titrated in difficulty according to the dynamic performance of the individual. For example, in a verbal working memory exercise, a patient may be tasked with quickly sorting words that appear on the screen into boxes that are labeled with different semantic categories (e.g., clothes, food). Higher levels of this exercise may reduce the time limit for sorting words or displaying unlabeled boxes, which would further challenge the patient to use working memory skills to mentally keep track of the categories. The optimal challenge level and reward contingencies that are conducive to treatment engagement and success in populations with mental illness is still a subject of debate. Preliminary research does suggest that CR facilitated by a therapist helps bolster engagement and self-efficacy in patients as therapists may monitor and address negative reactions to failures in real time.

In addition to drill-and-practice cognitive training, patients are taught *strategy monitoring*, that is, the process of bringing into awareness the problem-solving approaches used to tackle cognitive exercises. Once patients gain insight into their approaches, they may more readily adapt or switch strategies when environmental demands of the exercises change. Initially, therapists verbally reinforce, model, and shape flexible problem solving for CR recipients. In a group therapy setting, peers may further support each other by sharing similar stuck points and strategies. Patients are encouraged to work toward being independent in identifying their in-the-moment cognitive processes, evaluating their performance, and developing a repertoire of strategies from which they can experiment with and prune away strategies that are less effective for the given circumstances.

In the research setting, several facilitation modes of strategy monitoring have been documented. Some CR programs encourage patients to document their strategies and work with therapists to distinguish effective versus ineffective strategies. Other programs prompt patients to verbalize their thoughts as they work through cognitive training exercises. Our CR therapists have adopted communication styles of Socratic questioning and guided discovery when prompting patients to reflect on their strategies. After patients have a chance to work on the cognitive exercises, therapists start the dialogue with open-ended prompts (i.e., "What was your strategy?"), and if necessary, gradually provide more specific questions or examples that guide the patient in identifying any cognitive skills and behaviors that were used (i.e., "How were you using visual working memory skills in this exercise?"; "Tell me how you planned your actions"; "Some people find it helpful to use trial and error in sorting words into boxes; how do you think this relates to your approach?").

The rationale for strategy monitoring mirrors the theory of evidence-based psychotherapy models, which generally emphasize the development of metacognitive insight into the antecedents of dysfunction (i.e., systems of thoughts, feelings, and behaviors) before one can address presenting concerns. Along these lines, patients are exposed to challenging stages of cognitive training that may activate negative self-attributions and withdrawal from the treatment. These cognitive challenges are set up by therapists as opportunities to learn how to apply their thinking skills to manage stressful tasks. Patients are empowered to actively test out self-generated problem-solving strategies and build confidence in their cognitive abilities, which is something that troubles many with mental illness. By these means, strategy monitoring aims to maintain patient engagement with cognitive training in light of distressing challenges and thereby maximize treatment outcomes. Monitoring of cognitive processes has been found to be an important predictor of how well patients with mental illness utilize their thinking skills to support functioning in everyday life (Ladegaard, Larsen, Videbech, & Lysaker, 2014).

Transfer or "bridging" techniques are another important element of the restorative CR approach developed to facilitate the application of newly acquired cognitive and problem-solving skills to daily endeavors such as scheduling medical appointments or finding/maintaining employment. Traditionally, transfer techniques are discussion-based between peers (group therapy settings) or with a therapist. In these discussions, patients brainstorm ideas for how they may generalize cognitive skills and strategies drawn from drill-and-practice training to their daily lives. Typically, patients are prompted to keep in mind how their treatment gains can help them achieve individualized goals related to self-care, interpersonal functioning, recreational activities, and work (household and/or vocational).

Transfer techniques have been shown to have improvements in functional outcomes that are at most modest in effect size (Bell, Fiszdon, Greig, Wexler, & Bryson, 2007; Hodge et al., 2008; McGurk, Mueser, Feldman, Wolfe, & Pascaris, 2007; Medalia, Revheim, & Casey, 2001; Twamley et al., 2008). Thus, patient-specific characteristics may hinder functional improvements that are commensurate with cognitive gains. Since the benefits from bridging discussions are contingent on the amount of active participation, certain symptoms of mental disorders such as anxiety, low self-efficacy, and negative thinking patterns may become barriers to participation. For this reason, our team has devised a set of role-playing exercises through which patients can gain confidence in using their cognition to support their daily undertakings. Real-world settings are simulated with tangible props. For example, patients may be tasked with organizing a pantry of food items, and discussion of which strategies they learned from cognitive training exercises could be applied in this everyday life situation. We found these role-plays were successful in a psychiatric sample and led to improvements in everyday skill use and work functioning (Bowie, Milanovic, Tran, & Cassidy, 2017).

CR FOR DEPRESSION

A variety of cognitive-enhancing procedures in the treatment of major depressive disorder (MDD) have recently emerged. Individuals with MDD show significant, medium effect-size impairments in multiple cognitive domains, including executive function, memory, and attention, relative to healthy individuals (Rock, Roiser, Riedel, & Blackwell, 2014). Cognitive impairment in MDD is associated with reduced response to pharmacological interventions and psychotherapy (Dunkin et al., 2000). In addition, cognitive impairment is associated with poor psychosocial functioning (Jaeger, Berns, Uzelac, & Davis-Conway, 2006; Lam, Kennedy, McIntyre, & Khuller, 2014), even following remission of MDD symptoms (Woo, Rosenblat, Kakar, Bahk, & McIntyre, 2016). In comparison to the large body of literature available for brain injury and schizophrenia populations, the CR for MDD literature is small, but it is growing. For example, a recent meta-analysis of CCT interventions for MDD by Motter and colleagues (2016) reported on nine clinical trials and found medium effect-size improvements in attention and working memory, small effect-size improvements in symptom severity and daily functioning, and large effect-size improvements in global functioning (i.e., measures assessing comprehensive abilities across a wide range of cognitive domains). In contrast, nonsignificant effects were found for executive functioning and verbal memory, although these effects have been reported in some studies. Although studies in this meta-analysis allowed participants to be engaged in concurrent treatment for depressive symptoms (e.g., antidepressants, psychotherapy), this did not account for a large portion of the variance in the effect of CCTs on depressive symptoms, suggesting that CCTs alone may improve depressive symptomatology (Motter et al., 2016).

Consistent with Motter and colleagues' (2016) findings, the majority of work to date has investigated CCTs in the treatment of cognitive dysfunction among individuals with MDD (Alvarez, Sotres, Leon, Estrella, & Sosa, 2008; Bowie et al., 2013; Calkins, McMorran, Siegle, & Otto, 2015; Elgamel, McKinnon, Ramakrishnan, Joffe, & MacQueen, 2007; Lee et al., 2013; Meusel, Hall, Fougere, McKinnon, & MacQueen, 2013; Naismith et al., 2011; Owens, Koster, & Derakshan, 2013; Preiss, Shatil, Cermakova, Cimermanova, & Ram, 2013; Segrave, Arnold, Hoy, & Fitzgerald, 2014; Siegle et al., 2014; Trapp, Engel, Hajak, Lautenbacher, & Gallhofer, 2016). Very limited work has investigated noncomputerized approaches that emphasize the learning of compensatory strategies aimed at improving cognitive functioning in MDD (Gumport, Dong, Lee, & Harvey, 2018; Harvey et al., 2016). Interestingly, studies investigating top-down approaches in MDD have focused on enhancing outcomes for cognitive therapy rather than on improving cognitive functioning. Here, memory for contents of cognitive therapy treatment sessions was significantly higher, and improvements in functional impairment were significantly greater for those who had completed a memory support intervention (consisting of strategies for promoting learning memory) in addition to cognitive therapy, in comparison to those who received cognitive therapy alone at posttreatment and 6-month follow-up (Gumport et al., 2018; Harvey et al., 2016).

As the field moves toward studying cognitive remediation for MDD, it will be important to consider the lessons learned during the adaptation of CR for schizophrenia, to assess how characteristics that are predominant in MDD might affect treatment engagement and outcomes, and to formulate appropriate outcome measures. Early studies of CR in schizophrenia were often direct adaptations from neuropsychological rehabilitation for other conditions, as noted above. This failure to consider the unique issues related to schizophrenia led to a number of challenges in improving cognition and functioning outcomes. There are several aspects of how CR has evolved in schizophrenia that, when applied to MDD, will still need further modification. In the next sections, we review some potential issues and how we have developed a cognitive remediation program for MDD that includes new procedures that consider these challenges (see Table 18.1).

TABLE 18.1. Potential Issues in MDD That Might Limit Engagement and Success in Traditional CR

Issue	Potential methods to add to traditional CR
Low motivation to improve cognition	Goal setting
Negative beliefs about cognitive ability	Goal setting and strategy development
Reduced engagement with cognitively complex daily activities	Cognitive activation
Lack of confidence in using cognitive abilities in daily life	Role plays and engaging with real-life activities during treatment sessions

Issue 1: Low Motivation to Improve Cognition

Initiating and maintaining engagement with CR treatment can be challenging for patients with MDD. This may be due to motivational deficits that are a central component of the disorder. On clinical measures, MDD patients often report an impaired capacity to derive pleasure and enjoyment from hedonic experiences (termed *anhedonia symptoms*). Anhedonia in controlled experimental settings can be observed in MDD patients as a reduced reactivity to reward (e.g., monetary incentive for accurate task performance) and a reduced ability to make reward-specific behavioral changes to maximize future pleasurable experiences at the rate of healthy comparison groups (Pizzagalli, Iosifescu, Hallett, Ratner, & Fava, 2008; Pizzagalli, Jahn, & O'Shea, 2005). MDD patients also struggle with deciding whether to complete an effortful task, despite the greater reward that is offered in exchange for the work (for a review, see Culbreth, Moran, & Barch, 2018).

Experimental findings of blunted reward sensitivity and impaired reinforcement-based learning align with the motivation challenges we observe in our CR groups for MDD. Participants struggle with regular attendance of group sessions, and many drop out early in the course of treatment. A common reason our participants provide for premature withdrawal is a sudden recurrence of depressive symptoms that make it difficult to find the motivation to attend further sessions. In addition, CR participants often report low motivation and energy as barriers to completing prescribed at-home cognitive training exercises. Although these observations are anecdotal feedback, they contextualize experimental findings and suggest that motivation deficits in MDD hinder adaptive behavioral change that could lead to positive outcomes like improved cognitive functioning.

CR trials that have addressed indicators of treatment engagement reveal that low motivation, although a rate limiter of treatment success, can be malleable. In a CR program at an outpatient psychiatric clinic, participant-determined schedule of attendance was associated with greater cognitive improvement (Choi & Medalia, 2005). Our team found that the more time CR participants with treatment-resistant depression spent on online cognitive training exercises, the better their gains in cognitive functioning (Bowie et al., 2013). One study used a motivational interviewing procedure to connect cognitive training with clear, personalized goals and found that this method increased session attendance, task-specific intrinsic motivation, and treatment outcomes (Fiszdon, Kurtz, Choi, Bell, & Martino, 2016). This preliminary work highlights the importance of considering how we can address motivation issues in future iterations of CR programs for MDD.

Issue 2: Negative Beliefs about Cognitive Ability

As MDD patients often have internalized negative beliefs about self-worth, they may easily be harsh critics of their cognitive functioning and treatment prospects in CR. Depressed individuals self-report significantly higher and more frequent day-to-day cognitive problems than what is measured with objective neuropsychological assessment (Farrin, Hull, Unwin, Wykes, & David, 2003). Self-evaluations of cognitive impairment can also hinder performance on cognitively demanding tasks. For example, negative perceptions of cognitive abilities by MDD patients in one study affected performance on a standardized memory task, especially for patients with longer chronicity of depression (MacQueen,

Galway, Hay, Young, & Joffe, 2002). Similarly, on a computer-based sustained attention task, depressed individuals slowed their reaction times when they perceived their task performance was poor (e.g., after making errors; Farrin et al., 2003). This reaction to cognitive failure on the task was not observed in healthy comparison participants or brain-injured patients. In decision-making tasks, processes related to internally focused thinking (e.g., low self-efficacy, low concentration, and rumination) instead of external factors (e.g., preoccupation with task itself) were predictors of difficulties with decision making (van Randenborgh, de Jong-Meyer, & Hüffmeier, 2010). Taken together, MDD patients are vulnerable to negative attribution biases about one's cognitive abilities that may compromise the transfer of these abilities from training to real-world functional contexts.

Issue 3: Reduced Engagement in Cognitive Tasks

Many individuals with MDD appear to be averse to engaging in cognitive tasks and tend to withdraw from certain tasks or avoid them entirely when given a chance. For example, on a sustained working memory task, we found that participants with more severe depressive symptoms more frequently skipped trials (that is, they provided no response within the allotted time frame) when the task demands increased (Bowie, Milanovic, et al., 2017). In a recent study, MDD patients often chose to complete a lower cognitive effort task for less reward over a high-effort, high-reward option. This attenuated cognitive effort expenditure for reward was a significant predictor of functional disability (Tran, Hagen, Hollenstein, & Bowie, in press). Hershenberg and colleagues (2016) examined decisions to complete trial-by-trial number pair comparisons and increased the number of correct trials required before the participant could earn a reward. Depressed participants on this task were more likely to skip trials at lower success criteria than healthy comparisons. Thus, it appears that MDD patients are hesitant to both approach and persist at a cognitively challenging task. This can impede treatment success in CR, for learning from cognitive training exercises is contingent on seeking enough cognitive challenge to stimulate neuroplasticity.

Issue 4: Low Confidence in Cognitive Abilities

MDD patients tend to greatly underestimate the adequacy of their cognitive abilities to carry out the challenging roles and responsibilities encountered in day-to-day life. In a recent CR trial, our team recruited MDD participants who elected to enroll in the program due to self-reported cognitive difficulties. Neuropsychological assessments revealed that the global cognitive functioning of nearly 75% of CR-seeking individuals was within normal limits (Tran et al., in press). As MDD patients tend to have low endorsement of their own cognitive abilities, they may be prone to develop a heightened sense of disability in both cognitive and life functioning. Indeed, CR trials have found that even when cognitive functioning is intact or remediated, depressed individuals often have minimal or delayed improvements in everyday roles and activities (Bowie, Grossman, Gupta, Holshausen, & Best, 2017; Gupta et al., 2013; Naismith et al., 2011; Naismith, Redoblado-Hodge, Lewis, Scott, & Hickie, 2010). There is a need for an additional element to the traditional CR curriculum that would provide opportunities to succeed in cognitively challenging tasks so as to improve the confidence of depressed individuals in their own cognitive abilities.

ACTION-BASED CR

In an attempt to address the barriers to CR response in depressed individuals, action-based CR (ABCR) was designed. ABCR relies on the three traditional pillars of cognitive remediation, but also contains elements designed with consideration of the idiosyncrasies of depressive illness that may limit outcomes in cognitive remediation. In ABCR, *cognitive activation* (drill-and-practice cognitive exercises), *strategy monitoring*, and transfer/*generalization* are all conducted with additional considerations for the negative beliefs that characterize depression. In addition to these traditional cognitive remediation pillars, ABCR also includes *goal setting and activity scheduling* (to enhance motivation and activation), *simulations of real-life activities* (as opposed to verbal discussion to bridge cognitive skills to daily life), and *therapist intervention* (to help patients reevaluate negative beliefs and increase confidence to use cognitive abilities in daily life). An overview of the techniques used in ABCR is presented in Table 18.2.

Results from an open-label nonrandomized controlled trial support the efficacy of ABCR (Bowie, Milanovic, et al., 2017). Compared to a traditional discussion-based cognitive remediation program that lacked goal setting, real-world role plays, and activity scheduling, ABCR produced larger and more durable improvements in functional skills. Participants who received ABCR were also more likely to become competitively employed within 6 months (68% vs. 40%) and reported less job-related stress after treatment. Additionally, individuals who received ABCR reported greater improvements in their perceived competence to complete cognitively complex tasks than individuals who received traditional cognitive remediation. The ability of ABCR to decrease job-related stress and

TABLE 18.2. Therapy Techniques Used in ABCR

Pillars	Techniques	Targeted mechanisms
Didactic introduction	Psychoeducation Normalization	Motivation Orientation
Cognitive training	Drill and practice Repetitive exercise	Neuroplasticity Cognitive stimulation
Strategic monitoring	Identify strategies Develop new strategies Prune ineffective strategies	Metacognitive monitoring Flexible problem solving
Real-world simulation	Role play Transfer of skills	Planning activities Procedural learning
Cognitive activation planning	Goal setting Identifying homework tasks	Cognitive engagement Cognitive confidence

increase perceived competence suggests that the intervention is improving factors that are especially important to consider in depression. Finally, a critical finding of this trial was the dramatically larger retention in ABCR (83%) compared to traditional cognitive remediation (57%). Impairments in motivation and energy make it challenging to retain individuals with depression in treatment, so the fact that over three-quarters were retained in ABCR is an important achievement.

Given these promising results, it is also pertinent to consider whether delivering ABCR is feasible in routine clinical environments. Two PhD-level therapists working with a group of patients for two 2-hour sessions per week for 10 weeks may not be feasible. However, it will be important to evaluate the long-term cost savings if work and disability outcomes are maintained. Furthermore, implementing the elements of ABCR that successfully increased confidence, functioning, and treatment retention could be important for other cognitive-enhancing treatments for depression. The specific elements of ABCR and how they address the depression-related challenges that might limit engagement and success in cognitive enhancing therapies are discussed below.

Goal Setting

Throughout treatment but particularly early on, depression can interfere with motivation and energy levels to engage in cognitive remediation. For some patients, motivation may be initially high, but as life circumstances change the importance of treatment may be overshadowed by other priorities. Additionally, while many individuals report cognitive difficulties in their daily lives, it can be challenging for individuals with depression to identify how enhancing cognition could help them in daily life. Goal setting provides an opportunity for patients to identify personally relevant reasons for improving cognition, initiate engagement in treatment, access motivation for continued treatment adherence, and provide reasons for continuing treatment when life circumstances become difficult. Goal setting is often overlooked in cognitive-enhancing treatments, yet it is critical to motivate individuals with depression to engage and persist in treatment.

Goal setting is a collaborative process in which the therapist guides the patient in discovering their goals across several domains of functioning. Goal setting begins with developing a broad goal that is functionally relevant. Clinical experience and empirical evidence have suggested six domains of community functioning that are useful to consider in setting functional goals (see Figure 18.1).

For many individuals with depression, goals will initially be generic and ill defined such as "I want to feel better" or "I want my mood to improve." As part of the collaborative process, it is important to guide the individual to make this goal specific and behavioral. For example, the therapist could ask, "What sorts of things would you be doing if you were feeling better?" Through this collaborative process, patients develop a concrete list of goals that are personally relevant and functionally based. While it is not necessary for individuals to have goals in each of the functional domains in Figure 18.1, it can be useful to explore each domain with the individual.

Although some goals may be motivating in themselves, many goals are long-term events that may take significant time and resources to achieve (i.e., achieving new vocational training). In order to maintain motivation over the time it takes to achieve long-term

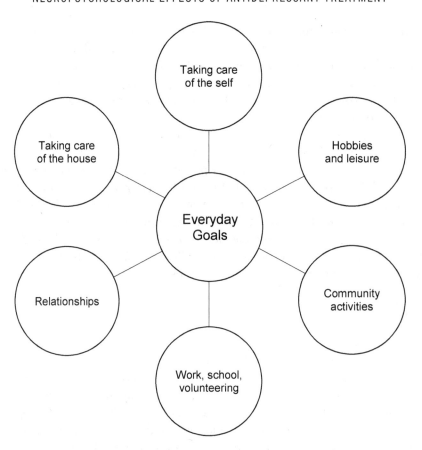

FIGURE 18.1. Broad domains of functioning for goal setting.

goals, it is important to break these larger goals into smaller steps that can be accomplished in a briefer time frame (i.e., searching the Internet to find a career counselor). Creating the sequence of small steps required to achieve the broader goal provides frequent opportunities for the individual to experience success and positive reinforcement, and to further increase motivation to continue pursuing the goal. When goal setting is done properly, the goals that are set up should be virtually impossible for the individual to "fail" at. For example, if an individual must take an exam to receive a new vocational certification, a typical goal that they might have would be to pass the exam. However, it is quite possible that they could fail the exam, which would strengthen the negative beliefs we are attempting to reframe in therapy. For someone with depression who experiences low motivation and negative beliefs about themselves, a better goal would be to *take the exam*. This goal is not linked to a specific outcome but to a behavior that they can control, which will serve to increase motivation for the next step toward the broader goal even if they fail the exam on this attempt.

To facilitate motivation to engage in cognitive remediation, it is critical to link individuals' goals (broad and specific) to their cognitive abilities. Most people are not used to thinking about their lives within a cognitive context, and thus links between cognitive abilities and goals are important to facilitate treatment engagement. For example, an individual whose goal is to take better care of the house by doing laundry and dishes more often could benefit from discussion surrounding which cognitive abilities might be especially important for these functional tasks. Memory might be important to remember to do the tasks, attention might be important to make sure that the task is done properly, and planning might be important to fit these chores into an otherwise busy life. Without a direct link being drawn between functional goals and cognitive abilities, the opportunity for individuals to access motivation to improve cognitive abilities is missed and individuals may not persist in treatment.

Individuals with depression may also experience hopelessness about their ability to achieve goals or improve their cognitive abilities. Goal setting provides an opportunity for the therapist to convey hope that the techniques used in cognitive remediation can improve cognitive abilities and help the individual achieve their goals. It is important not to overpromise the results of therapy. However, depression makes it challenging for individuals to be hopeful, and so it is critical for therapists to carry the hope for their patients until their patients are able to have successful experiences and see the benefits of treatment.

Since motivational impairments are a core feature of depression, goal setting is an important tool. However, if goal setting is only done at the beginning of treatment, it is likely to have limited results. Goals are the glue that hold therapy sessions together and provide an overarching reason for treatment from session to session. As a result, goals should be frequently revisited over the course of treatment, and any progress toward goals should also be acknowledged and praised. Frequent reinforcement of small successes will build motivation to continue treatment and to move on to the next step toward the broader goal.

Cognitive Activation

Symptoms of depression such as fatigue and diminished interest or pleasure in activities can make it challenging for individuals to engage in cognitively stimulating activities in daily life. Often when individuals with depression present for treatment, they are spending less time in vocational activities, have withdrawn from their social networks, and may not be readily engaged in activities of daily living. Individuals who have experienced depression for prolonged periods of time may be engaged in very little activity and are often actively avoiding any complex activities that require substantial cognitive effort.

Similar to how muscles weaken if they are not exercised, cognitive abilities can atrophy when they are not regularly used. Lack of cognitive stimulation can cause synaptic connections to weaken and neuronal tissue to decrease in volume. Cognitive activation is the process through which we help patients activate their cognitive abilities more frequently. Cognitive activation can be considered to consist of two components: *computerized cognitive training*, and *engagement with cognitively stimulating tasks in daily life*.

In addition to completing cognitive activation exercises in session, it can also be useful for individuals to practice the cognitive exercises outside of session to further increase neuroplasticity and to learn that they are capable of success without a therapist immediately present. Cognitive activation from computerized exercises is typically not sufficient to produce broad and sustained changes in everyday functioning. Thus, cognitive activation is likely to be most beneficial if it includes engagement in cognitively challenging activities in daily life. Scheduling cognitively challenging activities into the individual's day will increase the likelihood that they regularly engage in such activities. Cognitive activation should also be incorporated into goal setting, so that goals include engagement in cognitively stimulating daily activities. Examples of such goals could include learning a new skill, returning to work, increasing vocational training, or planning an event. Engagement in such cognitively stimulating activities can produce a cycle through which cognitive abilities improve through cognitive stimulation, which then make the activity easier to complete and thus more likely that the individual will engage in that activity in the future (Figure 18.2).

For many individuals with depression, negative beliefs will interfere with the breadth of exercises that are practiced. Parallel to the cognitive avoidance that occurs in the daily lives of individuals with depression, cognitive avoidance is likely to occur during the cognitive training exercises. While it can be helpful for individuals to have mastery experiences on exercises that they find less challenging, it is also important for individuals to practice the exercises that they find to be most challenging. Thus, an important role for the therapist is to encourage individuals to practice cognitively challenging exercises. While practicing these exercises, it is important to draw the individual's attention to every small success that they experience in order to develop a stronger sense of self-efficacy to complete challenging tasks.

Strategy Monitoring

Typical strategy monitoring in cognitive remediation provides an opportunity for individuals to metacognitively monitor the strategies they are using, flexibly develop new strategies, and prune away strategies that are consistently proving ineffective. In working with individuals experiencing depression, strategy monitoring also provides an opportunity to address negative beliefs that are activated while completing cognitive activation

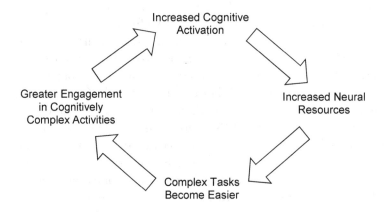

FIGURE 18.2. A feedback cycle through which cognitive activation facilitates engagement with cognitively stimulating activities.

exercises or role-play simulations. Individuals with depression will frequently report negative beliefs about their ability to complete the cognitive activation exercises, the role-play scenarios, and other tasks related to everyday functioning. If unaddressed, these beliefs can hinder therapy progress and potentially increase negative expectancies about cognitively complex tasks. For example, if an individual repeatedly struggles to achieve success at cognitive activation exercises, then beliefs such as "I'm stupid" or "I am incapable of doing even easy tasks" could be strengthened. When working with individuals experiencing depression, it is important to elicit these beliefs during cognitive activation and generalization exercises so that they can be evaluated. For example, these beliefs frequently become activated when individuals reach a level of difficulty on computerized cognitive exercises that they are initially unable to complete. In these situations, the individual's attention will become fixated on the level they were unable to complete. It is important to broaden the individual's perspective and remind them of their successes on previous levels of the computer exercises and to reevaluate any negative beliefs that have become activated. For example, "I am incapable of doing even easy tasks" could be reevaluated as "I have been successful so far, but this level is more difficult and I will need a new strategy to be successful at it."

Strategy monitoring also provides an opportunity to develop problem-solving skills. By practicing metacognitive awareness of the strategies being used, individuals learn to distance themselves from their experience and generate alternative strategies to complete tasks. Patients then have the opportunity to determine which strategies are working best for them and which strategies may be worth discontinuing. After using the strategy, individuals can then reevaluate the strategy and continuously refine it. Although this process can be used to solve problems in any domain of the patient's life, the cognitive remediation environment provides a safe environment for patients to practice the problem-solving process. It is also common that individuals will not immediately link strategy-monitoring techniques to other situations in their lives. Thus, it is critical to use the strategy-monitoring techniques to also develop strategies for everyday situations. The goal of using strategy monitoring in this way is to help patients to learn that there are no "automatic fail" situations and that they simply need to find the best strategy to approach a situation in order to succeed.

Role-Play Simulations of Everyday Activities

Transferring cognitive gains to improvement in real-world behavior is one of the biggest challenges for cognitive remediation. This challenge is amplified by the fact that many individuals with chronic mental disorders experience impairments in the ability to think abstractly about how skills developed in therapy could apply to novel situations found in everyday life. Similarly, depression is associated with impairments in verbal and working memory, which makes it more challenging for individuals to recall the skills learned in therapy and apply them in daily life. Thus, using discussion-based techniques to generalize learning in therapy to everyday activities may have limited efficacy. Interestingly, *procedural* learning and memory tend to be intact in depression. ABCR capitalizes on procedural learning through the use of role-play simulations to help bridge the gap between strategy monitoring during computerized exercises and the activities of daily life.

When designing role-play simulations, it is important to tailor the simulations to the idiosyncratic needs of the individual. This involves linking the simulations to activities that the individual actually performs, or wishes to perform, in their everyday life. Simulations that are not directly linked to activities the individual will encounter in daily life are unlikely to be effective methods of generalizing treatment response. Additionally, role-play simulations should be linked to the cognitive activation exercises that the individual is practicing. If a simulation is not linked to the strategies that are being developed during the cognitive activation exercises, then patients will not have the opportunity to test the new strategies that have been developed in the role-play simulation. An example of how a role-play simulation could bridge the gap between computerized exercise and real-world activity is presented in Table 18.3.

In ABCR, the real-world simulations were developed collaboratively with individuals who had lived experience of persistent mental disorders and employers who were routinely hiring from a vocational rehabilitation center. The simulations in ABCR focus on a broad range of skills that many individuals with mental health difficulties identify as areas they struggle with and as goals for treatment. Real-world simulations in ABCR include sorting items at a store, using public transit maps to plan a trip, and introductions with other people in which one must remember specific facts about them. While simulations should be tailored to the specific needs of the individual, it is also important to use simulations that address all of the broad domains of functioning included in Figure 18.1.

Although real-world simulations capitalize on intact procedural memory abilities, it is also important for patients to explicitly link how the strategies developed during the cognitive training exercises contributed to their performance in the simulation and how the strategies can be used in other areas of daily life. This link can initially be quite challenging to make, and it is important for therapists to guide patients in discovering these connections. Once patients have made the connection, it is important to test the strategies outside of session in daily life. After a strategy has been tested in daily life, it can be refined if it is effective or it can be pruned away if deemed ineffective. Given the lack of confidence in one's cognitive abilities and negative beliefs about the self that characterize depression, it is often challenging for clients to immediately apply the strategies from therapy to everyday life. The simulations serve as a safe environment to initially test strategies that can bridge treatment to the real world and increase the likelihood of individuals applying therapy skills in their daily lives.

TABLE 18.3. An Example of How Simulations Can Bridge the Gap between Computerized Exercises and the Real World

Computer exercise	Strategy	Role-play simulation	Strategy applied to simulation	Everyday life
Arrange rings on towers as efficiently as possible to match a template.	Plan out each step before making the move.	Everyone is out sick at work, and you have to quickly complete several different tasks.	Plan a strategy for each task you will need to complete before you actually start doing it.	Plan out all the tasks you need to get done at work and prioritize them before you actually start working on them.

CONCLUSION

The increasing research focus on the prevalence, severity, and functional implications of cognitive deficits in MDD has spurred a rapidly growing literature on efforts to improve cognition. Early studies using cognitive training or cognitive remediation have largely borrowed from treatment procedures used in schizophrenia. It is critical to continue to explore, with experimental studies, how cognitive deficits in MDD interact with other features of the illness, including motivation, negative self-attributions, and withdrawal. This is the best way to understand how to develop new strategies that will ensure that the treatment target addresses more than a performance-based cognitive deficit and that treatment outcomes affect daily life goals. Early work suggests that when we incorporate treatment principles from other cognitive and behavioral therapies into cognitive remediation, motivation increases lead to better engagement and retention, treatment effects are larger and more durable, and real-world behavior change is more likely.

REFERENCES

Alvarez, L. M., Sotres, J. F. C., Leon, S. O., Estrella, J., & Sosa, J. J. S. (2008). Computer program in the treatment for major depression and cognitive impairment in university students. *Computers in Human Behavior, 24*(3), 816–826.

Barlati, S., Deste, G., De Peri, L., Ariu, C., & Vita, A. (2013). Cognitive remediation in schizophrenia: Current status and future perspectives. *Schizophrenia Research and Treatment, 2013,* 156084.

Bell, M., Fiszdon, J., Greig, T., Wexler, B., & Bryson, G. (2007). Neurocognitive enhancement therapy with work therapy in schizophrenia: 6-month follow-up of neuropsychological performance. *Journal of Rehabilitation Research and Development, 44*(5), 761–770.

Best, M. W., & Bowie, C. R. (2017). A review of cognitive remediation approaches for schizophrenia: from top-down to bottom-up, brain training to psychotherapy. *Expert Review of Neurotherapeutics, 17*(7), 713–723.

Best, M. W., Gale, D., Tran, T., Haque, M. K., & Bowie, C. R. (2019). Brief executive function training for individuals with severe mental illness: Effects on EEG synchronization and executive functioning. *Schizophrenia Research, 203,* 32–40.

Best, M. W., Milanovic, M., Iftene, F., & Bowie, C. R. (2019) A randomized controlled trial of executive functioning training compared with perceptual training for schizophrenia spectrum disorders: Effects on neurophysiology, neurocognition, and functioning. *American Journal of Psychiatry, 176*(4), 297–306.

Bowie, C. R., Bell, M. D., Fiszdon, J. M., Johannesen, J. K., Lindenmayer, J. P., McGurk, S. R., et al. (2020). Cognitive remediation for schizophrenia: An expert working group white paper on core techniques. *Schizophrenia Research, 215,* 49–53.

Bowie, C. R., Grossman, M., Gupta, M., Holshausen, K., & Best, M. W. (2017). Action-based cognitive remediation for individuals with serious mental illnesses: Effects of real-world simulations and goal setting on functional and vocational outcomes. *Psychiatric Rehabilitation Journal, 40*(1), 53–60.

Bowie, C. R., Gupta, M., Holshausen, K., Jokic, R., Best, M., & Milev, R. (2013). Cognitive remediation for treatment-resistant depression: Effects on cognition and functioning and the role of online homework. *Journal of Nervous and Mental Disease, 201*(8), 680–685.

Bowie, C. R., McGurk, S. R., Mausbach, B., Patterson, T. L., & Harvey, P. D. (2012). Combined cognitive remediation and functional skills training for schizophrenia: effects on cognition, functional competence, and real-world behavior. *American Journal of Psychiatry, 169*(7), 710–718.

Bowie, C. R., Milanovic, M., Tran, T., & Cassidy, S. (2017). Disengagement from tasks as a function of cognitive load and depressive symptom severity. *Cognitive Neuropsychiatry, 22*(1), 83–94.

Calkins, A. W., McMorran, K. E., Siegle, G. J., & Otto, M. W. (2015). The effects of computerized cognitive control training on community adults with depressed mood. *Behavioural and Cognitive Psychotherapy, 43*(5), 578–589.

Choi, J., & Medalia, A. (2005). Factors associated with a positive response to cognitive remediation in a community psychiatric sample. *Psychiatric Services, 56*(5), 602–604.

Cicerone, K. D., Dahlberg, C., Malec, J. F., Langenbahn, D. M., Felicetti, T., Kneipp, S., et al. (2005). Evidence-based cognitive rehabilitation: Updated review of the literature from 1998 through 2002. *Archives of Physical Medicine and Rehabilitation, 86*(8), 1681–1692.

Culbreth, A. J., Moran, E. K., & Barch, D. M. (2018). Effort-cost decision-making in psychosis and depression: Could a similar behavioral deficit arise from disparate psychological and neural mechanisms? *Psychological Medicine, 48*(6), 889–904.

Dunkin, J. J., Leuchter, A. F., Cook, I. A., Kasl-Godley, J. E., Abrams, M., & Rosenberg-Thompson, S. (2000). Executive dysfunction predicts nonresponse to fluoxetine in major depression. *Journal of Affective Disorders, 60*(1), 13–23.

Eack, S. M., Hogarty, G. E., Cho, R. Y., Prasad, K. M., Greenwald, D. P., Hogarty, S. S., et al. (2010). Neuroprotective effects of cognitive enhancement therapy against gray matter loss in early schizophrenia: Results from a 2-year randomized controlled trial. *Archives of General Psychiatry, 67*(7), 674–682.

Elgamel, S., McKinnon, M. C., Ramakrishnan, K., Joffe, R. T., & MacQueen, G. (2007). Successful computer-assisted cognitive remediation therapy in patients with unipolar depression: A proof of principle study. *Psychological Medicine, 37*(9), 1229–1238.

Farrin, L., Hull, L., Unwin, C., Wykes, T., & David, A. (2003). Effects of depressed mood on objective and subjective measures of attention. *Journal of Neuropsychiatry and Clinical Neurosciences, 15*(1), 98–104.

Fiszdon, J. M., Kurtz, M. M., Choi, J., Bell, M. D., & Martino, S. (2016). Motivational interviewing to increase cognitive rehabilitation adherence in schizophrenia. *Schizophrenia Bulletin, 42*(2), 327–334.

Gumport, N. B., Dong, L., Lee, J. Y., & Harvey, A. G. (2018). Patient learning of treatment contents in cognitive therapy. *Journal of Behavior Therapy and Experimental Psychiatry, 58*, 51–59.

Gupta, M., Holshausen, K., Best, M. W., Jokic, R., Milev, R., Bernard, T., et al. (2013). Relationships among neurocognition, symptoms, and functioning in treatment-resistant depression. *Archives of Clinical Neuropsychology, 28*(3), 272–281.

Harvey, A. G., Lee, J., Smith, R. L., Gumport, N. B., Hollon, S. D., Rabe-Hesketh, S., et al. (2016). Improving outcome for mental disorders by enhancing memory for treatment. *Behaviour Research and Therapy, 81*, 35–46.

Hershenberg, R., Satterthwaite, T. D., Daldal, A., Katchmar, N., Moore, T. M., Kable, J. W., et al. (2016). Diminished effort on a progressive ratio task in both unipolar and bipolar depression. *Journal of Affective Disorders, 196*, 97–100.

Hodge, M. A. R., Siciliano, D., Withey, P., Moss, B., Moore, G., Judd, G., et al. (2008). A randomized controlled trial of cognitive remediation in schizophrenia. *Schizophrenia Bulletin, 36*(2), 419–427.

Jaeger, J., Berns, S., Uzelac, S., & Davis-Conway, S. (2006). Neurocognitive deficits and disability in major depressive disorder. *Psychiatry Research, 145*(1), 39–48.

Ladegaard, N., Larsen, E. R., Videbech, P., & Lysaker, P. H. (2014). Higher-order social cognition in first-episode major depression. *Psychiatry Research, 216*(1), 37–43.

Lam, R. W., Kennedy, S. H., McIntyre, R. S., & Khuller, A. (2014). Cognitive dysfunction in major depressive disorder: Effects on psychosocial functioning and implications for treatment. *Canadian Journal of Psychiatry, 59*(12), 649–654.

Lee, R. S. C., Redoblado-Hodge, M. A., Naismith, S. L., Hermens, D. F., Porter, M. A., & Hickie, I. B. (2013). Cognitive remediation improves memory and psychosocial functioning in first-episode psychiatric out-patients. *Psychological Medicine, 43*(6), 1161–1173.

MacQueen, G. M., Galway, T. M., Hay, J., Young, L. T., & Joffe, R. T. (2002). Recollection memory deficits in patients with major depressive disorder predicted by past depressions but not current mood state or treatment status. *Psychological Medicine, 32*(2), 251–258.

McGurk, S. R., Mueser, K. T., Feldman, K., Wolfe, R., & Pascaris, A. (2007). Cognitive training for supported employment: 2–3 year outcomes of a randomized controlled trial. *American Journal of Psychiatry, 164*(3), 437–441.

Medalia, A., & Choi, J. (2009). Cognitive remediation in schizophrenia. *Neuropsychology Review, 19*(3), 353.

Medalia, A., Revheim, N., & Casey, M. (2001). The remediation of problem-solving skills in schizophrenia. *Schizophrenia Bulletin, 27*(2), 259–267.

Meusel, L. A. C., Hall, G. B. C., Fougere, P., McKinnon, M. C., & MacQueen, G. M. (2013). Neural correlates of cognitive remediation in patients with mood disorders. *Psychiatry Research: Neuroimaging, 214*(2), 142–152.

Motter, J. N., Pimontel, M. A., Rindskopf, D., Devanand, D. P., Doraiswamy, P. M., & Sneed, J. R. (2016). Computerized cognitive training and functional recovery in major depressive disorder: A meta-analysis. *Journal of Affective Disorders, 189,* 184–191.

Naismith, S. L., Diamond, K., Carter, P. E., Norrie, L. M., Redoblado-Hodge, M. A., Lewis, S. J. G., et al. (2011). Enhancing memory in late-life depression: The effects of combined psychoeducation and cognitive training program. *American Journal of Geriatric Psychiatry, 19*(3), 240–248.

Naismith, S. L., Redoblado-Hodge, M. A., Lewis, S. J. G., Scott, E. M., & Hickie, I. B. (2010). Cognitive training in affective disorders improves memory: A preliminary study using the NEAR approach. *Journal of Affective Disorders, 121*(3), 258–262.

Owens, M., Koster, E. H., & Derakshan, N. (2013). Improving attention control in dysphoria through cognitive training: Transfer effects on working memory capacity and filtering efficiency. *Psychophysiology, 50*(3), 297–307.

Pizzagalli, D. A., Iosifescu, D., Hallett, L. A., Ratner, K. G., & Fava, M. (2008). Reduced hedonic capacity in major depressive disorder: Evidence from a probabilistic reward task. *Journal of Psychiatric Research, 43*(1), 76–87.

Pizzagalli, D. A., Jahn, A. L., & O'Shea, J. P. (2005). Toward an objective characterization of an anhedonic phenotype: A signal-detection approach. *Biological Psychiatry, 57*(4), 319–327.

Podd, M. H. (2011). *Cognitive remediation for brain injury and neurological illness: Real life changes.* New York: Springer Science & Business Media.

Preiss, M., Shatil, E., Cermakova, R., Cimermanova, D., & Ram, I. (2013). Personalized cognitive training in unipolar and bipolar disorder: A study of cognitive functioning. *Frontiers in Human Neuroscience, 7,* 108.

Rock, P. L., Roiser, J. P., Riedel, W. J., & Blackwell, A. D. (2014). Cognitive impairment in depression: A systematic review and meta-analysis. *Psychological Medicine, 44*(10), 2029–2040.

Segrave, R. A., Arnold, S., Hoy, K., & Fitzgerald, P. B. (2014). Concurrent cognitive control training augments the antidepressant efficacy of tDCS: A pilot study. *Brain Stimulation, 7*(2), 325–331.

Siegle, G. J., Price, R. B., Jones, N. P., Ghinassi, F., Painter, T., & Thase, M. E. (2014). You gotta work at it: Pupillary indices of task focus are prognostic for response to a neurocognitive intervention for rumination in depression. *Clinical Psychological Science, 2*(4), 455–471.

Subramaniam, K., Luks, T. L., Fisher, M., Simpson, G. V., Nagarajan, S., & Vinogradov, S. (2012). Computerized cognitive training restores neural activity within the reality monitoring network in schizophrenia. *Neuron, 73*(4), 842–853.

Tran, T., Hagen, A. E. F., Hollenstein, T., & Bowie, C. R. (in press). Physical and cognitive effort-based decision-making in depression: Relationships to symptoms and functioning. *Clinical Psychological Science.*

Trapp, W., Engel, S., Hajak, G., Lautenbacher, S., & Gallhofer, B. (2016). Cognitive remediation for depressed inpatients: Results of a pilot randomized controlled trial. *Australian and New Zealand Journal of Psychiatry, 50*(1), 46–55.

Twamley, E. W., Savla, G. N., Zurhellen, C. H., Heaton, R. K., & Jeste, D. V. (2008). Development and pilot testing of a novel compensatory cognitive training intervention for people with psychosis. *American Journal of Psychiatric Rehabilitation, 11*(2), 144–163.

van Randenborgh, A., de Jong-Meyer, R., & Hüffmeier, J. (2010). Decision making in depression: differences in decisional conflict between healthy and depressed individuals. *Clinical Psychology and Psychotherapy, 17*(4), 285–298.

Woo, Y. S., Rosenblat, J. D., Kakar, R., Bahk, W. M., & McIntyre, R. S. (2016). Cognitive deficits as a mediator of poor occupational function in remitted major depressive disorder patients. *Clinical Psychopharmacology and Neuroscience, 14*(1), 1–16.

Wykes, T., Brammer, M., Mellers, J., Bray, P., Reeder, C., Williams, C., et al. (2002). Effects on the brain of a psychological treatment: Cognitive remediation therapy: Functional magnetic resonance imaging in schizophrenia. *British Journal of Psychiatry, 181*(2), 144–152.

Wykes, T., Huddy, V., Cellard, C., McGurk, S. R., & Czobor, P. (2011). A meta-analysis of cognitive remediation for schizophrenia: Methodology and effect sizes. *American Journal of Psychiatry, 168*(5), 472–485

CHAPTER 19

Exercise

Tracy L. Greer
Hunter Small

While the terms *exercise* and *physical activity* are often used interchangeably, these concepts are distinct. Physical activity has been defined as bodily movement executed by the contraction of skeletal muscles, which results in increased caloric requirements beyond resting energy expenditure (American College of Sports Medicine [ACSM], 2009; Caspersen, Powell, & Christenson, 1985). Exercise is a subcategory of physical activity that involves planned, structured, and repetitive bodily movement carried out with the intention of maintaining or improving physical fitness (ACSM, 2009; Caspersen et al., 1985). Exercise is known to be important for overall health and well-being and is routinely recommended by clinical providers to target and reduce a variety of clinical symptoms and/or to prevent disease onset. The ACSM recommends that most adults engage in a minimum of 30 minutes of moderate intensity aerobic activity 5 days per week, or vigorous intensity aerobic exercise for a minimum of 20 minutes 3 days per week (ACSM, 2009). This regimen can be completed flexibly, with bouts of exercise of 10 minutes or more, and combinations of moderate and vigorous intensity. The ACSM also recommends that adults perform resistance exercises for each of the major muscle groups and neuromotor exercise (involving balance, agility, and coordination) 2–3 days per week, and flexibility exercises for each of the major muscle-tendon groups 2 or more days per week (ACSM, 2009; Garber et al., 2011). However, individuals who engage in exercise in order to reduce risk and/or symptoms of chronic disease or disability may benefit from exceeding the minimum recommended amounts (Haskell et al., 2007).

Engaging in exercise is associated with a reduced likelihood of depression, as well as many other psychiatric disorders, and may also have a preventative effect against disease development (Farmer et al., 1988; Galper, Trivedi, Barlow, Dunn, & Kampert, 2006; Goodwin, 2003). Exercise, whether alone or in combination with medication, reduces depressive symptoms in individuals with major depressive disorder (MDD), although recent meta-analyses have concluded that the most rigorously conducted trials are associated with lower effect sizes (Cooney et al., 2013; Krogh, Nordentoft, Sterne, & Lawlor,

2011; Lawlor & Hopker, 2001; Mead et al., 2009). Regardless, evidence is substantial enough to have prompted the inclusion of exercise in many treatment guidelines, including the American Psychiatric Association Practice Guidelines, which recommends exercise as a first-line treatment for mild MDD and an adjunctive treatment for all levels of depressive severity (American Psychiatric Association, 2019).

Exercise is also associated specifically with cognitive benefits in healthy individuals across the lifespan (Churchill et al., 2002; Cotman & Berchtold, 2002; Etnier et al., 1997; Sibley & Etnier, 2003). Exercise has a long history of association with reductions in age-associated cognitive decline (Government Office for Science, 2008), as well as cognitive improvements in association with a wide range of physical and mental disorders, including neurodegenerative disorders such as mild cognitive impairment, dementia, and Parkinson's disease, and psychiatric disorders such as schizophrenia (Firth et al., 2017; Murray, Sacheli, Eng, & Stoessl, 2014; ten Brinke et al., 2015). Observed cognitive improvements have been associated with a wide variety of exercise types, including aerobic exercise and mind–body interventions (Firth et al., 2017; Murray et al., 2014; ten Brinke et al., 2015).

While cognitive impairments are recognized as a critical aspect of many medical and psychiatric illnesses, the importance of cognitive impairments in depressive disorders has been much more slowly realized. It is encouraging that recent research has placed greater emphasis on cognitive and functional outcomes in depression to improve our understanding of how best to treat these symptoms, as they are of great importance to patients (Lam, Filteau, & Milev, 2011). A recent survey of practicing psychiatrists in six countries suggested that clinical awareness of the importance of cognition in MDD has also increased, although clinical detection and management of cognitive function in depression is still most often based on clinical interview rather than the use of objective assessments (El Hammi et al., 2014).

Despite the slow trajectory of emphasis on cognitive function in depression, it is well established that depressed individuals experience a wide variety of cognitive impairments that include psychomotor slowing and reduced attention and concentration, executive functioning and working memory, and visual and verbal learning and memory (Trivedi & Greer, 2014; Veiel, 1997). While these cognitive impairments are broad in scope, much previous research has concluded that these impairments are not as pronounced as in other disorders, such as schizophrenia or Alzheimer's disease (Lewis, 2004; Christensen, Griffiths, MacKinnon, & Jacomb, 1997). An alternative conclusion is that individuals with depression exhibit a greater degree of heterogeneity of cognitive impairments (i.e., some individuals with depression have more robust cognitive impairments than others; Gualtieri & Morgan, 2008). This heterogeneity is an important consideration when evaluating the impact of exercise on cognition in depressed individuals. Another important consideration is the relationship between cognitive impairments and depressive symptom severity. Evidence suggests that both can improve in conjunction with antidepressant treatment (McClintock, Husain, Greer, & Cullum, 2010), although cognitive impairments have been shown to persist even when symptomatic remission is achieved (Hasselbalch, Knorr, Hasselbalch, Gade, & Kessing, 2012; Weiland-Fiedler et al., 2004). This finding suggests some independence between symptom severity and cognitive function in depression and supports the need for identifying effective targeted treatments, such as exercise, that will directly improve cognition.

NEUROBIOLOGICAL EFFECTS OF EXERCISE

Before discussing clinical studies of exercise on cognitive outcomes in depressed individuals, it is important to highlight the numerous neurobiological effects of exercise that support cognitive benefits across disease states, including depression (Greer, Furman, & Trivedi, 2017). Exercise has been associated with increased volumetric changes in the brain globally, as well as in specific areas of the brain that are associated with particular cognitive abilities. Volumetric increases in both white and gray matter were observed in prefrontal and temporal cortices in healthy but sedentary older adults (ages 60–79) who participated in a 6-month aerobic exercise regimen, compared to those in a nonaerobic stretching program or sedentary younger individuals (ages 18–30; Colcombe et al., 2006). These results indicate that aerobic exercise may play a critical role in preserving and improving cognitive functioning and overall brain health in older adults (Colcombe et al., 2006). Substantial changes in white matter integrity in frontal and temporal lobes, as well as improvements in short-term memory, were observed for sedentary older adults (ages 55–80) participating in a one-year aerobic training program (involving 40-minute walking sessions), as compared to controls (stretching; Voss et al., 2013). However, the improvements in short-term memory were not linked to the changes in white matter integrity.

Several studies have also demonstrated increases in hippocampal volume in association with exercise in healthy adults (Erickson et al., 2009, 2011; Niemann, Godde, & Voelcker-Rehage, 2014; Thomas et al., 2016) as well as in clinical populations, including those with mild cognitive impairment (ten Brinke et al., 2015), multiple sclerosis (Leavitt et al., 2014), schizophrenia (Pajonk et al., 2010; Scheewe et al., 2013), and depression (Krogh et al., 2014). Such changes certainly support the benefit of exercise for declarative memory tasks, as hippocampal integrity is essential for performance on such tasks. Furthermore, exercise has been shown to increase cerebral blood flow (Ainslie et al., 2008), which is recognized as an important factor for increasing brain volume, as well as decreasing atrophy. The potential positive impact of these volumetric changes can be evaluated by looking at broader changes and function across brain networks. For example, exercise increases functional connectivity within the default mode network and frontal executive network, which are critical to the resting coherence of brain networks that enable optimal neurocognitive performance (Voss, Nagamatsu, Liu-Ambrose, & Kramer, 2011).

Several molecular changes associated with exercise (including normalization of monoaminergic neurotransmission and factors associated with stress and immune function) are likely mechanisms by which exercise has a positive impact on overall depression, as well as cognition specifically (Phillips & Fahimi, 2018). Exercise decreases several pro-inflammatory factors, such as tumor necrosis factor–alpha, interleukin 6, and interleukin 1 and may therefore mitigate inflammatory-induced cognitive impairments (Phillips & Fahimi, 2018). Exercise is also associated with increases in brain-derived neurotrophic factor (BDNF; Szuhany, Bugatti, & Otto, 2015), a protein implicated in neurogenesis, dendritic growth, and synaptic plasticity (Binder & Scharfman, 2004), all of which are associated with cognitive health. Exercise-induced increases in BDNF were greater in men and greater in aerobic exercise compared to anaerobic exercise, highlighting the potential importance of factors that may differentially impact our understanding of these relationships and their effect on cognitive function.

Novel approaches to engaging individuals in exercise, such as exergaming, have been examined, including the exer-tour and exer-score interventions used in the Aerobic and Cognitive Exercise Study (Anderson-Hanley et al., 2018). Data from this pilot study not only support neurobiological changes that occur in conjunction with cognitive improvements, but may also help with long-term adoption and engagement of individuals in an exercise program.

COGNITIVE BENEFITS OF EXERCISE FOR HEALTH AND DISEASE

Exercise has long been touted as important for general cognitive health (Cotman & Berchtold, 2002; Van Praag, 2009; Voss et al., 2011). Evidence also supports that age-associated cognitive decline can be slowed with exercise (Government Office for Science, 2008). Exercise is also key to healthy aging, as mild cognitive impairment (MCI), often thought to be a precursor of dementia, has been shown to improve with exercise. However, results examining such benefits have been variable across different cognitive domains and studies, and the strength of these results has been tempered by the heterogeneity of study designs that have examined this issue (Gates, Fiatarone Singh, Sachdev, & Valenzuela, 2013; Zheng, Xia, Zhou, Tao, & Chen, 2016).

More pronounced cognitive decline, such as that observed with Alzheimer's disease, has also been shown to be positively impacted by exercise across all stages of the disease (Colcombe & Kramer, 2003). Improvements have been noted with a variety of aerobic exercise programs in a wide variety of cognitive domains, including executive function as measured by the Clock Drawing Test (Ohman et al., 2016), general cognitive functions as measured by Alzheimer's Disease Assessment Scale—Cognition scores (Yang et al., 2015), and mental speed and attention as measured by the Symbol Digits Modalities Test (for participants who attended 80% or more of their exercise sessions; Hoffmann et al., 2016). Furthermore, two meta-analyses (Groot et al., 2016; Strohle et al., 2015) demonstrated global cognitive improvements in exercising individuals with Alzheimer's disease (and lesser improvements in those with MCI), with the greatest improvements realized by those who participated in aerobic exercise interventions.

Exercise has been used to improve cognition in other disorders, including Parkinson's disease, where the majority of improvements have been seen in executive functioning (Murray et al., 2014). Trials examining exercise interventions have shown executive function improvements as assessed by a variety of tasks, including the Wisconsin Card Sorting Task (Tanaka et al., 2009), the Spatial Working Memory test from the Cambridge Neuropsychological Test Automated Battery, and the verbal fluency test, in the absence of improvements in spatial and pattern recognition memory (Cruise et al., 2011). Importantly, many studies that yielded cognitive benefits associated with exercise in individuals with Parkinson's disease evaluated individuals who were early in the disease course. Therefore, the extent to which improvements may be sustained or achieved in those with more advanced disease may need further evaluation (Petzinger et al., 2013).

Cognitive outcomes in psychiatric disease, particularly schizophrenia, have also been shown to improve with exercise. A meta-analysis of aerobic exercise showed improvements in attention/vigilance, social cognition, and working memory domains, as well as global cognition among patients with schizophrenia (Firth et al., 2017). However, another meta-analysis failed to show the cognitive benefits of exercise on cognition in schizophrenia (Dauwan, Begemann, Heringa, & Sommer, 2016), perhaps due to being underpowered. A review of the impact of exercise on cognitive functioning in bipolar disorder highlighted the favorable neurocognitive benefits of exercise, including potential resolution of disrupted metabolic and neurobiological mechanisms that contribute to cognitive deficits in bipolar disorder (Kucyi, Alsuwaidan, Liauw, & McIntyre, 2010).

EXERCISE-ASSOCIATED COGNITIVE IMPROVEMENTS IN DEPRESSION

Two recent comprehensive reviews aimed to synthesize our understanding of the efficacy of exercise on cognition in depression. First, Brondino and colleagues (2017) included eight trials in a systematic review examining how exercise impacts cognition in adults with MDD. The included trials utilized assessments that examined specific cognitive domains, including attention/vigilance, processing speed, reasoning, verbal and visual memory, and working memory, as well as global cognition. The exercise interventions reviewed were very broad in scope, including anaerobic exercise, aerobic exercise, and mind–body interventions (e.g., yoga, tai-chi). Exercise was not associated with improvements in global cognition, nor any of the specific domains, even when exercise intensity, exercise adherence (number of sessions per week), and study duration were controlled for in the analyses. The authors noted the limitations of the review, including the breadth of cognitive domains and tasks included, as well as clinical heterogeneity, as the studies included both symptomatic and remitted depressed individuals.

Second, a subsequent meta-analysis by Sun, Lanctot, Herrmann, and Gallagher (2018) also failed to find a significant effect of exercise on global cognition (consisting of processing speed, attention/vigilance, working memory, verbal learning and memory, visual learning and memory, reasoning, and problem-solving domains) in individuals with MDD. As with the Brondino and colleagues (2017) study, the authors noted several limitations that may have contributed to the negative effect. These limitations include methodological issues in the studies that were included in the meta-analysis, such as lack of cognitive impairment at baseline and a lower than recommended mean duration of exercise (131 minutes per week compared to the recommended 150 minutes per week (ASCM, 2009). Additionally, the meta-analysis included uncontrolled studies that prevented concluding that the positive effects of exercise on specific cognitive domains were attributable to exercise as opposed to practice effects. Subgroup analyses indicated that interventions combining physical exercise and cognitive activity (e.g., mind–body interventions: yoga, tai-chi, cognitive training, and cardio training) improved global cognition ($N = 4$, $n = 150$, $p = .048$), with differences between subgroups (mind–body vs. physical exercise alone) not reaching statistical significance ($p = .077$).

While these syntheses of studies of exercise and cognitive function fail to support a benefit of exercise on cognition in MDD, their limitations are notable and should be considered with respect to the plethora of individual studies that display a significant benefit of exercise on specific cognitive domains. Table 19.1 highlights studies of aerobic exercise that have been associated with significant improvements in a variety of cognitive domains

TABLE 19.1. Cognitive Improvements Associated with Aerobic Exercise in MDD

Attention/concentration	Visual learning and memory	Executive functioning/working memory
• CANTAB BLC (Greer et al., 2015) • ST-CC (Vasques et al., 2011[a]) • ST-IC (Kubesch et al., 2003)	• CANTAB DMS (Greer et al., 2015) • CANTAB PRM (Greer et al., 2015) • RCFT (Krogh et al., 2012)	• CANTAB IED (Greer et al., 2015) • CANTAB SOC (Greer et al., 2015) • CANTAB SWM (Greer et al., 2015) • DSB (Berman et al., 2012) • GoNogo (Kubesch et al., 2003) • RCFT (Krogh et al., 2012) • ST-IC (Kubesch et al., 2003; Vasques et al., 2011[a]) • Stroop (Kubesch et al., 2003)

Note. BLC, Big Little Circle; CANTAB, Cambridge Neuropsychological Test Automated Battery; DMS, Delayed Matching to Sample; DSB, Digit Span Backwards; IED, Intra/Extra Dimensional Set Shifting; PRM, Pattern Recognition Memory; RCFT, Rey's Complex Figure Test; SOC, Stockings of Cambridge; ST-CC, Stroop Task—congruent condition; ST-IC, Stroop Task—incongruent condition; SWM, Spatial Working Memory.
[a]Uncontrolled study following acute exercise.

(utilizing a variety of representative tasks), and Table 19.2 represents similar benefits associated with mind–body interventions. However, there have also been several evaluations of studies that failed to find any cognitive benefits of exercise (Heissel et al., 2015; Krogh, Saltin, Gluud, & Nordentoft, 2009; Luttenberger et al., 2015). Furthermore, within studies demonstrating significant cognitive improvements, some hypothesized cognitive improvements failed to reach significance, and multiple outcomes from a task (e.g., reaction time and number of errors) may not all have reached significance. In addition, while the tables are intended to synthesize information regarding cognitive improvements with exercise in persons with MDD, they do not capture the variability seen within the results, including variability in associated effects based on duration, intensity, and type of exercise. As one would expect, adherence to the targeted dose/intensity/duration was important, so that the expected intervention was adequately received by the participants. In some instances, intent to treat analyses failed to achieve statistical significance, but subanalyses

TABLE 19.2. Cognitive Improvements Associated with Mind–Body Interventions in MDD

Attention/ concentration	Verbal learning and memory	Visual learning and memory	Psychomotor speed	Executive functioning/ working memory
• DVT (Chan et al., 2012) • LCT (Sharma et al., 2006)	• CVLT (Lavretsky et al., 2011)	• BVMT- R (Oertel-Knöchel et al., 2014)	• AN (Oertel-Knöchel et al., 2014) • LCT (Sharma et al., 2006) • TMT A (Oertel-Knöchel et al., 2014)	• DSB (Sharma et al., 2006) • WMS-III LNS (Oertel- Knöchel et al., 2014) • WMS-III SS (Oertel-Knöchel et al., 2014)

Note. AN, Animal Naming; BVMT-R, Brief Visuospatial Memory Test—Revised; CVLT, California Verbal Learning Test; DSB, Digit Span Backwards; DVT, Digit Vigilance Test; LCT, Letter Cancellation Test; LNS, Letter–Number Span; SS, Spatial Span; TMT A, Trail Making Test Part A; WMS-III, Wechsler Memory Scale—Third Edition.

that included only those receiving an adequate dose of exercise showed significant cognitive improvements. Another very important factor is variable use of antidepressant pharmacotherapy among participants and the stability of concomitant medication use during the study evaluation period. Some antidepressants may have deleterious effects on certain cognitive functions (see Rosenblat, Chapter 15, this volume). This may explain some instances in which lower doses and/or control groups exhibited worsened cognitive abilities over the study period (Greer, Grannemann, Chansard, Karim, & Trivedi, 2015).

CONCLUSIONS

There are many limitations to the evaluation of cognitive impairments and efficacy of treatments in addressing such impairments that are inherent in the field. These limitations include slow emphasis of cognitive outcomes as an aspect of treatment efficacy in depression; variability in expression of cognitive impairments in individuals with depression; the breadth of cognitive domains affected by depression; and the associated wealth of cognitive tasks available to assess these domains. These same issues have been noted as limitations to the interpretation of studies (and the synthesis of this literature) that have examined the impact of exercise on cognitive function in depressed individuals.

Despite the noted limitations and the need for additional research in this area, exercise has been associated with improved cognition in several studies of individuals with depression and should be considered as part of a targeted treatment approach. Aerobic exercise has shown the strongest evidence for improving cognition in depression, including greater neurobiological changes as well as efficacy in improving cognitive outcomes in other clinical populations. Future well-designed evaluations of exercise on cognitive outcomes in depressed individuals are greatly needed to better clarify how exercise can benefit cognitive health in depression and how exercise-associated neurobiological changes facilitate cognitive improvement. As is true of all exercise interventions, before a depressed patient initiates an exercise program, consideration should be given to overall health and any limitations or barriers to initiating exercise, and exercise should occur under the supervision of a physician and/or trained professional (Haskell et al., 2007). Furthermore, monitoring should occur to increase adherence and to evaluate and resolve any barriers related to ongoing exercise (Trivedi, Greer, Grannemann, Chambliss, & Jordan, 2006).

REFERENCES

Ainslie, P. N., Cotter, J. D., George, K. P., Lucas, S., Murrell, C., Shave, R., et al. (2008). Elevation in cerebral blood flow velocity with aerobic fitness throughout healthy human ageing. *Journal of Physiology, 586*, 4005–4010.

American College of Sports Medicine. (2009). Benefits and risks associated with physical activity. ACSM Guidelines for Exercise Testing and Prescription. Retrieved from *www.acsm.org/docs/default-source/publications-files/acsm-guidelines-download-10th-edabf32a97415a400e9b3be594a6cd7fbf.pdf?sfvrsn=aaa6d2b2_0*

American Psychiatric Association. (2019). American Psychiatric Association practice guidelines. Retrieved from *https://psychiatryonline.org/guidelines*

Anderson-Hanley, C., Barcelos, N. M., Zimmerman, E. A., Gillen, R. W., Dunnam, M., Cohen, B. D., et al. (2018). The aerobic and cognitive exercise study (ACES) for community-dwelling older adults with or at-risk for mild cognitive impairment (MCI): Neuropsychological, neurobiological and neuroimaging outcomes of a randomized clinical trial. *Frontiers in Aging Neuroscience, 10*, 76.

Berman, M. G., Kross, E., Krpan, K. M., Askren, M. K., Burson, A., Deldin, P. J., et al. (2012). Interacting with nature improves cognition and affect for individuals with depression. *Journal of Affective Disorders, 140*(3), 300–305.

Binder, D. K., & Scharfman, H. E. (2004). Brain-derived neurotrophic factor. *Growth Factors, 22*, 123–131.

Blackwood, S. K., MacHale, S. M., Power, M. J., Goodwin, G. M., & Lawrie, S. M. (1998). Effects of exercise on cognitive and motor function in chronic fatigue syndrome and depression. *Journal of Neurology, Neurosurgery and Psychiatry, 65*(4), 541–546.

Brondino, N., Rocchetti, M., Fusar-Poli, L., Codrons, E., Correale, L., Vandoni, M., et al. (2017). A systematic review of cognitive effects of exercise in depression. *Acta Psychiatrica Scandinavica, 135*(4), 285–295.

Caspersen, C. J., Powell, K. E., & Christenson, G. M. (1985). Physical activity, exercise, and physical fitness: Definitions and distinctions for health-related research. *Public Health Reports, 100*(2), 126.

Chan, A. S., Wong, Q. Y., Sze, S. L., Kwong, P. P., Han, Y. M., & Cheung, M. C. (2012). A Chinese Chan-based mind–body intervention for patients with depression. *Journal of Affective Disorders, 142*(1–3), 283–289.

Christensen, H., Griffiths, K., MacKinnon, A., & Jacomb, P. (1997). A quantitative review of cognitive deficits in depression and Alzheimer-type dementia. *Journal of the International Neuropsychological Society, 3*(6), 631–651.

Churchill, J. D., Galvez, R., Colcombe, S., Swain, R. A., Kramer, A. F., & Greenough, W. T. (2002). Exercise, experience and the aging brain. *Neurobiology of Aging, 23*(5), 941–955.

Colcombe, S. J., Erickson, K. I., Scalf, P. E., Kim, J. S., Prakash, R., McAuley, E., et al. (2006). Aerobic exercise training increases brain volume in aging humans. *Journals of Gerontology. Series A, Biological Sciences and Medical Sciences, 61*, 1166–1170.

Colcombe, S., & Kramer, A. F. (2003). Fitness effects on the cognitive function of older adults: a meta-analytic study. *Psychological Science, 14*, 125–130.

Cooney, G. M., Dwan, K., Greig, C. A., Lawlor, D. A., Rimer, J., Waugh, F. R., et al. (2013). Exercise for depression. *Cochrane Database of Systematic Reviews*, CD004366.

Cotman, C. W., & Berchtold, N. C. (2002). Exercise: A behavioral intervention to enhance brain health and plasticity. *Trends in Neurosciences, 25*(6), 295–301.

Cruise, K. E., Bucks, R. S., Loftus, A. M., Newton, R. U., Pegoraro, R., & Thomas, M. G. (2011). Exercise and Parkinson's: benefits for cognition and quality of life. *Acta Neurologica Scandinavica 123*, 13–19.

Dauwan, M., Begemann, M. J., Heringa, S. M., & Sommer I. E. (2016). Exercise improves clinical symptoms, quality of life, global functioning, and depression in schizophrenia: A systematic review and meta-analysis. *Schizophrenia Bulletin, 42*, 588–599.

El Hammi, E., Samp, J., Rémuzat, C., Auray, J. P., Lamure, M., Aballéa, S., et al. (2014). Difference of perceptions and evaluation of cognitive dysfunction in major depressive disorder patients across psychiatrists internationally. *Therapeutic Advances in Psychopharmacology, 4*(1), 22–29.

Erickson, K. I., Prakash, R. S., Voss, M. W., Chaddock, L., Hu, L., Morris, K. S., et al. (2009). Aerobic fitness is associated with hippocampal volume in elderly humans. *Hippocampus, 19*, 1030–1039.

Erickson, K. I., Voss, M. W., Prakash, R. S., Basak, C,. Szabo, A., Chaddock L., et al. (2011). Exercise training increases size of hippocampus and improves memory. *Proceedings of the National Academy of Science USA, 108*, 3017–3022.

Etnier, J. L., Salazar, W., Landers, D. M., Petruzzello, S. J., Han, M., & Nowell, P. (1997). The influence of physical fitness and exercise upon cognitive functioning: a meta-analysis. *Journal of Sport and Exercise Psychology, 19*, 249–277.

Farmer, M. E., Locke, B. Z., Mościcki, E. K., Dannenberg, A. L., Larson, D. B., & Radloff, L. S. (1988).

Physical activity and depressive symptoms: The NHANES I Epidemiologic Follow-up Study. *American Journal of Epidemiology, 128*(6), 1340–1351.

Firth, J., Stubbs, B., Rosenbaum, S., Vancampfort, D., Malchow, B., Schuch, F., et al. (2017). Aerobic exercise improves cognitive functioning in people with schizophrenia: A systematic review and meta-analysis. *Schizophrenia Bulletin, 43*(3), 546–556.

Galper, D. I., Trivedi, M. H., Barlow, C. E., Dunn, A. L., & Kampert, J. B. (2006). Inverse association between physical inactivity and mental health in men and women. *Medicine and Science in Sports and Exercise, 38*(1), 173–178.

Garber, C. E., Blissmer, B., Deschenes, M. R., Franklin, B. A., Lamonte, M. J., Lee, I. M., et al. (2011). American College of Sports Medicine position stand. Quantity and quality of exercise for developing and maintaining cardiorespiratory, musculoskeletal, and neuromotor fitness in apparently healthy adults: guidance for prescribing exercise. *Medicine and Science in Sports and Exercise, 43*(7), 1334–1359.

Gates, N., Fiatarone Singh, M. A., Sachdev, P. S. & Valenzuela, M. (2013). The effect of exercise training on cognitive function in older adults with mild cognitive impairment: A meta-analysis of randomized controlled trials. *American Journal of Geriatric Psychiatry, 21*, 1086–1097.

Goodwin, R. D. (2003). Association between physical activity and mental disorders among adults in the United States. *Preventive Medicine, 36*(6), 698–703.

Government Office for Science. (2008). *Foresight Mental Capital and Wellbeing Project. Final project report – Executive summary.* London: Author.

Greer, T. L., Furman, J. L., & Trivedi, M. H. (2017). Evaluation of the benefits of exercise on cognition in major depressive disorder. *General Hospital Psychiatry, 49*, 19–25.

Greer, T. L., Grannemann, B. D., Chansard, M., Karim, A. I., & Trivedi, M. H. (2015). Dose-dependent changes in cognitive function with exercise augmentation for major depression: Results from the TREAD study. *European Neuropsychopharmacology, 25*, 248–256.

Groot, C., Hooghiemstra, A. M., Raijmakers, P. G., van Berckel, B. N., Scheltens, P., Scherder, E. J., et al. (2016). The effect of physical activity on cognitive function in patients with dementia: A meta-analysis of randomized control trials. *Ageing Research Reviews, 25*, 13–23.

Gualtieri, C. T. & Morgan, D. W. (2008). The frequency of cognitive impairment in patients with anxiety, depression, and bipolar disorder: An unaccounted source of variance in clinical trials. *Journal of Clinical Psychiatry, 69*, 1122–1130.

Haskell, W. L., Lee, I. M., Pate, R. R., Powell, K. E., Blair, S. N., Franklin, B. A., et al. (2007). Physical activity and public health: updated recommendation for adults from the American College of Sports Medicine and the American Heart American Heart Association. *Circulation, 116*(9), 1081.

Hasselbalch, B. J., Knorr, U., Hasselbalch, S. G., Gade, A. & Kessing, L. V. (2012). Cognitive deficits in the remitted state of unipolar depressive disorder. *Neuropsychology 26*, 642–651.

Heissel, A., Vesterling, A., White, S. A., Kallies, G., Behr, D., Arafat, A. M., et al. (2015). Feasibility of an exercise program for older depressive inpatients. *GeroPsych, 28*, 163–171.

Hoffmann, K., Sobol, N. A., Frederiksen, K. S., Beyer, N., Vogel, A., Vestergaard, K., et al. (2016). Moderate-to-high intensity physical exercise in patients with Alzheimer's disease: A randomized controlled trial. *Journal of Alzheimer's Disease, 50*, 443–453.

Krogh, J., Nordentoft, M., Sterne, J. A. & Lawlor, D. A. (2011). The effect of exercise in clinically depressed adults: Systematic review and meta-analysis of randomized controlled trials. *Journal of Clinical Psychiatry, 72*, 529–538.

Krogh, J., Rostrup, E., Thomsen, C., Elfving, B., Videbech, P., & Nordentoft, M. (2014). The effect of exercise on hippocampal volume and neurotrophines in patients with major depression–a randomized clinical trial. *Journal of Affective Disorders, 165*, 24–30.

Krogh, J., Saltin, B., Gluud, C., & Nordentoft, M. (2009). The DEMO trial: A randomized, parallel-group, observer-blinded clinical trial of strength versus aerobic versus relaxation training for patients with mild to moderate depression. *Journal of Clinical Psychiatry, 70*, 790–800.

Krogh, J., Videbech, P., Thomsen, C., Gluud, C., & Nordentoft, M. (2012). DEMO-II trial. Aerobic exercise versus stretching exercise in patients with major depression—a randomised clinical trial. *PloS One, 7*(10), e48316.

Kubesch, S., Bretschneider, V., Freudenmann, R., Weidenhammer, N., Lehmann, M., Spitzer, M., et al. (2003). Aerobic endurance exercise improves executive functions in depressed patients. *Journal of Clinical Psychiatry, 64*(9), 1005–1012.

Kucyi, A., Alsuwaidan, M. T., Liauw, S. S., & McIntyre, R. S. (2010). Aerobic physical exercise as a possible treatment for neurocognitive dysfunction in bipolar disorder. *Postgraduate Medicine, 122*(6), 107–116.

Lam, R. W., Filteau, M. J., & Milev, R. (2011). Clinical effectiveness: The importance of psychosocial functioning outcomes. *Jounral of Affective Disorders, 132*(Suppl. 1), S9–S13.

Lavretsky, H., Alstein, L. L., Olmstead, R. E., Ercoli, L. M., Riparetti-Brown, M., Cyr, N. S. et al. (2011). Complementary use of tai chi augments escitalopram treatment of geriatric depression: A randomized controlled trial. *American Journal of Geriatric Psychiatry, 19*(10), 839–850.

Lawlor, D. A., & Hopker, S. W. (2001). The effectiveness of exercise as an intervention in the management of depression: Systematic review and meta-regression analysis of randomised controlled trials. *BMJ, 322*, 763–767.

Leavitt, V. M., Cirnigliaro, C., Cohen, A., Farag, A., Brooks, M., Wecht, J. M., et al. (2014). Aerobic exercise increases hippocampal volume and improves memory in multiple sclerosis: Preliminary findings. *Neurocase, 20*(6), 695–697.

Lewis, R. (2004). Should cognitive deficit be a diagnostic criterion for schizophrenia? *Journal of Psychiatry and Neuroscience, 29*(2):102–113.

Luttenberger, K., Stelzer, E. M., Först, S., Schopper, M., Kornhuber, J., & Book, S. (2015). Indoor rock climbing (bouldering) as a new treatment for depression: Study design of a waitlist-controlled randomized group pilot study and the first results. *BMC Psychiatry, 15*, 201.

McClintock, S. M., Husain, M. M., Greer, T. L. & Cullum, C. M. (2010). Association between depression severity and neurocognitive function in major depressive disorder: A review and synthesis. *Neuropsychology, 24*, 9–34.

Mead, G. E., Morley, W., Campbell, P., Greig, C. A., McMurdo, M., & Lawlor, D. A. (2009). Exercise for depression. *Cochrane Database of Systematic Reviews*, CD004366.

Murray, D. K., Sacheli, M. A., Eng, J. J., & Stoessl, A. J. (2014). The effects of exercise on cognition in Parkinson's disease: A systematic review. *Translational Neurodegeneration, 3*, 5.

Niemann, C., Godde, B., & Voelcker-Rehage, C. (2014). Not only cardiovascular, but also coordinative exercise increases hippocampal volume in older adults. *Frontiers in Aging Neuroscience, 6*, 170.

Oertel-Knöchel, V., Mehler, P., Thiel, C., Steinbrecher, K., Malchow, B., Tesky, V., et al. (2014). Effects of aerobic exercise on cognitive performance and individual psychopathology in depressive and schizophrenia patients. *European Archives of Psychiatry and Clinical Neuroscience, 264*(7), 589–604.

Ohman, H., Savikko, N., Strandberg, T. E., Kautiainen, H., Raivio, M. M., Laakkonen, M. L., et al. (2016). Effects of exercise on cognition: The Finnish Alzheimer disease exercise trial: A randomized, controlled trial. *Journal of the American Geriatrics Society, 64*, 731–738.

Pajonk, F. G., Wobrock, T., Gruber, O., Scherk, H., Berner, D., Kaizl, I., et al. (2010). Hippocampal plasticity in response to exercise in schizophrenia. *Archives of General Psychiatry, 67*(2), 133–143.

Petzinger, G. M., Fisher, B. E., McEwen, S., Beeler, J. A., Walsh, J. P., & Jakowec, M. W. (2013). Exercise-enhanced neuroplasticity targeting motor and cognitive circuitry in Parkinson's disease. *Lancet Neurology, 12*, 716–726.

Phillips, C., & Fahimi, A. (2018). Immune and neuroprotective effects of physical activity on the brain in depression. *Frontiers in Neuroscience, 12*, 498.

Scheewe, T. W., van Haren, N. E., Sarkisyan, G., Schnack, H. G., Brouwer, R. M., de Glint, M., et al. (2013). Exercise therapy, cardiorespiratory fitness and their effect on brain volumes: A randomised controlled trial in patients with schizophrenia and healthy controls. *European Neuropsychopharmacology, 23*, 675–685.

Sharma, V. K., Das, S., Mondal, S., Goswami, U., & Gandhi, A. (2006). Effect of Sahaj Yoga on neurocognitive functions in patients suffering from major depression. *Indian Journal of Physiology and Pharmacology, 50*(4), 375.

Sibley, B. A., & Etnier, J. L. (2003). The relationship between physical activity and cognition in children: A meta-analysis. *Pediatric Exercise Science, 15*(3), 243–256.

Strohle, A., Schmidt, D. K., Schultz, F., Fricke, N., Staden, T., Hellweg, R., et al. (2015). Drug and exercise treatment of Alzheimer disease and mild cognitive impairment: A systematic review and meta-analysis of effects on cognition in randomized controlled trials. *American Journal of Geriatric Psychiatry, 23*, 1234–1249.

Sun, M., Lanctot, K., Herrmann, N., & Gallagher, D. (2018). Exercise for cognitive symptoms in depression: A systematic review of interventional studies. *Canadian Journal of Psychiatry, 63*(2), 115–128.

Szuhany, K. L., Bugatti, M., & Otto, M. W. (2015). A meta-analytic review of the effects of exercise on brain-derived neurotrophic factor. *Journal of Psychiatric Research, 60*, 56–64.

Tanaka, K., Quadros, A. C., Jr., Santos, R. F., Stella, F., Gobbi, L. T., & Gobbi, S. (2009). Benefits of physical exercise on executive functions in older people with Parkinson's disease. *Brain and Cognition, 69*, 435–441.

ten Brinke, L. F., Bolandzadeh, N., Nagamatsu, L. S., Hsu, C. L., Davis, J. C., Miran-Khan, K., et al. (2015). Aerobic exercise increases hippocampal volume in older women with probable mild cognitive impairment: A 6-month randomised controlled trial. *British Journal of Sports Medicine, 49*, 248–254.

Thomas, A. G., Dennis, A., Rawlings, N. B., Stagg, C. J., Matthews, L., Morris, M., et al. (2016). Multimodal characterization of rapid anterior hippocampal volume increase associated with aerobic exercise. *Neuroimage, 131*, 162–170.

Trivedi, M. H., & Greer, T. L. (2014). Cognitive dysfunction in unipolar depression: implications for treatment. *Journal of Affect Disorders, 152–154*, 19–27.

Trivedi, M. H., Greer, T. L., Grannemann, B. D., Chambliss, H. O., & Jordan, A. N. (2006). Exercise as an augmentation strategy for treatment of major depression. *Journal of Psychiatric Practice, 12*(4), 205–213.

Van Praag, H. (2009). Exercise and the brain: something to chew on. *Trends in Neurosciences, 32*(5), 283–290.

Vasques, P. E., Moraes, H., Silveira, H., Deslandes, A. C., & Laks, J. (2011). Acute exercise improves cognition in the depressed elderly: The effect of dual-tasks. *Clinics, 66*(9), 1553–1557.

Veiel, H. O. (1997). A preliminary profile of neuropsychological deficits associated with major depression. *Journal of Clinical and Experimental Neuropsychology, 19*, 587–603.

Voss, M. W., Heo, S., Prakash, R. S., Erickson, K. I., Alves, H., Chaddock, L., et al. (2013). The influence of aerobic fitness on cerebral white matter integrity and cognitive function in older adults: Results of a one-year exercise intervention. *Human Brain Mapping, 34*(11), 2972–2985.

Voss, M. W., Nagamatsu, L. S., Liu-Ambrose, T., & Kramer, A. F. (2011). Exercise, brain, and cognition across the life span. *Journal of Applied Physiology, 111*(5), 1505–1513.

Weiland-Fiedler, P., Erickson, K., Waldeck, T., Luckenbaugh, D. A., Pike, D., Bonne O., et al. (2004). Evidence for continuing neuropsychological impairments in depression. *Journal of Affective Disorders, 82*, 253–258.

Yang, S. Y., Shan, C. L., Qing, H., Wang, W., Zhu, Y., Yin, M. M., et al. (2015). The effects of aerobic exercise on cognitive function of Alzheimer's disease patients. *CNS and Neurological Disorders—Drug Targets, 14*, 1292–1297.

Zheng, G., Xia, R., Zhou, W., Tao, J., & Chen L. (2016). Aerobic exercise ameliorates cognitive function in older adults with mild cognitive impairment: A systematic review and meta-analysis of randomised controlled trials. *British Journal of Sports Medicine 50*(23), 1443–1450.

CHAPTER 20

Electroconvulsive Therapy

Martha Finnegan
Declan M. McLoughlin

This chapter briefly summarizes the use of electroconvulsive therapy (ECT) for depression, including indications for the treatment, how it is administered, and a summary of evidence of its effectiveness. The chapter also explores the literature on the effects of ECT on cognition and the impact of recent developments in ECT practice on cognitive function.

ECT FOR DEPRESSION

Electroconvulsive therapy (ECT) is the most acutely effective treatment for treatment-resistant depression and can be lifesaving (UK ECT Review Group, 2003). Of those who experience nonresponse or partial response after two antidepressant medications, 44–70% can achieve remission with ECT (Kolshus, Jelovac, & McLoughlin, 2017; UK ECT Review Group, 2003). The Consortium for Research in ECT reported a 75% remission rate among depressed patients treated three times a week with ECT, the vast majority of which occurred in the first 4 weeks of treatment (Husain et al., 2004). A landmark meta-analysis reported a standardized effect size of –0.91 (95% confidence interval [CI] = –1.27 to –0.54) for ECT compared to sham ECT (n = 256 patients), and an effect size of –0.80 (95% CI = –1.29 to –0.29) for ECT compared to antidepressant pharmacotherapy (n = 1,144 patients; UK ECT Review Group, 2003). Early use of ECT is associated with shorter and less costly hospital stays (Markowitz, Brown, Sweeney, & Mann, 1987) and lower 30-day readmission (Slade, Jahn, Regenold, & Case, 2017). ECT has also been reported to enhance health-related quality of life in both the short and the long term (McCall, Prudic, Olfson, & Sackeim, 2006) and is associated with reduced all-cause mortality (Munk-Olsen, Laursen, Videbech, Mortensen, & Rosenberg, 2007; Prudic & Sackeim, 1999).

MECHANISM OF ACTION

There are many hypothesized explanations of ECT's antidepressant effect (McCall, Andrade, & Sienaert, 2014; Ryan & McLoughlin, 2018). The precise mechanism of action remains unknown, but there is evidence for multiple mechanisms involving neuroplasticity, neurotransmitters, neurotrophic factors, and epigenetic modification. Similarly, there is evidence of ECT's effects in systems involved in a variety of hypotheses of depression etiology such as hypothalamic–pituitary–adrenal axis dysfunction, immune dysfunction, and brain circuitry.

INDICATIONS FOR ECT

In the United States, the American Psychiatric Association recommends ECT as a first-line treatment for severe mental illness where rapid or high probability of response is required, such as severe major depressive disorder (MDD), acute mania, mood disorders with psychotic symptoms, and catatonia, or where ECT has previously been used to good effect. It is also recommended as a secondary treatment for treatment-resistant illness, such as treatment-resistant depression (TRD; American Psychiatric Association, 2001). ECT is cost-effective when compared to other treatments for depression such as repetitive transcranial magnetic stimulation (see Kavanaugh & Croarkin, Chapter 23, this volume) and antidepressant medications (see Rosenblat, Chapter 15, this volume; Knapp et al., 2008; Ross, Zivin, & Maixner, 2018). ECT is generally used to treat principal diagnostic indications, including MDD, bipolar disorder, and schizophrenia, and it may be used for other diagnostic indications, including psychiatric syndromes associated with medical conditions and medical disorders (American Psychiatric Association, 2010). The United Kingdom's National Institute for Health and Clinical Excellence (NICE; 2009) recommends the use of ECT for fast and short-term improvement of severe psychiatric symptoms after all other treatment options have failed in severe depressive illness, a prolonged or severe episode of mania, or catatonia.

ADMINISTRATION OF ECT

ECT involves administration of a short-acting anesthetic and muscle relaxant. An electrical charge is then passed through the brain via electrodes placed on the head either bilaterally (on both temples) or unilaterally on the right side (one electrode on the temple and one to the right of the vertex; see Figure 20.1). Bifrontal ECT is administered in some centers but has no clear advantage relative to bitemporal or right unilateral electrode placement (Dunne & McLoughlin, 2012). The electrical charge induces a modified generalized seizure, monitored by electroencephalogram (EEG). The minimal electrical dose necessary to elicit an adequate generalized seizure (e.g., ≥15 seconds of motor activity or ≥25 seconds on the EEG) is the "stimulus threshold" dose. This is established at the first ECT session, and subsequent treatments are given at a multiple of times of the stimulus

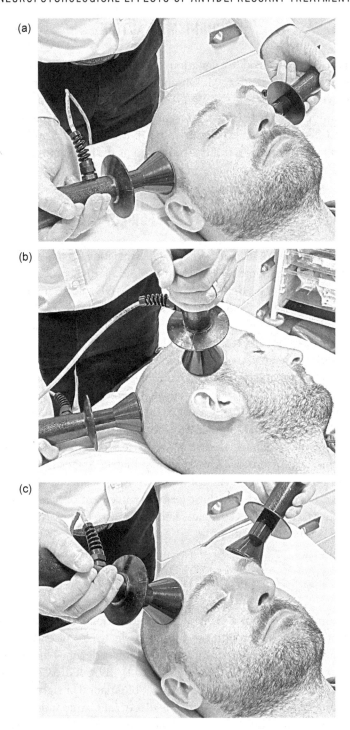

FIGURE 20.1. Electrode placement in (a) bitemporal, (b) right unilateral, and (c) bifrontal ECT.

threshold in order to produce antidepressant benefits. For bitemporal ECT, treatment is generally administered at 1.5 times the threshold dose, and for right unilateral ECT this is usually six times the threshold dose (Kolshus et al., 2017).

TREATMENT PARAMETERS

ECT is administered two or three times a week in a course of applications that can vary from 3 to 15 treatments, depending on patient antidepressant response. Twice weekly ECT is standard across Europe. In the United States and some Australian centers, however, ECT is performed three times a week. There is no clear advantage to either schedule, but administering ECT three times a week is associated with more acute cognitive side effects (Semkovska & McLoughlin, 2010).

Pulse width is also an important treatment parameter. The original sine-wave ECT has long been replaced by brief-pulse ECT (0.5–1.5-millisecond stimulus), which reduces cognitive adverse effects while maintaining antidepressant efficacy. In recent years, pulses of <0.5 millisecond (ultrabrief-pulse ECT) have been utilized. Ultrabrief-pulse ECT was found to reduce cognitive adverse effects, but antidepressant efficacy may be limited at this pulse width, with a meta-analysis of brief-pulse versus ultrabrief-pulse ECT showing a standardized mean difference of 0.25 (95% CI = 0.08 to 0.41; $p = .004$) in favor of brief-pulse unilateral ECT (Tor et al., 2015).

CONCERNS IN ECT PRACTICE

ECT is a medically safe procedure (Blumberger at al., 2017; Tørring et al., 2017; UK ECT Review Group, 2003). The main medical risks are related to the anesthesia and muscle relaxant required for a modified seizure. Mortality associated with ECT is 2.1 per 100,000 treatments, lower than that associated with surgical procedures under general anesthesia (3.4 per 100,000; Tørring, Sanghani, Petrides, Kellner, & Østergaard, 2017). Apart from raised intracranial pressure, there are few absolute contraindications to the administration of ECT, but patients must be fit for general anesthesia (Tess & Smetana, 2009). Arguably, the primary limiting factor in the use of ECT, then, is concern about cognitive side effects.

Another major concern is the risk of depressive relapse following successful ECT. Indeed, in the first 6 months following successful ECT, 37% of people relapse despite continuing antidepressant therapy, with the period of greatest risk being the first 3 months (Jelovac, Kolshus, & McLoughlin, 2013). These rates are similar to the relapse rates of patients who respond to pharmacological treatment only after three or more antidepressant steps and most likely reflect the recurrent nature of TRD (Rush et al., 2006). It has also been suggested that ECT studies are composed of increasingly treatment-resistant populations that are at high risk for relapse regardless of the modality of treatment (Sackeim, 2017). Taking antidepressants after ECT halved the risk (risk ratio = .49, $p < .0001$, number needed to treat = 3.3) for relapse at 6 months from nearly 80% (Jelovac et al.,

2013). In one trial, 84% of those on placebo pharmacotherapy relapsed upon discontinuation of ECT (Sackeim et al., 2001). Therefore, some form of continuation therapy is clearly essential. Continuation ECT provides some protection against relapse to those who have responded to ECT for acute depression (Kellner et al., 2006). A combination of continuation ECT and pharmacotherapy tailored to the patient's depressive symptoms may be superior to either alone (Kellner et al., 2016a, 2016b). However, in certain countries around the globe, continuation ECT is not currently recommended in clinical guidelines, and further research has been recommended (NICE, 2009).

There are local, regional, and global differences in ECT practice (Finnegan et al., 2018), including wider use of ECT for psychosis in India and other Asian and African countries (with good reported outcomes) than in Europe, Australia, or North America. Because of its effectiveness as an emergency treatment for acute illness, ECT is administered under involuntary conditions around the world (Finnegan at al., 2018; Leiknes, Schweder, & Høie, 2012). Jurisdictions differ widely in their approach to the provision and regulation of involuntary ECT, from total restriction to unregulated use of involuntary ECT. In the United States, where 1.5% of general hospital inpatients with severe mood disorder received ECT during their admission (Slade et al., 2017), there have been concerns about the underuse of the treatment and inequitable access to ECT (Sackeim, 2017).

Throughout its history, the use of ECT has attracted much debate. This chapter cannot address this history in comprehensive detail, but more information can be found in Abrams's *History of ECT* (2002). In its early years, ECT may have been administered indiscriminately in crude forms. These historical misuses and abuses are in stark contrast to current regulated and evidence-based practice of modern and advanced forms of ECT. Though historical abuses should be acknowledged, condemned, and remembered, it is important not to confound current debates about how to optimize modern ECT practice with historical information. Some aspects of the effect of ECT on cognitive function remain unclear, and mental health professionals, patients, and their families share concerns about this lack of clarity. However, these concerns must be viewed alongside the substantive robust evidence base for ECT's effectiveness in treating debilitating, often treatment-resistant, and sometimes life-threatening psychiatric illnesses. Focusing on elucidating the true effect of ECT on cognition and developing validated assessment instruments that can be used in clinical practice would be of major benefit in ensuring adequate treatment and health care for those with severe mental illness.

COGNITIVE EFFECTS OF ECT

Between 14 and 75% of patients report ECT-related anxiety, most commonly worrying about memory impairment or brain damage (Obbels, Verwijk, Bouckaert, & Sienaert, 2017). Although many factors are known to be associated with the cognitive effects of ECT, including clinical factors such as preexisting cognitive impairment, as well as treatment factors such as stimulus dose and electrode laterality (McClintock et al., 2014), there are few reliable predictors of the effects of ECT on cognition during and after treatment. One reason for the ongoing uncertainty about the severity and duration of cognitive effects of ECT is that the relative contributions of preexisting mood disorder, baseline cognition,

ECT treatment, and residual depressive symptoms to cognitive performance after ECT are not fully understood. Subtle or patchy cognitive impairments after ECT may have a great impact on quality of life, and currently available instruments may be inadequate to detect such impairments. Clearly, there is wide interindividual variability in the effects of ECT on cognition (Obbels et al., 2018), but without standardized instruments designed specifically for cognitive assessment during ECT, predicting those likely to experience negative effects remains a challenge.

TYPES OF ADVERSE COGNITIVE EFFECTS

Cognitive side effects can be described as immediate (just after treatment), subacute (during the treatment course), or longer-term (during and at the completion of a course of ECT). Retrograde amnesia is considered separately. (See Table 20.1.)

Immediate Cognitive Effects

Transient disorientation is expected immediately after the ECT session and rarely persists beyond 60 minutes (Sobin, Sackeim, Prudic, & Devanand, 1995). Impaired attention and amnesia for the time period in the ECT treatment and recovery are also common. Time to reorientation after ECT—the time at which correct responses to four out of five questions about orientation to person (name, date of birth, current age), place (name of hospital), and time (day of the week) are given after recommencing spontaneous breathing (Semkovska et al., 2016)—is a particularly important measure, for it is one of few available predictors of retrograde amnesia (Martin, Galvez, & Loo, 2015; Sobin et al., 1995). In one study, longer time to reorientation has also been associated with better antidepressant outcomes (Bjølseth et al., 2016). This simple measure therefore has great potential clinical utility and identifying those with longer time to reorientation could help guide treatment choices to minimize cognitive side effects.

TABLE 20.1. Cognitive Side Effects of ECT (Lezak, 2012)

- *Anterograde amnesia:* impaired ability to remember new information from the time of commencing ECT onward
- *Retrograde amnesia:* impaired ability to remember information learned before commencing ECT
- *Autobiographical amnesia:* impaired ability to remember events personally experienced at a particular time and place (episodic autobiographical memories, e.g., something that happened at a wedding you attended) and pieces of general information from one's own life (semantic autobiographical memories, e.g., year of graduation)
- *Subjective memory difficulty:* the experience of feeling as though one has a problem with one's memory, regardless of performance on objective memory testing
- *Impaired executive function:* impairment in higher-brain functions such as judgment, planning, and completing complex tasks

Electrode laterality and, in older people, the number of ECT treatments are associated with greater time of disorientation (Martin et al., 2015). Stimulus dosing and pulse width both affect time to reorientation but may be crucial to ECT's antidepressant effects. Higher stimulus doses and the use of brief-pulse (0.5–1.0 milliseconds) ECT are both associated with longer times to reorientation. Electrode laterality is also important in time to reorientation—median time to recovery of orientation was 19 minutes in those who were randomized to high-dose (six times threshold) right unilateral ECT compared to 26 minutes in those who received bitemporal ECT (1.5 times threshold; Semkovska et al., 2016). In meta-analysis, patients administered high-dose right unilateral ECT had an overall 8-minute shorter time of recovery of orientation than those who received bitemporal ECT (mean difference = –8.28, 95% CI = –12.86 to –3.70, p = .0004, Kolshus et al., 2017). Ultrabrief pulse ECT resulted in a significantly shorter time to reorientation after six ECT treatments in one randomized controlled trial, with a time to reorientation of 15.4 minutes in the ultrabrief pulse arm versus 22.3 minutes in the brief pulse arm (F = 8.08; p = .006). However, brief-pulse ECT is more effective than ultrabrief pulse (0.3 milliseconds) ECT for depression (Tor et al., 2015).

It is difficult to identify those patients who are likely to experience more than 90 minutes of disorientation after ECT, but they may be more likely to be older (Martin et al., 2015), have poorer cognitive function at baseline (Sobin et al., 1995), and have psychotic symptoms (Calev et al., 1991). Persistent disorientation (e.g., lasting more than 90 minutes) is more likely with bitemporal ECT, occurring in 13% of those with high-dose bitemporal ECT (at 2.5 times threshold) versus 2% of those having high-dose right unilateral ECT (at six times threshold; Sackeim et al., 2000).

Lithium and ECT

The mood stabilizer lithium, which has anticholinergic activity, has been proposed as a possible aggravating factor for cognitive impairment during and after ECT, with retrospective or observational reports of poorer cognition among those who have both ECT and lithium (Volpe & Tavares, 2012), as well as reports of prolonged seizure with this combination (Sartorius, Wolf, & Henn, 2005). Until more robust information is available, exercising caution in those with higher serum lithium levels (Thirthalli, Harish, & Gangadhar, 2011) and monitoring serum lithium levels among ECT patients is a sensible precaution.

Postictal Delirium

A minority of those who experience disorientation may present with postictal delirium. This acute confusional state can be differentiated from prolonged time to reorientation by the presence of severe disorientation and amnesia. Estimates vary from 12 to 65% of patients (Reti et al., 2014), with most estimates around 30–40% (Kikuchi, Yasui-Furukori, Fujii, Katagai, & Kaneko, 2009); those who have catatonic symptoms as well as longer seizure durations are more at risk (Kikuchi et al., 2009; Reti et al., 2014). Patients may present as restless and anxious and can often be managed with supportive health care. Those who are more agitated may benefit from further intravenous anesthetic or benzodiazepine to reduce risk of self-injury, but this treatment will result in a longer recovery due to the need for further airway monitoring. Persisting delirium beyond a few hours should be investigated for other possible underlying causes.

Subacute and Longer-Term Cognitive Effects

Cognitive functions that may be impaired during and immediately after the course of ECT include anterograde memory and executive function. Anterograde amnesia is common during and immediately after an ECT course, affecting verbal memory more than visual memory, and resolving within days or weeks after the last ECT session. This can result in challenges for patients, such as remembering names of staff, medications, ECT information, and appointment times. Practical supports can help patients to cope with anterograde amnesia, and providing education and advance information about the common occurrence of this problem aids preparedness for both patient and family member(s).

For the majority of patients, anterograde memory function will return to pre-ECT baseline or improve beyond baseline 2 or more weeks after completion of an ECT course (Semkovska & McLoughlin, 2010). Repeated courses of ECT or continuation of ECT have not been found to be associated with any cumulative cognitive impairment (Brus et al., 2017; Petrides, Tobias, Kellner, & Rudorfer, 2011; Russell et al., 2003; Smith et al., 2010). After recovery, those who continue ECT in order to prevent relapse and those who continue pharmacotherapy have comparable cognitive outcomes at 24 weeks, with modest improvement of anterograde memory observed at 12 weeks in both groups (Smith et al., 2010).

Nonmemory Cognitive Side Effects

Cognitive functions other than memory can be negatively affected by ECT (Table 20.2), but they generally improve, becoming the same as, or modestly better than, baseline performance following the end of the ECT course. For example, impairments in executive functions such as set shifting and phonemic fluency are present soon after completing an ECT course (Semkovska & McLoughlin, 2010), suggesting that these cognitive impairments are also present during the ECT course. However, in the same meta-analysis, performance on executive function tasks improved approximately 4–15 days post ECT compared with the pre-ECT baseline, with continuing improvements beyond 15-day follow-up.

Similarly, meta-analysis showed small to medium impairments in visual episodic memory (worse for delayed than for immediate visual recall) during the ECT course, with stabilization or modest improvement beyond baseline performance levels by approximately 15 days post-ECT (Semkovska & McLoughlin, 2010). In one small study ($n = 24$), impairments were identified in visual and visuospatial memory in people having ECT, with some of these impairments persisting after one month (Falconer, Cleland, Fielding, & Reid, 2010). However, ECT was administered at twice the seizure threshold, which likely amplified the cognitive problems. In another study, visual learning and memory improved during the ECT course, a finding that correlated with improvement in depression symptom severity (Maric et al., 2016). However, in that study, ECT was administered

TABLE 20.2. Effects of ECT on Cognitive Functions Other Than Verbal Memory

Cognitive function/test	Effect of ECT	Outcome	Summary	Reference
Phonemic fluency	Impairment present soon after completing ECT course	Test performance improved post-ECT compared with pre-ECT baseline	Impaired and improved	Semkovska & McLoughlin (2010)
Set shifting	Impairment present soon after completing ECT course	Test performance improved post-ECT compared with pre-ECT baseline	Impaired and improved	Semkovska & McLoughlin (2010)
Visual episodic memory (visual recall)	Impairment present during ECT course	Test performance stabilized or improved post-ECT compared with pre-ECT baseline	Impaired and improved	Semkovska & McLoughlin (2010)
Visual/visuospatial memory	Impairment present during ECT course and soon after completing course	Test performance remained impaired post-ECT compared with pre-ECT baseline	Impaired, did not improve	Falconer, Cleland, Fielding, & Reid (2010)
Visual learning and memory	No significant impairment present during or soon after ECT course	Test performance improved post-ECT compared with pre-ECT baseline	Not impaired but improved	Maric et al. (2016)
Working memory	No significant impairment present soon after ECT course	Test performance improved post-ECT compared with pre-ECT baseline	Not impaired but improved	Semkovska & McLoughlin (2010)

three times per week, and the finding may not be generalizable. Working memory (as measured by the Backward Digit Span Test) was not impaired at 0–3 days posttreatment and improved relative to pre-ECT baseline at follow-up more than 15 days posttreatment (Semkovska & McLoughlin, 2010). As with anterograde memory, there is little to no evidence of cumulative impairment of nonmemory cognitive functions with repeated ECT courses. Factors affecting long-term cognitive performance include age (Sackeim et al., 2007), severity of depression at the time of testing, and number of days since the last ECT session (Semkovska & McLoughlin, 2010).

Although objective testing has provided no evidence of long-lasting impairment in nonmemory cognitive functions after ECT, some case reports and reviews have described severe and persistent difficulties (Fink, 2007). It is important to acknowledge the limitations of current assessment schedules in understanding this discrepancy between observed versus experienced findings. For example, as cognitive function was not routinely assessed in healthy comparison populations in many ECT studies, it remains unclear whether the cognitive improvement seen after ECT represents a return to a pre-depression, pre-ECT level of cognitive function. It is also possible that faint or erratic impairments in executive function cannot be identified by current cognitive instruments; that is, they lack ecological validity, but they are noted by the person experiencing them.

RETROGRADE AMNESIA

ECT research over the past three decades has focused mostly on autobiographical retrograde amnesia, possibly due both to the lack of clarity regarding severity and duration of this form of amnesia after ECT, and to the significant distress associated with the difficulty in remembering events from one's own life (Rose, Fleischmann, Wykes, Leese, & Bindman, 2003). Retrograde amnesia is associated with a higher number of ECT treatments, bitemporal ECT (vs. high-dose right unilateral ECT; Kolshus et al., 2017), and brief-pulse ECT (compared with ultrabrief-pulse ECT; Tor et al., 2015). However, while unilateral ECT has both superior cognitive outcomes and equivalent depression outcomes as bitemporal ECT, ultrabrief-pulse ECT (when compared with brief-pulse ECT) has only a cognitive advantage and does not maintain antidepressant efficacy (depending on how it is dosed). In addition to ECT treatment factors, patient factors also affect the risk of retrograde amnesia. Premorbid IQ, age (Sackeim et al., 2007), global cognitive function at baseline (Sobin et al., 1995), and longer time to reorientation (Martin et al., 2015) all confer increased risk of the presence and magnitude of retrograde amnesia for autobiographical information. A temporal gradient is observed in retrograde amnesia, with more recent memories being more vulnerable to loss during ECT than, for example, older memories such as those from childhood (Lisanby, Maddox, Prudic, Devanand, & Sackeim, 2000).

As outlined above in relation to subjective memory difficulty, there is a discrepancy between the reported findings of large observational studies, which show no evidence of persistent retrograde amnesia following ECT, and case reports of individual experiences of severe, sometimes profound autobiographical memory impairment after ECT (Fink, 2007). Understanding this gap between observed and experienced cognitive effects is difficult, for the assessment of retrograde memory with precision is hampered by an absence of standardized and psychometrically sound assessment instruments for retrograde amnesia in ECT (Semkovska & McLoughlin, 2013).

SUBJECTIVE MEMORY DIFFICULTY

Subjective memory difficulty after ECT is not associated with performance on current instruments for cognitive testing, but it should not be underestimated. Indeed, such reported memory difficulty by patients is both common (reported by up to one-third of patients (Rose et al., 2003) and serious, with subjective memory difficulty often outweighing patients' perceptions of any benefit from ECT (NICE, 2009). Little is known about this experience; it is suggested that subjective memory difficulty is a form of misattribution of the effects of age, mood, somatic complaints on memory (Fink, 2007), or a symptom of anxiety (Andrade, Arumugham, & Thirthalli, 2016).

Instruments like the Squire Subjective Memory Assessment (Squire, Wetzel, & Slater, 1979) and the Subjective Assessment of Memory Impairment (Kumar, Han, Tiller, Loo, & Martin, 2016) have been used to investigate this occurrence in ECT populations. The experience of subjectively reported memory difficulty without corresponding objective evidence is associated with depression severity, and while younger, female patients are more at risk, those who remit from depression after ECT are less likely to report subjective memory difficulty (Brus et al., 2017). Persisting objective retrograde memory impairment is associated with worse subjective memory difficulty (Berman, Prudic, Brakemeier, Olfson, & Sackeim, 2008).

COGNITIVE ASSESSMENT

Clinicians are advised to assess individual risks (including risk of cognitive impairment) and benefits for patients considering ECT (American Psychiatric Association, 2010; NICE, 2009). The U.S. Food and Drug Administration recently recommended that clinical ECT practice should incorporate cognitive assessments of attention, executive function, and memory. However, there currently exist no specifically designed recommended instruments for cognitive testing in ECT practice that would aid such a baseline assessment of risk (see Table 20.3). Meta-analytic evidence showed that most cognitive impairments most likely should resolve within 15 days post-ECT (Semkovska & McLoughlin, 2010), suggesting that cognitive impairments apparent for more than one month should be further investigated with formal neuropsychological testing. Currently available instruments are imperfect, but evidence supports performing at least a global cognitive assessment pre-ECT, during the course of ECT (e.g., after six treatments), at a set time after ECT (e.g., within 3 days after the last ECT treatment), and after 1–2 months.

How should such a global cognitive assessment be performed? Such an assessment would preferably measure multiple cognitive functions, including immediate and delayed verbal recall, attention, working memory, autobiographical memory, and at least one aspect of executive function (e.g., cognitive flexibility). No specific single instrument exists to cover all the needs of clinicians for monitoring patients' cognitive function during ECT. Detailed cognitive assessment such as that performed for research purposes is unlikely to be practical for severely unwell patients or busy clinical environments. The CANTAB (cognitive assessment software, Cambridge Cognition, 2017) is highly sensitive and provides detailed results but is unlikely to be feasible in routine practice (Falconer et al., 2010; Fray, Robbins & Sahakian, 1996; Tsaltas et al., 2011). Screening batteries have been suggested (Martin et al., 2013), but commonly used screening tools such as the standardized Mini-Mental State Examination (sMMSE; Molloy, Alemayehu, & Roberts, 1991) are inadequate for this purpose as they were initially developed for dementia screening. In particular, the sMMSE lacks a measure of executive function and can only detect substantial versus modest impairment (Tombaugh & McIntyre, 1992). Other global cognitive assessments such as the Montreal Cognitive Assessment (MoCA; Nasreddine et al., 2005) and Addenbrooke's Cognitive Assessment Version III (ACE-III; Hodges & Larner, 2017; Hsieh, Schubert, Hoon, Mioshi, & Hodges, 2013) have the advantage of sensitivity to change as well as mild cognitive impairment. The MoCA has been reported to be more sensitive to a range of cognitive impairments than the MMSE at both pre-ECT and post-ECT assessments (Moirand et al., 2018). Since September 2020, access to the MoCA has been restricted to those who have completed an online training program (*mocatest. org*). No specialized training is required for the ACE-III, which is publicly available and

TABLE 20.3. Characteristics of Highlighted Cognitive Assessment Tools in ECT

Instrument	Advantages	Disadvantages	Reference
Cognitive screening[a]			
sMMSE	• Widely and freely available • No training required • Quick to administer	• No test of executive function • Poor sensitivity • Parallel versions not available	Molloy et al. (1991)
MoCA	• Sensitive to impairment • Includes executive function • Freely available • Parallel versions available • Quick to administer	• Training recommended	Nasreddine et al. (2005)
CANTAB	• Sensitive to impairment • Sensitive to change • Includes executive function • Detailed results provided	• Not freely available • Training recommended • Lengthy, challenging for subject • Not designed for routine clinical practice	Cambridge Cognition (*www. cambridgecognition. com*)
ACE-III	• Sensitive to impairment • Sensitive to change • Includes executive function • Parallel versions available • No training required • Freely available	• Requires more time than sMMSE or MoCA	Hodges & Larner (2017); Hseih et al. (2013)
Retrograde amnesia[a]			
CUAMI, CUAMI-SF	• Predominant instrument used in ECT literature • Sensitive to group-level differences between treatment modalities • Short form available	• Normative data not available for comparison • Not suited to assessing for change due to floor effect • No separate scores for episodic and semantic recall • Lengthy, challenging for subject	McElhiney et al. (1995, 2001); Sackeim et al. (2000)
K-AMI	• Widely used in ECT literature • Normative data available for comparison • Separate scores for episodic and semantic recall	• May not be sufficiently sensitive for ECT purposes • No measure of consistency of recall • Lengthy, challenging for subject	Kopelman et al. (1989)

Note. sMMSE, Standardized Mini-Mental State Examination; MoCA, Montreal Cognitive Assessment; CANTAB, Cambridge Neuropsychological Test Automated Battery; ACE-III, Addenbrooke's Cognitive Examination, Version III; CUAMI-SF, Columbia University Autobiographical Memory Interview—Short Form; K-AMI, Kopelman Autobiographical Memory Interview.
[a]Several other assessment tools for retrograde amnesia are available and have been used in ECT populations but are not discussed here. For further discussion, see Jelovac et al. (2016).

highly sensitive, though it takes longer to administer than the MoCA. Both instruments are available in a variety of languages and in parallel validated versions for retesting during and after ECT.

RETROGRADE AMNESIA ASSESSMENT

Assessing retrograde memory in people with depression is hindered by an absence of an ideal instrument and the impact of both time and mood symptoms on performance in retrograde memory assessments. Healthy nondepressed people experience memory decay, showing a declining ability to retrieve autobiographical information over time. Some reduction in consistency of recall can therefore be perceived as "normal" and is seen in healthy controls even after an interval of 2 months (Semkovska, Noone, Carton, & McLoughlin, 2012). Therefore, reduced consistency of autobiographical recall over time is nonspecific to depressed people or to depressed people who receive ECT, with estimates of normal rate of loss of autobiographical memories ranging from 27% after 6 weeks (Talarico & Rubin, 2003) to 31–42% after 2 months (Anderson, Cohen, & Taylor, 2000). In addition to the confounding impact of normal loss of autobiographical memories over time, depressed people in particular display a difficulty in identification of separate incidents from their own autobiographical memory, a phenomenon known as reduced specificity or overgeneralization. This is a robust finding across different types of assessment in depression (Jelovac, O'Connor, McCarron, & McLoughlin, 2016). Furthermore, when depressed people do manage to identify separate events, they recall few specific details. Depressed people are likely to have poor scores on episodic autobiographical memory assessments (where scores are provided for specific events and associated details). This is the case even when they have no impaired semantic autobiographical memory (remembering, for example, an address from childhood), because of the reduced specificity associated with depression (Verwijk et al., 2015). When compared with healthy nondepressed controls, both those depressed people who have responded to ECT and those who have not responded continued to display reduced specificity of autobiographical memories at 3 months after ECT (Jelovac et al., 2016). This is important because many instruments for assessment of retrograde amnesia measure consistency of recall, asking the subject to recount information provided on initial testing and scoring the percentage of baseline information recalled on retesting. Where very little information was provided by a depressed person experiencing reduced specificity at baseline testing, full recall of only a few items at retesting will result in a score that does not reflect change in autobiographical memory that may be present, that is, a floor effect. Interindividual variability in autobiographical memory is common (Obbels et al., 2018), and instruments need to be able to identify both improvement and disimprovement.

To understand the effect of ECT on loss of autobiographical memories, we first need to understand the effects of time and change in depressive symptoms on the loss of autobiographical memories. This requires that the instruments used for assessment of retrograde memory in ECT populations would have available normative information on non-depressed people and depressed people having treatment other than ECT, which is inconsistently the case. For both clinicians and patients, an ideal instrument to assess retrograde autobiographical amnesia would be short, comprehensive, and simple to administer, providing a score for memory detail (semantic and episodic) as well as a consistency score for retesting. These scores could be compared with normative information from the general population. Arguably no currently available instrument—for example, the Columbia University Autobiographical Memory Interview (CUAMI) or the short form (CUAMI-SF; McElhiney et al., 1995; McElhiney, Moody, & Sackeim, 2001) and the Kopelman Autobiographical Memory Interview (K-AMI; Kopelman, Wilson, & Baddeley, 1989)—meets these ideal clinical practice criteria.

The CUAMI-SF (Sackeim et al., 2000) was the predominant instrument for assessment of autobiographical amnesia in ECT research and has been used to show differences in retrograde amnesia associated with different ECT treatment modalities, such as electrode placement and pulse width (Kolshus et al., 2017; Sackeim et al., 2000, 2008), which led to refinements in ECT practice to reduce cognitive side effects. It is not an ideal instrument, for it lacks publicly available normative data and psychometric properties for comparison of both healthy controls and depressed people not having ECT (Sackeim, 2014; Semkovska & McLoughlin, 2013). As the instrument relies on consistency of autobiographical recall, the floor effect, as related above, limits its usefulness because positive change, such as that suggested by interindividual variability, cannot be detected. That is, performance on the instrument can only remain stable or worsen; it cannot improve. This is in stark contrast to other cognitive instruments that allow for a wide range of performance, albeit worsened, stable, or improved. The CUAMI-SF does not provide separate scores for episodic and semantic recall and, as with many autobiographical memory assessments, it is long (the short form takes approximately 20–25 minutes to administer).

The K-AMI is also widely used, although it was not originally designed for ECT research (Sienaert, Vansteelandt, Demyttenaere, & Peuskens, 2010). The K-AMI may be insufficiently sensitive for ECT-related autobiographical amnesia (Jelovac et al., 2016) and is also lengthy in regard to administration and scoring (approximately 25+ minutes). Unlike the CUAMI, the K-AMI does not provide a measure of consistency of recall but does provide separate scores for both semantic and episodic autobiographical memory. In addition, the K-AMI is psychometrically sound, and some normative data on the performance of healthy controls and other clinical populations are available via the test publisher. Importantly, unlike the CUAMI, the K-AMI allows for improvement of scores on retesting should memory improve during or after a course of ECT.

MINIMIZATION AND PREVENTION OF ADVERSE COGNITIVE EFFECTS

Electrode placement, stimulus dose, pulse width, and treatment frequency can all be managed to help optimize cognitive outcomes after ECT. Clinicians should balance the importance of rapidity and the reliability of the antidepressant effect and impact on cognitive function on a case-by-case basis (e.g., personalized medicine). For example, higher electrical stimulus is associated with greater cognitive side effects but is important for antidepressant response to treatment (Sackeim et al., 1993). ECT is administered three times a week (vs. twice a week; see Lerer et al., 1995), and now-obsolete sine-wave stimuli are both associated with greater cognitive impairment (vs. brief-pulse stimuli; Sackeim et al., 2007).

The choice of electrode placement should be made in collaboration with patients where possible. High-dose right unilateral ECT has equivalent antidepressant efficacy to bitemporal ECT but has less impact on cognition (Sackeim et al., 1993, 2007) when administered at six times stimulus threshold (Kolshus et al., 2017). While bifrontal ECT may have a cognitive advantage over bitemporal ECT (slightly less decline in MMSE score; Dunne & McLoughlin, 2012), there is insufficient evidence to recommend its routine use.

Modification of pulse width presents another opportunity to optimize cognitive outcomes. Ultrabrief pulse ECT results in clearly improved cognitive outcomes (recovery of orientation, global cognitive function, anterograde memory (learning and recall), and retrograde memory) compared with brief pulse ECT (Tor et al., 2015; Verwijk et al., 2012). The advantage may come at a price, with a significantly less robust antidepressant effect, requiring more treatments to achieve remission (Tor et al., 2015). However, some evidence suggests that right unilateral ultrabrief-pulse ECT in elderly adults has robust antidepressant benefits (Kellner et al., 2016a, 2016b) and minimal cognitive adverse effects (Lisanby et al., 2020).

Primary Prevention of Adverse Cognitive Effects

Identification of those patients most at risk (e.g., older patients with baseline cognitive impairment or a history of cognitive difficulties after ECT) allows clinicians to initiate treatment with parameters that have relatively less adverse impact on cognition. For example, in a severely unwell patient who is at high risk for cognitive side effects but requires a rapid response to treatment, brief-pulse high-dose right unilateral ECT should be considered as the initial treatment setting. In patients whose risk for cognitive side effects is of greater concern than need for rapid recovery, clinicians could prescribe ultra-brief-pulse right unilateral ECT. Though not guided by specific evidence, it is pragmatic to avoid additional possible sources of transient cognitive impairment such as any unnecessary anticholinergic agents (e.g., atropine) during the treatment. Where the clinical situation permits, it is common to optimize medical health prior to any physical treatment such as ECT. In addition, cardiovascular, cerebrovascular, and respiratory risk factors should be considered to prevent further exacerbation of cognitive impairment by concurrent chronic medical illness.

Premature discontinuation of an ECT course because of distress related to cognitive side effects should be avoided wherever possible. Therefore, possibly the most useful thing clinicians can do to limit the impact of cognitive side effects of ECT is to educate patients and families about what to expect during ECT. For example, during the consent process, clinicians should inform the patient (and their family, if involved) about the prevalence of cognitive side effects despite best treatment and how this may manifest in daily activities during the ECT course. Mental health professionals of all disciplines can help by providing practical support to patients (and their family) overcome difficulties they face during the ECT course if cognitive effects materialize. Patients should be informed that they should not drive during the ECT course and should be directed to any available local law or policy on this point.

Secondary Prevention of Adverse Cognitive Effects

For patients who present with cognitive impairment during ECT, the above treatment factors can also be modified during ECT to limit the impact on cognitive function. Currently, sources of guidance are unavailable for clinicians as to when and which treatment changes should be made. Further research on reducing the effect of ECT on cognition has been conducted with a variety of potential methods, including ketamine anaesthesia for ECT (McGirr et al., 2017) and augmentation of ECT with cognitive training (Choi, Wang, Feng & Prudic, 2017), but these interventions failed to improve cognitive outcomes. One area that remains under investigation is the use of acetylcholinesterase inhibitors during ECT, which has resulted in improved cognitive outcomes. Studies are highly heterogeneous (Henstra et al., 2017), however, and at present this intervention remains experimental.

SUMMARY

- ECT is a safe, effective treatment used around the world for severe mental illness.
- Its use is limited by concerns about cognitive side effects—predominantly anterograde amnesia, retrograde amnesia, and nonmemory cognitive functions.
- Cognitive impairment is common during and immediately after the course of ECT, but many cognitive functions improve to beyond baseline after finishing ECT.
- Acute disorientation is common and is usually managed by supportive care alone, but time to reorientation is an important predictor of retrograde amnesia and should therefore be routinely assessed.
- Retrograde amnesia remains difficult to assess, and there are no standardized, psychometrically sound instruments designed specifically to assess cognitive function in ECT.
- Repeated courses of ECT do not appear to confer any cumulative cognitive impairment.
- Identifying patients who are more at risk of cognitive impairment and modifying treatment factors such as electrode placement, pulse width, and stimulus dose can help to minimize cognitive side effects.
- Clinicians should consider use of high-dose right unilateral ECT as it maintains antidepressant efficacy, but it has fewer cognitive effects relative to bitemporal ECT.
- Ultra-brief-pulse ECT also has been found to reduce cognitive side effects relative to brief pulse ECT, but findings have been mixed regarding its rate and speed of antidepressant response and remission
- Cognitive function should be routinely assessed before, during, and after ECT, where possible, considering the use of global cognitive function screening measures such as the MoCA or ACE-III.

REFERENCES

Abrams, R. (2002). *History of ECT* (4th ed.). New York: Oxford University Press.

American Psychiatric Association. (2001). *The practice of electroconvulsive therapy: recommendations for treatment, training, and privileging.* Washington, DC: American Psychiatric Press.

American Psychiatric Association. (2010). *Practice guideline for the treatment of patients with major depressive disorder* (3rd ed.). Arlington, VA: Author.

Anderson, S. J., Cohen, G., & Taylor, S. (2000). Rewriting the past: Some factors affecting the variability of personal memories. *Applied Cognitive Psychology, 14*(5), 435–454.

Andrade, C., Arumugham, S., & Thirthalli, J. (2016). Adverse effects of electroconvulsive therapy. *Psychiatric Clinics of North America, 39*(3), 513–530.

Berman, R. M., Prudic, J., Brakemeier, E. L., Olfson, M., & Sackeim, H. A. (2008). Subjective evaluation of the therapeutic and cognitive effects of electroconvulsive therapy. *Brain Stimulation, 1*(1), 16–26.

Bjølseth, T. M., Engedal, K., Benth, J. Š., Bergsholm, P., Dybedal, G. S., Gaarden, T. L., et al. (2016). Speed of recovery from disorientation may predict the treatment outcome of electroconvulsive therapy (ECT) in elderly patients with major depression. *Journal of Affective Disorders, 190,* 178–186.

Blumberger, D. M., Seitz, D. P., Herrmann, N., Kirkham, J. G., Ng, R., Reimer, C., et al. (2017). Low medical morbidity and mortality after acute courses of electroconvulsive therapy in a population-based sample. *Acta Psychiatrica Scandinavica, 136*(6), 583–593.

Brus, O., Nordanskog, P., Båve, U., Cao, Y., Hammar, Å., Landén, M., et al. (2017). Subjective memory immediately following electroconvulsive therapy. *Journal of ECT, 33*(2), 96–103.

Calev, A., Cohen, R., Tubi, N., Nigal, D., Shapira, B., Kugelmass, S., et al. (1991). Disorientation and bilateral moderately suprathreshold titrated ECT. *Journal of ECT, 7*(2), 99–110.

Choi, J., Wang, Y., Feng, T., & Prudic, J. (2017). Cognitive training to improve memory in individuals undergoing electroconvulsive therapy: Negative findings. *Journal of Psychiatric Research, 92,* 8–14.

Dunne, R. A., & McLoughlin, D. M. (2012). Systematic review and meta-analysis of bifrontal electroconvulsive therapy versus bilateral and unilateral electroconvulsive therapy in depression. *World Journal of Biological Psychiatry, 13*(4), 248–258.

Falconer, D., Cleland, J., Fielding, S., & Reid, I. C. (2010). Using the Cambridge Neuropsychological Test Automated Battery (CANTAB) to assess the cognitive impact of electroconvulsive therapy on visual and visuospatial memory. *Psychological Medicine, 40*(6), 1017–1025.

Fink, M. (2007). Complaints of loss of personal memories after electroconvulsive therapy: evidence of a somatoform disorder? *Psychosomatics, 48*(4), 290–293.

Finnegan, M., Bayazit, H., Cronin, T., Guler, K., Galligan, T., Karababa, F. I., et al. (2018). Towards international standards: East meets west. *Journal of ECT, 34*(1), 1–2.

Finnegan, M., O'Connor, S., & McLoughlin, D. M. (2018). Involuntary and voluntary electroconvulsive therapy: A case-control study. *Brain Stimulation, 11*(4), 860–862.

Fray, P. J., Robbins, T. W., & Sahakian, B. J. (1996). Neuropsychiatric applications of CANTAB. *International Journal of Geriatric Psychiatry, 11*(4), 329–336.

Henstra, M. J., Jansma, E. P., Velde, N., Swart, E. L., Stek, M. L., & Rhebergen, D. (2017). Acetylcholinesterase inhibitors for electroconvulsive therapy-induced cognitive side effects: A systematic review. *International Journal of Geriatric Psychiatry, 32*(5), 522–531.

Hodges J. R., & Larner A. J. (2017). Addenbrooke's Cognitive Examinations: ACE, ACE-R, ACE-III, ACEapp, and M-ACE. In A. Larner (Ed.), *Cognitive screening instruments* (pp. 109–137). New York: Springer.

Hsieh, S., Schubert, S., Hoon, C., Mioshi, E., & Hodges, J. R. (2013). Validation of the Addenbrooke's Cognitive Examination III in frontotemporal dementia and Alzheimer's disease. *Dementia and Geriatric Cognitive Disorders, 36*(3–4), 242–250.

Husain, M. M., Rush, A. J., Fink, M., Knapp, R., Petrides, G., Rummans, T., et al. (2004). Speed of response and remission in major depressive disorder with acute Electroconvulsive therapy (ECT): A consortium for research in ECT (CORE) report. *Journal of Clinical Psychiatry, 65*(4), 485–491.

Jelovac, A., Kolshus, E., & McLoughlin, D. M. (2013). Relapse following successful electroconvulsive therapy for major depression: A meta-analysis. *Neuropsychopharmacology, 38*(12), 2467–2474.

Jelovac, A., O'Connor, S., McCarron, S., & McLoughlin, D. M. (2016). Autobiographical memory specificity in major depression treated with electroconvulsive therapy. *Journal of ECT, 32*(1), 38–43.

Kellner, C. H., Husain, M. M., Knapp, R. G., McCall, W. V., Petrides, G., Rudorfer, M. V., et al. (2016a). Right unilateral ultrabrief pulse electroconvulsive therapy (ECT) in geriatric depression: Phase 1 of the PRIDE Study. *American Journal of Psychiatry, 173*(11), 1101–1109.

Kellner, C. H., Husain, M. M., Knapp, R. G., McCall, W. V, Petrides, G., Rudorfer, M. W., et al. (2016b). A novel strategy for continuation ECT in geriatric depression: Phase 2 of the PRIDE study. *American Journal of Psychiatry, 173*(11), 1110–1118.

Kellner, C. H., Knapp, R. G., Petrides, G., Rummans, T. A., Husain, M. M., Rasmussen, K., et al. (2006). Continuation electroconvulsive therapy vs. pharmacotherapy for relapse prevention in major depression: a multisite study from the Consortium for Research in Electroconvulsive Therapy (CORE). *Archives of General Psychiatry, 63*(12), 1337–1344.

Kikuchi, A., Yasui-Furukori, N., Fujii, A., Katagai, H., & Kaneko, S. (2009). Identification of predictors of post-ictal delirium after electroconvulsive therapy. *Psychiatry and Clinical Neurosciences, 63*(2), 180–185.

Knapp, M., Romeo, R., Mogg, A., Eranti, S., Pluck, G., Purvis, R., et al. (2008). Cost-effectiveness of transcranial magnetic stimulation vs. electroconvulsive therapy for severe depression: a multicentre randomised controlled trial. *Journal of Affective Disorders, 109*(3), 273–285.

Kolshus, E., Jelovac, A., & McLoughlin, D. M. (2017). Bitemporal v. high-dose right unilateral electroconvulsive therapy for depression: A systematic review and meta-analysis of randomized controlled trials. *Psychological Medicine, 47*(3), 518–530.

Kopelman, M., Wilson, B., & Baddeley, A. (1989). The autobiographical memory interview: a new assessment of autobiographical and personal semantic memory in amnesic patients. *Journal of Clinical and Experimental Neuropsychology, 11*(5), 724–744.

Kumar, D. R., Han, H. K., Tiller, J., Loo, C. K., & Martin, D. M. (2016). A brief measure for assessing patient perceptions of cognitive side effects after electroconvulsive therapy: The subjective assessment of memory impairment. *Journal of ECT, 32*(4), 256–261.

Leiknes, K. A., Schweder, L. J. V., & Høie, B. (2012). Contemporary use and practice of electroconvulsive therapy worldwide. *Brain and Behavior, 2*(3), 283–344.

Lerer, B., Shapira, B., Calev, A., Tubi, N., Drexler, H., & Kindler, S. (1995). Antidepressant and cognitive effects of twice- versus three-times-weekly ECT. *American Journal of Psychiatry, 152*(4), 564.

Lezak, M. D. (2012). *Neuropsychological Assessment* (5th ed.). Oxford, UK: Oxford University Press.

Lisanby, S. H., Maddox, J. H., Prudic, J., Devanand, D., & Sackeim, H. A. (2000). The effects of electroconvulsive therapy on memory of autobiographical and public events. *Archives of General Psychiatry, 57*(6), 581–590.

Lisanby, S. H., McClintock, S. M., Alexopoulos, G., Bailine, S. H., Bernhardt, E., Briggs, M. C., et al. (2020). Neurocognitive effects of combined electroconvulsive therapy (ECT) and venlafaxine in geriatric depression: Phase 1 of the PRIDE study. *American Journal of Geriatric Psychiatry, 28*(3), 304–316.

Maric, N. P., Stojanovic, Z., Andric, S., Soldatovic, I., Dolic, M., & Spiric, Z. (2016). The acute and medium-term effects of treatment with electroconvulsive therapy on memory in patients with major depressive disorder. *Psychological Medicine, 46*(4), 797–806.

Markowitz, J., Brown, R., Sweeney, J. & Mann, J. J. (1987). Reduced length and cost of hospital stay for major depression in patients treated with ECT. *American Journal of Psychiatry, 144*(8), 1025.

Martin, D. M., Gálvez, V., & Loo, C. K. (2015). Predicting retrograde autobiographical memory changes following electroconvulsive therapy: Relationships between individual, treatment, and early clinical factors. *International Journal of Neuropsychopharmacology, 18*(12), pyv067.

Martin, D. M., Katalinic, N., Ingram, A., Schweitzer, I., Smith, D. J., Hadzi-Pavlovic, D., et al. (2013). A new early cognitive screening measure to detect cognitive side-effects of electroconvulsive ther-apy? *Journal of Psychiatric Research, 47*(12), 1967–1974.

McCall, W. V., Andrade, C., & Sienaert. P. (2014). Searching for the mechanism (s) of ECT's therapeutic effect. *Journal of ECT, 30*(2), 87–89.

McCall, W. V., Prudic, J., Olfson, M., & Sackeim, H. (2006). Health-related quality of life following ECT in a large community sample. *Journal of Affective Disorders, 90*(2–3), 269–274.

McClintock, S. M., Choi, J., Deng, Z.-D., Appelbaum, L. G., Krystal, A. D., & Lisanby, S. H. (2014). Multifactorial determinants of the neurocognitive effects of electroconvulsive therapy. *Journal of ECT, 30*(2), 165–176.

McElhiney, M., Moody, B., & Sackeim, H. A. (2001). *Manual for administration and scoring the Colum-bia University Autobiographical Memory Interview—Short form (Version 3)*. New York: New York State Psychiatric Institute.

McElhiney, M. C., Moody, B. J., Steif, B. L., Prudic, J., Devanand, D., Nobler, M. S., et al. (1995). Autobiographical memory and mood: effects of electroconvulsive therapy. *Neuropsychology, 9*(4), 501–504.

McGirr, A., Berlim, M. T., Bond, D. J., Chan, P. Y., Yatham, L. N.& Lam, R. W. (2017). Adjunctive ket-amine in electroconvulsive therapy: Updated systematic review and meta-analysis. *British Journal of Psychiatry, 210*(6), 403–447.

Moirand, R., Galvao, F., Lecompte, M., Poulet, E., Haesebaert, F., & Brunelin, J. (2018). Usefulness of the Montreal Cognitive Assessment (MoCA) to monitor cognitive impairments in depressed patients receiving electroconvulsive therapy. *Psychiatry Research, 259*, 476–481.

Molloy, D., Alemayehu, E., & Roberts, R. (1991). A standardized Mini-Mental State Examination (SMMSE): Improved reliability compared to the traditional MMSE. *American Journal of Psychia-try, 148*, 102–105.

Munk-Olsen, T., Laursen, T. M., Videbech, P., Mortensen, P. B., & Rosenberg, R. (2007). All-cause mor-tality among recipients of electroconvulsive therapy: Register-based cohort study. *British Journal of Psychiatry, 190*(5), 435–439.

Nasreddine, Z. S., Phillips, N. A., Bédirian, V., Charbonneau, S., Whitehead, V., Collin, I., et al. (2005). The Montreal Cognitive Assessment, MoCA: A brief screening tool for mild cognitive impairment. *Journal of the American Geriatrics Society, 53*(4), 695–699.

National Institute for Health and Care Excellence. (2009). Guidance on the use of electroconvulsive therapy (NICE Technology Appraisal Guidance [TA59]). Retrieved October 13, 2021, from *www.nice.org.uk/guidance/ta59*

Obbels, J., Verwijk, E., Bouckaert, F., & Sienaert, P. (2017). ECT-related anxiety: A systematic review. *Journal of ECT, 33*(4), 229–236.

Obbels, J., Verwijk, E., Vansteelandt, K., Dols, A., Bouckaert, F., Schouws, S., et al. (2018). Long-term neurocognitive functioning after electroconvulsive therapy in patients with late-life depression. *Acta Psychiatrica Scandinavica, 138*(3), 223–231.

Petrides, G., Tobias, K. G., Kellner, C. H., & Rudorfer, M. V. (2011). Continuation and maintenance electroconvulsive therapy for mood disorders: Review of the literature. *Neuropsychobiology, 64*(3), 129–140.

Prudic, J., & Sackeim, H. A. (1999). Electroconvulsive therapy and suicide risk. *Journal of Clinical Psy-chiatry, 60*(Suppl. 2), 104–110.

Reti, I. M., Krishnan, A., Podlisky, A., Sharp, A., Melinda, W., Neufeld, K. J. et al. (2014). Predictors of electroconvulsive therapy postictal delirium. *Psychosomatics, 55*(3), 272–279.

Rose, D., Fleischmann, P., Wykes, T., Leese, M., & Bindman, J. (2003). Patients' perspectives on electro-convulsive therapy: Systematic review. *British Medical Journal, 326*(7403), 1363.

Ross, E. L., Zivin, K., & Maixner, D. F. (2018). Cost-effectiveness of electroconvulsive therapy vs. phar-macotherapy/psychotherapy for treatment-resistant depression in the United States. *Journal of the American Medical Association: Psychiatry, 75*(7), 713–722.

Rush, A. J., Trivedi, M. H., Wisniewski, S. R., Nierenberg, A. A., Stewart, J. W., Warden, D., et al. (2006). Acute and longer-term outcomes in depressed outpatients requiring one or several treatment steps: A STAR* D report. *American Journal of Psychiatry, 163*(11), 1905–1917.

Russell, J. C., Rasmussen, K. G., O'Connor, M. K., Copeman, C. A., Ryan, D. A., & Rummans, T. A. (2003). Long-term maintenance ECT: A retrospective review of efficacy and cognitive outcome. *Journal of ECT, 19*(1), 4–9.

Ryan, K. M., & McLoughlin, D. M. (2018). From molecules to mind: Mechanisms of action of electroconvulsive therapy. *Acta Psychiatrica Scandinavica, 138*(3), 177–179.

Sackeim, H. A. (2014). Autobiographical memory and electroconvulsive therapy: Do not throw out the baby. *Journal of ECT, 30*(3), 177–186.

Sackeim, H. A. (2017). Modern electroconvulsive therapy: Vastly improved yet greatly underused. *Journal of the American Medical Association: Psychiatry, 74*(8), 779–780.

Sackeim, H. A., Haskett, R. F., Mulsant, B. H., Thase, M. E., Mann, J. J., Pettinati, H. M., et al. (2001). Continuation pharmacotherapy in the prevention of relapse following electroconvulsive therapy: A randomized controlled trial. *Journal of the American Medical Association, 285*(10), 1299–1307.

Sackeim, H. A., Prudic, J., Devanand, D., Kiersky, J. E., Fitzsimons, L., Moody, B. J., et al. (1993). Effects of stimulus intensity and electrode placement on the efficacy and cognitive effects of electroconvulsive therapy. *New England Journal of Medicine, 328*(12), 839–846.

Sackeim, H. A., Prudic, J., Devanand, D., Nobler, M. S., Lisanby, S. H., Peyser, S., et al. (2000). A prospective, randomized, double-blind comparison of bilateral and right unilateral electroconvulsive therapy at different stimulus intensities. *Archives of General Psychiatry, 57*(5), 425–434.

Sackeim, H. A., Prudic, J., Fuller, R., Keilp, J., Lavori, P. W., & Olfson, M. (2007). The cognitive effects of electroconvulsive therapy in community settings. *Neuropsychopharmacology 32*(1), 244–254.

Sackeim, H. A., Prudic, J., Nobler, M. S., Fitzsimons, L., Lisanby, S. H., Payne, N., et al. (2008). Effects of pulse width and electrode placement on the efficacy and cognitive effects of electroconvulsive therapy. *Brain Stimulation, 1*(2), 71–83.

Sartorius, A., Wolf, J., & Henn, F. A. (2005). Lithium and ECT–concurrent use still demands attention: three case reports. *World Journal of Biological Psychiatry, 6*(2), 121–124.

Semkovska, M., Landau, S., Dunne, R., Kolshus, E., Kavanagh, A., Jelovac, A., et al. (2016). Bitemporal versus high-dose unilateral twice-weekly electroconvulsive therapy for depression (EFFECT-Dep): A pragmatic, randomised, non-inferiority trial. *American Journal of Psychiatry, 173*(4), 408–417.

Semkovska, M., & McLoughlin, D. M. (2010). Objective cognitive performance associated with electroconvulsive therapy for depression: A systematic review and meta-analysis. *Biological Psychiatry, 68*(6), 568–577.

Semkovska, M., & McLoughlin, D. M. (2013). Measuring retrograde autobiographical amnesia following electroconvulsive therapy: Historical perspective and current issues. *Journal of ECT, 29*(2), 127–133.

Semkovska, M., Noone, M., Carton, M., & McLoughlin, D. M. (2012). Measuring consistency of autobiographical memory recall in depression. *Psychiatry Research, 197*(1–2), 41–48.

Sienaert, P., Vansteelandt, K., Demyttenaere, K., & Peuskens, J. (2010). Randomized comparison of ultra-brief bifrontal and unilateral electroconvulsive therapy for major depression: Cognitive side-effects. *Journal of Affective Disorders, 122*(1–2), 60–67.

Slade, E. P., Jahn, D. R., Regenold, W. T., & Case, B. G. (2017). Association of electroconvulsive therapy with psychiatric readmissions in US hospitals. *Journal of the American Medical Association: Psychiatry, 74*(8), 798–804.

Smith, G. E., Rasmussen Jr, K. G., Cullum, C. M., Felmlee-Devine, M. D., Petrides, G., Rummans, T. A., et al. (2010). A randomized controlled trial comparing the memory effects of continuation electroconvulsive therapy versus continuation pharmacotherapy: Results from the Consortium for Research in ECT (CORE) study. *Journal of Clinical Psychiatry, 71*(2), 185–193.

Sobin, C., Sackeim, H. A., Prudic, J., & Devanand, D. (1995). Predictors of retrograde amnesia following ECT. *American Journal of Psychiatry, 152*(7), 995–1001.

Squire, L., Wetzel, C., & Slater, P. (1979). Memory complaint after electroconvulsive therapy: Assessment with a new self-rating instrument. *Biological Psychiatry, 14*(5), 791–801.

Talarico, J. M., & Rubin, D. C. (2003). Confidence, not consistency, characterizes flashbulb memories. *Psychological Science, 14*(5), 455–461.

Tess, A. V., & Smetana, G. W. (2009). Medical evaluation of patients undergoing electroconvulsive therapy. *New England Journal of Medicine, 360*(14), 1437–1444.

Thirthalli, J., Harish, T., & Gangadhar, B. N. (2011). A prospective comparative study of interaction between lithium and modified electroconvulsive therapy. *World Journal of Biological Psychiatry, 12*(2), 149–155.

Tombaugh, T. N., & McIntyre, N. J. (1992). The Mini-Mental State Examination: A Comprehensive Review. *Journal of the American Geriatrics Society, 40*(9), 922–935.

Tor, P.-C., Bautovich, A., Wang, M.-J., Martin, D., Harvey, S. B., & Loo, C. (2015). A Systematic Review and Meta-Analysis of Brief Versus Ultrabrief Right Unilateral Electroconvulsive Therapy for Depression. *Journal of Clinical Psychiatry, 76*(9), 1132–1133.

Tørring, N., Sanghani, S. N., Petrides, G., Kellner, C. H., & Østergaard, S. D. (2017). The mortality rate of electroconvulsive therapy: A systematic review and pooled analysis. *Acta Psychiatrica Scandinavica, 35*(5), 388–397.

Tsaltas, E., Kalogerakou, S., Papakosta, V.-M., Kontis, D., Theochari, E., Koutroumpi, M., et al. (2011). Contrasting patterns of deficits in visuospatial memory and executive function in patients with major depression with and without ECT referral. *Psychological Medicine, 41*(5), 983–995.

UK ECT Review Group. (2003). Efficacy and safety of electroconvulsive therapy in depressive disorders: A systematic review and meta-analysis. *Lancet, 361*(9360), 799–808.

Verwijk, E., Comijs, H. C., Kok, R. M., Spaans, H.-P., Stek, M. L., & Scherder, E. J. (2012). Neurocognitive effects after brief pulse and ultrabrief pulse unilateral electroconvulsive therapy for major depression: A review. *Journal of Affective Disorders, 140,* 233–243.

Verwijk, E., Spaans, H.-P., Comijs, H. C., Kho, K. H., Sienaert, P., Bouckaert, F., et al. (2015). Relapse and long-term cognitive performance after brief pulse or ultrabrief pulse right unilateral electroconvulsive therapy: A multicenter naturalistic follow up. *Journal of Affective Disorders, 184,* 137–144.

Volpe, F. M., & Tavares, A. R. (2012). Lithium plus ECT for mania in 90 cases: Safety issues. *Journal of Neuropsychiatry and Clinical Neurosciences, 24*(4), 33.

CHAPTER 21

Magnetic Seizure Therapy

Jeena Thomas
Zhi-De Deng
Shriya Awasthi
Sarah H. Lisanby

Electroconvulsive therapy (ECT; see Finnegan & McLoughlin, Chapter 20, this volume for additional information) is known as the most effective and rapidly acting antidepressant treatment for severe depression. It has evolved considerably since its first introduction more than 80 years ago, with each step in that evolution not only making the treatment more feasible, but also improving its risk/benefit ratio by lowering the adverse impact on neurocognitive function. Magnetic seizure therapy (MST), the most recent step in that evolution, refers to the intentional use of repetitive transcranial magnetic stimulation (rTMS; see Kavanaugh & Croarkin, Chapter 23, this volume, for additional information), under anesthesia, to induce a seizure for the treatment of depression.

MST was designed to retain the antidepressant therapeutic aspects of ECT, which are hypothesized to be attributed to the induced seizure, while minimizing or eliminating the adverse cognitive effects of ECT potentially attributable to the administered electric field. ECT applies electricity directly to the scalp to induce a seizure. Due to the impedance of the scalp and skull, ECT exposes the brain to nonfocal electric fields that affect large regions of the brain. Magnetic stimulation, which is unimpeded by the scalp and skull, is substantially more focal than ECT and allows the induction of a seizure with very low levels of electric field exposure to the brain. Studies to date show that MST, relative to ECT, possesses antidepressant effects with substantially lower cognitive side effects. In this chapter, we describe the rationale and development of MST, emphasizing the focal electric field induction achieved through MST. The enhanced focality achieved with MST is thought to be responsible for its minimal neurocognitive side effects. This chapter also focuses on neurocognitive and other effects that result from MST, in comparison to ECT.

RATIONALE FOR MST

Although ECT is the most effective antidepressant treatment for major depressive disorder (MDD; American Psychiatric Association, 2001), it has a number of side effects, including adverse effects on cognition (Lisanby, Maddox, Prudic, Devanand, & Sackeim, 2000; McClintock, Tirmizi, Chansard, & Husain, 2011; Squire, Slater, & Chace, 1975). MST was developed with the goal of reducing these cognitive adverse effects while preserving the efficacy of ECT by sparing brain regions associated with the adverse cognitive side effects from exposure to the electric field and resultant seizure (Sackeim, 1994).

Conventional ECT is administered at a fixed pulse amplitude of 800 or 900 mA (milliamperes) and results in stimulation of up to 100% of the brain (Lee, Deng, Laine, Lisanby, & Peterchev, 2011). Not only is conventional ECT nonfocal, it stimulates the brain with field strengths that are more than six-fold higher than necessary for inducing neuronal depolarization (Lee et al., 2011). The nonfocal stimulation, coupled with the excessively strong neural activation, has been hypothesized to contribute to the adverse side effects reported with ECT, such as retrograde amnesia, and maladaptive neuroplasticity in brain regions related to cognitive function such as the hippocampus (e.g., mossy fiber sprouting and cellular proliferation). Depending on the type of ECT, retrograde amnesia has been reported to extend for months to years, and although recovery takes place gradually over time, it may be incomplete (Lisanby et al., 2000; Squire, Slater, & Miller, 1981; Weiner, 2000). Retrograde amnesia for autobiographical memories has been associated with increased left frontotemporal electroencephalography (EEG) theta power (Luber et al., 2000; Nobler et al., 2000). While the functional changes in prefrontal regions may be important for ECT's therapeutic antidepressant effects, the amnestic effects of ECT may be related to the functional change observed in the medial temporal lobe (Chen, Shin, Duman, & Sanacora, 2001; Gombos, Spiller, Cottrell, Racine, & McIntyre Burnham, 1999; Lisanby, Sackeim, et al., 2003). Despite these changes to brain function; there is no evidence of ECT associated anatomical brain damage (Agelink et al., 2001; Coffey et al., 1991; Devanand, Dwork, Hutchinson, Bolwig, & Sackeim, 1994; Dwork et al., 2004).

It has been hypothesized that improving the spatial precision of the applied electric field and resultant seizure by focusing them on structures important for efficacy (e.g., prefrontal cortex) and sparing regions related to cognitive side effects (e.g., temporal regions), may be a powerful means of retaining the ECT-induced antidepressant efficacy while reducing the cognitive side effects (Lisanby, 2002; Lisanby, Morales, et al., 2003; Lisanby, Schlaepfer, Fisch, & Sackeim, 2001). ECT uses radial currents, which pass through deep brain structures. In contrast, MST avoids scalp and skull impedance and produces an electric field that is localized to the superficial cortex and tangential to the surface of the brain (Cretaz, Brunoni, & Lafer, 2015). Additionally, MST minimizes direct stimulation of deeper brain structures, like the hippocampus (Lee et al., 2011; Lisanby, Moscrip, et al., 2003; Moscrip, Terrace, Sackeim, & Lisanby, 2006) and avoids the medial temporal structures implicated in the amnestic side effects of ECT; yet it retains the antidepressant effects (Kayser et al., 2011).

The superficial electrical currents and focal seizures produced through MST result in antidepressant effects similar to those produced by ECT, while reducing the adverse cognitive effects associated with ECT (Fitzgerald et al., 2018). A recent pairwise meta-analysis reported that MST was comparable to a moderate and high dose of right unilateral ECT (Mutz et al., 2019). The same study included a network meta-analysis that used data from published MST studies and found that MST was more efficacious than sham treatment. Despite the small sample size, there was a high odds ratio (5.55) that favored MST over sham treatment (Mutz et al., 2019). In comparison, there is a 2.74 odds ratio for low- to moderate-dose right unilateral ECT, a 7.27 odds ratio for high dose right unilateral ECT, and a 3.17 odds ratio for high-frequency repetitive TMS (Mutz et al., 2019). While these results are positive for MST, Mutz and colleagues (2019) advocated for additional MST research that would include sham controlled conditions to allow for a better understanding of the antidepressant effect size.

Overall, results for cognitive tests that assess the functionality of deeper temporal structures were superior following MST when compared to ECT, whereas cognitive outcomes were relatively similar for tests that engaged prefrontal cortex brain regions (Cretaz et al., 2015; Kallioniemi, McClintock, Deng, Husain, & Lisanby, 2019; Lisanby, Luber, Schlaepfer, & Sackeim, 2003). Few case reports have indicated temporary manic symptoms following MST, which were then resolved within 2 weeks (Noda et al., 2015). Consistent with the differential impact on aspects of cognition, computational techniques to model the intracranial currents support the hypothesis that MST relative to ECT is more superficial and focused and induces less current in temporal lobe structures (Lee, Lisanby, Laine, & Peterchev, 2017).

HOW DOES MST WORK?

MST Procedure and Device

As with ECT, MST is administered by a psychiatrist, an anesthesiologist, and the nursing staff. The treatment is performed under anesthesia in an ECT procedure room with an anesthesia station and available safety equipment (e.g., crash cart). Anesthesiologists administer anesthetic agents that result in transient unconsciousness and muscular paralysis. Earplugs and a bite block are required for patients' hearing protection and dental protection, respectively (Lisanby, Schlaepfer, et al., 2001).

MST devices (see Figure 21.1) make use of biphasic sinusoidal magnetic pulses and require a higher-power output compared to standard rTMS devices (Lisanby, Luber, Finck, Schroeder, & Sackeim, 2001; Lisanby, Schlaepfer, et al., 2001). The induction of a seizure is assessed using a two-channel frontotemporal scalp EEG and motor seizure expression observed in the leg, which is cuffed prior to administration of the muscle relaxant. MST is typically administered at 100% maximal device output at a frequency that ranges up to 100 Hz (Lisanby & Peterchev, 2007). However, the optimal parameters for seizure induction and optimizing antidepressant efficacy are still under investigation.

MST Coil Configurations

Commercial transcranial magnetic stimulation coils (see Plate 21.1 in the color insert) are typically unable to induce seizures under anesthesia unless either a wider pulse width and/or a higher frequency of pulses in long stimulation trains is given (Lisanby, Luber, Sackeim,

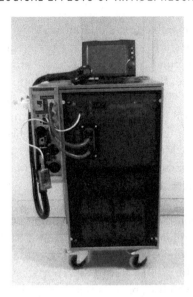

FIGURE 21.1. Example of an MST device. This is the Magstim theta that used a circular coil to provide MST. The theta was created by the Magstim Company, Ltd. (Spring Gardens, United Kingdom) and was used in MST research.

Finck, & Schroeder, 2001). The correlation of the maximum induced electric field strength relative to threshold showed that the double-cone (DCONE) coil was more focal than the H-coil (Deng, Lisanby, & Peterchev, 2013b). The DCONE was found to be a strong coil with a slightly deeper electric field and is the most focal, whereas the circular (CIRC) MST coil was found to be a weak coil with the most superficial electric field that resulted in the smallest activated brain volume (Deng, Lisanby, et al., 2013b; Lee et al., 2011). The cap (CAP) MST coil activates the largest brain volume, and simulations of the generated electric fields indicate that the CAP MST coil has the worst intrinsic focality. This relationship between maximum induced electric field strength relative to threshold also demonstrates the elevated efficiency of the DCONE coil, with the CIRC coil proving to be the least efficient and the CAP coil the second most efficient (Deng, Lisanby, et al., 2013b).

The anatomy of the brain and head also influence the effects of MST. The head diameter of a patient has the most impact on the MST-induced electric field (Deng, Lisanby, & Peterchev, 2015). The CAP and CIRC MST coils were found to be more sensitive to anatomical variability than the DCONE MST coil based on the induced electric fields (Deng et al., 2015). Compared to ECT, the induced field strength of MST is not as dependent on anatomical variations in the tissue's conductivity (Deng, Lisanby, & Peterchev, 2013a). Adjustments in MST current amplitude require less than a 12% change, compared to as much as a 68% adjustment for ECT when administered to patients with different head anatomies (Deng, Lisanby, et al., 2013a). Subsequently, the need to individualize current amplitude in seizure therapy is more necessary when administering ECT than it is for MST, and yet the standard practice in ECT is to not individualize pulse amplitude. In a later study, Lee and colleagues (2017) demonstrated that individualizing the current amplitude reduced stimulation focality variation between patients by 40–53% among those who received ECT and 26% for those who received MST. These results indicated that while individualizing current amplitude is crucial for the administration of ECT and plays a less important role in MST administration, individualization of amplitude for MST is important to consider in future developments of the MST procedure.

While MST is significantly more focal and less dependent on anatomical variation than ECT, it is important to note that MST requires a large amount of current in the coil to induce the desired current in the brain (Deng, Lisanby, et al., 2013a). The technology behind MST is much more complex than ECT as it requires greater power in the MST device to produce suprathreshold electric fields in the brain than for ECT.

Focality

The spatial precision of MST has been shown to reduce the adverse cognitive side effects of ECT. Magnetic fields penetrate high-resistance structures, like the scalp and skull, without impedance (Barker, Jalinous, & Freeston, 1985; Deng, McClintock, Oey, Luber, & Lisanby, 2015). Magnetic induction, compared to the electrical induction used in ECT, reduces the strength of scalp currents (Deng, Lisanby, et al., 2015; Deng, McClintock, et al., 2015). According to simulations conducted on a spherical head model, MST produces an electric field that is three to six times weaker and 10–60 times more focal than conventional ECT (Deng, Lisanby, & Peterchev, 2011). The stark differences between the characteristics of MST and ECT demonstrated on spherical head models provides general principles and patterns that differentiate the two treatments. Lee, Lisanby, Laine, and Peterchev (2016) observed the differences of ECT and MST on a head model created from magnetic resonance imaging. That study emphasized the ability of MST to induce weaker and more focal seizures. Even at lower amplitudes, ECT relative to MST induces stronger stimulation of the brain (Lee et al., 2016).

Compared to ECT, MST uses a significantly reduced stimulation strength. ECT produces a maximum stimulation strength that is up to 15 times greater than what is induced by MST (Lee et al., 2016). The conventional electrode configuration of ECT at a current of just 233 mA or more stimulates a larger volume of the brain than MST (Deng, Lisanby, et al., 2013a). The CIRC MST coil has been shown to induce more focal stimulation than all ECT electrode placements, such that relative to ECT, MST stimulation is three to nine times weaker and two to five times more focal (Lee et al., 2016). More specifically, frontomedial and bifrontal ECT electrode placements generally induce a median stimulation strength that is 2.0 to 5.8 times threshold, while the CIRC MST coil can produce a stimulation strength that ranges from only 0.3 to 0.8 times the threshold (Lee et al., 2016).

Dosing of MST

The optimal guidelines for MST dosing, including parameters such as frequency, coil selection, and site of stimulation are still fully unknown. Currently, MST treatment is dosed in a manner similar to ECT dosing strategies, whereby trains of pulses are administered in increasing numbers every 20 seconds until a seizure is induced in a single anesthesia session. The subsequent MST sessions are conducted at a specific percentage above the seizure threshold in order to confer antidepressant efficacy. Studies in nonhuman primate preclinical models have indicated that titrating in the pulse amplitude domain, rather than by increasing the total number of pulses in the train, induces seizures at significantly lower amplitudes than what is conventionally used (Peterchev, Krystal, Rosa, & Lisanby, 2015). These results demonstrate the importance of exploring and utilizing individualized dose titration in MST pulse amplitude, and potentially using motor threshold titrations to predict the seizure threshold (Peterchev et al., 2015). Since both the efficacy and side effects of ECT are dose related (Lisanby et al., 2000; Sackeim et al., 2000, 2008), optimizing the various MST dosing aspects may be central to enhancing its clinical impact.

Even at high frequency (i.e., 100 Hz), MST has demonstrated a relatively benign cognitive side-effect profile (Cretaz et al., 2015; Daskalakis et al., 2020; Fitzgerald et al., 2013). Several study participants who received high-frequency MST were reported to awake fully oriented post-MST, which relative to ECT indicated quicker reorientation (Fitzgerald et al., 2013; Kirov et al., 2008). Compared to patients treated with ECT, those who received high-frequency MST had shorter motor seizures, which further supported the focality of MST (Fitzgerald et al., 2013). MST appears to be more efficient in inducing seizures at lower frequencies (i.e., 25 Hz) than higher (i.e., 100 Hz) frequency MST (Cretaz et al., 2015; Kayser et al., 2015; Kayser & Wagner, 2018). Nevertheless, patients who received high-frequency relative to low-frequency MST had better clinical and cognitive outcomes (Cretaz et al., 2015; Kayser et al., 2015).

Physiological Response

The seizure expression of MST is generally similar to ECT (Kayser, Bewernick, Hurlemann, Soehle, & Schlaepfer, 2013), but comparisons of the two treatments found that the seizures induced by MST have reduced seizure amplitude, less postictal suppression in the theta, alpha, and beta frequency bands, and shorter seizure duration (Cretaz et al., 2015; Cycowicz, Luber, Spellman, & Lisanby, 2008, 2009; Cycowicz, Rowny, Luber, & Lisanby, 2018; Kayser et al., 2011). Using EEG data to create topographical visualizations of seizure induction by ECT and MST, Deng, Peterchev, and colleagues (2013) analyzed the delta, theta, alpha, and beta EEG frequency bands. The analysis of EEG frequency bands showed an increase of EEG power compared to baseline in all frequencies observed during the early and mid-ictal periods during ECT-induced seizures and a decrease of EEG power during the postictal period compared to baseline. By contrast, seizures induced by MST relative to baseline had minimal change in EEG power during the ictal and postictal periods.

High-frequency MST elicits a significant amount of postictal suppression, which is correlated with a significant reduction in depression symptom severity (Backhouse et al., 2018; Kayser & Wagner, 2018). The focality of MST seizure induction seems to correspond with ictal activity that begins later than the onset of less focal seizures (Kayser et al., 2011). The differences in seizure induction, as seen by the uniqueness of the EEG frequency bands that resulted from the seizures induced by MST and ECT, highlight the variation in the mechanism and the depth of seizure activation that result from each treatment.

Recently, Backhouse and colleagues (2018) compared the EEG of patients who received MST with different stimulation frequencies. Specifically, MST-induced seizures administered at 25 Hz, 50 Hz, and 100 Hz were evaluated for various EEG attributes of the seizure, and the results were compared to the evaluation of seizures found in published

ECT studies. The different MST stimulation frequencies resulted in varying ictal EEG characteristics, where 100-Hz MST-induced seizures were less adequate and weaker in global seizure strength than those seizures induced by 25- or 50-Hz MST (Backhouse et al., 2018). The cognitive benefits of MST may not be attributed to just the focality of MST, but also the MST-induced EEG effects. Based on the characteristics of patients' EEG, MST-induced seizures seem to result in different clinical outcomes because of what could be a different mechanism of seizure induction compared to the mechanism of ECT-induced seizures (Backhouse et al., 2018).

Using fluorodeoxyglucose while patients with treatment-resistant depression (TRD) had positron emission tomography (PET) scans to measure glucose levels before and after MST treatments, Hoy and colleagues (2013) observed how brain glucose metabolism was affected by 100-Hz MST. Depression symptom severity scores of the 10 patients studied significantly decreased following MST, and cognitive function remained stable. The pre- and post-MST PET scans showed increased glucose metabolism primarily on the left side of the brain. Additionally, metabolism significantly increased in the basal ganglia and orbital frontal cortex, and less significantly increased in the medial frontal cortex and dor-solateral prefrontal cortex (PFC). Increased glucose metabolism in these areas indicated that MST upregulates the metabolism in the frontolimbic regions of the brain, regions that are dysregulated in patients with depression.

Brain Dynamics: Network and Resting-State Dynamics

Resting-state EEG and the characteristics of seizures further elucidate the differences between MST and ECT. The fluctuations in resting-state EEG recordings are studied for patterns that repeat, which, in turn, are an indication of entropy over time. Complexity increases when there are fewer self-similar temporal patterns (Costa, Goldberger, & Peng, 2005). During a fine timescale, a shorter timescale with fewer fluctuations is observed, and a course timescale highlights a longer period of time that will have greater fluctuations. A reduction in the complexity of fine timescales has been observed following the successful administration of antidepressant treatments (Farzan et al., 2017).

When comparing the resting states at baseline and after an MST or ECT course, the complexity during fine timescales is significantly reduced after ECT and MST treatments (Farzan et al., 2017). Such a reduction in fine timescale complexity, especially in the fron-tocentral and parieto-occipital regions, has been found to be correlated with decreased depression severity (Farzan et al., 2017). A difference between the two seizure therapies was observed with an increase in coarse timescale complexity of those who responded with ECT compared to a decrease in complexity of coarse timescale in those who responded with MST (Farzan et al., 2017). In addition, the entropy observed in resting-state brain dynamics following MST is more localized than the entropy observed following ECT. Farzan and colleagues (2017) inferred that the effects of ECT seen in patients' resting-state EEG recordings were associated with the cognitive impairment characteristic of ECT.

Microstate analysis is the combination of EEG and functional brain network dynam-ics whereby brain state dynamics are measured over time. Recent microstate analysis has mapped out brain state dynamics with four microstates, labeled A, B, C, and D (Atluri et al., 2018), that were associated with microstate maps derived from resting-state functional magnetic resonance imaging (fMRI; Britz, Van De Ville, & Michel, 2010). These micro-states were observed as a measure for the length in brain network stability in a particular state before the brain transitions to another state. By incorporating resting-state fMRI data with microstates, prior studies have mapped microstates to specific brain networks (Britz et al., 2010; Musso, Brinkmeyer, Mobascher, Warbrick, & Winterer, 2010; Yuan, Zotev, Phillips, Drevets, & Bodurka, 2012).

The negative blood-oxygen-level-dependent (BOLD) activations correlated with microstate A in the bilateral superior and middle temporal gyri mapped connectivity that plays a significant role in phonological processing (Britz et al., 2010). Microstate B is asso-ciated with negative activation in the bilateral extrastriate visual areas (Britz et al., 2010). Microstate C correlates with positive BOLD activation in the fronto-insular cortex, which is associated with the salience network (Britz et al., 2010). Finally, microstate D is linked to the ability to distinguish stimuli associated with behavior and the ability to change and refocus attention because of negative ventral and dorsal frontoparietal BOLD activa-tion (Britz et al., 2010). The networks associated with microstates C and D appear to be impaired in patients with depression (Atluri et al., 2018; Hamilton et al., 2011; Mulders, van Eijndhoven, Schene, Beckmann, & Tendolkar, 2015).

Atluri and colleagues (2018) observed the effect of ECT and MST on brain network dynamics and how differences affected antidepressant effects. ECT changed global brain network dynamics, whereas changes influenced by MST were specific to neither select brain networks nor antidepressant outcomes. While ECT resulted in patients experienc-ing a longer period of microstate A and a decrease in microstates B, C, and D frequen-cies, MST specifically showed an association between improvement in cognition and a decrease in microstate B. The baseline measures of all four microstate dynamics following MST influenced the prediction of MST's therapeutic ability to reduce suicidal ideation in patients. Following MST, patients also demonstrated activation of the posterior cingulate cortex and the precuneus in all four microstates. These two regions are specifically associ-ated with the default-mode network and, subsequently, indicated that MST has the ability to target and treat the impairment of a network, that is, the default-mode network, associ-ated with TRD (Atluri et al., 2018).

SAFETY AND FEASIBILITY:
FIRST-IN-ANIMAL AND FIRST-IN-HUMAN STUDIES

MST was first successfully used for seizure induction in *Macaca mulatta*, which was chosen as a nonhuman primate (NHP) model because of head size anatomic compatibil-ity with pediatric round TMS coils and cognitive task performance compatibility with humans (Lisanby, Luber, Finck, et al., 2001). A Magstim rTMS device was customized to increase the maximum frequency and pulse width, which allowed for the successful induction of a seizure under anesthesia. MST was feasible when either ketamine hydro-chloride or methohexital was used for anesthesia, and succinylcholine chloride was used as a muscle relaxant (Lisanby, Luber, Finck, et al., 2001).

Lisanby, Schlaepfer, and colleagues (2001) later demonstrated the feasibility of MST in humans in an adult patient with MDD, who had no benefit from several pharmacological interventions. The patient received four MST treatments, during which succinylcholine was used as the muscle relaxant and either etomidate or thiopental was used as the anesthetic agent. For administration of MST, a customized Magstim stimulator with a higher maximum pulse width and frequency was used, with either a double-cone coil targeted to the vertex or a figure-8 coil targeted to the right PFC. All MST sessions resulted in successful seizure induction, based on EEG recordings and motor observations. Following treatment with MST, depression severity decreased and global cognitive function remained intact.

Lisanby, Luber, and colleagues (2003) went on to conduct the first clinical trial of MST in the United States, which was also the first randomized control trial to compare MST and ECT in a within-subject study design. This study compared the acute neurocognitive effects of MST and ECT in 10 adult patients with MDD. MST was successfully used to induce seizures in all 10 patients, with no acute adverse events, no significant modifications in anesthesia dosing, and compared to ECT, no substantial differences in physiological effects. Overall, patients performed significantly better after MST sessions than ECT sessions on cognitive measures. Patients had quicker time to orientation after both threshold and suprathreshold MST relative to ECT sessions. Following the threshold MST relative to ECT condition, patients recognized more affective faces. Following the suprathreshold MST relative to the ECT condition, patients also showed better performance on measures of neutral face recognition and sentence recognition.

Larger clinical trials, detailed below in our discussion of the side effects of MST, have provided additional evidence for the limited cognitive side effects of MST compared to ECT, even when MST was administered at a higher frequency (Fitzgerald et al., 2013) and with an accelerated MST course (Wang et al., 2019). There is minimal evidence of anterograde or retrograde amnesia immediately following MST. In contrast, for ECT, anterograde amnesia may last up to a month following treatment, and retrograde amnesia may last 6 months or longer (McClintock et al., 2011).

Neuropathology

In preclinical NHP models, neither MST nor ECT produced neuropathological lesions (Dwork et al., 2004). ECT resulted in greater immunoreactivity for glial fibrillary acidic protein in various NHP brain regions, which implied broad astrocytic activation with ECT that was unseen with MST (Dwork et al., 2004). There has been no observed histological damage or cell loss in the NHPs' post-MST-induced seizures (Dwork et al., 2009). From unpublished data, the same observed increased cell proliferation in NHPs who received ECT, but not in those who received MST, was found in areas of the hippocampal gyrus. ECT is reported to result in mossy fiber sprouting in the dentate gyrus, an effect that is not observed with antidepressant medications. In animal seizure models, mossy-fiber sprouting has been found to affect the normal functioning of the hippocampus by producing cognitive impairment (Chen et al., 2001; Gombos et al., 1999; Lisanby, Sackeim, et al., 2003). In contrast, MST produces no significant mossy-fiber sprouting, which is further indication that MST has no impact on medial temporal lobe structures (Lisanby, Sackeim, et al., 2003). The lack of mossy-fiber sprouting in patients treated with MST may indicate minimal physiological and structural changes in the hippocampus, consistent with less impact on cognitive functions subserved by the hippocampus (Chen et al., 2001; Gombos et al., 1999; Lisanby, Sackeim, et al., 2003).

NHP Cognition

In preclinical models, reorientation was found to be much faster after MST than after ECT (Moscrip et al., 2006). The subjects who received ECT also proved to have less accuracy in task performance compared to those who received MST or sham. Moscrip and colleagues (2006) observed consistency in completion time and accuracy during the learning and anterograde memory tasks for both the MST and sham conditions. However, after the ECT condition, subjects took longer to complete the same tasks and performed with less accuracy after completion of the session compared to subjects' baseline performance, and after both the MST and sham conditions. Although there was slight impairment in performance on the serial learning test for recall of the newly learned list after the MST and ECT conditions relative to sham, only the ECT condition significantly impaired the serial learning test for recalling old lists.

In a study that compared NHPs that received daily ECT for 5 weeks, 100-Hz MST, and a sham, time to complete the orientation test significantly increased only after the ECT condition (Spellman et al., 2008). In fact, the moderate-dose MST (2.5 times the seizure threshold) and the high-dose MST (six times the seizure threshold) conditions both resulted in similar neurocognitive task completion times that were similar to baseline. In addition, the anterograde memory, retrograde memory, and task completion times were significantly slower in the ECT condition relative to the high-dose MST condition. Accuracy across all cognitive tasks remained stable after the high-dose MST condition.

In both the Moscrip and colleagues (2006) and Spellman and colleagues (2008) studies, subjects' neurocognitive function was measured using a computerized cognitive battery that was designed to assess time to orientation (through recall of previously over-learned picture), anterograde amnesia (through recall of newly learned list of pictures), and retrograde amnesia (through recall of previously learned list of pictures). Spellman and colleagues used this computerized cognitive battery and added more cognitive measures that assessed spatial and serial working memory. Subjects after the ECT relative to the high-dose MST or sham conditions were significantly deficient when they completed the serial working memory task. The high-dose MST and sham conditions resulted in similar accuracy rates on the serial and spatial working memory measures, though following ECT, accuracy decreased on both measures (Spellman et al., 2008).

Stereotypy is understood as a cognitive component process that is essential to spatial working memory performance. McClintock and colleagues (2013) compared the stereotypy of NHPs after the high-dose MST, ECT, and sham conditions. The results showed that stereotypy remained constant after the MST condition; however, ECT disrupted stereotypy. Compared to the MST and sham treatments, after ECT there was less association between actual and prediction positions of the spatial working memory task, and time to task completion significantly increased. Ultimately, when testing for the ability to process spatial information, ECT significantly decreased pattern formation, accuracy, and efficiency.

CLINICAL EVIDENCE

Side Effects

Studies that have compared the side effects produced by MST and ECT have found that MST produces significantly fewer overall side effects than ECT (Kayser et al., 2013; Kosel, Frick, Lisanby, Fisch, & Schlaepfer, 2003; Polster, Kayser, Bewernick, Hurlemann, & Schlaepfer, 2015). Lisanby, Luber, and colleagues (2003) compared ECT and MST interventions and documented the occurrence and severity of subject side effects. In that study, patients tolerated the MST sessions well with no serious adverse events. Patients who received MST relative to ECT in the threshold and suprathreshold conditions were found to have lower physical side effects (e.g., headache, muscle ache).

ECT has been found to produce a surge in prolactin levels, which is caused when the seizure spreads through the diencephalic region (Abrams & Swartz, 1985; Fink, 1986; Ohman, Walinder, Balldin, & Wallin, 1976; Swartz & Abrams, 1984). In a study that compared the effects of ECT and MST on serum prolactin levels in preclinical and clinical models, MST relative to ECT had a nonsignificant prolactin surge (Morales, Luber, & Kwon, 2003). The difference between the resulting MST and ECT prolactin levels is consistent with MST's limited seizure spread to the diencephalic region due to enhanced focality (Morales et al., 2003).

Anesthetic and Cardiac Safety of MST

In both MST and ECT sessions, patients generally receive succinylcholine as the mode for muscle relaxation. MST treatments produce a weaker seizure, compared to ECT treatments, as seen in the EEG tracings acquired during either session (Backhouse et al., 2018; Cretaz et al., 2015; Cycowicz et al., 2008, 2009, 2018; Deng, Peterchev, et al., 2013; Kayser et al., 2011; Kayser & Wagner, 2018; White et al., 2006). Having induced a less robust seizure, a small dose of succinylcholine is required in MST to protect the body from the motor convulsion (White et al., 2006). Rowny and colleagues (2009) observed more changes in heartrate following ECT in NHPs compared to MST, indicating that MST resulted in a significantly less sympathetic and parasympathetic response than ECT because MST minimizes penetration of deeper brain structures. Additionally, administration of MST relative to ECT also resulted in patients having less cardiovascular responsivity (e.g., change in blood pressure; White et al., 2006). As such, administration of anitcholinergic and antihypertensive medications, like labetalol or nicardipine, are significantly reduced in dosage in MST.

Neurocognitive Effects of MST

A clinical study demonstrated that patients who received high-dose MST (100 Hz) reoriented significantly faster compared to reorientation after ECT (Kirov et al., 2008). More specifically, patients tended to take on average 7 minutes to reorient following a MST session whereas it took on average about 26 minutes to reorient after an ECT session (Kirov et al., 2008). Another clinical study tested the therapeutic effects of MST paired with psychotropic medications in patients with TRD (Kayser et al., 2011). That study showed that of all the cognitive and neurocognitive assessments administered, patients who received

100-Hz MST compared to those who received ECT performed significantly better on the geometric shapes portion of the Visual Neglect Test (Kayser et al., 2011).

Daskalakis and colleagues (2020) studied and compared the effects of high-frequency (100-Hz), medium-frequency (50- or 60-Hz), and low-frequency (25-Hz) MST. Of 140 screened patients, 86 of them completed at least 8 MST sessions and 47 completed the study protocol. Patients showed significantly improved visuospatial learning and memory. All patients who received an adequate course of MST or who completed the protocol showed decreased autobiographical memory consistency. There was an average of 19% consistency loss among the patients who received at least eight treatments of MST. This finding is comparable to pharmacotherapy and less than an average of 27% consistency loss that results from ECT (Kessler et al., 2014). The moderate-frequency MST group had a significantly greater consistency loss than the low- and high- frequency MST groups (Daskalakis et al., 2020).

Efficacy

Studies to date suggest that the antidepressant efficacy of MST is comparable to that of ECT, though additional clinical controlled research is warranted with sufficiently powered samples to provide a strong test of noninferiority. Comparing 10 patients who received MST and 10 who received ECT, 60% and 40% of patients treated with MST and ECT showed clinical response, respectively (Kayser et al., 2011). Of the responders, half achieved remission in MST, while 100% of ECT responders went into remission.

MST also proved effective in treating patients experiencing suicidal ideation, whereby 67% of patients with TRD and suicidal ideation had a 53% remission rate (Sun et al., 2016). Sun and colleagues (2018) studied the effects of MST on suicidal ideation in patients with TRD using the Scale for Suicidal Ideation. After patients completed the MST course relative to baseline, 44.4% of them no longer had suicidal ideation. This change in suicidal ideation was significantly associated with decreased long-interval cortical inhibition (LICI) in the dorsolateral PFC. Such effects of MST on LICI substantiate the treatment's influence on the neuroplasticity that results from long-term potentiation–like mechanisms. This finding replicated earlier work by Sun and colleagues (2016), who showed that measures of LICI in the dorsolateral PFC could also be used as a predictor for how patients may respond, specifically regarding remission of suicidal ideation, after completing an MST course.

A recent small-case series on three patients with MDD who received accelerated MST (aMST), administered at 100 Hz for 6 consecutive days, showed positive results that encouraged further study in this particular treatment delivery paradigm (Wang et al., 2019). Generally, MST is administered no more than three times a week, and this was the first study that examined the effects of daily MST sessions. The first patient went into remission, and both the second and third patients showed antidepressant clinical response. None of the patients reported delirium or prolonged confusion at any point during the aMST course. Each patient showed positive outcomes in their neurocognitive assessments, and only one patient reported muscle pain after the first two sessions. While these results appear promising, larger clinical trials are needed to fully assess the safety and feasibility of aMST.

Fitzgerald and colleagues (2018) studied the effects of ECT and 100-Hz MST treatments on 37 patients and found that the therapeutic effects of both treatments remained consistent across all clinical outcome measures. Patients in both ECT and MST groups received up to 15 antidepressant treatments, and the number of treatments was similar between both groups, where 12.4 ± 2.7 treatments were given to the MST group and 12.4 ± 2.3 treatments were given to the ECT group. All patients received 12 treatments, and both treatment conditions produced relatively similar antidepressant changes. While ECT showed significant improvement in one cognitive inhibition task, following MST, patients showed significantly improved processing speed and memory.

High-frequency (100-Hz) MST proved to have the largest response rate of 41.7%, compared to low-frequency (33.3% response rate; 25Hz) and moderate-frequency (26.9% response rate; 50 Hz or 60 Hz) MST among patients who had at least eight MST sessions (Daskalakis et al., 2020). Patients receiving high-frequency MST also had the highest rate of remission (33.3%), which was significantly higher than low-frequency MST (11.1%). Patients who completed the protocol and received high-frequency MST also had the highest response rate (60%) compared to low- (57.9%) and moderate-frequency (53.8%) MST. Study protocol completers who received high-frequency MST also had the highest remission rate (53.3%) compared to the other MST frequencies and was significantly higher than low-frequency MST (21.1% remission rate).

Effect of MST on Other Clinical Indications

While MST's therapeutic effects are used primarily for patients with MDD, MST has recently been demonstrated to be feasible and safe for use in patients with schizophrenia (Jiang et al., 2018; Tang et al., 2018). Tang and colleagues (2018) led the first study that observed the clinical effects of MST in eight patients with treatment-resistant schizophrenia. Four patients completed the protocol and four dropped out. All eight patients showed significant improvement in psychotic symptoms, which significantly decreased by the end of the protocol, and there was a statistically significant improvement in quality of life. All patients were found to have significant improvement in clinical outcome and quality of life, and equally important, overall cognitive function remained stable.

In a case report on the first reported administration of MST on an adolescent with refractory bipolar depression, Noda and colleagues (2014) observed the therapeutic effects of MST in treatment-resistant bipolar depression. An 18-year-old male patient with bipolar II disorder received a total of 27 MST sessions over the span of approximately 5 months. After 12 MST sessions, depression symptom severity decreased by approximately 40%, and by the 18th MST session, the patient showed remission. Aside from minimally reduced autobiographical memory recall, overall cognitive abilities remained stable. The patient did experience nausea and elongated seizures after the first MST session, both of which were resolved with 1 mg of granisetron (or 4 mg of odansetron) and 1 or 2 mg of midazolam, respectively (Noda et al., 2014). Noda and colleagues reported that the patient experienced remission for at least 11 months.

The minimal cognitive implications resulting from MST make it worth studying in populations with special concern regarding cognition, including children and adolescents, elderly adults, and those with neuropsychiatric illnesses such as traumatic brain injury and neurodegenerative disease (e.g., Alzheimer's disease, Parkinson's disease; Luber, McClintock, & Lisanby, 2013). Further study is required to assess the therapeutic effects MST may have on vulnerable populations (Kayser, Bewernick, Wagner, & Schlaepfer, 2019); studies to date have provided strong evidence for the feasibility, safety, and efficacy of MST.

TABLE 21.1. Summary of Clinical Investigations Testing the Feasibility, Safety, and Efficacy of MST

Study	Sample size and diagnosis	Study description	Device	MST coil targeting and ECT electrode placement	Study design	Main outcomes and significance
Lisanby et al. (2001)	$N = 1$: TRD	First in human study for MST	Customized Magstim	Double-cone coil centered over vertex or figure-8 coil centered over right prefrontal cortex	Single-subject open-label case report	1. First case report to demonstrate the feasibility of inducing seizures under anesthesia using a modified rTMS coil
Lisanby et al. (2003)	$N = 10$: MDD	Investigate the safety and feasibility of MST compared to ECT	• MST: 50-Hz customized Magstim • ECT: Mecta 5000Q	• MST: figure-8, double-cone, or round coil centered over RUL site, midline frontal site, or vertex • ECT: RUL or BL electrode placements	Double-blinded crossover between MST and ECT	1. First study comparing MST and ECT 2. MST was superior to ECT for neurocognitive outcomes 3. Shorter seizure duration for MST compared to ECT
Kosel et al. (2003)	$N = 1$: MDD	Report efficacy and cognitive outcomes following MST for patient with MDD	50-Hz customized Magstim	Butterfly coil centered over vertex	Open-label case report	1. Patient achieved remission after 12 MST treatments 2. Recovery time following MST treatment was significantly shorter than the expected recovery time for ECT 3. Improvements in verbal learning and memory test scores following MST treatment compared to baseline scores
White et al. (2006)	$N = 20$: MDD	Larger study focusing on anesthetic parameters for MST and ECT	• MST: 50-Hz customized Magstim • ECT: Mecta 5000Q	• MST: Double-cone coil centered over midline prefrontal cortex or cap coil centered over vertex • ECT: BF electrode placement	Open parallel design case-controlled between MST and ECT	1. Faster reorientation times, better neurocognitive outcomes, and lower cardiovascular and electroencephalographic bispectral index values for MST treatment group compared to ECT treatment group 2. MST associated with decreased requirement for muscle relaxant 3. Reduction in HDRS scores after both MST and ECT, although reductions were significantly greater following ECT

Study	Sample	Purpose	Device	Coil/placement	Design	Findings
Kirov et al. (2008)	N = 11: MDD	Pilot study examining clinical and neurocognitive outcomes of high-dose MST (HD-MST) at 100 Hz instead of 50 Hz	100-Hz modified Magstim	Round coil centered over vertex or frontal cortex	Double-blinded crossover between MST and ECT	1. Similar antidepressant efficacy of MST and ECT 2. Faster reorientation times for MST patients compared to ECT (7 min 12 sec reorientation time for MST vs. 26 min 35 sec for ECT) 3. HD-MST was generally safe with only significant side effects being myoclonic movements
Kayser et al. (2011)	N = 20: TRD	Compare outcomes of ECT and MST with pharmacological treatment	• MST: 100-Hz MagVenture • ECT: Thymatron IV	• MST: Twin coil centered over vertex • ECT: RUL electrode placement	Double-blinded randomized trial with MST and ECT	1. No statistically significant difference in clinical efficacy between MST and ECT based on MADRS scores 2. Better performance in visual neglect cognitive assessment following MST when compared to ECT 3. Improvements in neurocognitive test scores from baseline following MST
Kayser et al. (2013)	N = 7: 6 MDD, 1 BP-II	Compare seizure parameters for ECT and MST	• MST: 100-Hz MagVenture • ECT: Thymatron IV	• MST: Twin coil centered over vertex • ECT: RUL or BL electrode placement	Open-label trial including ECT nonresponders	1. MST and ECT seizure parameters were similar based on EEG data, suggesting similar physiological processes underlying seizure induction and antidepressant mechanism 2. Shorter reorientation time after MST compared to ECT
Hoy et al. (2013)	N = 10: MDD	Explore effects of MST on brain glucose metabolism	100-Hz MagVenture	Twin coil centered over vertex	Open-label	1. Significant changes in glucose metabolism based on PET data in several brain regions following MST 2. 57% response rate to MST based on changes in MADRS scores
Fitzgerald et al. (2013)	N = 13: MDD	Assess safety and clinical efficacy of high-frequency 100-Hz MST	100-Hz MagVenture	Twin coil centered over vertex	Open-label	1. 100-Hz MST was safe and resulted in negligible cognitive side effects 2. 38% of patients responded to high-frequency MST

(continued)

TABLE 21.1. *(continued)*

Study	Sample size and diagnosis	Study description	Device	MST coil targeting and ECT electrode placement	Study design	Main outcomes and significance
Noda et al. (2014)	$N = 1$: Refractory bipolar disorder	Case study for use of MST in adolescent depression	100-Hz MagVenture	Twin coil centered over frontal cortex	Open-label trial, which is currently ongoing	1. Full remission after 18 MST treatments based on HDRS scores 2. No cognitive decline following MST other than autobiographical memory impairment 3. First documented usage of MST to successfully treat an adolescent with refractory bipolar depression
Noda et al. (2015)	$N = 2$: MDD	Case report for development of mania following MST	100-Hz MagVenture	Twin coil centered over midline prefrontal cortex	Open-label	1. Both subjects achieved remission after MST treatments 2. Both subjects developed post-MST mania that resolved within 2 weeks
Polster et al. (2015)	$N = 20$: MDD $N = 10$: Healthy controls	Compare and contrast effects of MST and ECT on memory retrieval	• MST: 100-Hz MagVenture • ECT: Thymatron IV	• MST: Twin coil centered over vertex • ECT: RUL electrode placement	Open-label	1. Delayed recall observed in patients after ECT but not MST based on posttreatment cognitive assessments
Kayser et al. (2015)	$N = 26$: TRD	Assess effects of MST on brain glucose metabolism in conjunction with clinical and cognitive outcomes	100-Hz MagVenture	Twin coil centered bilaterally over vertex	Randomized design for 10 patients, open-label design for 16 patients	1. 46% remission rate and 69% response rate for MST treatment 2. No adverse cognitive effects of MST based on pre- and posttreatment assessments of language, working memory, attention, visual perception, and others 3. Based on PET scans, increased brain glucose metabolic rate in frontal cortex and decreased metabolic rate within left striatum
Sun et al. (2016)	$N = 33$: TRD	Assess effect of MST on suicidal ideations in patients with TRD;	100-Hz MagVenture	Twin coil centered over frontal cortex	Open-label	1. Significant decline in suicidal ideation after MST based on SSI scores 2. Overall remission rate of 53% 3. Pretreatment measures of N100 and

Author	N: population	Aim	Device	Coil/electrode placement	Design	Findings
		correlate TMS-EEG measures with likelihood of remission				LICI in frontal cortex predicted remission with ~89% accuracy
Farzan et al. (2017)	$N = 34$: TRD	Explore whether MST and ECT antidepressant mechanisms are based on modulation of complexity of the resting state EEG signal	MST: 100-Hz MagVenture ECT: Mecta 5000Q	• MST: Twin coil centered over frontal cortex • ECT: RUL or BT electrode placement	Open-label	1. Reduction in complexity within central and parieto-occipital regions at fine timescales predicts decline in depression severity 2. Increases in complexity within parieto-central regions at course timescales predicts declines in test scores measuring autobiographical memory
Tang (2018)	$N = 8$: Schizophrenia	Assess safety and feasibility of MST for treatment resistant schizophrenia	100-Hz MagVenture	Twin coil centered over frontal cortex	Open-label	1. Improvements in symptoms observed in the 4/8 patients who completed the study 2. No neurocognitive changes after MST other than decline in autobiographical memory test scores
Sun et al. (2018)	$N = 23$: TRD	Assess whether MST changes SSI scores and overall neuroplasticity using TMS-EEG	100-Hz MagVenture	Twin coil centered over frontal cortex	Open-label	1. Larger study supporting findings of Sun (2016) related to reductions in SSI scores and decline of long interval cortical inhibition following MST
Fitzgerald et al. (2018)	$N = 37$: MDD	Compare clinical and cognitive outcomes of MST and RUL-ECT	MST: 100-Hz MagVenture ECT: Thymatron IV	• MST: Dual-cone coil centered over vertex • ECT: RUL electrode placement	Double-blinded and randomized between ECT and MST	1. In MST, posttreatment improvements in neurocognitive tests of psychomotor speed, verbal memory, and cognitive inhibition 2. In ECT, observed posttreatment improvement in performance for one cognitive task 3. No decline in cognitive scores for any assessments given 4. No difference in clinical efficacy between MST and ECT based on HDRS scores, although overall response rate was low for both

(continued)

TABLE 21.1. *(continued)*

Study	Sample size and diagnosis	Study description	Device	MST coil targeting and ECT electrode placement	Study design	Main outcomes and significance
Jiang et al. (2018)	$N = 8$: Schizophrenia	Investigate safety and feasibility of adding MST to standard course schizophrenia treatment	25-Hz MagVenture	Twin coil centered over vertex	Open-label	1. 6/10 patients completed all MST treatments, 5/10 experienced reductions in symptoms, and 3/10 responded to MST treatment 2. Improved delayed recall and immediate memory test scores after MST treatments
Backhouse et al. (2018)	$N = 61$: Unipolar depression	Correlate seizure characteristics with efficacy of MST at different stimulation frequencies	25-, 50-, or 100-Hz MagVenture	Twin coil centered over frontal cortex	Open-label	1. Seizure characteristics differed across stimulation frequencies 2. Seizure characteristics predicted likelihood of clinical response to MST 3. Low-frequency stimulation at 25 and 50 Hz was better for inducing seizures compared to 100-Hz stimulation
Athuri et al. (2018)	$N = 75$: TRD $N = 55$: Healthy controls	Explore effects of ECT and MST on brain network dynamics at various stimulation frequencies	25-, 50-, 60-, or 100-Hz MagVenture MST	Twin coil centered over frontal cortex	Not specified	1. First study demonstrating that MST and ECT modulate global brain network dynamics
Kayser et al. (2019)	$N = 38$: MDD, bipolar I, or bipolar II	Identify demographic and clinical predictors of MST response	100-Hz MagVenture	Twin coil centered over vertex	Open-label	1. 68% response rate for MST based on HDRS scores 2. Several clinical correlates of MST response, including depression severity,

						Findings
						number of depressive episodes, length of depressive episodes, number of failed treatments, and presence of melancholic or anxiety symptoms 3. Several demographic predictors of MST response, such as family history of depression
Wang et al. (2019)	$N = 3$: TRD	Assess safety and clinical efficacy of accelerated MST administered on consecutive days	100-Hz Magstim stimulator	Circular coil centered over vertex	Open-label	1. No severe adverse events after accelerated MST 2. 2/3 patients responded to accelerated MST 3. Improvement in cognitive test performance observed after MST treatments in all patients
Daskalakis et al. (2020)	$N = 86$: MDD	Assess the therapeutic efficacy and neurocognitive effects of MST at varying frequencies over the prefrontal cortex, within a comparatively larger sample size	25-, 50-, 60-, or 100-Hz MagPro MST	Twin coil centered over prefrontal cortex	Open-label	1. EEG seizure duration did not vary significantly for MST administered at different frequencies 2. Highest response rate (41.7%), highest remission rate (33.3%), and shortest reorientation time (3.99 min) for high-frequency 100-Hz MST 3. Across all MST groups, improvements in visuospatial memory test scores and reductions in autobiographical memory test scores; performance on all other cognitive assessments remained stable, supporting safety of MST for all frequencies tested

Note. RUL, right unilateral; BL, bilateral; BF, bifrontal; BT, bitemporal; HDRS, Hamilton Depression Rating Scale; MADRS, Montgomery–Åsberg Depression Rating Scale.v

CONCLUSIONS

Growing evidence supports MST as a promising antidepressant treatment that may retain the efficacy of ECT but with little to no adverse clinical, subjective, or neurocognitive effects. Using electromagnetic induction, MST induces seizures with great focality, such that only regions of the superficial brain cortex are activated. With demonstrated antidepressant effects and neurocognitive safety, MST may represent an appealing treatment for MDD, TRD, and potentially other psychiatric disorders (e.g., schizophrenia) across the lifespan. An adequately powered noninferiority trial is currently underway (Confirmatory Efficacy and Safety Trial of Magnetic Seizure Therapy for Depression, 2017), the results of which will be a powerful test of whether MST will eventually become part of the neuropsychiatric armamentarium. Overall, preclinical and clinical investigations (summarized in Table 21.1 on pages 396–401) have supported the feasibility, safety, and efficacy of MST. Future research will continue to inform and refine administrative paradigms to ensure optimal antidepressant benefit with concordant cognitive safety.

ACKNOWLEDGMENTS

We would like to thank Ms. Brigit S. Sullivan, National Institutes of Health Library, for reviewing the manuscript of this chapter.

REFERENCES

Abrams, R., & Swartz, C. M. (1985). Electroconvulsive therapy and prolactin release: effects of stimulus parameters. *Convulsion Therapy, 1*(2), 115–119.

Agelink, M. W., Andrich, J., Postert, T., Wurzinger, U., Zeit, T., Klotz, P., et al. (2001). Relation between electroconvulsive therapy, cognitive side effects, neuron specific enolase, and protein S-100. *Journal of Neurology, Neurosurgery and Psychiatry, 71*(3), 394–396.

American Psychiatric Association. (2001). *The practice of electroconvulsive therapy: Recommendations for treatment, training, and privileging. A task force report of the American Psychiatric Association*. Washington, DC: Author.

Atluri, S., Wong, W., Moreno, S., Blumberger, D. M., Daskalakis, Z. J., & Farzan, F. (2018). Selective modulation of brain network dynamics by seizure therapy in treatment-resistant depression. *Neuroimage: Clinical, 20*, 1176–1190.

Backhouse, F. A., Noda, Y., Knyahnytska, Y., Farzan, F., Downar, J., Rajji, T. K., et al. (2018). Characteristics of ictal EEG in magnetic seizure therapy at various stimulation frequencies. *Clinical Neurophysiology, 129*(8), 1770–1779.

Barker, A. T., Jalinous, R., & Freeston, I. L. (1985). Non-invasive magnetic stimulation of human motor cortex. *Lancet, 1*(8437), 1106–1107.

Britz, J., Van De Ville, D., & Michel, C. M. (2010). BOLD correlates of EEG topography reveal rapid resting-state network dynamics. *Neuroimage, 52*(4), 1162–1170.

Chen, A. C., Shin, K. H., Duman, R. S., & Sanacora, G. (2001). ECS-Induced mossy fiber sprouting and BDNF expression are attenuated by ketamine pretreatment. *Journal of ECT, 17*(1), 27–32.

Coffey, C. E., Weiner, R. D., Djang, W. T., Figiel, G. S., Soady, S. A., Patterson, L. J., et al. (1991). Brain anatomic effects of electroconvulsive therapy. A prospective magnetic resonance imaging study. *Archives of General Psychiatry, 48*(11), 1013–1021.

Confirmatory efficacy and safety trial of magnetic seizure therapy for depression (CREST-MST). (2017). Retrieved March 14, 2019, from *https://clinicaltrials.gov/ct2/show/NCT03191058*.

Costa, M., Goldberger, A. L., & Peng, C. K. (2005). Multiscale entropy analysis of biological signals. *Physical Review E: Statistical, Nonlinear, and Soft Matter Physics, 71*(2, Pt. 1), 021906.

Cretaz, E., Brunoni, A. R., & Lafer, B. (2015). Magnetic seizure therapy for unipolar and bipolar depression: A systematic review. *Neural Plasticity, 2015*, 521398.

Cycowicz, Y. M., Luber, B., Spellman, T., & Lisanby, S. H. (2008). Differential neurophysiological effects of magnetic seizure therapy (MST) and electroconvulsive shock (ECS) in non-human primates. *Clinical EEG and Neuroscience, 39*(3), 144–149.

Cycowicz, Y. M., Luber, B., Spellman, T., & Lisanby, S. H. (2009). Neurophysiological characterization of high-dose magnetic seizure therapy: Comparisons with electroconvulsive shock and cognitive outcomes. *Journal of ECT, 25*(3), 157–164.

Cycowicz, Y. M., Rowny, S. B., Luber, B., & Lisanby, S. H. (2018). Differences in seizure expression between magnetic seizure therapy and electroconvulsive shock. *Journal of ECT, 34*(2), 95–103.

Daskalakis, Z. J., Dimitrova, J., McClintock, S. M., Sun, Y., Voineskos, D., Rajji, T. K., et al. (2020). Magnetic seizure therapy (MST) for major depressive disorder. *Neuropsychopharmacology, 45*(2), 276–282.

Deng, Z. D., Lisanby, S. H., & Peterchev, A. V. (2011). Electric field strength and focality in electroconvulsive therapy and magnetic seizure therapy: A finite element simulation study. *Journal of Neural Engineering, 8*(1), 016007.

Deng, Z. D., Lisanby, S. H., & Peterchev, A. V. (2013a). Controlling stimulation strength and focality in electroconvulsive therapy via current amplitude and electrode size and spacing: comparison with magnetic seizure therapy. *Journal of ECT, 29*(4), 325–335.

Deng, Z. D., Lisanby, S. H., & Peterchev, A. V. (2013b). Electric field depth-focality tradeoff in transcranial magnetic stimulation: Simulation comparison of 50 coil designs. *Brain Stimulation, 6*(1), 1–13.

Deng, Z. D., Lisanby, S. H., & Peterchev, A. V. (2015). Effect of anatomical variability on electric field characteristics of electroconvulsive therapy and magnetic seizure therapy: A parametric modeling study. *IEEE Transactions on Neural Systems and Rehabilitation Engineering, 23*(1), 22–31.

Deng, Z. D., McClintock, S. M., Oey, N. E., Luber, B., & Lisanby, S. H. (2015). Neuromodulation for mood and memory: From the engineering bench to the patient bedside. *Current Opinion in Neurobiology, 30*, 38–43.

Deng, Z. D., Peterchev, A. V., Krystal, A. D., Luber, B., McClintock, S. M., Husain, M. M., et al. (2013). *Topography of seizures induced by electroconvulsive therapy and magnetic seizure therapy.* Paper presented at the International IEEE/EMBS Conference on Neural Engineering.

Devanand, D. P., Dwork, A. J., Hutchinson, E. R., Bolwig, T. G., & Sackeim, H. A. (1994). Does ECT alter brain structure? *American Journal of Psychiatry, 151*(7), 957–970.

Dwork, A. J., Arango, V., Underwood, M., Ilievski, B., Rosoklija, G., Sackeim, H. A., et al. (2004). Absence of histological lesions in primate models of ECT and magnetic seizure therapy. *American Journal of Psychiatry, 161*(3), 576–578.

Dwork, A. J., Christensen, J. R., Larsen, K. B., Scalia, J., Underwood, M. D., Arango, V., et al. (2009). Unaltered neuronal and glial counts in animal models of magnetic seizure therapy and electroconvulsive therapy. *Neuroscience, 164*(4), 1557–1564.

Farzan, F., Atluri, S., Mei, Y., Moreno, S., Levinson, A. J., Blumberger, D. M., et al. (2017). Brain temporal complexity in explaining the therapeutic and cognitive effects of seizure therapy. *Brain, 140*(4), 1011–1025.

Fink, M. (1986). Neuroendocrine predictors of electroconvulsive therapy outcome. Dexamethasone suppression test and prolactin. *Annals of the New York Academy of Sciences, 462*, 30–36.

Fitzgerald, P. B., Hoy, K. E., Elliot, D., McQueen, S., Wambeek, L. E., Chen, L., et al. (2018). A pilot study of the comparative efficacy of 100 Hz magnetic seizure therapy and electroconvulsive therapy in persistent depression. *Depression and Anxiety, 35*(5), 393–401.

Fitzgerald, P. B., Hoy, K. E., Herring, S. E., Clinton, A. M., Downey, G., & Daskalakis, Z. J. (2013). Pilot study of the clinical and cognitive effects of high-frequency magnetic seizure therapy in major depressive disorder. *Depression and Anxiety, 30*(2), 129–136.

Gombos, Z., Spiller, A., Cottrell, G. A., Racine, R. J., & McIntyre Burnham, W. (1999). Mossy fiber sprouting induced by repeated electroconvulsive shock seizures. *Brain Research, 844*(1–2), 28–33.

Hamilton, J., Furman, D., Chang, C., Thomason, M., Dennis, E., & Gotlib, I. (2011). Default-mode and task-positive network activity in major depressive disorder: implications for adaptive and maladaptive rumination. *Journal of Biological Psychiatry, 70*(4), 327–333.

Hoy, K. E., Thomson, R. H., Cherk, M., Yap, K. S., Daskalakis, Z. J., & Fitzgerald, P. B. (2013). Effect of magnetic seizure therapy on regional brain glucose metabolism in major depression. *Psychiatry Research, 211*(2), 169–175.

Jiang, J., Li, Q., Sheng, J., Yang, F., Cao, X., Zhang, T., et al. (2018). 25 Hz magnetic seizure therapy is feasible but not optimal for chinese patients with schizophrenia: A case series. *Frontiers in Psychiatry, 9*, 224.

Kallioniemi, E., McClintock, S. M., Deng, Z. D., Husain, M. M., & Lisanby, S. H. (2019). Magnetic seizure therapy: Towards personalized seizure therapy for major depression. *Personalized Medicine in Psychiatry, 17–18*, 37–42.

Kayser, S., Bewernick, B. H., Grubert, C., Hadrysiewicz, B. L., Axmacher, N., & Schlaepfer, T. E. (2011). Antidepressant effects, of magnetic seizure therapy and electroconvulsive therapy, in treatment-resistant depression. *Journal of Psychiatric Research, 45*(5), 569–576.

Kayser, S., Bewernick, B. H., Hurlemann, R., Soehle, M., & Schlaepfer, T. E. (2013). Comparable seizure characteristics in magnetic seizure therapy and electroconvulsive therapy for major depression. *European Neuropsychopharmacology, 23*(11), 1541–1550.

Kayser, S., Bewernick, B. H., Matusch, A., Hurlemann, R., Soehle, M., & Schlaepfer, T. E. (2015). Magnetic seizure therapy in treatment-resistant depression: Clinical, neuropsychological and metabolic effects. *Psychological Medicine, 45*(5), 1073–1092.

Kayser, S., Bewernick, B. H., Wagner, S., & Schlaepfer, T. E. (2019). Clinical predictors of response to magnetic seizure therapy in depression: A preliminary report. *Journal of ECT, 35*(1), 48–52.

Kayser, S., & Wagner, S. (2018). Stimulation frequency of magnetic seizure therapy contributes to the adequacy of seizures. *Clinical Neurophysiology, 129*(8), 1718–1719.

Kessler, U., Schoeyen, H. K., Andreassen, O. A., Eide, G. E., Malt, U. F., Oedegaard, K. J., et al. (2014). The effect of electroconvulsive therapy on neurocognitive function in treatment-resistant bipolar disorder depression. *Journal of Clinical Psychiatry, 75*(11), 1306–1313.

Kirov, G., Ebmeier, K., Scott, A., Atkins, M., Khalid, N., Carrick, L., et al. (2008). Quick recovery of orientation after magnetic seizure therapy for major depressive disorder. *British Journal of Psychiatry, 193*(2), 152–155.

Kosel, M., Frick, C., Lisanby, S. H., Fisch, H. U., & Schlaepfer, T. E. (2003). Magnetic seizure therapy improves mood in refractory major depression. *Neuropsychopharmacology, 28*(11), 2045–2048.

Lee, W. H., Deng, Z. D., Laine, A. F., Lisanby, S. H., & Peterchev, A. V. (2011). Influence of white matter conductivity anisotropy on electric field strength induced by electroconvulsive therapy. *Conference Proceedings of the IEEE Engineering in Medicine and Biology Society, 2011*, 5473–5476.

Lee, W. H., Lisanby, S. H., Laine, A. F., & Peterchev, A. V. (2016). Comparison of electric field strength and spatial distribution of electroconvulsive therapy and magnetic seizure therapy in a realistic human head model. *European Psychiatry, 36*, 55–64.

Lee, W. H., Lisanby, S. H., Laine, A. F., & Peterchev, A. V. (2017). Minimum electric field exposure for seizure induction with electroconvulsive therapy and magnetic seizure therapy. *Neuropsychopharmacology, 42*(6), 1192–1200.

Lisanby, S. H. (2002). Update on magnetic seizure therapy: A novel form of convulsive therapy. *Journal of ECT, 18*(4), 182–188.

Lisanby, S. H., Luber, B., Finck, A. D., Schroeder, C., & Sackeim, H. A. (2001). Deliberate seizure induction with repetitive transcranial magnetic stimulation in nonhuman primates. *Archives of General Psychiatry, 58*(2), 199–200.

Lisanby, S. H., Luber, B., Sackeim, H. A., Finck, A., & Schroeder, C. (2001). Deliberate seizure induction with repetitive transcranial magnetic stimulation in nonhuman primates. *Archives of General Psychiatry, 58*(2), 199–200.

Lisanby, S. H., Luber, B., Schlaepfer, T. E., & Sackeim, H. A. (2003). Safety and feasibility of magnetic seizure therapy (MST) in major depression: randomized within-subject comparison with electroconvulsive therapy. *Neuropsychopharmacology, 28*(10), 1852–1865.

Lisanby, S. H., Maddox, J. H., Prudic, J., Devanand, D. P., & Sackeim, H. A. (2000). The effects of electroconvulsive therapy on memory of autobiographical and public events. *Archives of General Psychiatry, 57*(6), 581–590.

Lisanby, S. H., Morales, O., Payne, N., Kwon, E., Fitzsimons, L., Luber, B., et al. (2003). New developments in electroconvulsive therapy and magnetic seizure therapy. *CNS Spectrum, 8*(7), 529–536.

Lisanby, S. H., Moscrip, T., Morales, O., Luber, B., Schroeder, C., & Sackeim, H. (2003). Neurophysiological characterization of magnetic seizure therapy (MST) in non-human primates. *Supplements in Clinical Neurophysiology, 56,* 81–99.

Lisanby, S. H., & Peterchev, A. V. (2007). Magnetic seizure therapy for the treatment of depression. In M. A. Marcollin & F. Padberg (Eds.),*Transcranial brain stimulation for treatment of psychiatric disorders* (pp. 155–171). Basel, Switzerland: Karger.

Lisanby, S. H., Sackeim, H. A., Dwork, A. J., Underwood, M., Wang, X., Kassir, S., et al. (2003). Effects of electroconvulsive shock and magnetic seizure therapy on mossy fiber sprouting and cellular proliferation in the primate hippocampus. *Biological Psychiatry, 53*(Suppl.), 173S.

Lisanby, S. H., Schlaepfer, T. E., Fisch, H. U., & Sackeim, H. A. (2001). Magnetic seizure therapy of major depression. *Archives of General Psychiatry, 58*(3), 303–305.

Luber, B., McClintock, S. M., & Lisanby, S. H. (2013). Applications of transcranial magnetic stimulation and magnetic seizure therapy in the study and treatment of disorders related to cerebral aging. *Dialogues in Clinical Neuroscience, 15*(1), 87–98.

Luber, B., Nobler, M. S., Moeller, J. R., Katzman, G. P., Prudic, J., Devanand, D. P., et al. (2000). Quantitative EEG during seizures induced by electroconvulsive therapy: Relations to treatment modality and clinical features. II. Topographic analyses. *Journal of ECT, 16*(3), 229–243.

McClintock, S. M., DeWind, N. K., Husain, M. M., Rowny, S. B., Spellman, T. J., Terrace, H., et al. (2013). Disruption of component processes of spatial working memory by electroconvulsive shock but not magnetic seizure therapy. *International Journal of Neuropsychopharmacology, 16*(1), 177–187.

McClintock, S. M., Tirmizi, O., Chansard, M., & Husain, M. M. (2011). A systematic review of the neurocognitive effects of magnetic seizure therapy. *International Review of Psychiatry, 23*(5), 413–423.

Morales, O., Luber, B., & Kwon, E. (2003). Prolactin response to convulsive therapy: Magnetic seizure therapy (MST) versus electroconvulsive shock (ECS) in nonhuman primates (abstract). *Journal of ECT, 19,* 58A.

Moscrip, T. D., Terrace, H. S., Sackeim, H. A., & Lisanby, S. H. (2006). Randomized controlled trial of the cognitive side-effects of magnetic seizure therapy (MST) and electroconvulsive shock (ECS). *International Journal of Neuropsychopharmacology, 9*(1), 1–11.

Mulders, P. C., van Eijndhoven, P., Schene, A., Beckmann, C., & Tendolkar, I. (2015). Resting-state functional connectivity in major depressive disorder: A review. *Journal of Neuroscience, 56,* 330–344.

Musso, F., Brinkmeyer, J., Mobascher, A., Warbrick, T., & Winterer, G. (2010). Spontaneous brain activity and EEG microstates. A novel EEG/fMRI analysis approach to explore resting-state networks. *Neuroimage, 52*(4), 1149–1161.

Mutz, J., Vipulananthan, V., Carter, B., Hurlemann, R., Fu, C. Y., & Young, A. H. (2019). Comparative efficacy and acceptability of non-surgical brain stimulation for the acute treatment of major depressive episodes in adults: Systematic review and network meta-analysis. *BMJ, 364,* l1079.

Nobler, M. S., Luber, B., Moeller, J. R., Katzman, G. P., Prudic, J., Devanand, D. P., et al. (2000). Quantitative EEG during seizures induced by electroconvulsive therapy: Relations to treatment modality and clinical features. I. Global analyses. *Journal of ECT, 16*(3), 211–228.

Noda, Y., Daskalakis, Z. J., Downar, J., Croarkin, P. E., Fitzgerald, P. B., & Blumberger, D. M. (2014). Magnetic seizure therapy in an adolescent with refractory bipolar depression: A case report. *Neuropsychiatric Disease and Treatment, 10,* 2049–2055.

Noda, Y., Daskalakis, Z. J., Fitzgerald, P. B., Downar, J., Rajji, T. K., & Blumberger, D. M. (2015). Magnetic seizure therapy-induced mania: A report of 2 cases. *Journal of ECT, 31*(1), e4–e6.

Ohman, R., Walinder, J., Balldin, J., & Wallin, L. (1976). Prolactin response to electroconvulsive therapy. *Lancet, 2,* 936–937.

Peterchev, A. V., Krystal, A. D., Rosa, M. A., & Lisanby, S. H. (2015). Individualized low-amplitude seizure therapy: Minimizing current for electroconvulsive therapy and magnetic seizure therapy. *Neuropsychopharmacology, 40*(9), 2076–2084.

Polster, J. D., Kayser, S., Bewernick, B. H., Hurlemann, R., & Schlaepfer, T. E. (2015). Effects of electroconvulsive therapy and magnetic seizure therapy on acute memory retrieval. *Journal of ECT, 31*(1), 13–19.

Rowny, S. B., Cycowicz, Y. M., McClintock, S. M., Truesdale, M. D., Luber, B., & Lisanby, S. H. (2009). Differential heart rate response to magnetic seizure therapy (MST) relative to electroconvulsive therapy: A nonhuman primate model. *Neuroimage, 47*(3), 1086–1091.

Sackeim, H. A. (1994). Magnetic stimulation therapy and ECT. *Convulsion Therapy, 10*(4), 255–258.

Sackeim, H. A., Prudic, J., Devanand, D. P., Nobler, M. S., Lisanby, S. H., Peyser, S., et al. (2000). A prospective, randomized, double-blind comparison of bilateral and right unilateral electroconvulsive therapy at different stimulus intensities. *Archives of General Psychiatry, 57*(5), 425–434.

Sackeim, H. A., Prudic, J., Nobler, M. S., Fitzsimons, L., Lisanby, S. H., Payne, N., et al. (2008). Effects of pulse width and electrode placement on the efficacy and cognitive effects of electroconvulsive therapy. *Brain Stimulation, 1*(2), 71–83.

Spellman, T., McClintock, S. M., Terrace, H., Luber, B., Husain, M. M., & Lisanby, S. H. (2008). Differential effects of high-dose magnetic seizure therapy and electroconvulsive shock on cognitive function. *Biological Psychiatry, 63*(12), 1163–1170.

Squire, L. R., Slater, P. C., & Chace, P. M. (1975). Retrograde amnesia: temporal gradient in very long term memory following electroconvulsive therapy. *Science, 187*, 77–79.

Squire, L. R., Slater, P. C., & Miller, P. L. (1981). Retrograde amnesia and bilateral electroconvulsive therapy. Long-term follow-up. *Archives of General Psychiatry, 38*(1), 89–95.

Sun, Y., Blumberger, D. M., Mulsant, B. H., Rajji, T. K., Fitzgerald, P. B., Barr, M. S., et al. (2018). Magnetic seizure therapy reduces suicidal ideation and produces neuroplasticity in treatment-resistant depression. *Translational Psychiatry, 8*(1), 253.

Sun, Y., Farzan, F., Mulsant, B. H., Rajji, T. K., Fitzgerald, P. B., Barr, M. S., et al. (2016). Indicators for remission of suicidal ideation following magnetic seizure therapy in patients with treatment-resistant depression. *JAMA Psychiatry, 73*(4), 337–345.

Swartz, C., & Abrams, R. (1984). Prolactin levels after bilateral and unilateral ECT. *British Journal of Psychiatry, 144*, 643–645.

Tang, V. M., Blumberger, D. M., McClintock, S. M., Kaster, T. S., Rajji, T. K., Downar, J., et al. (2018). Magnetic seizure therapy in treatment-resistant schizophrenia: A pilot study. *Frontiers in Psychiatry, 8*, 310–310.

Wang, J., Vila-Rodriguez, F., Jiang, W., Ren, Y. P., Wang, C. M., & Ma, X. (2019). Accelerated magnetic seizure therapy for treatment of major depressive disorder: A report of 3 cases. *Journal of ECT, 35*(2), 135–138.

Weiner, R. D. (2000). Retrograde amnesia with electroconvulsive therapy: Characteristics and implications. *Archives of General Psychiatry, 57*(6), 591–592.

White, P. F., Amos, Q., Zhang, Y., Stool, L., Husain, M. M., Thornton, L., et al. (2006). Anesthetic considerations for magnetic seizure therapy: A novel therapy for severe depression. *Anesthesia and Analgesia, 103*(1), 76–80, table of contents.

Yuan, H., Zotev, V., Phillips, R., Drevets, W., & Bodurka, J. (2012). Spatiotemporal dynamics of the brain at rest—exploring EEG microstates as electrophysiological signatures of BOLD resting state networks. *Neuroimage, 60*(4), 2062–2072.

CHAPTER 22

Implantable Neurostimulation Devices for Depression
Vagus Nerve Stimulation and Deep Brain Stimulation

Scott T. Aaronson
Alik S. Widge

In the growing field of neurostimulation for psychiatric conditions, the implantable devices vagus nerve stimulation (VNS) and deep brain stimulation (DBS) are unique. The treatment paradigm offered by these devices is dramatically different from that of all other mental health interventions. This is due to the relatively high cost (approximately $35,000 for VNS and $250,000 for DBS), the need for surgical implantation, the target population including patients with significant treatment refractory major depressive disorder (MDD), and a cumulative antidepressant response pattern that grows over months and years rather than weeks. The study designs for evaluating these devices and protocols for their use in clinical care thus need to be considered carefully and will differ from other noninvasive neuromodulation interventions (e.g., transcranial magnetic stimulation).

While VNS and DBS devices have been used in clinical trials that investigated their feasibility, safety, and efficacy in severely treatment-resistant MDD, the majority of their clinical use has been for neurological conditions (e.g., epilepsy, Parkinson's disease). At least 90% of the 50,000 VNS implantations worldwide have been for medication refractory epilepsy, and most of the DBS implantations have been performed to treat Parkinsonism. The entire dataset of patients implanted with these devices was used to inform the consideration of how they may effect cognitive function. A summary of the particulars of VNS and DBS appears in Table 22.1.

VAGUS NERVE STIMULATION

Overview of VNS

Vagus nerve stimulation was first developed and approved by the United States Food and Drug Administration (FDA) in 1997 for the treatment of intractable epilepsy. Observations

TABLE 22.1. Summary of DBS and VNS Information

	DBS	VNS
US FDA label and availability	Approved for Parkinsonism, dystonia, essential tremor. Humanitarian use exemption for OCD. No insurance coverage for depression	Approved for treatment-resistant epilepsy and TRD. Very limited insurance coverage for TRD (pending Medicare trial).
Target psychiatric population	Severe TRD, OCD, schizophrenia. Under investigation for other neuropsychiatric diseases.	Severe TRD both unipolar and bipolar depression.
Efficacy in depression	One positive RCT (VCVS target), two negative RCTs (VCVS and SCC targets), open-label evidence at multiple targets.	Very large open-label trial highly supportive. Two RCTs suggestive of efficacy, but negative (due to short time to response and low-dose stimulation effective).
Time to response	Generally 3–6 months, but newer paradigms may have a much shorter time to benefit.	6–12 months.
Brain targets	Multiple strategies. Three current areas of investigation: SCC, medial forebrain bundle, ventral internal capsule/ventral striatum.	Afferent fibers of left vagus nerve with stimulation ascending through the nucleus tractus solitarius to multiple brain regions.
Neurocognitive effects	Transient postsurgical impairment, likely no long-term negative effect, some possible cognitive enhancement as found in some studies.	Some positive cognitive effects, which may not be separate from depressive symptom improvement.
Side effects	Transient, dose-dependent agitation, hypomania, and possible suicidality.	Voice alteration when device is stimulating.

Note. US FDA, United States Food and Drug Administration; OCD, obsessive–compulsive disorder; TRD, treatment-resistant depression; RCT, randomized controlled trial; VCVS, ventral capsule ventral striatum; SCC, subgenual cingulate cortex.

made by investigators and clinicians supported the notion of mood improvement in patients with epilepsy treated with VNS (Elger, Hoppe, Falkai, Rush, & Elger, 2000). This finding led to a series of studies in patients with treatment-resistant depression (TRD). Those studies led to eventual clearance by the FDA for the use of VNS as an antidepressant treatment in patients with TRD who found no benefit from at least four antidepressant medications. This approval by the FDA occurred despite the findings from a randomized clinical trial (RCT) that did not meet its primary outcome measure (Rush et al., 2005).

The current VNS device marketed by LivaNova PLC (London, United Kingdom) consists of a titanium-encased lithium battery that is implanted under the skin in the upper chest wall and then connected to pig-tailed electrodes that are wrapped around the left vagus nerve by a lead wire that is tunneled under the skin (see Figure 22.1). The device is implanted under general or local anesthesia in approximately 1–2 hours. Two weeks following the surgery, the device is activated, and stimulation parameters are programmed by a wand that is connected wirelessly to a handheld programming tablet. The telemetric programming wand sets the four stimulation parameters for the device, including the current (from 0.25 to 3.0 mA), frequency of stimulation (from 20 to 50 Hz), pulse width (from 130 to 500 msec), and the duty cycle (adjustable from the usual settings of 30 seconds on and 5 minutes off). The initial parameter settings are gradually titrated up, usually over the first 2 weeks of treatment, as tolerated by the patient.

While the mechanism of action is unclear, several preclinical studies and clinical neuroimaging studies demonstrated that clinical improvement after chronic treatment was related to increased limbic activity and changes in neurochemistry (Yuan, Li, Sun, Arias-Carrion, & Machado, 2016). VNS demonstrates gradually improved efficacy that

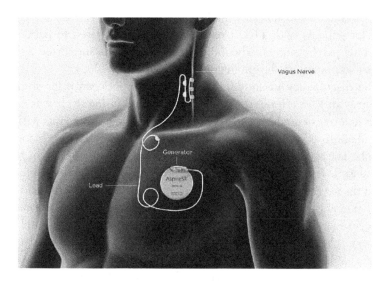

FIGURE 22.1. Example of a vagus nerve stimulator. The device is implanted in the upper chest with leads tunneled under the skin and wrapped around the left vagus nerve just below the branch of the recurrent laryngeal nerve. Figure courtesy of LivaNova USA, Inc.

onsets about 3–6 months into treatment and grows over time. Studies have found improved antidepressant outcomes at 1 and 2 years after long-term treatment (Nahas et al., 2005; Sackeim et al., 2007).

Efficacy of VNS in TRD

VNS has been studied in patients with highly treatment-resistant MDD. The first open-label studies comprised a total of 60 patients with both unipolar and bipolar depression (Rush et al., 2000). The average number of adequate failed antidepressant trials in those studies was at least two and averaged between four and five. The antidepressant response rates at 10–12 weeks were between 30 and 40%, and the remission rates were 14–17%, respectively. Remarkably, naturalistic long-term follow-up of these study participants demonstrated continued antidepressant improvement at 1 and 2 years of chronic treatment, with response rates at 44 and 42% and remission rates at 27 and 22%, respectively (Nahas et al., 2005).

A subsequent VNS RCT was conducted that enrolled 235 patients and included a 12-week sham controlled phase, followed by a long-term observation phase (Rush et al., 2005). Relative to the initial study, the participants in this study had a higher level of treatment resistance as on average they failed at least four antidepressant medication trials inclusive of monotherapy and adjunctive psychotropic agents. At the end of the 12-week sham treatment phase, the antidepressant outcomes between those randomized to active or sham stimulation was insignificant. Indeed, both the active and sham stimulation groups showed approximately 15% response and 10% remission rates. However, follow-up observations again demonstrated a cumulative antidepressant improvement in response and remission with response rates between 27 and 34%, depending on the depression symptom severity outcome measure and a remission rate of 16% at 1-year follow-up. Importantly, for patients with TRD treated with VNS compared to patients with TRD treated with only psychotropic medications, longer-term data supported a decline in suicide attempts and psychiatric hospitalizations (Nahas et al., 2005).

Given the discrepancy in antidepressant outcome between prior studies and findings of benefits with VNS after chronic use, a VNS dose finding study was conducted that compared three levels of double-blinded stimulation in 331 participants with highly TRD (Aaronson et al., 2013). Over 97% of the participants failed at least six previous antidepressant treatments. The acute phase treatment lasted 22 weeks, after which the output current could be increased. The participants were followed longitudinally for up to 50 weeks. At completion of the acute phase at 22 weeks, the three dosing treatment conditions showed similar significant antidepressant effects as measured on the primary depression severity outcome measure (a clinician-rated Inventory of Depressive Symptomatology [IDS-C]). In the long-term phase, the mean change in the IDS-C total scores showed continued improvement; that is, participants continued to show antidepressant improvements.

An analysis of those participants who had an antidepressant response in the acute phase demonstrated significantly greater durability of the response with both medium and high relative to low VNS doses. Overall, the response rates and remission rates at 22 weeks were 20% and 10%, respectively. At 50 weeks, the overall response rates varied from 27 to 53%, and the remission rates ranged from 15 to 23%, which were dependent on the depression severity metric and assigned dose group. The percentage of participants with an acute antidepressant response who continued to maintain antidepressant response at 50 weeks varied from 77 to 92% in both the medium- and high-dose groups compared to 44–69% in the low-dose group (Aaronson et al., 2013).

The largest and longest study published to date in TRD compared 494 patients who were implanted with VNS to 301 patients receiving treatment as usual (TAU) at the same specialty clinics (Aaronson et al., 2017). The study reported on the cumulative response rates over approximately 5 years in this large clinical patient population. The average number of antidepressant treatment failures for the study population was 7.9, which was far higher than the two treatment failures considered to diagnose TRD. The cumulative response rate was significantly higher for those patients treated with VNS relative to TAU (67.6% vs. 40.9%, respectively). The superior antidepressant outcomes for patients treated with VNS was also seen in multiple subanalyses, including patients with a history of ECT response or nonresponse, presence of bipolar symptoms, or history of significant anxiety at baseline (Aaronson et al., 2017). Collectively, the available evidence supports the antidepressant benefits with appropriately dosed (e.g., medium dose, high dose) chronic VNS therapy.

Side Effects and Tolerability

There is a large safety database for VNS given that the majority of implantations were conducted to control epilepsy. The VNS device is well tolerated, and the retention of subjects through the studies that examined its anti-epileptic and antidepressant effects has been very high. The major adverse events are primarily related to the surgery for implantation, which tends to be self-limited or associated with when the device was in the stimulation part of the duty cycle. The electrode for the VNS is typically wrapped around the left vagus nerve near the superior and recurrent laryngeal nerves. During stimulation, this can cause voice alterations, hoarseness, or coughing, which are all frequently seen. Bradyarrhythmias and sleep apnea were rare side effects. The rate of stimulation-induced mania or hypomania was low, and adjustment of treatment parameters likely reduced such symptoms.

Interpretation of Study Results

Several difficulties have impacted the development of VNS as an antidepressant therapy for TRD. The evidence demonstrates that it took at minimum 6 months, but possibly more, to see significant antidepressant outcome differences between participants treated with active and sham stimulation. As the first major VNS trial had a priori set 12 weeks from implantation as its primary depression severity outcome measure timepoint, the double-blind phase was too short to demonstrate significant separation between active and sham. In the dose-finding study, the low-dose arm (at 0.25 mA and a pulse width of 125 msec) was intended to be a surrogate for sham treatment. As it turned out, however, even this low-dose condition demonstrated significant antidepressant response compared to the in-group baseline. As such, while the low-dose relative to the medium- and high-dose treated patients had a significantly less durable antidepressant response, the study failed to meet the a priori established primary depression severity outcome criteria. The most recent observational study provided evidence of antidepressant efficacy in a large persistently and severely ill patient population. However, the significance of the results is tempered by the fact that an observational study does not carry the impact of a randomized sham controlled trial. Nonetheless, for patients with TRD, VNS is a feasible and safe antidepressant therapy.

VNS and Cognitive Function: Safety

A review article from 2014 that reported on the effect of VNS on cognitive function (Vonck et al., 2014) underscored the small size of the database that included only one study with 27 participants with TRD (Sackeim et al., 2001) and the rest of the studies involved patients with epilepsy or Alzheimer's disease. Several problems limit the applicability of the larger VNS dataset. The cognitive problems often seen in chronic TRD, relative to those of epilepsy or Alzheimer's disease, create a very different cognitive profile at baseline. Equally important, the VNS device settings for most acute effect studies were well below target dose ranges for adequate management of depressive symptoms (0.5 mA for the short-term studies vs. 1.0 mA for depression).

The Sackeim and colleagues (2001) study sought to determine if VNS, as an antidepressant therapy, could have adverse cognitive effects. Twenty-seven patients with TRD who were implanted with a VNS device completed a neuropsychological battery at two timepoints, including 2–4 weeks before surgery and 12 weeks after surgery (after 8 weeks at the target VNS stimulation dose). Relative to baseline cognitive test performance, significant improvements were found in motor speed, word fluency, psychomotor functioning, and executive functioning cognitive domains. These cognitive improvements were significantly correlated with depression severity improvement but were unrelated with VNS current output. Due to the small sample size, it was unclear whether the improved cognitive performance was only a manifestation of the improvement in depressive symptoms or if it represented an independent change secondary to VNS therapy. Importantly, as there was no indication of cognitive worsening, the study provided evidence that VNS therapy was cognitively safe. In patients with VNS therapy for indications other than TRD, there has been modest improvement in aspects of verbal memory and stability of cognitive performance throughout chronic stimulation provision (Vonck et al., 2014).

VNS and Cognitive Function: Possible Mechanism of Action

While VNS exerts a wide range of effects on the central nervous system, including increased c-fos expression in multiple brain regions, increased ΔFos B immunoreactivity (both of which are markers for increased neuronal activity and sensitivity), and decreased proinflammatory cytokine synthesis (Carreno & Frazer, 2017), it is more likely that the effect on cognitive function may be mediated by its effect on biogenic amines. VNS stimulation is largely conducted afferently through the nucleus tractus solitarius, with an excitatory effect on the locus coeruleus (LC). This then increases noradrenergic activity in the many brain structures that the LC projects to, such as the hippocampus, thalamus, hypothalamus, amygdala, dorsal raphe nucleus, cerebellum, and cerebral cortex (Vonck et al., 2014). VNS has also been shown to facilitate long-term potentiation in the dentate gyrus, which is hypothesized to exert some memory-enhancing effects and involve LC-mediated activation of beta-noradrenergic neurons (Zuo, Smith, & Jensen, 2007). Currently, the mechanisms of action underlying VNS's effects on cognitive function remain unclear.

The Future of VNS as an Antidepressant Therapy

For over a decade (2007–2019), VNS remained uncovered by most insurance companies given the noncoverage determination (NCD) made by the Centers for Medicare and Medicaid Services (CMS) in 2006. The strength of a large observational study (Aaronson et al., 2017; Conway et al., 2018) led to CMS rescinding its NCD and supporting VNS therapy coverage with evidence development in 2019. This policy shift will likely lead both to more third-party coverage of VNS therapy for TRD as well as more opportunities to further understand the effects of VNS on cognitive function.

DEEP BRAIN STIMULATION

Overview and Clinical Efficacy

DBS is an emerging device-based treatment for MDD. Like VNS, DBS is a surgical treatment that requires implanted electronic hardware. The difference is that in DBS, stimulation is applied directly to brain regions believed to govern depressive symptoms. Multiple DBS systems are labeled for Parkinson's disease and other movement disorders, but all share a common architecture (see Figure 22.2), including an implanted brain electrode (often called a "lead") whose electrical connections then tunnel subcutaneously through the neck to a subclavicular controller and implanted pulse generator. As recently reviewed (in Widge, Malone, & Dougherty, 2018), three different brain locations have been tested as DBS targets in MDD, following three different theories of depressive neurobiology.

The subgenual cingulate cortex (SCC) was identified as a "hot spot" on neuroimaging that became more active when patients and healthy volunteers experienced highly sad or negative moods. It was targeted for DBS following an early theory (which is now not well supported) that applying DBS to a hyperactive region of cerebral cortex would create a "virtual lesion" and suppress such activity. In open-label studies of both MDD and bipolar depression, SCC DBS led to response rates as high as 92% (11 of 12) in patients with highly treatment-refractory depression (Holtzheimer et al., 2012). In the only published RCT to date; however, SCC DBS and sham treatment (namely, DBS system implantation without electrical pulse delivery) showed similar antidepressant outcomes (Holtzheimer et al., 2017). Since then, the originators of SCC DBS have performed additional neuroimaging which suggested that the actual target is not the SCC gray matter, but a confluence of white matter tracts that often runs next to SCC. Prospective targeting of that confluence, based on patient-specific tractographic imaging, had a similarly high antidepressant

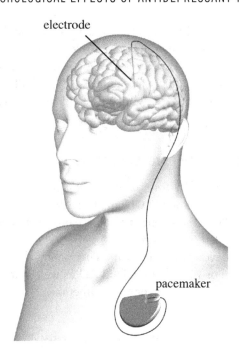

FIGURE 22.2. Example of a deep brain stimulator. The figure illustrates electrode placement into central/deep structures not reachable with noninvasive techniques and connection of that electrode to a battery and pulse generator in the chest. Actual implants are usually bilateral, with one electrode and one pulse generator for each hemisphere. In newer conceptions, multiple electrodes are connected to each pulse generator to stimulate a network. Figure adapted from Wikimedia Commons sources under CC-Attribution license.

response rate of 80% at 1 year (Riva-Posse et al., 2018). Response rates are somewhat lower outside the original authors' group (Ramasubbu et al., 2020), but the patient-specific imaging approach still offers great promise for an era of more personalized antidepressant treatment.

The medial forebrain bundle (MFB) is a deep white matter bundle, just superior to the oculomotor tracts, that is strongly involved in perceptions of reward and pleasure. Schlaepfer, Bewernick, Kayser, Mädler, and Coenen (2013) theorized that stimulating this bundle might therefore be specifically effective in highly anhedonic MDD. Like the SCC, the MFB must be identified and targeted through patient-specific neuroimage-guided tractography, as white matter bundle locations have significant interindividual variability (Makris et al., 2016; Schlaepfer et al., 2013). In an open-label study, six of seven MFB-stimulated patients with MDD experienced antidepressant response, defined as a 50% decrease on the Montgomery–Åsberg Depression Rating Scale (MADRS) total score (Schlaepfer et al., 2013). In a phenomenon that appears to be unique to the MFB target, improvement was very rapid, as four of seven of the study participants achieved antidepressant response in less than a week of stimulation. Although the target was proposed specifically for anhedonia, response was actually driven by improvement on multiple MADRS depression subscales. Furthermore, like SCC, it remains unclear if MFB DBS can separate from a well-designed surgical placebo. In a small study conducted in the United States, at 1-month postimplant with no active stimulation, two of four patients met antidepressant response criteria (Fenoy et al., 2016). Very similar results were seen in a larger study that was conducted in Germany. Specifically, patients with and without stimulation showed nearly identical depression severity improvement trajectories, with rapid antidepressant response that was achieved within approximately 2 weeks (Coenen et al., 2019).

Last, but not least, the ventral internal capsule–ventral striatum (VCVS) target was discovered serendipitously. This brain target was originally stimulated to treat obsessive–compulsive disorder (OCD) in hopes of disrupting a presumed hyperactivity in capsular loops that connected the cortex, thalamus, and striatum (Dougherty et al., 2018). In those early studies of the VCVS target, investigators noted that patients' mood improved before they reported a change in OCD-related behavioral ratings. The subsequent testing of VCVS in many ways resembled what was found with the SCC and MFB targets. In an open-label study, eight of 15 patients (50%) achieved antidepressant response by 3 months (Malone et al., 2009). However, in a double-blind RCT, there was no significant difference in antidepressant outcome between active DBS and an inactive implant at the end of a 16-week comparison period (Dougherty et al., 2015).

For the VCVS, however, a separate group of investigators tested an alternate study design in parallel (Bergfeld et al., 2016). Rather than randomizing whether patients received stimulation immediately after implant, they provided all participants with a year of open-label active treatment, then conducted a blinded crossover discontinuation. In that open-label year, 40% (10 of 25 participants) responded. For the 9 responders who agreed to participate in the blind discontinuation, all (100%) relapsed during their sham period. This was the first and to date the only RCT of DBS in psychiatry to reach its prospective endpoint. Similar to VNS, the antidepressant effects of DBS appear to incrementally build up over time.

DBS and Cognitive Function: No Evidence for Neurocognitive Decline

The initial literature on the effects of DBS on cognitive function focused on safety and on ruling out harm. The actual brain tissue disruption from the surgical placement of the lead is very small, but it is sufficient to cause improvements in psychiatric symptoms on its own, without electrical stimulation (Bergfeld et al., 2016; Dougherty et al., 2015; Fenoy et al., 2016; Holtzheimer et al., 2017). Therefore, it stood to reason that there might also be subtle deleterious cognitive effects. At all three tested brain targets; however, adverse cognitive effects of DBS have been largely ruled out. In both open-label (Bewernick, Kayser, Sturm, & Schlaepfer, 2012; Holtzheimer et al., 2012; Malone et al., 2009; Schlaepfer et al., 2013) and larger blinded studies (Bergfeld et al., 2017; Coenen et al., 2019; Holtzheimer et al., 2017), no significant declines have been found from the pre-DBS baseline across a variety of neurocognitive metrics across time up to one year. The one exception was the study of the VCVS target, which found a small negative effect on an unspecified response-inhibition metric (Dougherty et al., 2015). The clinical significance of that isolated finding remains unclear and seems likely to be minimal, given that this finding has failed to be replicated in other DBS studies.

Although persistent cognitive decline is not a side effect of DBS, there is strong evidence for transient cognitive impairment. Mayberg and colleagues describe a "rough patch" that can occur after about 3 months of SCC DBS, which is characterized by emotional dysregulation and impulsivity (Crowell, Garlow, Riva-Posse, & Mayberg, 2015). Similarly, the MFB (Coenen et al., 2019) and VCVS (Bergfeld et al., 2016; Dougherty et al., 2015) DBS brain targets can cause hypomania, usually in a voltage-dependent and rapidly reversible fashion. In some reports, the incidence of DBS-induced hypomania has been found to be up to 50% (Widge et al., 2015). All of these impairments appear to be completely transient, but they demonstrate that all known DBS targets engage circuits that govern both mood and cognitive function. This phenomenon of overlapping circuits has been well known from DBS in Parkinson's disease. The subthalamic nucleus (STN), a common target for Parkinson's disease DBS, is divisible into motor, associative (cognitive), and limbic subterritories, based on the projection to different cortical regions. Spread of the electric field outside of the motor STN can cause significant emotional and cognitive changes, including impulsive and hypomanic syndromes that resemble the effects of VCVS DBS (Kurtis, Rajah, Delgado, & Dafsari, 2017). Some investigators have even attempted to leverage this effect to develop STN DBS as a treatment for "low-impulsivity" disorders such as OCD, with promising initial results that require replication (Tyagi et al., 2019).

DBS and Cognition: Cognitive Enhancement as Mechanism of Action?

More recently, emphasis has shifted from ruling out cognitive decline after psychiatric DBS to considering whether this therapy could actually enhance cognitive function, and whether this might in part be the mechanism that leads to therapeutic outcomes (Bilge, Gosai, & Widge, 2018). Clinicians working with patients receiving DBS therapy have frequently commented on the patients' increased ability to engage with and benefit from evidence-based psychotherapies (cognitive-behavioral therapy [CBT]) that require new behavioral learning. In OCD, one study specifically documented an augmenting interaction between VCVS DBS and CBT (Mantione, Nieman, Figee, & Denys, 2014). DBS applied to the SCC (Holtzheimer et al., 2012; Moreines, McClintock, Kelley, Holtzheimer, & Mayberg, 2014) and MFB (Coenen et al., 2019) has also been found to modestly improve cognitive flexibility and verbal intellectual ability, respectively. These results are difficult to interpret because they represent change from a severely depressed baseline, which for some patients may involve preexisting cognitive inefficiency and impairment. That is, it is unclear whether DBS improved patients' mood by enhancing their cognitive abilities, or whether, instead, an improved mood unmasked their expected level of performance on neuropsychological testing. This is again a situation in which there are strong parallels between DBS and VNS.

Recent results from our lab (Widge et al., 2019) may help clarify the above chicken-and-egg problem. We tested for acute performance changes on a set-shifting task as a cohort of VCVS DBS patients performed that task with stimulation ON and OFF. Acute withdrawal of chronic DBS slowed patients' performance and diminished prefrontal electroencephalography (EEG) activity that is classically associated with set shifting and response inhibition. Furthermore, the degree of EEG change was predictive of patients' ultimate clinical outcome. This suggested that DBS, at least within VCVS, does have acute and beneficial cognitive effects.

THE FUTURE OF DBS IN DEPRESSION

Our group (Widge et al., 2017) is now working to transform the prior positive research findings into "closed-loop" feedback-driven algorithms. Traditionally, DBS settings are determined manually, through a trial-and-error process. A closed-loop approach determines settings based directly on a readout of brain activity, for example, a physiologic biomarker. In our case, we hypothesize that brain-based markers of cognitive function can be read out or "decoded" in real time by a suitably configured implant. Other groups are attempting similar approaches for real-time stimulation control to enhance memory function (Ezzyat et al., 2018) or mood (Sani et al., 2018, Scangos et al., 2021). In fact, brain implants capable of this recording and real-time stimulation are already marketed for epilepsy and are available for investigational use in other disorders (Lo & Widge, 2017). While closed-loop technology is still in development and remains several years away from the clinic, the vast growth of this research effort highlights a growing understanding of the critical role that cognitive function plays in the response to emotional events. A focus on specific domains of cognitive function also aligns clinical DBS with basic neuroscience research, as proposed by the National Institute of Mental Health Research Domain Criteria initiative. These developing brain implant technologies hold great promise for the use of neuromodulation in MDD, TRD, and a wide variety of other disorders (Bilge et al., 2018; Lo & Widge, 2017; Widge et al., 2018).

REFERENCES

Aaronson, S. T., Carpenter, L. L., Conway, C. R., Reimherr, F. W., Lisanby, S. H., Schwartz, T. L., et al. (2013). Vagus nerve stimulation therapy randomized to different amounts of electrical charge for treatment-resistant depression: acute and chronic effects. *Brain Stimul, 6*(4), 631–640.

Aaronson, S. T., Sears, P., Ruvuna, F., Bunker, M., Conway, C. R., Dougherty, D. D., et al. (2017). A 5-year observational study of patients with treatment-resistant depression treated with vagus nerve stimulation or treatment as usual: Comparison of response, remission, and suicidality. *American Journal of Psychiatry, 174*(7), 640–648.

Bergfeld, I. O., Mantione, M., Hoogendoorn, M. L. C., Ruhé, H. G., Horst, F., Notten, P., et al. (2017). Impact of deep brain stimulation of the ventral anterior limb of the internal capsule on cognition in depression. *Psychological Medicine, 47*(9), 1647–1658.

Bergfeld, I. O., Mantione, M., Hoogendorn, M. L., Ruhé, H. G., Notten, P., van Laarhoven, J., et al. (2016). Deep brain stimulation of the ventral anterior limb of the internal capsule for treatment-resistant depression: A randomized clinical trial. *JAMA Psychiatry, 73*(5), 456–464.

Bewernick, B. H., Kayser, S., Sturm, V., & Schlaepfer, T. E. (2012). Long-term effects of nucleus accumbens deep brain stimulation in treatment-resistant depression: Evidence for sustained efficacy. *Neuropsychopharmacology, 37*(9), 1975–1985.

Bilge, M. T., Gosai, A., & Widge, A. S. (2018). Deep brain stimulation in psychiatry: Mechanisms, models, and next-generation therapies. *Psychiatric Clinics of North America, 41*(3), 373–383.

Carreno, F. R., & Frazer, A. (2017). Vagal nerve stimulation for treatment-resistant depression. *Neurotherapeutics, 14*(3), 716–727.

Coenen, V. A., Bewernick, B. H., Kayser, S., Kilian, H., Boström, J., Greschus, S., et al. (2019). Supero-lateral medial forebrain bundle deep brain stimulation in major depression: A gateway trial. *Neuropsychopharmacology, 44*(7), 1224–1232.

Conway, C. R., Kumar, A., Xiong, W., Bunker, M., Aaronson, S. T., & Rush, A. J. (2018). Chronic vagus nerve stimulation significantly improves quality of life in treatment-resistant major depression. *Journal of Clinical Psychiatry, 79*(5), 18m12178.

Crowell, A. L., Garlow, S. J., Riva-Posse, P., & Mayberg, H. S. (2015). Characterizing the therapeutic response to deep brain stimulation for treatment-resistant depression: A single center long-term perspective. *Frontiers in Integrative Neuroscience, 9,* 41.

Dougherty, D. D., Brennan, B., Stewart, S. E., Wilhelm, S., Widge, A. S., & Rauch, S. L. (2018). Neuro-scientifically informed formulation and treatment planning for patients with obsessive-compulsive disorder: A review. *JAMA Psychiatry, 75*(10), 1081–1087.

Dougherty, D. D., Rezai, A. R., Carpenter, L. L., Howland, R. H., Bhati, M. T., O'Reardon, J. P., et al. (2015). A randomized sham-controlled trial of deep brain stimulation of the ventral capsule/ventral striatum for chronic treatment-resistant depression. *Biological Psychiatry, 78*(4), 240–248.

Elger, G., Hoppe, C., Falkai, P., Rush, A. J., & Elger, C. E. (2000). Vagus nerve stimulation is associated with mood improvements in epilepsy patients. *Epilepsy Research, 42*(2–3), 203–210.

Ezzyat, Y., Wanda, P. A., Levy, D. F., Kadel, A., Aka, A., Pedisich, I., et al. (2018). Closed-loop stimulation of temporal cortex rescues functional networks and improves memory. *Nature Communications, 9*(1), 365.

Fenoy, A. J., Schulz, P., Selvaraj, S., Burrows, C., Spiker, D., Cao, B., et al. (2016). Deep brain stimulation of the medial forebrain bundle: Distinctive responses in resistant depression. *Journal of Affective Disorders, 203,* 143–151.

Holtzheimer, P. E., Husain, M. M., Lisanby, S. H., Taylor, S. F., Whitworth, L. A., McClintock, S., et al. (2017). Subcallosal cingulate deep brain stimulation for treatment-resistant depression: A multisite, randomised, sham-controlled trial. *Lancet Psychiatry, 4,* 839–849.

Holtzheimer, P. E., Kelley, M. E., Gross, R. E., Filkowski, M. M., Garlow, S. J., Barrocas, A., et al. (2012). Subcallosal cingulate deep brain stimulation for treatment-resistant unipolar and bipolar depression. *Archives of General Psychiatry, 69*(2), 150–158.

Kurtis, M. M., Rajah, T., Delgado, L. F., & Dafsari, H. S. (2017). The effect of deep brain stimulation on the non-motor symptoms of Parkinson's disease: A critical review of the current evidence. *NPJ Parkinson's Disease, 3,* 16024.

Lo, M.-C., & Widge, A. S. (2017). Closed-loop neuromodulation systems: Next-generation treatments for psychiatric illness. *International Review of Psychiatry, 29*(2), 191–204.

Makris, N., Rathi, Y., Mouradian, P., Bonmassar, G., Papadimitriou, G., Ing, W. I., et al. (2016). Variability and anatomical specificity of the orbitofrontothalamic fibers of passage in the ventral capsule/ventral striatum (VC/VS): Precision care for patient-specific tractography-guided targeting of deep brain stimulation (DBS) in obsessive compulsive disorder (OCD). *Brain Imaging and Behavior, 10*(4), 1054–1067.

Malone, D. A., Dougherty, D. D., Rezai, A. R., Carpenter, L. L., Friehs, G. M., Eskandar, E. N., et al. (2009). Deep brain stimulation of the ventral capsule/ventral striatum for treatment-resistant depression. *Biological Psychiatry, 65*(4), 267–275.

Mantione, M., Nieman, D. H., Figee, M., & Denys, D. (2014). Cognitive-behavioural therapy augments the effects of deep brain stimulation in obsessive–compulsive disorder. *Psychological Medicine, 44*(16), 3515–3522.

Moreines, J. L., McClintock, S. M., Kelley, M. E., Holtzheimer, P. E., & Mayberg, H. S. (2014). Neuropsychological function before and after subcallosal cingulate deep brain stimulation in patients with treatment-resistant depression. *Depression and Anxiety, 31*(8), 690–698.

Nahas, Z., Marangell, L. B., Husain, M. M., Rush, A. J., Sackeim, H. A., Lisanby, S. H., et al. (2005). Two-year outcome of vagus nerve stimulation (VNS) for treatment of major depressive episodes. *Journal of Clinical Psychiatry, 66*(9), 1097–1104.

Ramasubbu, R., Clark, D. L., Golding, S., Dobson, K. S., Mackie, A., Haffenden, A., & Kiss, Z. H. (2020).

Long versus short pulse width subcallosal cingulate stimulation for treatment-resistant depression: A randomised, double-blind, crossover trial. *Lancet Psychiatry, 7*(1), 29–40.

Riva-Posse, P., Choi, K. S., Holtzheimer, P. E., Crowell, A. L., Garlow, S. J., Rajendra, J. K., et al. (2018). A connectomic approach for subcallosal cingulate deep brain stimulation surgery: Prospective targeting in treatment-resistant depression. *Molecular Psychiatry, 23*, 843–849.

Rush, A. J., George, M. S., Sackeim, H. A., Marangell, L. B., Husain, M. M., Giller, C., et al. (2000). Vagus nerve stimulation (VNS) for treatment-resistant depressions: A multicenter study. *Biological Psychiatry, 47*(4), 276–286.

Rush, A. J., Marangell, L. B., Sackeim, H. A., George, M. S., Brannan, S. K., Davis, S. M., et al. (2005). Vagus nerve stimulation for treatment-resistant depression: A randomized, controlled acute phase trial. *Biological Psychiatry, 58*(5), 347–354.

Sackeim, H. A., Brannan, S. K., Rush, A. J., George, M. S., Marangell, L. B., & Allen, J. (2007). Durability of antidepressant response to vagus nerve stimulation (VNS). *International Journal of Neuropsychopharmacology, 10*(6), 817–826.

Sackeim, H. A., Keilp, J. G., Rush, A. J., George, M. S., Marangell, L. B., Dormer, J. S., et al. (2001). The effects of vagus nerve stimulation on cognitive performance in patients with treatment-resistant depression. *Neuropsychiatry, Neuropsychology, and Behavioral Neurology, 14*(1), 53–62.

Sani, O. G., Yang, Y., Lee, M. B., Dawes, H. E., Chang, E. F., & Shanechi, M. M. (2018). Mood variations decoded from multi-site intracranial human brain activity. *Nature Biotechnology, 36*, 954–961.

Scangos, K. W., Khambhati, A. N., Daly, P. M., Makhoul, G. S., Sugrue, L. P., Zamanian, H., et al. (2021). Closed-loop neuromodulation in an individual with treatment-resistant depression. *Nature Medicine, 27*(10), 1696–1700.

Schlaepfer, T. E., Bewernick, B. H., Kayser, S., Mädler, B., & Coenen, V. A. (2013). Rapid effects of deep brain stimulation for treatment-resistant major depression. *Biological Psychiatry, 73*(12), 1204–1212.

Tyagi, H., Apergis-Schoute, A. M., Akram, H., Foltynie, T., Limousin, P., Drummond, L. M., et al. (2019). A randomised trial directly comparing ventral capsule and anteromedial subthalamic nucleus stimulation in obsessive compulsive disorder: Clinical and imaging evidence for dissociable effects. *Biological Psychiatry, 85*(9), 726–734.

Vonck, K., Raedt, R., Naulaerts, J., De Vogelaere, F., Thiery, E., Van Roost, D., et al. (2014). Vagus nerve stimulation . . . 25 years later! What do we know about the effects on cognition? *Neuroscience and Biobehavioral Reviews, 45*, 63–71.

Widge, A. S., Ellard, K. K., Paulk, A. C., Basu, I., Yousefi, A., Zorowitz, S., et al. (2017). Treating refractory mental illness with closed-loop brain stimulation: Progress towards a patient-specific transdiagnostic approach. *Experimental Neurology, 287*(4), 361–472.

Widge, A. S., Licon, E., Zorowitz, S., Corse, A., Arulpragasam, A. R., Camprodon, J. A., et al. (2015). Predictors of hypomania during ventral capsule/ventral striatum deep brain stimulation. *Journal of Neuropsychiatry and Clinical Neurosciences, 28*(1), 38–44.

Widge, A. S., Malone, D. A. J., & Dougherty, D. D. (2018). Closing the loop on deep brain stimulation for treatment-resistant depression. *Frontiers in Neuroscience, 12*, 175.

Widge, A. S., Zorowitz, S., Basu, I., Paulk, A. C., Cash, S. S., Eskandar, E. N., et al. (2019). Deep brain stimulation of the internal capsule enhances human cognitive control and prefrontal cortex function. *Nature Communications, 10*, 1536.

Yuan, T. F., Li, A., Sun, X., Arias-Carrion, O., & Machado, S. (2016). Vagus nerve stimulation in treating depression: A tale of two stories. *Current Molecular Medicine, 16*(1), 33–39.

Zuo, Y., Smith, D. C., & Jensen, R. A. (2007). Vagus nerve stimulation potentiates hippocampal LTP in freely-moving rats. *Physiology and Behavior, 90*(4), 583–589.

CHAPTER 23

Transcranial Magnetic Stimulation

Brian Kavanaugh
Paul Croarkin

Transcranial magnetic stimulation (TMS) was first described by Barker and colleagues in 1985, when the authors utilized the device to noninvasively stimulate the human motor cortex (Barker, Jalinous, & Freeston, 1985). As originally described by Barker, TMS consists of a magnetic stimulator and the placement of an electromagnetic coil on the scalp (Barker et al., 1985; George, Lisanby, & Sackeim, 1999). The magnetic stimulator discharges electrical current in rapid on-and-off pulses through the stimulating coil. This electrical current creates a time-varying magnetic field in the coil, which then induces electrical current and neuronal depolarization (if at appropriate strength) in the neural tissue (George et al., 1999; Kobayashi & Pascual-Leone, 2003; Lisanby, Luber, Perera, & Sackeim, 2000). Unlike other methods of stimulation, TMS is noninvasive, requires no direct contact with the brain or anesthesia/analgesics, and when delivered safely, is associated with no adverse effects other than transient mild headaches and discomfort. TMS is particularly appealing as a method of cortical stimulation, given its ability to bypass the skull and target specific cortical regions. This method of cortical stimulation was originally examined as inducing contralateral motor movements at the motor cortex (Barker et al., 1985). However, research quickly progressed to examining the effects of TMS at nonmotor regions, most notably the dorsolateral prefrontal cortex (DLPFC), and its possible effects in a range of neurological and psychiatric symptomology (George et al., 1999; Kobayashi & Pascual-Leone, 2003; Lisanby et al., 2000). Relatedly, TMS can be utilized as an experimental probe, while repetitive TMS (rTMS) is the application of TMS at a regular frequency, often utilized in a therapeutic manner (Lisanby et al., 2000). While rTMS has been investigated across various psychiatric disorders, the majority of TMS-related research and treatment has focused on major depressive disorder (MDD).

ORIGINAL rTMS-MDD STUDIES

Systematic investigation into the antidepressant effects of rTMS in patients with MDD began with an original study by Hoflich, Kasper, Hufnagel, Ruhrmann, and Moller (1993) that administered 10 sessions of TMS to two patients with medication-resistant MDD with psychosis. No antidepressant effect was found in one patient, but a slight improvement in depression severity was seen in the other patient. George and colleagues (1995) then found that at least 1 week of daily high-frequency (HF) rTMS (20 Hz at left DLPFC) significantly improved depression severity in six patients with medication-resistant depression during psychiatric hospitalization. These findings were followed by Pascual-Leone and Rubio (1996), who utilized a randomized crossover design study showing that the left DLPFC rTMS had a significant effect on depression in 17 patients with medication-resistant MDD of psychotic type.

Following their original findings, George and colleagues (1997) conducted a randomized, crossover design study that examined 2 weeks of HF rTMS (20 Hz at left DLPFC) compared to 2 weeks of sham in 12 patients with depression. Active compared to sham rTMS significantly improved depressive symptoms, with a decrease of 5 depression scale score points in active rTMS and a 3-point increase in scale score points during sham rTMS. In a similar study, Kolbinger, Hoflich, Hufnagel, Moller, and Kasper (1995) found significant depression improvement after 1 week of active rTMS (250 transcranial magnetic stimuli/session) compared to sham rTMS in a sample of 15 patients with depression. Of note, the stimulation "below threshold" (i.e., motoric threshold minus 0.3 tesla) showed a stronger depression effect than the simulation "above threshold" (i.e., motoric threshold plus 0.3 tesla). A later open-label study of 50 patients with refractory depression found a 42% response rate to rTMS (10 Hz), with response observed in 56% of young adult patients, but only 23% of elderly adult patients (Figiel, 1998). Preliminary findings were followed by two multisite, randomized, sham-controlled trials of 3–5 weeks of daily HF rTMS at left DLPFC in adults with treatment-resistant depression (George et al., 2010; O'Reardon et al., 2007). The study results indicated the statistically significant and clinically meaningful antidepressant efficacy of rTMS, with remission rates of 13–17.4% and response rates of 23.9–24.5%. Later trials and studies facilitated the development of multiple TMS platforms for clinical use (McClintock et al., 2018; Perera et al., 2016).

rTMS ANTIDEPRESSANT EFFICACY

Numerous meta-analyses have examined the efficacy of HF rTMS to the left DLPFC, the most commonly utilized site of stimulation for antidepressant treatment (Anderson, Hoy, Daskalakis, & Fitzgerald, 2016; Berlim, van den Eynde, & Daskalakis, 2013; Berlim, van den Eynde, Tovar-Perdomo, & Daskalakis, 2014; Brunoni et al., 2017; Gaynes et al., 2014). For HF rTMS at the left DLPFC, remission/response rates have ranged from 18.6 to 53.8% for remission and from 29 to 62% for response (Berlim, Neufeld, & van den Eynde, 2013; Berlim et al., 2014; Fitzgerald, Hoy, Anderson, & Daskalakis, 2016; Gaynes et al., 2014), along with accompanying odds ratios (OR) of 2.42–3.3 for remission and 1.9–3.3 for response (Berlim, Neufeld, et al., 2013; Berlim et al., 2014). Such meta-analyses found a 57% reduction (Fitzgerald et al., 2016) and a 4+ point raw score reduction (Gaynes et al., 2014) in depression rating scale total scores. rTMS was equally effective as a monotherapy compared to use as an augmentative therapy (Berlim et al., 2014), although less severe baseline depression (i.e., lower severity at baseline, shorter depressive episode), history of multiple prior depressive episodes, and higher stimulation intensity were associated with greater likelihood of response (Fitzgerald et al., 2016). Low-frequency (LF) rTMS to the right DLPFC shows an equal response/remission profile to HF rTMS, with one meta-analysis finding a 34.6% remission rate (OR = 4.76) and a 38.2% response rate (OR = 3.35) after ~12 rTMS sessions (Berlim, van den Eynde, et al., 2013). The study authors additionally noted that monotherapy and >1,200 total pulses were possibly associated with higher rates of treatment response (Berlim, van den Eynde, et al., 2013). While there is ongoing research focused on identifying clinical variables or dosing parameters that enhance response or remission, most of this work has been inconclusive (Fitzgerald et al., 2020). This is a critical area of focus for future research and clinical practice.

Brunoni and colleagues (2017) capitalized on the accelerating amount of meta-analyses to conduct a network meta-analysis of 81 prior studies that included 4,233 patients. (Table 23.1 lists targeted regions for different protocols.) The results indicated that priming low frequency (OR = 4.66), bilateral (OR = 3.96), HF (OR = 3.07), intermittent theta burst stimulation (iTBS; OR = 2.54), and LF (OR = 2.37) rTMS were more effective than sham for both response and remission rates (with only iTBS not showing a remission effect). Alternatively, accelerated, deep, and synchronized rTMS were not more effective than sham for response/remission rates. Priming rTMS had a lower dropout rate than HF, LF, synchronized, and sham TMS, and while priming and bilateral rTMS had higher relative ranking efficacy, direct comparisons were unable to be conducted.

Additional meta-analyses have further examined specific subsamples or rTMS protocols. Of note, Razza and colleagues (2018) identified a large placebo response effect in a meta-analysis of 61 prior studies (1,328 patients), additionally finding that placebo response

TABLE 23.1. Target of Different TMS Protocols

	Left DLPFC	Right DLPFC
HF-rTMS	✓	
LF-rTMS		✓
Bilateral	✓	✓
iTBS	✓	
cTBS		✓
aTMS	✓	
pTMS		✓
dTMS	✓	
sTMS	✓	

Note. HF, high frequency; LF, low frequency; iTBS, intermittent TBS; cTBS, continuous TBS; aTMS, accelerated HF-rTMS; pTMS, priming LF-rTMS; dTMS, deep TMS; sTMS, low-field synchronized TMS.

was associated with active rTMS response (positively associated), severity of depression (negatively associated), and publication year (higher rate in recent publications; not due to publication bias, but potentially due to changes in sham stimulation methodology, especially for newer protocols). Additional meta-analyses have identified similar rates of remission/response for left HF (response: 43.1%) versus right LF (response: 32.8%) and bilateral (response: 47.2%; remission: 35.1%) versus unilateral (response: 46%; remission: 33.3%) rTMS (J. Chen et al., 2013; J. J. Chen et al., 2014). While electroconvulsive therapy (ECT) may be more efficacious than rTMS, rTMS is associated with fewer treatment-associated side effects; LF rTMS is more tolerated and bilateral rTMS may possess the most optimal efficacy/acceptability combination (Chen et al., 2014). Importantly, as rTMS parameters/protocols have advanced, the efficacy of rTMS has improved over time (Gross, Nakamura, Pascual-Leone, & Fregni, 2007). Furthermore, in HF rTMS, Teng and colleagues (2017) found efficacy directly related to total sessions and per-day pulses, with efficacy steadily improving from 5 (standardized mean difference [SMD] = –0.43), 10 (SMD = .60), 15 (SMD = –1.13), and 20 (SMD = –2.74) sessions. Additionally, 1,200–1,500 pulses obtained the maximum effect, compared to higher (1,600–1,800; 2,000–3,000) and lower (<1,000) number of pulses. Although the majority of research focused on adult patient cohorts,

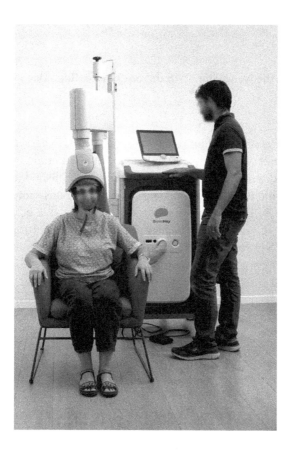

FIGURE 23.1. Image of the BrainsWay Deep TMS device. Reproduced with permission from BrainsWay.

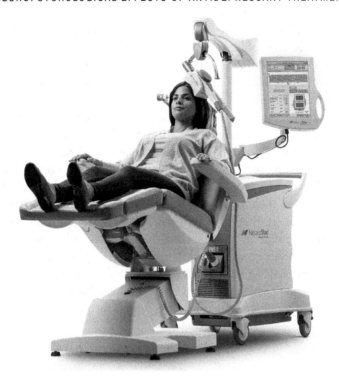

FIGURE 23.2. Image of the NeuroStar TMS therapy device. Reproduced with permission from Neuronetics.

antidepressant efficacy has been found in adolescents (15–21 years; L. Yang et al., 2017; X. R. Yang et al., 2014) and older adults (60–84 years; Conelea et al., 2017). Most relevant to clinical care, the antidepressant efficacy has also been established in naturalistic, clinical practice settings, with clinician- and patient-assessed response rates of 41.5–60.3% and remission rates of 26.5–37.1% (Carpenter et al., 2012; Conelea et al., 2017). While HF-rTMS at the left DLPFC was predominantly utilized in these naturalistic studies (>90%), bilateral and LF-rTMS at right DLPFC were also utilized (Carpenter et al., 2012).

Multiple devices/protocols are now approved by the U.S. Food and Drug Administration (FDA) as clinical treatments, for MDD, including the 10-Hz protocol utilizing the figure-8 coil, the 18-Hz protocol utilizing the H1 coil, and the 3-minute iTBS protocol utilizing the figure-of-eight coil (see Figures 23.1 and 23.32 for example devices). Furthermore, while not yet a clinical treatment, combining rTMS with concurrent psychotherapy sessions has shown promising effects that should continue to be examined (Donse, Padberg, Sack, Rush, & Arns, 2018; Russo, Tirrell, Busch, & Carpenter, 2018).

rTMS FOR DEPRESSION ACROSS THE LIFESPAN

Recent work has examined the role of rTMS as a treatment for MDD in adolescents. The existing literature includes case reports and unblinded, open trials with small sample sizes (Donaldson, Gordon, Melvin, Barton, & Fitzgerald, 2014). In general, these studies have simply adapted protocols from adult studies, and rTMS was typically applied as an adjunctive treatment. Existing experience is encouraging, but caution is warranted as at present adequately powered randomized controlled trials are lacking. One challenge inherent in these protocols is defining treatment-resistant depression in adolescent samples. Prior expert consensus guidelines have suggested that therapeutic rTMS should only be utilized in youth with a compelling clinical need (Rossi, Hallett, Rossini, Pascual-Leone, & Safety of TMS, 2009). As with any off-label intervention, caution is warranted, and a careful risk/benefit ratio analysis needs to be computed. Two lucid commentaries have discussed the potential risks associated with applying brain stimulation treatments to developing youth (Davis, 2014; Geddes, 2015), which include the unknown effects and side effects of stimulation on the developing brain, the lack of clear intensity/dosing guidelines, and more generally, the limited translation of adult findings to children. Recently, a large multicenter randomized controlled trial of 10-Hz rTMS for adolescents ages 12–21 with major depressive disorder was completed (Neuronetics, 2018). Although adolescent patients treated with 10-Hz rTMS had an improvement in depressive symptom, there was no difference compared to sham stimulation. Treatment with rTMS was well tolerated by adolescents, and no new safety concerns were identified (Croarkin et al., 2021).

Major depressive disorder is common in elderly adults and is often treatment-resistant (Blumberger, Hsu, & Daskalakis, 2015). Although other antidepressant therapies (ECT, combined medication and psychotherapy) often play a key role in managing severe late-life depression, many elderly adults often struggle with relapse after successful antidepressant treatment and ongoing functional impairment. The cognitive effects associated with ECT as well as medication–medication interaction side effects can be problematic. As such, rTMS could provide a safe and useful antidepressant treatment option. Early research with TMS in late-life depression contended that treatment may have been less effective due to increased distance between the TMS coil and the cortex given the relative cortical atrophy associated with age (Pallanti et al., 2012). Due to concerns which have now been found to be incorrect, elderly adult participants were often excluded from large clinical trials of rTMS for MDD. Contemporary research that has focused on interventional rTMS for late-life depression has reported much more promising antidepressant outcome results. Recent studies have argued that advanced age is not associated with decreased efficacy for depression (Berlim et al., 2014). Equally important, ongoing work has suggested that rTMS is safe for the elderly adult population (Janicak et al., 2008). Given the clinical need and lack of other available effective treatments, TMS will likely continue to be a valuable clinical intervention for late-life depression.

NEUROBIOLOGY OF ANTIDEPRESSANT EFFICACY

A comprehensive review of the neuroimaging findings underlying the depressive efficacy of rTMS is beyond the scope of this chapter, as multiple review papers have comprehensively examined this topic (Anderson et al., 2016; Noda et al., 2015; Philip, Barredo, Aiken, & Carpenter, 2018; Taib et al., 2018). Unfortunately, the variability in study methodology prevents a coherent synthesis of the findings (Noda et al., 2015; Philip et al., 2018; Taib et al., 2018). The methodological variability relates to the various rTMS protocols/parameters (e.g., 5 vs. 10 Hz), neuroimaging approaches (e.g., functional magnetic resonance imaging vs. electroencephalography [EEG]), and statistical/data analyses (e.g., networks vs. regions; negative vs. positive correlations). Despite such variability, a few findings have been reported regarding the underlying neurobiologic mechanisms of rTMS-associated antidepressant effects.

Pre/post-changes following rTMS in structure and/or function have been identified in the anterior cingulate cortex (ACC; including subgenual and perigenual ACC), frontal regions (including DLPFC, superior medial frontal gyrus, bilateral middle frontal gyri, dorsomedial prefrontal cortex, right orbitofrontal cortex), temporoparietal regions (including middle temporal cortex, hippocampus, precuneus), insula, and subcortical structures (including putamen, thalami; Taib et al., 2018). A large portion of the structures are directly involved in the neurobiology of depression (e.g., DLPFC, hippocampus), further highlighting the association of these structures to antidepressant clinical outcomes. Beyond individual regions, neural network alterations, particularly related to the default mode network (DMN), central executive network (CEN), and salience network (SN), have been identified in the literature (Anderson et al., 2016; Philip et al., 2018). DMN changes have been among the most consistent findings, particularly related to its connectivity to other networks (e.g., CEN), whereas the effect on the CEN has been found to be inconsistent across studies (Anderson et al., 2016; Philip et al., 2018). More generally, alterations to dysfunctional connectivity between DMN, CEN, and SN are part of a leading hypothesis for neurobiological causes of clinical efficacy. Although less work has examined EEG-related changes underlying antidepressant efficacy, promising findings related to neural oscillatory activity have been reported (Leuchter, Cook, Jin, & Phillips, 2013), particularly given the alpha band frequency of 10 Hz rTMS and the theta band frequency of iTBS.

THE USE OF rTMS IN RELATED NEUROPSYCHIATRIC CONDITIONS

There has been increased attention regarding the possible efficacy of rTMS in treatment of additional neuropsychiatric conditions, notably obsessive–compulsive disorder (OCD), schizophrenia, and posttraumatic stress disorder (PTSD). In an original meta-analysis of available psychiatric disorders, rTMS administered to the left or right DLPFC was not found to produce substantial effects of OCD symptomology (Slotema, Blom, Hoek, & Sommer, 2010). Of note, only three studies that investigated OCD were available at that time. Since then, three additional meta-analyses for rTMS in OCD have been published, with at least 18 randomized clinical trials (RCTs) conducted in OCD (Berlim, Neufeld, et al., 2013; Ma & Shi, 2014; Rehn, Eslick, & Brakoulias, 2018). These meta-analyses found medium-large effects (Hedges' $g = 0.59$–0.79) of active rTMS on OCD symptomology (measured by the Yale–Brown Obsessive Compulsive Scale). The response rate was reported at 35% (compared to 13% for sham rTMS), with a 2.65 increased odds ratio for response in active rTMS (Berlim, Neufeld, et al., 2013; Ma, 2014; Rehn et al., 2018). With regard to intensity, low-frequency and high-frequency protocols were both superior to sham, yet low-frequency rTMS was more effective than high-frequency rTMS (Rehn et al., 2018). With regard to location, the supplemental motor area (SMA) was superior to

DLPFC and orbitofrontal cortex (OFC). While left DLPFC and OFC efficacy was originally reported (Berlim, Neufeld, et al., 2013), a recent meta-analysis (with eight additional RCTs) found no superiority of left DLPFC and OFC to sham (Rehn, 2018). Alternatively, right DLPFC, bilateral DLPFC, and SMA were superior to sham, with effect sizes of g = 0.58, 1.18, and 1.68, respectively (Rehn et al., 2018). Based on the results of a randomized controlled trial of 100 patients, including a 38% response rate (compared to 11% response rate to sham TMS), the 20 Hz protocol with the H-1 coil became FDA approved for OCD in 2018 (FDA, 2018).

The effect of TMS on schizophrenia symptoms has been slightly inconsistent. A significant medium effect size on auditory verbal hallucinations (AVHs; MWES = 0.54) without an effect on negative symptoms (effect size = 0.39) was reported in an original meta-analysis by Slotema and colleagues (2010). When targeting the left or right DLPFC, the efficacy of active rTMS on negative symptoms has slightly varied. In the meta-analysis, a small, insignificant effect was reported (Slotema et al., 2010), yet a significant, small-to-medium effect was noted in another meta-analysis, most notably with medium effects at high frequency rTMS (Dlabac-de Lange, Knegtering, & Aleman, 2010). Although negative symptoms have largely targeted the DLPFC, AVH interventions have targeted the primary auditory cortex, with rTMS coil placement at the temporoparietal junction. Two other meta-analyses (Slotema, Aleman, Daskalakis, & Sommer, 2012; Slotema, Blom, van Lutterveld, Hoek, & Sommer, 2014) have identified a small-medium effect (MWES = 0.33–0.44) for rTMS on AVH. The strongest effects were found at the temporoparietal junction (MWES = 0.44–0.63), particularly the left temporoparietal junction at 1-Hz frequency (MWES = 0.63).

The research on PTSD remains less well established than other conditions, although two meta-analyses with positive findings have been conducted (Karsen, Watts, & Holtzheimer, 2014; Yan, Xie, Zheng, Zou, & Wang, 2017). The most recent meta-analysis examined 11 prior studies (Yan et al., 2017) and found large effects of LF (SMD = 0.92) and HF (SMD = 3.24) rTMS on PTSD symptomology. Subanalysis for HF studies found large effects of HF on reexperiencing (SMD = 1.77), avoidance (SMD = 1.57), and hyperarousal (SMD = 1.32; Yan et al., 2017).

THE NEUROCOGNITIVE EFFECTS OF TMS

Neurocognitive function was originally utilized to assess the overall safety of rTMS clinical studies. A prior meta-analysis of clinical trial data for various neuropsychiatric disorders found no negative neurocognitive side effects of rTMS across global, executive, attention, working memory, processing speed, memory, and visuospatial domains (Martin, McClintock, Forster, & Loo, 2016). Since then, there has been and continues to be growing interest in the possible neurocognitive-enhancing effects of rTMS in depression treatment. The interest in possible neurocognitive effects is at least in part related to the fact that neurocognitive dysfunction is a core, transdiagnostic component of psychopathology (Millan et al., 2012), and is a core domain in MDD diagnostic criteria according to the fifth edition of the *Diagnostic and Statistical Manual of Mental Disorders* (American Psychiatric Association, 2013; see Salem, Soares, & Selvaraj, Chapter 1, this volume, for additional information). Additionally, the primary site of rTMS administration, the DLPFC, is a core region of the frontoparietal central executive network (CEN), the neural network that subserves multiple aspects of neurocognition (e.g., working memory). The relationship between CEN, rTMS, and depression led to the hypothesis that rTMS may exert its antidepressant effects through modulation of CEN and related control processes. Neurocognitive results have been mixed and suggest that depression efficacy is likely not solely modulated by neurocognition. However, important neurocognitive effects have been identified.

While 60+ studies have identified TMS-related neurocognitive enhancement effects (Luber & Lisanby, 2014), only recently have meta-analyses more systematically examined the possible neurocognitive effects of TMS. The first meta-analysis (Brunoni & Vanderhasselt, 2014) examined the possible working memory effects of HF rTMS and transcranial direct current stimulation (tDCS) at the DLPFC. Although tDCS (see Martin, Moffa, & Nikolin, Chapter 24, this volume, for additional information) resulted in an isolated effect on working memory response time (RT), rTMS was associated with significant effects for both RT and accuracy (as noted by correct responses and error responses). A small cognitive improvement effect was found in healthy participants, but a medium effect was found in clinical samples (i.e., MDD, Parkinson's disease, schizophrenia). Martin and colleagues (Martin et al., 2016; Martin, McClintock, Forster, Lo, & Loo, 2017) utilized two meta-analyses to examine rTMS effects across multiple aspects of neurocognition in neuropsychiatric conditions. The first meta-analysis examined 30 studies across neuropsychiatric conditions and found no evidence of generalized neurocognitive improvement (Martin et al., 2016). An isolated working memory improvement was observed, with trend level significance in the overall sample attributed to a moderate effect size improvement in schizophrenia. A follow-up meta-analysis (Martin et al., 2017) examined the test-specific effects across 18 depression studies. Modest effects of rTMS were identified on the Trail Making Test (TMT) Parts A and B, a set of tests that measure psychomotor speed, visual scanning, and set shifting. Such cognitive effects were independent of mood improvement. As the authors noted, one significant limitation of the prior research to date is the heterogeneity in the specific neurocognitive tests utilized in studies. The TMT Part B had the second most studies available for analysis ($n = 13$), but half the tests had less than 10 studies available to the meta-analysis.

One recent analysis examined the possible effects of TBS (Lowe, Manocchio, Safati, & Hall, 2018). As expected, continuous theta burst stimulation (cTBS) had a reliable effect on executive function (EF), particularly left DLPFC, in that cTBS resulted in a small, attenuating effect on EF task performance (overall effect across multiple EF subdomains). With regard to iTBS, a quantitative analysis of effects could not be conducted given the limited sample size. However, 75% of studies found EF-enhancing effects, with 100% ($n = 4$) of studies that examined working memory finding a positive effect of iTBS on working memory performance. In another review that examined the possible rTMS effects of EF in depression (Ilieva et al., 2018), the study authors identified medium effect-size improvement in overall EF and response inhibition, but not in cognitive flexibility. Such EF improvements directly correlated to depression symptom severity improvement, rather than only to a direct effect of rTMS. Relatedly, another review found that five (out of 31) studies of rTMS in depression, schizophrenia, and Alzheimer's disease found a significant improvement in EF after treatment rTMS (Iimori et al., 2018). These studies all utilized high-frequency TMS ($n = 4$; 15–30 Hz) or iTBS ($n = 1$) during a multiweek protocol. While promising, these studies utilized a heterogeneous range of EF tests (e.g., Stroop Test, TmT, Wisconsin Card Sorting Test) that prevents a direct analysis of specific EF subdomains/tests.

Only one study to date has examined the possible neurocognitive effects of rTMS in adolescents with depression (Wall et al., 2013). That open-label study of HF rTMS found a significant improvement in the initial encoding and delayed recall of verbal information. There were no other effects on EF or other aspects of learning and memory. Moving beyond MDD studies, open-label studies of children/adolescents with neurodevelopmental disorders (e.g., autism, attention-deficit/hyperactivity disorder) have found EF effects in sustained attention/response inhibition and cognitive flexibility. Most of those studies utilized 1-Hz TMS applied to the left DLPFC or bilateral DLPFC (Casanova et al., 2012; Sokhadze, El-Baz, Sears, Opris, & Casanova, 2014; Sokhadze, El-Baz, Tasman, et al., 2014), while one study utilized iTBS applied to the right DLPFC (Abujadi, Croarkin, Bellini, Brentani, & Marcolin, 2018). The initial results of open-label studies provide support for possible positive TMS-associated effects on EF, though large, sham-controlled clinical trials are needed to confirm such findings.

In summary, rTMS is unlikely to induce global cognitive enhancement in neuropsychiatric populations. However, the majority of research to date provides promise for the possible beneficial effect of rTMS on working memory and other EF subdomains (e.g., response inhibition).

ETHICAL ISSUES

Clinical practice and research with rTMS has a promising future. However, clinicians and researchers have a duty and responsibility to maintain a fair degree of humility, caution, and equipoise with regard to clinical practice and future research endeavors. The advancement and clinical use of brain stimulation technologies are most likely outpacing systematic data and thorough ethical analyses. Systematically studied dosing patterns of rTMS are most suitable for application in clinical practice. The ethics of applying off-label treatments in terms of dosing and indication should be considered by individual clinicians in conjunction with transparent, comprehensive discussions with patients. In terms of research, the quality and replicability of rTMS research need to be considered carefully in the future. Further systematic study guided by existing guidelines in special populations is particularly important (McClintock et al., 2018; Rossi et al., 2009). The field of neuroethics is evolving and is particularly well suited to consider concerns related to the advancement and application of brain stimulation modalities such as rTMS.

CONCLUSION

Prior research and clinical practice have demonstrated that rTMS is a valuable clinical and research tool for major depressive disorder. Large multicenter trials and multiple meta-analytic studies have demonstrated the safety and antidepressant efficacy of rTMS for adult populations. Prior work suggests that standard rTMS protocols are safe with respect to neurocognition. Further research with TMS may demonstrate more specific and possibly therapeutic effects with respect to working memory and other EF domains. Broadly, future research will likely provide information on the safety and efficacy of novel dosing patterns of rTMS and its utility for additional neuropsychiatric indications. Ethical considerations need to be considered in research and clinical practice with brain stimulation modalities such as rTMS.

REFERENCES

Abujadi, C., Croarkin, P. E., Bellini, B. B., Brentani, H., & Marcolin, M. A. (2018). Intermittent theta-burst transcranial magnetic stimulation for autism spectrum disorder: An open-label pilot study. *Revista Brasileira de Psiquiatria, 40*(3), 309–311.

American Psychiatric Association. (2013). *Diagnostic and statistical manual of mental disorders* (5th ed.). Arlington, VA: Author.

Anderson, R. J., Hoy, K. E., Daskalakis, Z. J., & Fitzgerald, P. B. (2016). Repetitive transcranial magnetic stimulation for treatment resistant depression: Re-establishing connections. *Clinical Neurophysiology, 127*(11), 3394–3405.

Barker, A. T., Jalinous, R., & Freeston, I. L. (1985). Non-invasive magnetic stimulation of human motor cortex. *Lancet*, 1106–1107.

Berlim, M. T., Neufeld, N. H., & van den Eynde, F. (2013). Repetitive transcranial magnetic stimulation (rTMS) for obsessive-compulsive disorder (OCD): An exploratory meta-analysis of randomized and sham-controlled trials. *Journal of Psychiatric Research, 47*(8), 999–1006.

Berlim, M. T., van den Eynde, F., & Daskalakis, Z. J. (2013). Clinically meaningful efficacy and acceptability of low-frequency repetitive transcranial magnetic stimulation (rTMS) for treating primary major depression: A meta-analysis of randomized, double-blind and sham-controlled trials. *Neuropsychopharmacology, 38*(4), 543–551.

Berlim, M. T., van den Eynde, F., Tovar-Perdomo, S., & Daskalakis, Z. J. (2014). Response, remission and drop-out rates following high-frequency repetitive transcranial magnetic stimulation (rTMS) for treating major depression: A systematic review and meta-analysis of randomized, double-blind and sham-controlled trials. *Psychological Medicine, 44*(2), 225–239.

Blumberger, D. M., Hsu, J. H., & Daskalakis, Z. J. (2015). A review of brain stimulation treatments for late-life depression. *Current Treatment Options in Psychiatry, 2*(4), 413–421.

Brunoni, A. R., Chaimani, A., Moffa, A. H., Razza, L. B., Gattaz, W. F., Daskalakis, Z. J., et al. (2017). Repetitive transcranial magnetic stimulation for the acute treatment of major depressive episodes: A systematic review with network meta-analysis. *JAMA Psychiatry, 74*(2), 143–152.

Brunoni, A. R., & Vanderhasselt, M. A. (2014). Working memory improvement with non-invasive brain stimulation of the dorsolateral prefrontal cortex: A systematic review and meta-analysis. *Brain and Cognition, 86*, 1–9.

Carpenter, L. L., Janicak, P. G., Aaronson, S. T., Boyadjis, T., Brock, D. G., Cook, I. A., et al. (2012). Transcranial magnetic stimulation (TMS) for major depression: A multisite, naturalistic, observational study of acute treatment outcomes in clinical practice. *Depression and Anxiety, 29*(7), 587–596.

Casanova, M. F., Baruth, J. M., El-Baz, A., Tasman, A., Sears, L., & Sokhadze, E. (2012). Repetitive transcranial magnetic stimulation (rTMS) modulates event-related potential (ERP) indices of attention in autism. *Translational Neuroscience, 3*(2), 170–180.

Chen, J., Zhou, C., Wu, B., Wang, Y., Li, Q., Wei, Y., et al. (2013). Left versus right repetitive transcranial magnetic stimulation in treating major depression: A meta-analysis of randomised controlled trials. *Psychiatry Research, 210*(3), 1260–1264.

Chen, J. J., Liu, Z., Zhu, D., Li, Q., Zhang, H., Huang, H., et al. (2014). Bilateral vs. unilateral repetitive transcranial magnetic stimulation in treating major depression: A meta-analysis of randomized controlled trials. *Psychiatry Research, 219*(1), 51–57.

Conelea, C. A., Philip, N. S., Yip, A. G., Barnes, J. L., Niedzwiecki, M. J., Greenberg, B. D., et al. (2017). Transcranial magnetic stimulation for treatment-resistant depression: Naturalistic treatment outcomes for younger versus older patients. *Journal of Affective Disorders, 217,* 42–47.

Croarkin, P. E., Elmaadawi, A. Z., Aaronson, S. T., Schrodt, G. R., Jr., Holbert, R. C., Verdoliva, S., et al. (2021). Left prefrontal transcranial magnetic stimulation for treatment-resistant depression in adolescents: A double-blind, randomized, sham-controlled trial. *Neuropsychopharmacology, 46*(2), 462–469.

Davis, N. J. (2014). Transcranial stimulation of the developing brain: A plea for extreme caution. *Frontiers in Human Neuroscience, 8,* 600.

Dlabac-de Lange, J. J., Knegtering, R., & Aleman, A. (2010). Repetitive transcranial magnetic stimulation for negative symptoms of schizophrenia: Review and meta-analysis. *Journal of Clinical Psychiatry, 71*(4), 411–418.

Donaldson, A. E., Gordon, M. S., Melvin, G. A., Barton, D. A., & Fitzgerald, P. B. (2014). Addressing the needs of adolescents with treatment resistant depressive disorders: A systematic review of rTMS. *Brain Stimulation, 7*(1), 7–12.

Donse, L., Padberg, F., Sack, A. T., Rush, A. J., & Arns, M. (2018). Simultaneous rTMS and psychotherapy in major depressive disorder: Clinical outcomes and predictors from a large naturalistic study. *Brain Stimulation, 11*(2), 337–345.

Figiel, G. S., Epstein, C., McDonald, W. M., Amazon-Leece, J., Figiel, L., Saldivia, A., Glover, S. (1998). The use of rapid-rate transcranial magnetic stimulation (rTMS) in refractory depressed patients. *Journal of Neuropsychiatry and Clinical Neurosciences, 10,* 20–25.

Fitzgerald, P. B., Hoy, K. E., Anderson, R. J., & Daskalakis, Z. J. (2016). A study of the pattern of response to rTMS treatment in depression. *Depression and Anxiety, 33*(8), 746–753.

Fitzgerald, P. B., Hoy, K. E., Reynolds, J., Singh, A., Gunewardene, R., Slack, C., et al. (2020). A pragmatic randomized controlled trial exploring the relationship between pulse number and response to repetitive transcranial magnetic stimulation treatment in depression. *Brain Stimulation, 13*(1), 145–152.

Gaynes, B. N., Lloyd, S. W., Lux, L., Gartlehner, G., Hansen, R. A., Brode, S., et al. (2014). Repetitive transcranial magnetic stimulation for treatment-resistant depression: A systematic review and meta-analysis. *Journal of Clinical Psychiatry, 75*(5), 477–489; quiz 489.

Geddes, L. (2015). Brain stimulation in children spurs hope—and concern. *Nature, 525,* 436–437.

George, M. S., Lisanby, S. H., Avery, D., McDonald, W. M., Durkalski, V., Pavlicova, M., et al. (2010). Daily left prefrontal transcranial magnetic stimulation therapy for major depressive disorder. *Archives of General Psychiatry, 67*(5), 507–516.

George, M. S., Lisanby, S. H., & Sackeim, H. A. (1999). Transcranial magnetic stimulation: Applications in neuropsychiatry. *Archives of General Psychiatry, 56,* 300–311.

George, M. S., Wassermann, E. M., Kimbrell, T. A., Little, J. T., Williams, W. E., Danielson, A. L., et al. (1997). Mood improvement following daily left prefrontal repetitive transcranial magnetic stimulation in patients with depression: A placebo-controlled crossover trial. *American Journal of Psychiatry, 154,* 1752–1756.

George, M. S., Wassermann, E. M., Williams, W. A., Callahan, A., Ketter, T. A., Basser, P., et al. (1995). Daily repetitvie transcranial magnetic stimulation (rTMS) improves mood in depression. *Neuroreport, 6,* 1853–1856.

Gross, M., Nakamura, L., Pascual-Leone, A., & Fregni, F. (2007). Has repetitive transcranial magnetic stimulation (rTMS) treatment for depression improved? A systematic review and meta-analysis comparing the recent vs. the earlier rTMS studies. *Acta Psychiatrica Scandinavica, 116*(3), 165–173.

Hoflich, G., Kasper, S., Hufnagel, A., Ruhrmann, S., & Moller, H.-J. (1993). Application of transcranial magnetic stimulation in treatment of drug-resistant major depression—A report of two cases. *Human Psychopharmacology, 8,* 361–365.

Iimori, T., Nakajima, S., Miyazaki, T., Tarumi, R., Ogyu, K., Wada, M., et al. (2018). Effectiveness of the prefrontal repetitive transcranial magnetic stimulation on cognitive profiles in depression, schizophrenia, and Alzheimer's disease: A systematic review. *Progress in Neuropsychopharmacology and Biological Psychiatry, 88,* 31–40.

Ilieva, I. P., Alexopoulos, G. S., Dubin, M. J., Morimoto, S. S., Victoria, L. W., & Gunning, F. M. (2018). Age-related repetitive transcranial magnetic stimulation effects on executive function in depression: A systematic review. *American Journal of Geriatric Psychiatry, 26*(3), 334–346.

Janicak, P. G., O'Reardon, J. P., Sampson, S. M., Husain, M. M., Lisanby, S. H., Rado, J. T., et al. (2008). Transcranial magnetic stimulation in the treatment of major depressive disorder: A comprehensive summary of safety experience from acute exposure, extended exposure, and during reintroduction treatment. *Journal of Clinical Psychiatry, 69*, 222–232.

Karsen, E. F., Watts, B. V., & Holtzheimer, P. E. (2014). Review of the effectiveness of transcranial magnetic stimulation for post-traumatic stress disorder. *Brain Stimulation, 7*(2), 151–157.

Kobayashi, M., & Pascual-Leone, A. (2003). Transcranial magnetic stimulation in neurology. *Lancet Neurology, 2*(3), 145–156.

Kolbinger, H. M., Hoflich, G., Hufnagel, A., Moller, H.-J., & Kasper, S. (1995). Transcranial magnetic stimulation (TMS) in the treatment of major depression—A pilot study. *Human Psychopharmacology, 10*, 305–310.

Leuchter, A. F., Cook, I. A., Jin, Y., & Phillips, B. (2013). The relationship between brain oscillatory activity and therapeutic effectiveness of transcranial magnetic stimulation in the treatment of major depressive disorder. *Frontiers in Human Neuroscience, 7*, 37.

Lisanby, S. H., Luber, B., Perera, T., & Sackeim, H. A. (2000). Transcranial magnetic stimulation: Applications in basic neuroscience and neuropsychopharmacology. *International Journal of Neuropsychopharmacology, 3*, 259–-273.

Lowe, C. J., Manocchio, F., Safati, A. B., & Hall, P. A. (2018). The effects of theta burst stimulation (TBS) targeting the prefrontal cortex on executive functioning: A systematic review and meta-analysis. *Neuropsychologia, 111*, 344–359.

Luber, B., & Lisanby, S. H. (2014). Enhancement of human cognitive performance using transcranial magnetic stimulation (TMS). *Neuroimage, 85*(Pt. 3), 961–970.

Ma, Z.-R., & Shi, L.-J. (2014). Repetitive transcranial magnetic stimulation (rTMS) augmentation of selective serotonin reuptake inhibitors (SSRIs) for SSRI-resistant obsessive-compulsive disorder (OCD): A meta-analysis of randomized controlled trials. *Internal Journal of Clinical and Experimental Medicine, 7*(12), 4897–4905.

Martin, D. M., McClintock, S. M., Forster, J. J., Lo, T. Y., & Loo, C. (2017). Cognitive enhancing effects of rTMS administered to the prefrontal cortex in patients with depression: A systematic review and meta-analysis of individual task effects. *Depression and Anxiety, 34*(11), 1029–1039.

Martin, D. M., McClintock, S. M., Forster, J., & Loo, C. K. (2016). Does therapeutic repetitive transcranial magnetic stimulation cause cognitive enhancing effects in patients with neuropsychiatric conditions? A systematic review and meta-analysis of randomised controlled trials. *Neuropsychology Review, 26*(3), 295–309.

McClintock, S. M., Reti, I. M., Carpenter, L. L., McDonald, W. M., Dubin, M., Taylor, S. F., et al. (2018). Consensus recommendations for the clinical application of repetitive transcranial magnetic stimulation (rTMS) in the treatment of depression. *Journal of Clinical Psychiatry, 79*(1),16cs10905.

Millan, M. J., Agid, Y., Brune, M., Bullmore, E. T., Carter, C. S., Clayton, N. S., et al. (2012). Cognitive dysfunction in psychiatric disorders: Characteristics, causes and the quest for improved therapy. *Nature Reviews: Drug Discovery, 11*(2), 141–168.

Neuronetics. (2018). Safety and effectiveness of NeuroStar transcranial magnetic stimulation (TMS) therapy in depressed adolescents. Retrieved from *https://clinicaltrials.gov/ct2/show/NCT02586688*

Noda, Y., Silverstein, W. K., Barr, M. S., Vila-Rodriguez, F., Downar, J., Rajji, T. K., et al. (2015). Neurobiological mechanisms of repetitive transcranial magnetic stimulation of the dorsolateral prefrontal cortex in depression: A systematic review. *Psychological Medicine, 45*(16), 3411–3432.

O'Reardon, J. P., Solvason, H. B., Janicak, P. G., Sampson, S., Isenberg, K. E., Nahas, Z., et al (2007). Efficacy and safety of transcranial magnetic stimulation in the acute treatment of major depression: A multisite randomized controlled trial. *Biological Psychiatry, 62*(11), 1208–1216.

Pallanti, S., Di Rollo, A., Antonini, S., Cauli, G., Hollander, E., & Quercioli, L. (2012). Low-frequency rTMS over right dorsolateral prefrontal cortex in the treatment of resistant depression: Cognitive improvement is independent from clinical response, resting motor threshold is related to clinical response. *Neuropsychobiology, 65*(4), 227–235.

Pascual-Leone, A., & Rubio, B. (1996). Rapid-rate transcranial magnetic stimulation of left dorsolateral prefrontal cortex in drug-resistant depression. *Lancet, 348*(9022).

Perera, T., George, M. S., Grammer, G., Janicak, P. G., Pascual-Leone, A., & Wirecki, T. S. (2016). The clinical TMS society consensus review and treatment recommendations for TMS therapy for major depressive disorder. *Brain Stimulation, 9*(3), 336–346.

Philip, N. S., Barredo, J., Aiken, E., & Carpenter, L. L. (2018). Neuroimaging mechanisms of therapeutic transcranial magnetic stimulation for major depressive disorder. *Biological Psychiatry, Cognitive Neuroscience and Neuroimaging, 3*(3), 211–222.

Razza, L. B., Moffa, A. H., Moreno, M. L., Carvalho, A. F., Padberg, F., Fregni, F., et al. (2018). A systematic review and meta-analysis on placebo response to repetitive transcranial magnetic stimulation for depression trials. *Progress in Neuropsychopharmacology and Biological Psychiatry, 81*, 105–113.

Rehn, S., Eslick, G. D., & Brakoulias, V. (2018). A meta-analysis of the effectiveness of different cortical targets used in repetitive transcranial magnetic stimulation (rTMS) for the treatment of obsessive–compulsive disorder (OCD). *Psychiatric Quarterly, 89*(3), 645–665.

Rossi, S., Hallett, M., Rossini, P. M., Pascual-Leone, A., & Safety of TMS Consensus Group. (2009). Safety, ethical considerations, and application guidelines for the use of transcranial magnetic stimulation in clinical practice and research. *Clinical Neurophysiology, 120*(12), 2008–2039.

Russo, G. B., Tirrell, E., Busch, A., & Carpenter, L. L. (2018). Behavioral activation therapy during transcranial magnetic stimulation for major depressive disorder. *Journal of Affective Disorders, 236*, 101–104.

Slotema, C. W., Aleman, A., Daskalakis, Z. J., & Sommer, I. E. (2012). Meta-analysis of repetitive transcranial magnetic stimulation in the treatment of auditory verbal hallucinations: Update and effects after one month. *Schizophrenia Research, 142*(1–3), 40–45.

Slotema, C. W., Blom, J. D., Hoek, H. W., & Sommer, I. E. (2010). Should we expand the toolbox of psychiatric treatment methods to include repetitive transcranial magnetic stimulation (rTMS)? A meta-analysis of the efficacy of rTMS in psychiatric disorders. *Journal of Clinical Psychiatry, 71*(7), 873–884.

Slotema, C. W., Blom, J. D., van Lutterveld, R., Hoek, H. W., & Sommer, I. E. (2014). Review of the efficacy of transcranial magnetic stimulation for auditory verbal hallucinations. *Biological Psychiatry, 76*(2), 101–110.

Sokhadze, E. M., El-Baz, A. S., Sears, L. L., Opris, I., & Casanova, M. F. (2014). rTMS neuromodulation improves electrocortical functional measures of information processing and behavioral responses in autism. *Frontiers in Systems Neuroscience, 8*, 134.

Sokhadze, E. M., El-Baz, A. S., Tasman, A., Sears, L. L., Wang, Y., Lamina, E. V., et al. (2014). Neuromodulation integrating rTMS and neurofeedback for the treatment of autism spectrum disorder: An exploratory study. *Applied Psychophysiology and Biofeedback, 39*(3–4), 237–257.

Taib, S., Arbus, C., Sauvaget, A., Sporer, M., Schmitt, L., & Yrondi, A. (2018). How does repetitive transcranial magnetic stimulation influence the brain in depressive disorders?: A review of neuroimaging magnetic resonance imaging studies. *Journal of ECT, 34*(2), 79–86.

Teng, S., Guo, Z., Peng, H., Xing, G., Chen, H., He, B., et al. (2017). High-frequency repetitive transcranial magnetic stimulation over the left DLPFC for major depression: Session-dependent efficacy: A meta-analysis. *European Psychiatry, 41*, 75–84.

U.S. Food and Drug Administration. (2018). FDA permits marketing of transcranial magnetic stimulation for treatment of obsessive compulsive disorder [Press release]. Retrieved from *www.fda.gov/news-events/press-announcements/fda-permits-marketing-transcranial-magnetic-stimulation-treatment-obsessive-compulsive-disorder*

Wall, C. A., Croarkin, P. E., McClintock, S. M., Murphy, L. L., Bandel, L. A., Sim, L. A., et al. (2013). Neurocognitive effects of repetitive transcranial magnetic stimulation in adolescents with major depressive disorder. *Frontiers in Psychiatry, 4*, 165.

Yan, T., Xie, Q., Zheng, Z., Zou, K., & Wang, L. (2017). Different frequency repetitive transcranial magnetic stimulation (rTMS) for posttraumatic stress disorder (PTSD): A systematic review and meta-analysis. *Journal of Psychiatric Research, 89,* 125–135.

Yang, L., Zhou, X., Zhou, C., Zhang, Y., Pu, J., Liu, L., et al. (2017). Efficacy and acceptability of cognitive behavioral therapy for depression in children: A systematic review and meta-analysis. *Academic Pediatrics, 17*(1), 9–16.

Yang, X. R., Kirton, A., Wilkes, T. C., Pradhan, S., Liu, I., Jaworska, N., et al. (2014). Glutamate alterations associated with transcranial magnetic stimulation in youth depression: A case series. *Journal of ECT, 30*(3), 242–247.

CHAPTER 24

Transcranial Direct Current Stimulation

Donel M. Martin
Adriano Moffa
Stevan Nikolin

T he use of electrical stimulation as a treatment for clinical conditions can be traced back
to the 18th century. Since then, the technique has reemerged, first in early clinical
trials under the term *brain polarization* and now as *transcranial direct current stimulation
(tDCS)*, in subsequent modern trials conducted since the early 2000s. As of the year
2020, tDCS remains in development and has no regulatory approval for the treatment of
a neuropsychiatric disorder by the U.S. Food and Drug Administration. Interestingly, in
parallel with the modern clinical trials in depression, evidence emerged that tDCS could
produce acute and potentially long-lasting neurocognitive effects. Such neurocognitive
effects have potential relevance both for the antidepressant mechanisms of tDCS and for
broader therapeutic benefits when used to treat major depressive disorder (MDD). In this
chapter, we describe the modern use of tDCS, review its clinical efficacy in early and
modern trials in patients with MDD, and provide an overview and discussion of studies
that examined both acute and cumulative neurocognitive effects.

OVERVIEW OF tDCS

A tDCS machine is a small, battery-powered device that delivers a constant unidirectional electrical current of between 0 and 3 mA (milliamperes). The device is typically
connected to two rubber electrodes, a positively charged anode and a negatively charged
cathode, which are placed on the scalp (see Plate 24.1 in the color insert). The electrodes
drive an electrical current of negatively charged ions from the cathode to the anode, and
positively charged ions that flow in the opposite direction toward the cathode. A sponge
soaked in saline solution (a mixture of water and sodium chloride) is typically placed as
an intermediary between the scalp and the stimulating electrodes to facilitate current
flow and prevent localized areas of increased current density. With the use of modern

stimulation parameters and appropriate safety precautions, tDCS has been found to be safe and is associated with only minimal and transient side effects (e.g., tingling and itching (Bikson et al., 2016).

MECHANISMS OF ACTION

tDCS neuromodulatory effects are the result of electrical changes to the neuronal resting membrane potential. The direct current causes depolarization of the membrane potential, which involves lowering the threshold required to propagate a signal, and hyperpolarization, which involves inhibition of action potentials. Overall, tDCS neuromodulatory effects (i.e., excitatory or inhibitory) are dependent on the orientation of stimulated neurons relative to the electric field (see Plate 24.2 in the color insert). Importantly, tDCS involves a *subthreshold* stimulus of insufficient strength to directly induce neuronal firing. Rather, tDCS causes relatively low changes in the resting membrane potential (i.e., 0.2–0.5 mV) that alters the probability that a neuron will propagate an incoming signal (Stagg, Antal, & Nitsche, 2018).

A series of seminal studies conducted in the early 2000s demonstrated that tDCS produces after-effects that can outlast the duration of stimulation by several minutes and even hours (Nitsche & Paulus, 2000, 2001). These after-effects are similar to long-term potentiation and long-term depression processes, which are mediated by changes to synaptic plasticity (Kronberg, Bridi, Abel, Bikson, & Parra, 2017). The magnitude and duration of these after-effects are dependent on several factors, including the duration and intensity of the stimulus.

Importantly, tDCS induces no neuroplastic after-effects in the absence of ongoing cellular activity (Bikson & Rahman, 2013). Although tDCS stimulates large regions of the brain and may, therefore, be considered spatially imprecise, a recent study showed that tDCS effects indeed have neurophysiological functional specificity, selectively enhancing only the active neural networks following stimulation (Pisoni et al., 2018).

STIMULATION PARAMETERS

The stimulus parameters of a tDCS protocol strongly influence outcomes, which include current intensity, duration, and direction (i.e., electrode placements). Attempts to determine the optimal current intensity for inducing tDCS after-effects to date have been mixed (e.g., Chew, Ho, & Loo, 2015; Jamil et al., 2017). However, recent work has provided evidence in favor of an inverted-U-shaped dose–response curve, with a peak centered near 1 mA (Nikolin, Martin, Loo, & Boonstra, 2018). Further research is needed to empirically determine whether this curve differs between participant cohorts (e.g., healthy vs. depressed) and between individuals, although an examination of the literature has suggested this to be the case. Longer stimulation durations can produce longer lasting effects, although there is evidence of a limit beyond which there may be a reversal of effects (Monte-Silva et al., 2013). For this reason, most tDCS research employs a stimulation duration of 15–25 minutes (Bikson et al., 2016).

The electric field density generated by tDCS in the brain is influenced by several factors, such as electrode shape, size, number, placement (termed the "montage"), and individual physiological differences, including the skull and neuroanatomy. Electrode size generally ranges from 3.5 to 100 cm², although most research is conducted with electrodes of 25–35 cm². There is some evidence that larger electrodes can produce a greater increase in cortical excitation (Ho et al., 2016), although the optimal electrode size remains unclear. The number of electrodes used can also influence the electric field pattern. Most commonly, tDCS is delivered, using a pair of electrodes (an anode and cathode), and is termed *low density*. However, more complex montages of multiple anodes and cathodes can be used to further refine and guide the current flow to desired target regions, which is termed *high density*. Finally, the location of electrode placement determines which brain regions are preferentially excited or inhibited using tDCS. Electrodes placed close together increase the proportion of shunting of current across the scalp and therefore limit the amount penetrating the skull to stimulate neuronal tissue. Conversely, increasing the interelectrode distance stimulates a larger volume of the brain and reduces the degree of shunting through the scalp.

Many tDCS trials have placed the stimulating electrodes on the scalp with the assumption that the cortical tissue directly below the electrode will be preferentially modulated. Simulations of electric field density in which computational models estimate current pathways using high-resolution magnetic resonance imaging (MRI) and finite element method models have suggested that the electric fields are maximal in the region between the electrodes (Datta et al., 2009). Individual variations in the skull and neuroanatomy, including the individual pattern of cortical folding and the subsequent orientation of neurons relative to the tDCS electric field (whether they are tangential or radial to current flow), can also modulate tDCS-induced effects (Radman, Ramos, Brumberg, & Bikson, 2009).

A final aspect of the tDCS technique, which is particularly relevant to research, is the blinding procedure. Adequate blinding is critically important for randomized controlled trials to avoid bias and minimize nonspecific effects. Standard sham protocols ramp the current intensity up to 1–2 mA over several seconds, which is then gradually ramped back down before the tDCS device is turned off (Gandiga, Hummel, & Cohen, 2006). This procedure elicits paraesthetic sensations similar to those experienced during active tDCS and ensures that participants are unable to differentiate between the condition/s to which they have been randomized. Nevertheless, it is important to note that multiple variations of this procedure have been reported in the literature. Furthermore, built-in "sham modes" in modern tDCS devices vary with regard to procedure and stimulation output. Due to the potential biological effects of using some sham conditions (Nikolin et al., 2018), accurate reporting of the sham parameters is important for reproducibility among studies.

EARLY CLINICAL TRIALS IN DEPRESSION

Between 1964 and 1974, one pilot study and eight clinical trials were conducted that examined the clinical efficacy of "brain polarization." Although this technique is similar to modern tDCS, it typically uses lower current intensities (i.e., <0.5 mA), longer-session durations (e.g., >3 hours), and a montage with two anodes in the frontal region and one extracephalic cathode, usually over the leg.

Motivated by preclinical studies that showed stimulation of the exposed cortex by low-magnitude current could produce alterations in the ongoing neuronal firing rate, Lippold and Redfearn (1964) conducted a double-blind clinical trial with 32 subjects with mild depression and reported that anodal polarization increased alertness, motor activity, and elevated mood, whereas cathodal polarization induced silence and apathy. Costain, Redfearn, and Lippold (1964) presented what was considered the first double-blind, sham-controlled, randomized clinical trial (RCT) to use brain polarization for the treatment of depression. In that study, they also used the Lippold and Redfearn montage with two anodal electrodes placed over the eyebrows and the cathode placed over one knee. Nurses and psychiatrists evaluated the patients and observed a significant improvement of anxiety, agitation, and somatic symptoms with the active treatment.

Additional open-label trials have also found that direct current stimulation was efficacious for improving depressive symptoms (Baker, 1970; Carney, Cashman, & Sheffield, 1970; Herjanic & Moss-Herjanic, 1967; Ramsay & Schlagenhauf, 1966). Nevertheless, these findings should be interpreted with caution due to potential bias from the absence of a sham group. Indeed, a double-blind, sham-controlled clinical trial observed no differences in antidepressant activity between conditions (Arfai, Theano, Montagu, & Robin, 1970).

These inconsistent results in human clinical trials can be at least partially explained by variability in subjects' clinical characteristics, lack of standardized psychiatric measurement scales (which were not in widespread use in prior research), the use of tDCS devices with rudimentary control of the injected current strength, and significant variations in the stimulation parameters (e.g., current intensity varied from 0.02 to 0.5 mA, duration from 2 minutes to 11 hours a day, with variable numbers of repeated sessions). Possibly due to these mixed results and the introduction of new psychotropic medications, tDCS was largely forgotten between the mid-1970s until the turn of the century.

MODERN CLINICAL TRIALS FOR DEPRESSION

By the end of the 1990s, more precise methods and systematic observations started to be used, leading with the seminal experiment of Priori and colleagues (1998) and extending to the modern era of tDCS. Advances in neurosciences that broadened knowledge regarding functioning of the central nervous system, combined with the development of equipment that stored and discharged electricity more safely and accurately, propelled a new stage in the development of the tDCS technique. Compared to the brain polarization studies, modern tDCS studies used higher current intensities (between 1 and 2.5 mA), shorter session durations (from 20 to 30 minutes), a single anode placed over the left dorsolateral prefrontal cortex (DLPFC), and a cathode placed over the right cephalic region (supraorbital/Fp2, frontotemporal/F8 or DLPFC/F4).

The first two RCTs of tDCS, conducted in 2006, recruited, respectively, 10 and 18 antidepressant-medication free participants who received active (1 mA, 20 minutes every other day for 5 sessions) or simulated (sham) stimulation (Fregni, Boggio, Nitsche,

Marcolin, et al., 2006; Fregni, Boggio, Nitsche, Rigonatti, & Pascual-Leone, 2006). There was a significant mood improvement in the active group compared to baseline (mean reduction of 60% in depression scores versus 12% in the sham group), and these findings were replicated in the second RCT (Fregni, Boggio, Nitsche, Rigonatti, & Pascual-Leone, 2006). In 2008, two other positive RCTs (Boggio et al., 2008; Rigonatti et al., 2008) were conducted that used similar montages, but with higher current strength (2 mA) and a more intensive treatment regimen (one treatment a day for 10 days).

Following these positive results, unfortunately three other studies reported negative findings. Loo and colleagues (2010) recruited 40 patients with MDD and administered tDCS over five sessions (20 minutes every other day), with the active arm receiving 1 mA of current intensity. Palm and colleagues (2012) randomized 22 patients with depression to one of three groups: active 1 mA, active 2 mA, or sham for 2 weeks (10 daily sessions of 20 minutes each). Finally, Blumberger, Tran, Fitzgerald, Hoy, and Daskalakis (2012) randomized 24 patients with refractory MDD to receive 2 mA active tDCS or sham for 20 minutes and 15 sessions. In all of these RCTs, no significant difference in mood outcomes was observed between the active and sham conditions.

With the use of larger samples and assessment across a longer course of stimulation compared to the prior studies, the following two RCTs showed positive clinical outcomes. Loo and colleagues (2012) randomized 64 patients to sham or active tDCS (2 mA, 15 sessions over 3 weeks), and their study found significantly greater mood improvement with active compared to sham treatment. The Sertraline versus Electrical Current Therapy for Treating Depression Clinical Trial (SELECT; Brunoni, Valiengo, et al., 2013) randomized 120 subjects with MDD in a factorial design (four arms) to receive sertraline/placebo and active/sham tDCS, with the aim of assessing the safety and efficacy of the stimulation combined with antidepressant medication in comparison to tDCS only, medication only, and double placebo. A current of 2 mA was administered for 30 minutes in a total of 12 sessions. At the end of the 6-week trial, the combined tDCS + sertraline treatment effect differed in a statistically significant way from the effect for the other three groups. The authors concluded that the combination of tDCS and sertraline increased the efficacy of each treatment, but that the efficacy and safety of sertraline and tDCS were indifferent.

Considering the mixed results of the tDCS technique, Brunoni and colleagues (2016) conducted a systematic review and individual patient data (IPD) meta-analysis to clarify tDCS efficacy in depression and to explore individual predictors of antidepressant response. Six RCTs that involved 289 patients were used and showed that tDCS was significantly superior to sham for response, remission, and depression symptom severity improvement (see Figure 24.1). These effect sizes of tDCS, though small to medium, were comparable to those reported for transcranial magnetic stimulation (TMS; see Kavanaugh & Croarkin, Chapter 23, this volume, for additional information on TMS) and for antidepressant drug treatments (see Rosenblat, Chapter 15, this volume, for additional information on psychotropic medications) in primary care. In 2019, a new systematic review and an IPD meta-analysis were conducted (Moffa et al., 2020) with the addition of three new clinical trials (Brunoni et al., 2017; Loo et al., 2018; Pereira Junior Bde et al., 2015) confirming those results and presenting similar effect sizes.

In 2015, to overcome the limitations of the SELECT study (sertraline dose was low, and the study was not designed for noninferiority), the Escitalopram versus Electric

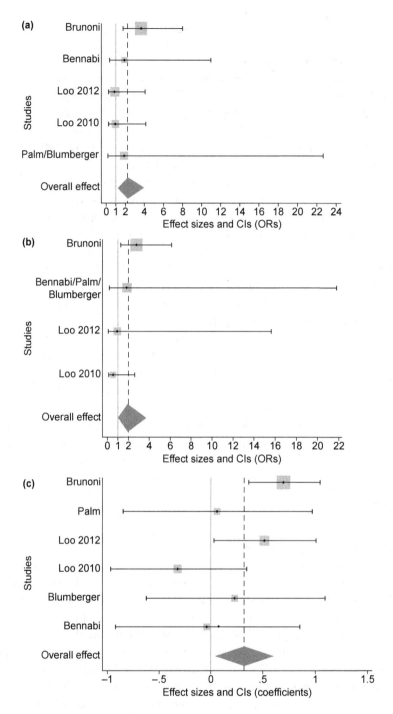

FIGURE 24.1. Individual patient data meta-analysis comparing active versus sham transcranial direct current stimulation (tDCS) in terms of (a) response; (b) remission and (c) depression improvement. Forest plots graphically illustrating the comparative efficacy of active with sham tDCS. For each study the relative strength of treatment effects is represented, the square represents the relative weight of each study, and the vertical bar is the 95% confidence interval. The rhombus represents the overall effect. Values >1 and >0 versus <1 and <0 represent positive and negative effects of active versus sham tDCS for categorical and continuous outcomes, respectively. From Brunoni et al. (2016). Copyright © 2016 Royal College of Psychiatrists; published by Cambridge University Press. Reprinted by permission.

Current Therapy to Treat Depression Clinical Study (ELECT-TDCS; Brunoni et al., 2017) was conducted. Its primary objective was to compare the efficacy of tDCS with the maximum dose of an antidepressant (escitalopram 20 mg/day) in a noninferiority design. A total of 245 patients with MDD were randomized to one of three groups: active tDCS and placebo pill; sham tDCS and escitalopram; and sham tDCS and placebo pill. Twenty-two sessions of tDCS (2 mA, 30 minutes) were delivered for 3 weeks over 15 consecutive days (no weekends) and then once a week until week 10. Even though both escitalopram and tDCS were found to be superior to placebo, the study findings could not claim noninferiority.

In the first international multicenter RCT, Loo and colleagues (2018) examined the efficacy of tDCS in patients with both unipolar ($N = 91$) and bipolar ($N = 39$) depression. Participants were randomized to active or sham tDCS, for twenty 2.5 mA, 30-minute sessions, administered over 4 weeks. Mood improved significantly in both unipolar and bipolar groups, with more remitters in the sham group among the unipolar patients and no difference between active and sham stimulation in the bipolar sample. These results were interpreted as potential improvement due to the placebo response in both conditions, or due to the "sham" stimulation as administered (two current ramps up to 1.0 and 0.5 mA, and a constant, low-intensity current of 0.034 mA for 30 minutes) was biologically active. This trial prompted a proof-of-concept study on tDCS dosage that supported the possibility that this minimal intensity of stimulation may have neuromodulatory effects (Nikolin et al., 2018).

EFFICACY IN MAJOR DEPRESSION

The recent clinical guidelines from the Canadian Network for Mood and Anxiety Treatments group (Milev et al., 2016) and European experts (Lefaucheur et al., 2017) considered tDCS to be probably effective for treatment of acute-phase MDD. Nevertheless, due to both modest clinical effects and mixed efficacy results, further research was recommended to establish the antidepressant effects of tDCS. For these reasons, tDCS for the treatment of MDD should be considered as being currently in development. The main goals of future studies are to optimize the parameters of stimulation, identify clinical or other features associated with improved antidepressant efficacy, and determine whether the technique should be used as either monotherapy or in combination with medication or some activity (e.g., cognitive training, meditation, cognitive behavioural therapy). Furthermore, the efficacy and safety of remotely supervised home-administered tDCS warrant study due to the potential translational implications.

OVERVIEW OF tDCS ACUTE COGNITIVE EFFECTS

The earliest explorations into the acute effects of a single tDCS session on cognitive function were made in the mid-2000s. These attempts used tDCS as an investigative tool to determine the relevance of the prefrontal cortex (PFC) for subserving specific cognitive functions such as probabilistic classification learning (Kincses, Antal, Nitsche, Bártfai, & Paulus, 2004) and working memory (Fregni et al., 2005). In those studies, tDCS was administered concurrently "online" during task performance. "Offline" stimulation instead refers to tDCS administered prior to task performance.

Following these pioneering efforts, research into tDCS acute cognitive effects saw an exponential increase, encompassing all aspects of cognitive functioning, including language, attention/perception, executive functioning, memory, and others (Jacobson, Koslowsky, & Lavidor, 2012). Despite this initial enthusiasm, a recent meta-analysis that included only controlled studies that used a crossover experimental design (i.e., to minimize interindividual differences) and that administered tDCS to the PFC (i.e., to minimize heterogeneity between studies) found only a small-sized effect on reaction time (Dedoncker, Brunoni, Baeken, & Vanderhasselt, 2016). Another issue has been that findings between different study labs have been mixed (Horvath, Forte, & Carter, 2015). Correspondingly, this has led to skepticism in the field regarding the utility and effectiveness of tDCS for producing acute cognitive effects. However, the most likely explanation for these modest effects and mixed outcomes has been the substantial heterogeneity in stimulation parameters and methodologies between studies. Furthermore, the use of primarily healthy samples may have limited the potential for observing enhancement effects. Interestingly, research in neuropsychiatric populations has tended to show greater consistency across studies (Berryhill & Martin, 2018).

To date, there have been several promising investigations of acute cognitive enhancement in clinical samples. For example, Hoy, Arnold, Emonson, Daskalakis, and Fitzgerald (2014) investigated the effect of "offline" anodal 1 mA, 2 mA, and sham tDCS over the left DLPFC (L-DLPFC) on working memory performance in patients with schizophrenia and found that only the highest current intensity improved accuracy. Similarly, Boggio and colleagues (2006) tested three current intensities (1 mA, 2 mA, and sham) and showed that 2 mA "online" stimulation of the L-DLPFC, but not the motor cortex, improved working memory in patients with idiopathic Parkinson's disease. In older patients with mild cognitive impairment, a single session of "online" anodal 1 mA tDCS over the left ventral inferior frontal gyrus improved semantic fluency and decreased task-related prefrontal hyperactivity, as assessed using functional magnetic resonance imaging (Meinzer et al., 2015). While these preliminary results demonstrated some potential cognitive benefits of tDCS across neuropsychiatric populations, replication is nevertheless required. Similar to the use of tDCS in healthy samples, further optimization of the approach, including determination of the optimal stimulus parameters (i.e., for particular neurocognitive effects and/or clinical conditions), will likely be warranted to improve and replicate cognitive benefit.

ACUTE COGNITIVE EFFECTS IN DEPRESSION

The early studies that found acute cognitive effects in healthy samples provided a rationale for investigating such effects in patients with MDD. As noted across multiple diagnostic criteria, MDD is characterized by deficits in neurocognitive function and emotion regulation, which are considered to be associated with key symptomology, including difficulties with concentration and rumination, as well as poor functional outcomes (Jaeger, Berns, Uzelac, & Davis-Conway, 2006). The L-DLPFC has been identified as a key node within the neural circuitry responsible for these deficits (Mayberg, 1997; Williams, 2017). Hence, it has been a focus for other noninvasive neurostimulation therapies for depression, including repetitive transcranial magnetic stimulation (rTMS; see Kavanaugh & Croarkin, Chapter 23, this volume). As described earlier, early modern controlled trials that used tDCS found that repeated treatments with the anode placed over this region produced antidepressant effects (Boggio et al., 2008; Fregni, Boggio, Nitsche, Marcolin, et al., 2006). Taken together, this research raised the possibility that tDCS acute cognitive effects could be related to antidepressant outcomes.

The first study to investigate acute cognitive effects in MDD was one of the first modern controlled clinical trials (Boggio et al., 2007). In that study, 26 patients with MDD were randomized to receive a single session of "offline" active tDCS, with the anode placed either over the L-DLPFC or occipital cortex or sham tDCS administered over the L-DLPFC, in a parallel-group design. Behavioral effects were examined using an affective go/no go task that had previously been found to be sensitive to rTMS stimulation of the DLPFC in patients with depression (Bermpohl et al., 2006). Significant performance improvements on the task only occurred with active L-DLPFC stimulation, and secondary analyses revealed that this improvement was limited to stimuli that showed positive emotional content (e.g., a couple holding hands). Participants in each condition then continued to receive active or sham tDCS over 10 consecutive days. Acute neurocognitive improvements; however, were unassociated with subsequent antidepressant outcomes. Given similar findings for acute effects of other antidepressant treatments on affective-based tasks (e.g., Bermpohl et al., 2006; Harmer, Hill, Taylor, Cowen, & Goodwin, 2003), the results provided an important foundation for further investigation of acute cognitive effects in patients with MDD.

Consequently, larger clinical trials similarly incorporated neurocognitive testing both to investigate potential acute cognitive effects and to establish the safety of this novel treatment. In a double-blind sham-controlled clinical trial that involved 64 patients with depression, Loo and colleagues (2012) administered the Symbol Digit Modalities Test (SDMT) as well as a simple and choice reaction test immediately prior to and following the first active or sham tDCS treatment session. Similar to Boggio and colleagues (2007), the anode was placed over the L-DLPFC, although the cathode was instead placed over F8. Results showed that only participants who received active tDCS significantly improved acute attention and working memory, as measured by the SDMT. No effects were found on the reaction time measures. This result provided further support for the acute neurocognitive effects with tDCS. Interestingly, the acute improvement observed in attention was consistent with participants' subjective reports of improved concentration with active stimulation assessed immediately after each treatment (unpublished data).

Subsequent work has provided further support for acute tDCS effects on both affective processing and cognitive function (see Table 24.1). With regard to affective processing, several different behavioral measures that involved emotional stimuli (i.e., words, pictures, faces) have been used in various experimental paradigms. Wolkenstein and Plewnia (2013), for example, investigated acute effects on a working memory task designed to assess "cognitive control" over distracting positive and negative valanced pictures. During active stimulation only, participants improved in both accuracy and reaction time, and showed

TABLE 24.1. Summary of Studies Investigating the Acute Effects of a Single tDCS Session in Depressed Samples

Study	Design	On/offline	Montage (A/C)	Current density (mA/cm²)	Sham setting	Task	Performance effect
Boggio et al. (2007)	Parallel	Offline	F3/RSO	0.057	On for 20 sec (max. 2 mA), then off.	Affective go/no go	Improved correct responses
Loo et al. (2012)	Parallel	Offline	F3/F8	0.057	On for 30 sec (max. 1 mA), then left on.	SDMT, SRT, CRT	Improved correct responses on SDMT
Brunoni et al. (2013b)	Parallel	Online	F3/F4	0.080	On for 60 sec (max. 2 mA), then off.	PCL	Absence of practice effect
Oliveira et al. (2013)	Parallel	Online	F3/F4	0.080	On for 60 sec (max. 2 mA), then off.	2-back	Improved correct responses
Wolkenstein & Plewnia (2013)	Crossover	Online	F3/EX	0.029	On for 40 sec (max. 1 mA), then sham setting.	DWM	Faster reaction times
Brunoni et al. (2014)	Parallel	Online	F3/F4	0.080	On for 60 sec (max. 2 mA), then off.	WEST	Faster reaction times
Moreno et al. (2015)	Parallel	Offline	OLE	0.080	On for 30 sec (max. 2 mA), then unknown.	2-back, IST	Improved residual score change on 2-back; faster switch cost on emotion IST
Gogler et al. (2016)	Parallel	Offline	F3/RSO	0.057	On for 45 sec (max. 2 mA), then sham setting.	TVA	Increased elements processed/sec
Brennan et al. (2017)	Crossover	Online and offline	F3/RSO	0.043	On for 60 sec (max. 1.5 mA), then unknown.	TT, TMT, DST, ERT	Improved recognition of anger and happy on ERT

Note. Anode (A) and cathode (C) sites using the 10–20 system for EEG. EX, extracephalic (right deltoid muscle); CRT, choice reaction time; DST, Digit Span Test; DWM, Delayed-Response Working Memory Task; ERT, Emotion Recognition Test; IST, Internal Shift Task; PCL, Probabilistic Classification Learning Task; SDMT, Symbol Digit Modalities Test; SRT, simple reaction time; TMT, Trail Making Test; TT, Tapping Test; TVA, theory of visual attention; WEST, Word Emotional Stroop Task.

amelioration of the poorer performance observed when they instead received sham stimulation. Consistent with an improvement in "cognitive control," Brunoni and colleagues (2014) similarly showed improved performance on an emotional Stroop task with "online" anodal tDCS, but not with sham stimulation administered over the same region.

For cognitive functioning, several studies have further demonstrated acute neurocognitive effects across other abilities subserved in part by the L-DLPFC, including working memory (Oliveira et al., 2013) and visual attention (Gogler et al., 2017). Notwithstanding, the results have not always been positive (e.g., Brennan et al., 2017; Brunoni, Zanao, et al. 2013).

COGNITIVE EFFECTS OF REPEATED SESSIONS IN DEPRESSION

Clinical trials of tDCS have indicated that multiple repeated treatments are necessary to produce antidepressant effects (Brunoni et al., 2016). A typical tDCS treatment course for depression involves patients attending daily sessions to receive tDCS over the course of several weeks, with the stimulation given while the patients are sitting at rest. Therapeutic effects are thus most likely the result of cumulative brain changes from repeated sessions. Studies that used the motor cortex to investigate tDCS-induced physiological changes indeed have suggested cumulative changes in cortical excitability (Alonzo, Brassil, Taylor, Martin, & Loo, 2012) and lasting changes in neuroplasticity (Player et al., 2014) with repeated treatments. Given such therapeutic and physiological effects with repeated sessions, it is therefore of interest to examine whether a treatment course relative to a single session may additionally produce neurocognitive benefit. The potential to cause cumulative or lasting neurocognitive improvement has important therapeutic implications due to the adverse impact of cognitive deficits on overall patient functioning and quality of life (Jaeger et al., 2006).

A small, early, double-blind, controlled clinical trial provided preliminary evidence for the potential cumulative neurocognitive benefits of tDCS (Fregni, Boggio, Nitsche, Rigonatti, et al., 2006). Eighteen participants with depression who were antidepressant free were randomized to receive five sessions of active (1 mA for 20 minutes, alternate days) or sham tDCS (stimulator turned off after 5 seconds), with the anode placed over the L-DLPFC and cathode positioned over the contralateral supraorbital area. A battery of neuropsychological tests was administered before and immediately after the last treatment day. While there was no difference in outcomes for the majority of cognitive tasks, a significant difference in improvement between conditions was found for the Digit Span Forward and Digit Span Backward tasks, with greater improvement in the active compared to the sham stimulation condition. This suggested that tDCS had positive effects for auditory simple attention and working memory. The cognitive improvement was unrelated to antidepressant effects. Although the sample size in the study was small, the study provided encouraging preliminary evidence to support further investigation of the potential benefit from repeated tDCS sessions.

Unfortunately, subsequent larger studies were unable to replicate that earlier finding. In two double-blind sham-controlled clinical studies, Loo and colleagues (2010, 2012) investigated neurocognitive effects following a tDCS treatment course with neuropsychological batteries sensitive to executive functioning. There were no differences between the active and sham conditions on the executive function measures, and thus they provided no evidence of cognitive benefit. In these studies, anodal tDCS was similarly administered to the L-DLPFC, and the cathode was placed over F8, with sessions similarly given over 5 alternate days (Loo et al., 2010) or over 15 daily sessions (Loo et al., 2012). One potentially important methodological difference between these and the study by Fregni, Boggio, Nitsche, Marcolin, and colleagues (2006), however, was that, in the sham condition in the Loo studies, the machine was not turned off after an initial ramp up and down. Thus, the sham conditions that involved the delivery of a constant very low-level current (0.016 mA) for the duration of each session may have had biological effects. In addition, unlike in the study by Fregni and colleagues, the majority of participants were taking concomitant antidepressant medications during treatment, which may have interacted with stimulation effects (McLaren, Nissim, & Woods, 2018).

An individual patient data meta-analysis that included data from seven double-blind sham-controlled studies sought to determine whether repeated tDCS sessions have neurocognitive benefits (Martin, Moffa, et al., 2018). The analysis included data from 478 patients (260 of whom received active tDCS and 218 of whom received sham) and investigated the effects on analogous neurocognitive outcomes (e.g., global cognition, verbal learning and delayed recall, verbal fluency) across studies. Consistent with the majority of individual trials however, no benefit with active tDCS was found compared to sham after controlling for mood effects. Unexpectedly, active tDCS was found to be associated with less cognitive improvement compared to sham on a measure of processing speed and attention, though this effect was largely driven by one study (ELECT trial: Brunoni et al., 2017). This meta-analysis thus provided strong evidence for no neurocognitive benefit from repeated active tDCS sessions when administered using this methodology. Nevertheless, given evidence for delayed antidepressant effects following repeated tDCS treatment (Loo et al., 2018), the potential for delayed neurocognitive benefits following the treatment course cannot be ruled out. Furthermore, given recent evidence for interactions between genotype (*BDNF* Val66Met and *COMT* Val158Met polymorphisms) and dose (McClintock et al., 2020), the potential for neurocognitive benefits in a subset of patients requires further research.

An additional caveat to the above research is that in those clinical trials, participants were given repeated tDCS sessions while sitting at rest (e.g., "offline" treatment). Preclinical studies have found that ongoing neural activity during tDCS is necessary to produce neuroplastic changes (Fritsch et al., 2010; Kronberg et al., 2017). Therefore, the failure to standardize brain activity during the depression treatment trials is both a potential source of interindividual variability and a possible rate-limiting factor for tDCS efficacy (Pisoni et al., 2018). Accordingly, several recent studies have investigated the potential for enhanced therapeutic effects when repeated tDCS is administered during training tasks that involve concurrent activation of targeted stimulated regions (Brunoni, Boggio, et al., 2014; Martin, Teng, et al., 2018; Segrave, Arnold, Hoy, & Fitzgerald, 2014). That is, the patient would actively work on a task that activates the L-DLPFC while concurrently being treated with tDCS applied to the L-DLPFC.

In a pilot study, Segrave and colleagues (2014) investigated the clinical and cognitive effects of tDCS combined with cognitive control training (CCT) administered during anodal stimulation of the L-DLPFC. Participants were randomized to one of three groups—active tDCS + CCT, sham tDCS + CCT, or active tDCS + sham CCT—and involved five daily repeated sessions. CCT included training on an attention task and completing a difficult adaptive working memory task (Paced Auditory Serial Addition Test). Interestingly, the results at the 3-week follow-up visit found that only the active tDCS + CCT group showed both significant mood and cognitive improvement on an affective working memory task. A subsequent larger controlled trial then utilized a similar approach with a larger sample, although active tDCS + CCT or sham tDCS + CCT was given instead over 10 consecutive weekdays (Brunoni, Boggio, et al., 2014). Similar to the study by Segrave and colleagues (2014), the clinical outcomes were examined at 2-week follow-up after the intervention. In contrast to the above positive study findings, active tDCS + CCT provided no significant clinical advantage with regard to mood effects. Importantly, however, potential cumulative neurocognitive benefits were not examined. Using an alternative approach, Martin, Teng, and colleagues (2018) examined the therapeutic effects of administering anodal tDCS over the L-DLPFC during cognitive emotional training over 18 sessions in an open-label pilot study that involved 20 participants. Both clinical and cognitive outcomes were examined following the 6-week intervention. While significant mood effects were found, there were no significant cognitive benefits. Unlike the other combined treatment studies, this study included no follow-up assessment.

Although research to date using this combined "online" approach has been limited and the results have been mixed, the potential for enhanced neurocognitive benefits relative to tDCS given alone cannot be ruled out at this stage. Further larger controlled trials with innovative tDCS paradigms are thus required to clarify this issue.

CONCLUSION AND FUTURE DIRECTIONS FOR NEUROCOGNITIVE ENHANCEMENT WITH tDCS IN DEPRESSION

The last decade has seen tDCS emerge as a promising new treatment for depression, with relative advantages for clinical translation, including minimal side effects, low cost, and potential for medically supervised home-based treatment application. While evidence to date suggests that a single tDCS session has acute neurocognitive effects, for example, on attention and emotion regulation, research using current methodologies has provided only limited evidence for more sustained neurocognitive benefits following repeated sessions. In terms of acute effects, future research would be of benefit to delineate optimal stimulation parameters for particular effects, the duration of effect following stimulation, and the interindividual factors (e.g., physiological) that are associated with outcomes. Furthermore, it remains to be determined whether acute neurocognitive effects may somehow be related to antidepressant effects. With regard to potentially cumulative or lasting neurocognitive benefits from repeated treatments, further research is required to determine whether using current treatment methodologies may have potential delayed neurocognitive benefits, whether there is a "dose" effect (e.g., related to stimulation intensity or total delivered charge), and whether benefits may be enhanced if tDCS is instead given with a concurrent activity or training.

REFERENCES

Alonzo, A., Brassil, J., Taylor, J. L., Martin, D., & Loo, C. K. (2012). Daily transcranial direct current stimulation (tDCS) leads to greater increases in cortical excitability than second daily transcranial direct current stimulation. *Brain Stimulation, 5*(3), 208–213.

Arfai, E., Theano, G., Montagu, J. D., & Robin, A. A. (1970). A controlled study of polarization in depression. *British Journal of Psychiatry, 116*(533), 433–434.

Baker, A. P. (1970). Brain stem polarization in the treatment of depression. *South Afrrican Medical Journal, 44*(16), 473–475.

Bermpohl, F., Fregni, F., Boggio, P. S., Thut, G., Northoff, G., Otachi, P. T., et al. (2006). Effect of low-frequency transcranial magnetic stimulation on an affective go/no-go task in patients with major depression: Role of stimulation site and depression severity. *Psychiatry Research, 141*(1), 1–13.

Berryhill, M. E., & Martin, D. (2018). Cognitive effects of transcranial direct current stimulation in healthy and clinical populations: An overview. *Journal of ECT, 34*(3), e25–e35.

Bikson, M., Grossman, P., Thomas, C., Zannou, A. L., Jiang, J., Adnan, T., et al. (2016). Safety of transcranial direct current stimulation: Evidence based update 2016. *Brain Stimulation, 9*(5), 641–661.

Bikson, M., & Rahman, A. (2013). Origins of specificity during tDCS: Anatomical, activity-selective, and input-bias mechanisms. *Frontiers in Human Neuroscience, 7*, 688.

Blumberger, D. M., Tran, L. C., Fitzgerald, P. B., Hoy, K. E., & Daskalakis, Z. J. (2012). A randomized double-blind sham-controlled study of transcranial direct current stimulation for treatment-resistant major depression. *Frontiers in Psychiatry, 3*, 74.

Boggio, P. S., Bermpohl, F., Vergara, A. O., Muniz, A. L., Nahas, F. H., Leme, P. B., et al. (2007). Go-no-go task performance improvement after anodal transcranial DC stimulation of the left dorsolateral prefrontal cortex in major depression. *Journal of Affective Disorders, 101*(1–3), 91–98.

Boggio, P. S., Ferrucci, R., Rigonatti, S. P., Covre, P., Nitsche, M., Pascual-Leone, A., et al. (2006). Effects of transcranial direct current stimulation on working memory in patients with Parkinson's disease. *Journal of the Neurological Sciences, 249*(1), 31–38.

Boggio, P. S., Rigonatti, S. P., Ribeiro, R. B., Myczkowski, M. L., Nitsche, M. A., Pascual-Leone, A., et al. (2008). A randomized, double-blind clinical trial on the efficacy of cortical direct current stimulation for the treatment of major depression. *International Journal of Neuropsychopharmacology, 11*(2), 249–254.

Brennan, S., McLoughlin, D. M., O'Connell, R., Bogue, J., O'Connor, S., McHugh, C., et al. (2017). Anodal transcranial direct current stimulation of the left dorsolateral prefrontal cortex enhances emotion recognition in depressed patients and controls. *Journal of Clinical and Experimental Neuropsychology, 39*(4), 384–395.

Brunoni, A. R., Boggio, P. S., De Raedt, R., Bensenor, I. M., Lotufo, P. A., Namur, V., et al. (2014). Cognitive control therapy and transcranial direct current stimulation for depression: A randomized, double-blinded, controlled trial. *Journal of Affective Disorders, 162*, 43–49.

Brunoni, A. R., Moffa, A. H., Fregni, F., Palm, U., Padberg, F., Blumberger, D. M., et al. (2016). Transcranial direct current stimulation for acute major depressive episodes: Meta-analysis of individual patient data. *British Journal of Psychiatry, 208*(6), 522–531.

Brunoni, A. R., Moffa, A. H., Sampaio-Junior, B., Borrione, L., Moreno, M. L., Fernandes, R. A., et al. (2017). Trial of electrical direct-current therapy versus escitalopram for depression. *New England Journal of Medicine, 376*(26), 2523–2533.

Brunoni, A. R., Valiengo, L., Baccaro, A., Zanao, T. A., de Oliveira, J. F., Goulart, A., et al. (2013a). The sertraline vs. electrical current therapy for treating depression clinical study: Results from a factorial, randomized, controlled trial. *JAMA Psychiatry, 70*(4), 383–391.

Brunoni, A. R., Zanao, T. A., Ferrucci, R., Priori, A., Valiengo, L., de Oliveira, J. F., et al. (2013b). Bifrontal tDCS prevents implicit learning acquisition in antidepressant-free patients with major depressive disorder. *Progress in Neuro-Psychopharmacology and Biological Psychiatry, 43*, 146–150.

Brunoni, A. R., Zanao, T. A., Vanderhasselt, M. A., Valiengo, L., De Oliveira, J. F., Boggio, P. S., et al. (2014). Enhancement of affective processing induced by bifrontal transcranial direct current stimulation in patients with major depression. *Neuromodulation, 17*(2), 138–141.

Carney, M. W., Cashman, M. D., & Sheffield, B. F. (1970). Polarization in depression. *British Journal of Psychiatry, 117*(539), 474–475.

Chew, T., Ho, K. A., & Loo, C. K. (2015). Inter- and Intra-individual variability in response to transcranial direct current stimulation (tDCS) at varying current intensities. *Brain Stimulation, 8*(6), 1130–1137.

Costain, R., Redfearn, J. W., & Lippold, O. C. (1964). A controlled trial of the therapeutic effect of polarization of the brain in depressive illness. *British Journal of Psychiatry, 110*, 786–799.

Datta, A., Bansal, V., Diaz, J., Patel, J., Reato, D., & Bikson, M. (2009). Gyri-precise head model of transcranial direct current stimulation: Improved spatial focality using a ring electrode versus conventional rectangular pad. *Brain Stimulation, 2*(4), 201–207, e201.

Dedoncker, J., Brunoni, A. R., Baeken, C., & Vanderhasselt, M.-A. (2016). A systematic review and meta-analysis of the effects of transcranial direct current stimulation (tDCS) over the dorsolateral prefrontal cortex in healthy and neuropsychiatric samples: Influence of stimulation parameters. *Brain Stimulation, 9*(4), 501–517.

Fregni, F., Boggio, P. S., Nitsche, M., Bermpohl, F., Antal, A., Feredoes, E., et al. (2005). Anodal transcranial direct current stimulation of prefrontal cortex enhances working memory. *Experimental Brain Research, 166*(1), 23–30.

Fregni, F., Boggio, P. S., Nitsche, M. A., Marcolin, M. A., Rigonatti, S. P., & Pascual-Leone, A. (2006). Treatment of major depression with transcranial direct current stimulation. *Bipolar Disorders, 8*(2), 203–204.

Fregni, F., Boggio, P. S., Nitsche, M. A., Rigonatti, S. P., & Pascual-Leone, A. (2006). Cognitive effects of repeated sessions of transcranial direct current stimulation in patients with depression. *Depression and Anxiety, 23*(8), 482–484.

Fritsch, B., Reis, J., Martinowich, K., Schambra, H. M., Ji, Y., Cohen, L. G., et al. (2010). Direct current stimulation promotes BDNF-dependent synaptic plasticity: potential implications for motor learning. *Neuron, 66*(2), 198–204.

Gandiga, P. C., Hummel, F. C., & Cohen, L. G. (2006). Transcranial DC stimulation (tDCS): A tool for double-blind sham-controlled clinical studies in brain stimulation. *Clinical Neurophysiology, 117*(4), 845–850.

Gogler, N., Willacker, L., Funk, J., Strube, W., Langgartner, S., Napiorkowski, N., et al. (2017). Single-session transcranial direct current stimulation induces enduring enhancement of visual processing speed in patients with major depression. *European Archives of Psychiatry and Clinical Neuroscience, 267*(7), 671–686.

Harmer, C. J., Hill, S. A., Taylor, M. J., Cowen, P. J., & Goodwin, G. M. (2003). Toward a neuropsychological theory of antidepressant drug action: Increase in positive emotional bias after potentiation of norepinephrine activity. *American Journal of Psychiatry, 160*(5), 990–992.

Herjanic, M., & Moss-Herjanic, B. (1967). Clinical report on a new therapeutic technique: polarization. *Canadian Psychiatric Association Journal, 12*(4), 423–424.

Ho, K.-A., Taylor, J. L., Chew, T., Gálvez, V., Alonzo, A., Bai, S., et al. (2016). The effect of transcranial direct current stimulation (tDCS) electrode size and current intensity on motor cortical excitability: Evidence from single and repeated sessions. *Brain Stimulation, 9*(1), 1–7.

Horvath, J. C., Forte, J. D., & Carter, O. (2015). Quantitative review finds no evidence of cognitive effects in healthy populations from single-session transcranial direct current stimulation (tDCS). *Brain Stimulation, 8*(3), 535–550.

Hoy, K. E., Arnold, S. L., Emonson, M. R., Daskalakis, Z. J., & Fitzgerald, P. B. (2014). An investigation into the effects of tDCS dose on cognitive performance over time in patients with schizophrenia. *Schizophrenia Research, 155*(1–3), 96–100.

Jacobson, L., Koslowsky, M., & Lavidor, M. (2012). tDCS polarity effects in motor and cognitive domains: A meta-analytical review. *Experimental Brain Research, 216*(1), 1–10.

Jaeger, J., Berns, S., Uzelac, S., & Davis-Conway, S. (2006). Neurocognitive deficits and disability in major depressive disorder. *Psychiatry Research, 145*(1), 39–48.

Jamil, A., Batsikadze, G., Kuo, H. I., Labruna, L., Hasan, A., Paulus, W., et al. (2017). Systematic evaluation of the impact of stimulation intensity on neuroplastic after-effects induced by transcranial direct current stimulation. *Journal of Physiology, 595*(4), 1273–1288.

Kincses, T. Z., Antal, A., Nitsche, M. A., Bártfai, O., & Paulus, W. (2004). Facilitation of probabilistic classification learning by transcranial direct current stimulation of the prefrontal cortex in the human. *Neuropsychologia, 42*(1), 113–117.

Kronberg, G., Bridi, M., Abel, T., Bikson, M., & Parra, L. C. (2017). Direct current stimulation modulates LTP and LTD: Activity dependence and dendritic effects. *Brain Stimulation, 10*(1), 51–58.

Lefaucheur, J. P., Antal, A., Ayache, S. S., Benninger, D. H., Brunelin, J., Cogiamanian, F., et al. (2017). Evidence-based guidelines on the therapeutic use of transcranial direct current stimulation (tDCS). *Clinical Neurophysiology, 128*(1), 56–92.

Lippold, O. C., & Redfearn, J. W. (1964). Mental changes resulting from the passage of small direct currents through the human brain. *British Journal of Psychiatry, 110*, 768–772.

Loo, C. K., Alonzo, A., Martin, D., Mitchell, P. B., Galvez, V., & Sachdev, P. (2012). Transcranial direct current stimulation for depression: 3-week, randomised, sham-controlled trial. *British Journal of Psychiatry, 200*(1), 52–59.

Loo, C. K., Husain, M. M., McDonald, W. M., Aaronson, S., O'Reardon, J. P., Alonzo, A., et al. (2018). International randomized-controlled trial of transcranial direct current stimulation in depression. *Brain Stimulation, 11*(1), 125–133.

Loo, C. K., Sachdev, P., Martin, D., Pigot, M., Alonzo, A., Malhi, G. S., et al. (2010). A double-blind, sham-controlled trial of transcranial direct current stimulation for the treatment of depression. *International Journal of Neuropsychopharmacology, 13*(1), 61–69.

Martin, D. M., Moffa, A., Nikolin, S., Bennabi, D., Brunoni, A. R., Flannery, W., et al. (2018). Cognitive effects of transcranial direct current stimulation treatment in patients with major depressive disorder: An individual patient data meta-analysis of randomised, sham-controlled trials. *Neuroscience and Biobehavioral Reviews, 90*, 137–145.

Martin, D. M., Teng, J. Z., Lo, T. Y., Alonzo, A., Goh, T., Iacoviello, B. M., et al. (2018). Clinical pilot study of transcranial direct current stimulation combined with cognitive emotional training for medication resistant depression. *Journal of Affective Disorders, 232*, 89–95.

Mayberg, H. S. (1997). Limbic-cortical dysregulation: A proposed model of depression. *Journal of Neuropsychiatry and Clinical Neuroscience, 9*(3), 471–481.

McClintock, S. M., Martin, D. M., Lisanby, S. H., Alonzo, A., McDonald, W. M., Aaronson, S. T., et al. (2020). Neurocognitive effects of transcranial direct current stimulation (tDCS) in unipolar and bipolar depression: Findings from an international randomized controlled trial. *Depression and Anxiety, 37*(3), 261–272.

McLaren, M. E., Nissim, N. R., & Woods, A. J. (2018). The effects of medication use in transcranial direct current stimulation: A brief review. *Brain Stimulation, 11*(1), 52–58.

Meinzer, M., Lindenberg, R., Phan, M. T., Ulm, L., Volk, C., & Floel, A. (2015). Transcranial direct current stimulation in mild cognitive impairment: Behavioral effects and neural mechanisms. *Alzheimer's and Dementia, 11*(9), 1032–1040.

Milev, R. V., Giacobbe, P., Kennedy, S. H., Blumberger, D. M., Daskalakis, Z. J., Downar, J., et al. (2016). Canadian network for mood and anxiety treatments (CANMAT) 2016 Clinical guidelines for the management of adults with major depressive disorder: Section 4. Neurostimulation treatments. *Canadian Journal of Psychiatry, 61*(9), 561–575.

Moffa, A. H., Martin, D., Alonzo, A., Bennabi, D., Blumberger, D. M., Benseñor, I. M., et al. (2020). Efficacy and acceptability of transcranial direct current stimulation (tDCS) for major depressive disorder: An individual patient data meta-analysis. *Progress in Neuro-Psychopharmacology and Biological Psychiatry, 99*, 109836.

Monte-Silva, K., Kuo, M.-F., Hessenthaler, S., Fresnoza, S., Liebetanz, D., Paulus, W., et al. (2013). Induction of late LTP-like plasticity in the human motor cortex by repeated non-invasive brain stimulation. *Brain Stimulation, 6*(3), 424–432.

Moreno, M. L., Vanderhasselt, M. A., Carvalho, A. F., Moffa, A. H., Lotufo, P. A., Bensenor, I. M., et al.

(2015). Effects of acute transcranial direct current stimulation in hot and cold working memory tasks in healthy and depressed subjects. *Neuroscience Letters, 591,* 126–131.

Nikolin, S., Martin, D., Loo, C. K., & Boonstra, T. W. (2018). Effects of TDCS dosage on working memory in healthy participants. *Brain Stimulation, 11*(3), 518–527.

Nitsche, M. A., & Paulus, W. (2000). Excitability changes induced in the human motor cortex by weak transcranial direct current stimulation. *Journal of Physioloby, 527*(Pt 3), 633–639.

Nitsche, M. A., & Paulus, W. (2001). Sustained excitability elevations induced by transcranial DC motor cortex stimulation in humans. *Neurology, 57*(10), 1899–1901.

Oliveira, J. F., Zanao, T. A., Valiengo, L., Lotufo, P. A., Bensenor, I. M., Fregni, F., et al. (2013). Acute working memory improvement after tDCS in antidepressant-free patients with major depressive disorder. *Neuroscience Letters, 537,* 60–64.

Palm, U., Schiller, C., Fintescu, Z., Obermeier, M., Keeser, D., Reisinger, E., et al. (2012). Transcranial direct current stimulation in treatment resistant depression: A randomized double-blind, placebo-controlled study. *Brain Stimulation, 5*(3), 242–251.

Pereira Junior Bde, S., Tortella, G., Lafer, B., Nunes, P., Bensenor, I. M., Lotufo, P. A., et al. (2015). The Bipolar Depression Electrical Treatment Trial (BETTER): Design, rationale, and objectives of a randomized, sham-controlled trial and data from the pilot study phase. *Neural Plasticity, 2015,* 684025.

Pisoni, A., Mattavelli, G., Papagno, C., Rosanova, M., Casali, A. G., & Romero Lauro, L. J. (2018). Cognitive enhancement induced by anodal tDCS drives circuit-specific cortical plasticity. *Cerebral Cortex, 28*(4), 1132–1140.

Player, M. J., Taylor, J. L., Weickert, C. S., Alonzo, A., Sachdev, P. S., Martin, D., et al. (2014). Increase in PAS-induced neuroplasticity after a treatment course of transcranial direct current stimulation for depression. *Journal of Affective Disorders, 167,* 140–147.

Priori, A., Berardelli, A., Inghilleri, M., Pedace, F., Giovannelli, M., & Manfredi, M. (1998). Electrical stimulation over muscle tendons in humans. Evidence favouring presynaptic inhibition of Ia fibres due to the activation of group III tendon afferents. *Brain, 121*(Pt. 2), 373–380.

Radman, T., Ramos, R. L., Brumberg, J. C., & Bikson, M. (2009). Role of cortical cell type and morphology in subthreshold and suprathreshold uniform electric field stimulation in vitro. *Brain Stimulation, 2*(4), 215–228.

Ramsay, J. C., & Schlagenhauf, G. (1966). Treatment of depression with low voltage direct current. *Southern Medical Journal, 59*(8), 932–934.

Rigonatti, S. P., Boggio, P. S., Myczkowski, M. L., Otta, E., Fiquer, J. T., Ribeiro, R. B., et al. (2008). Transcranial direct stimulation and fluoxetine for the treatment of depression. *European Psychiatry, 23*(1), 74–76.

Segrave, R. A., Arnold, S., Hoy, K., & Fitzgerald, P. B. (2014). Concurrent cognitive control training augments the antidepressant efficacy of tDCS: A pilot study. *Brain Stimulation, 7*(2), 325–331.

Stagg, C. J., Antal, A., & Nitsche, M. A. (2018). Physiology of transcranial direct current stimulation. *Journal of ECT, 34*(3), 144–152.

Williams, L. M. (2017). Defining biotypes for depression and anxiety based on large-scale circuit dysfunction: A theoretical review of the evidence and future directions for clinical translation. *Depression and Anxiety, 34*(1), 9–24.

Wolkenstein, L., & Plewnia, C. (2013). Amelioration of cognitive control in depression by transcranial direct current stimulation. *Biological Psychiatry, 73*(7), 646–651.

Index

Note. An *f* or a *t* following a page number indicate a figure or a table.